Cancer Imaging: A Clinical Perspective

Cancer Imaging: A Clinical Perspective

Edited by Heath Howard

hayle
medical

New York

Hayle Medical,
750 Third Avenue, 9th Floor,
New York, NY 10017, USA

Visit us on the World Wide Web at:
www.haylemedical.com

ISBN: 978-1-63241-693-3

Cataloging-in-Publication Data

Cancer imaging : a clinical perspective / edited by Heath Howard.
    p. cm.
Includes bibliographical references and index.
ISBN 978-1-63241-693-3
1. Cancer--Imaging. 2. Cancer--Imaging--Instruments. 3. Imaging systems in medicine.
4. Diagnostic imaging. I. Howard, Heath.
RC270.3.D53 C35 2019
616.994 075 4--dc23

Contents

Chapter 26

Chapter 27

Chapter 28

Chapter 29

Chapter 30

Chapter 31

Preface

The world is advancing at a fast pace like never before. Therefore, the need is to keep up with the latest developments. This book was an idea that came to fruition when the specialists in the area realized the need to coordinate together and document essential themes in the subject. That's when I was requested to be the editor. Editing this book has been an honour as it brings together diverse authors researching on different streams of the field. The book collates essential materials contributed by veterans in the area which can be utilized by students and researchers alike.

Most cancers are diagnosed either due to the appearance of signs and symptoms, or via screening. Some signs that are symptomatic of a cancer include a lump, unexplained weight loss, prolonged cough, abnormal bleeding, etc. Tissue from the area under suspicion is examined using x-rays, blood tests, endoscopy and contrast CT scans. Imaging techniques such as magnetic resonance imaging (MRI) and positron emission tomography (PET) are routinely used for diagnosis and detection of cancer. Immunohistochemistry and cytogenetics are some other kinds of tissue tests. Diagnosis of the tissue through a biopsy allows insight into the kind of proliferating cell, the associated genetic abnormalities, histological grade, etc. These tests allow information about molecular changes in fusion genes, chromosome number and mutations, thus enabling better assessment or prognosis and good treatment. This book is compiled in such a manner, that it will provide a clinical perspective of cancer imaging. It covers in detail some existing techniques and innovative practices concerning cancer imaging. As this field is emerging at a rapid pace, the elaborate content of this book will help the readers understand the modern concepts of the subject.

Each chapter is a sole-standing publication that reflects each author's interpretation. Thus, the book displays a multi-facetted picture of our current understanding of application, resources and aspects of the field. I would like to thank the contributors of this book and my family for their endless support.

Editor

Evaluation of tumor recurrences after radical prostatectomy using 18F-Choline PET/CT and 3T multiparametric MRI without endorectal coil: a single center experience

Felipe Couñago[1]*[iD], Manuel Recio[2], Antonio Maldonado[3], Elia del Cerro[1], Ana Aurora Díaz-Gavela[1], Israel J. Thuissard[4], David Sanz-Rosa[4], Francisco José Marcos[1], Karmele Olaciregui[5], María Mateo[6] and Laura Cerezo[7]

Abstract

Background: To evaluate and compare the utility of 18F-fluorocholine (18F-CH) PET/CT versus 3-Tesla multiparametric MRI (mpMRI) without endorectal coil to detect tumor recurrences in patients with biochemical relapse following radical prostatectomy (RP). Secondarily, to identify possible prognostic variables associated with mpMRI and 18F-CH PET/CT findings.

Methods: Retrospective study of 38 patients who developed biochemical recurrence after RP between the years 2011 and 2015 at our institution. PET/CT and mpMRI were both performed within 30 days of each other in all patients. The PET/CT was reviewed by a nuclear medicine specialist while the mpMRI was assessed by a radiologist, both of whom were blinded to outcomes.

Results: The median prostate-specific antigen (PSA) value pre-MRI/PET-CT was 0.9 ng/mL (interquartile range 0.4–2.2 ng/mL). There were no differences in the detection rate between 18F-CH PET/CT and mpMRI for local recurrence (LR), lymph node recurrence (LNR) and bone metastases (BM). Separately, mpMRI and 18F-CH PET/CT were positive for recurrence in 55.2% and 52.6% of cases, respectively, and in 65.7% of cases when findings from both modalities were considered together. The detection of LR was better with combined mpMRI and choline PET/CT versus choline PET/CT alone (34.2% vs 18.4%, $p = 0.04$). Salvage treatment was modified in 22 patients (57.8%) based on the imaging findings. PSA values on the day of biochemical failure were significantly associated with mpMRI positivity (adjusted odds ratio (OR): 30.9; 95% confidence interval (CI): 1.5–635.8). Gleason score > 7 was significantly associated with PET/CT positivity (OR: 13.9; 95% CI: 1.5–125.6). A significant association was found between PSA doubling time (PSADT) (OR: 1.3; 95% CI: 1.0–1.7), T stage (OR: 21.1; 95% CI: 1.6–272.1), and LR.

Conclusions: Multiparametric MRI and 18F-CH PET/CT yield similar detection rates for LR, LNR and pelvic BM. The combination of both imaging techniques provides a better LR detection versus choline PET/CT alone. The initially planned salvage treatment was modified in 57.8% of patients due to imaging findings. In addition to PSA values, Gleason score, T stage, and PSADT may provide valuable data to identify those patients that are most likely to benefit from undergoing both imaging procedures.

Keywords: Prostate cancer, Radical prostatectomy, Biochemical failure, Multiparametric MRI, 18F-Choline PET/CT

* Correspondence: fcounago@gmail.com
[1]Department of Radiation Oncology, Hospital Universitario Quiron Madrid, Calle Diego de Velazquez, 1, 28223, Pozuelo de Alarcón, Madrid, Spain
Full list of author information is available at the end of the article

Background

After radical prostatectomy (RP), 20–50% of patients with prostate cancer (PCa) will develop a tumor recurrence within ten years [1]. In patients with recurrent disease, accurate identification of the site of recurrence is crucial because the type of salvage treatment administered depends on whether the patient presents pelvic recurrence: local recurrence (LR) with or without pelvic lymph node recurrence (LNR) and/or bone metastases (BM), or extrapelvic distant metastases [2]. Currently, multiparametric magnetic resonance imaging (mpMRI) and 11C or 18F-choline (18F-CH) PET/CT are considered the diagnostic imaging tests of choice in this patient population [2]. However, in recent years prostate-specific membrane antigen (PSMA)-ligand imaging has shown promising results in detecting recurrences after RP, and for this reason use of this approach has become increasingly common [for a Review, see 3].

Multiparametric MRI has proven useful in the detection of LR in the prostate gland, even in patients with low prostate-specific antigen (PSA) levels (<0.5 ng/mL) [4], although few studies have assessed the value of mpMRI to LNR or pelvic bone BM [2, 5]. By contrast, 18F-CH PET/CT has proven effective in detecting LNR and BM after RP, primarily in patients with PSA >1 ng/mL or with PSA doubling time (PSADT) < 6 months [6]. The utility of 18F-CH PET/CT to detect LR has received only scant attention [1, 7].

Panebianco et al. compared mpMRI with endorectal coil, dynamic contrast enhanced (DCE), and spectroscopy to 18F-CH PET/CT [7], finding that mpMRI was more reliable at detecting LR. Another study recently compared mpMRI with endorectal coil to 11C-choline PET/CT to detect pelvic recurrences [8], finding that mpMRI was more accurate in detecting LR whereas 11C-PET/CT yielded better results in detecting LNR. Both methods presented similar detection rates for bone metastases. Other studies evaluating the role of PET/CT and mpMRI in PCa staging have found that the sensitivity of mpMRI to detect nodal metastases is similar to, or slightly lower than, that of choline PET/CT [9–11]. A recent meta-analysis found that mpMRI had a higher sensitivity and a lower specificity than choline PET/CT in the diagnosis of BM [12]. To our knowledge, no studies have been conducted to date to directly compare 3T-mpMRI without endorectal coil with diffusion weighted imaging (DWI) and DCE to 18F-CH PET/CT in the detection of pelvic recurrences after RP.

Given this context, the aim of the present study was to compare 18F-CH PET/CT to 3T mpMRI with a phased-array torso coil to determine their relative capabilities to detect pelvic LR, LNR, and BM after RP and to assess their impact on salvage therapy. Secondarily, we analyzed numerous clinical variables to determine potential predictors of positive findings on the imaging studies.

Methods

Study population

This was a retrospective, observational study of a cohort of 59 patients diagnosed with PCa who underwent 18F-FCH PET/CT at the Nuclear Medicine Department of the Hospital Universitario Quiron in Madrid between November 2011 and July 2015. Of these 59 patients, 21 were excluded from the study due to the following: staging 18F-CH PET/CT performed prior to the initial treatment ($n = 5$); biochemical failure after radical radiotherapy ($n = 10$); missing mpMRI ($n = 3$); lost to follow-up ($n = 3$). Therefore, all patients who presented a biochemical recurrence (defined as two consecutive elevations of PSA >0.2 ng/mL) after RP and also underwent mpMRI without endorectal coil and 18F-CH PET/CT within a maximum of 30 days of each other were included in the study ($n = 38$). The PSA values assessed prior to mpMRI and PET/CT imaging were statistically not significantly different. Patients who received salvage RT and/or androgen-deprivation therapy (ADT) after RP ($n = 11$) were also included. The study was approved by our institution's ethics committee.

Multiparametric magnetic resonance imaging protocol

The mpMRI protocol has been described in detail elsewhere [3, 13, 14]. Briefly, a 3T MRI was used (Signa HDxt 3.0 T G.E. Healthcare; Milwaukee, WI, USA) with a gradient strength of 33 mT/m and a gradient slew rate of 120 T/m/s. An 8-channel surface coil was used (Torso phased array). Morphological imaging included T1- and T2-weighted sequences and functional studies included DWI and DCE imaging. The apparent diffusion coefficient (ADC) map was calculated while using DWI and b-values of 0 and 1000 s/mm2 were used. DCE imaging was performed with gadolinium contrast. For DCE, a qualitative review was performed and uptake patterns of relapse-suspected lesions were classified as follows: type 1 curve (slow and progressive uptake), type 2 curve (initial uptake followed by a plateau), or type 3 curve (intense initial uptake followed by washout).

18F-choline PET/CT protocol

Patient preparation for PET-CT consisted of 4–6 h of fasting. All patients received an intravenous injection of 18F-fluoromethylcholine (4 MBq/kg) supplied by the Instituto Tecnologico PET (ITP) in Madrid. Whole body scan was started 60–90 min after injection of 18F-CH. Early dynamic images were not obtained. We just acquired late imaging. The whole-body acquisition was performed in the three dimensional mode, using 2 min per bed position from the base of the skull to the mid-thigh (six or seven bed positions). Images were reconstructed with a standard reconstruction ordered-subset expectation maximization iterative algorithm (two iterative steps) and reformatted into transverse, coronal and sagittal views. Diagnostic CT protocols (oral and intravenous contrasts) were applied. Furosemide was not used in this study. PET-CT scanning was performed using a Biograph 6 True Point HD LSO integrated device (Siemens Healthcare Molecular Imaging; Knoxville, Tennessee, USA) with an intrinsic axial resolution of 4.1 mm FWHM and iterative reconstruction. The CT scan (130–136 keV; 60–90 mAs) was taken in direct proportion to the patient's weight, followed by a PET scan (performed in the same parameter range) for 3 min per bed (approximately 6–7 min). The PET data were processed with iterative reconstruction and converted into PET images (based on CT) with and without attenuation correction. Acquired images were examined on an LCD monitor as both attenuation-corrected and uncorrected multiplanar PET, CT, and PET/CT fusion cross-sections (maximum intensity projection = MIP), using the eSOFT software (Siemens, USA).

Image analysis

A radiologist and a nuclear physician, both experts in uro-oncology, retrospectively reviewed the mpMRI and 18F-CH PET/CT images. These specialists performed the analysis independently of each other and both were blinded to outcomes. Radiological findings were scored from 1 to 3, as follows: a score of 1 indicated a negative finding (absence of recurrence), 2 was considered indeterminate, and 3 indicated positive findings (presence of recurrence). This same scoring approach was used to assess LR and bone and nodal metastases. All lesions with a score of 1 or 2 were considered negative for the purposes of the present study. The image analyses were performed as follows:

mpMRI

The diffusion sequence and the dynamic contrast-enhanced study were processed in a workstation (Advantage Workstation 4.3; GE Healthcare, Milwaukee, WI, USA). T2 and DWI sequences included the whole pelvis and iliac crests. DCE imaging was performed only in the prostate bed. LR was measured using the T2, DWI and DCE sequences while LNR and BM were assessed with T2 and DWI sequences. There is no validated scoring system to define a recurrence after RP on mpMRI [5]; consequently, we used the following mpMRI criteria for LR: presence of a soft tissue nodule on T2-weighted images in or around the prostatectomy bed in T2-weighted images; the presence of an area or hyperintense nodular lesion on the diffusion map, and a hypointense lesion on the ADC map with low ADC values and a DCE image showing an intense, early enhancement with plateau (type 2 curve) or posterior washing (type 3 curve). LR was positive considered when two or more sequences were abnormal. LNR were considered pathological when the short axis

diameter was longer than 8 mm, the MRI signal was heterogeneous, and the contour was irregular. BM was considered pathological when abnormalities were evident on T2 and DWI.

18F-CH PET/CT

18F-CH deposits with higher-than background activity not explained by physiological phenomena were considered positive. Semi-quantitative analysis of the abnormal radiotracer uptake was performed by using the maximum standardized uptake value (SUVmax). This value was obtained automatically.

Salvage treatment

Patients who presented post-RP biochemical recurrence without visible evidence of a tumor on the imaging techniques were treated with rescue RT (70–74 Gy) to the prostate bed. In patients with LR, the dose was increased to 76 Gy. Patients with a pelvic LNR received RT to the pelvic lymph nodes (52.8 Gy at 1.6 Gy/fraction) and the prostatectomy bed (66 Gy at 2 Gy/fraction), together with a simultaneous integrated boost (SIB) to affected lymph nodes (72.6 Gy at 2.2 Gy/fraction). The pelvic BMs were also included within the RT treatment volume with SIB (72.6 Gy at 2.2 Gy/fraction). In patients who had been previously treated with prostate bed RT and later developed pelvic LNR and/or BM, stereotactic fractionated body radiotherapy (SBRT) was prescribed to this localization (excluding the pelvis) as follows: BM: 27–35 Gy in 3 or 5 fractions; LNR: 30–37.5 Gy in 3 or 5 fractions. In oligometastatic (<5 metastases) patients with distant metastases, each lesion was treated with SBRT. ADT was added to the RT prescription at the discretion of the treating physician. However, patients with multiple distant metastases were treated with ADT alone.

Statistical analysis

Quantitative variables are given as medians with interquartile range (IQR) or as a mean ± standard deviation (SD). For qualitative variables, absolute and relative frequencies are given in percentages. The chi-square test was used to analyze qualitative variables. The student's T test or the Mann–Whitney U Test were used, as appropriate, to analyze significant differences among the quantitative variables.

McNemar's test was used to analyze differences between mpMRI and 18F-CH PET/CT in detection rates. A per patient analysis was performed. A Venn's diagram was used to show the distribution of LR and LNR [15].

A univariate/multivariate logistic regression analysis was performed to identify independent variables associated with the imaging findings. The statistical analysis was performed using SPSS, v. 21.0 (IBM Corp; Armonk,

NY; USA), with $p < 0.05$ considered significant for all analyses.

Results

The clinical characteristics and the variables related to the treatment of the 38 patients included in this study are detailed in Table 1. Treatment before 18F-CH PET/CT and mpMRI imaging consisted of the following: in 27 patients (71.1%), RP alone; in 4 patients (10.5%), RP

Table 1 Clinical, pathologic and treatment related characteristics

	ALL
	$n = 38$
Age, years	62,9 ± 7,2
Preoperative PSA, ng/mL	7,4 [9,8]
Pathologic T stage	
T2	25 (65,8)
T3	13 (34,2)
Pathologic N stage	
N0	16 (42,1)
Nx	22 (57,9)
Pathologic Gleason score	
≤7	28 (73,7)
>7	10 (26,3)
Positive surgical margin	
Yes	16 (42,1)
No	22 (57,9)
Perineural Invasion	
Yes	17 (44,7)
No	21 (55,3)
Lymphatic vessel invasion	
Yes	4 (10,5)
No	34 (89,5)
PSA levels, ng/mL	
Post radical prostatectomy	0,1 [0,3]
On day of biochemical failure	0,4 [0,7]
On day of choline PET/CT and mpMRI	0,9 [1,8]
Lowest PSA level after surgery	0,1 [0,3]
Treatment before mpMRI/choline PET/CT	
Radical prostatetcomy only	27 (71,1)
Radical prostatectomy and hormonotherapy	4 (10,5)
Radical prostatectomy and radiotherapy	7 (18,4)
Time from prostatectomy, months	
To first PSA recurrence	10,5 [22,3]
To mpMRI/PET/CT	27,5 [54,0]
PSA doubling time, months	4,5 [8,3]

Mean ± standard deviation; Median [interquartile range]; n (%)

plus ADT; and in 7 patients (18.4%), RP plus salvage RT. The median time relapsed from RP to mpMRI and 18F-CH PET/CT was 27.5 months [54]. Median age was 62.9 years [7.2]. In 13 cases (34.2%), the tumour stage was pT3. The Gleason score was >7 in 10 (26.3%) patients. Sixteen patients (42.1%) had positive surgical margins. The median PSA value prior to imaging was 0.9 ng/mL (interquartile range 0.4–2.2).

Separately, mpMRI and 18F-CH PET/CT were positive for recurrence in 55.2% (21/38 patients) and 52.6% (20/38 patients) of cases, respectively. When combined findings were considered, 65.7% (25/38 patients) of cases were positive for recurrence (Fig. 1). The combination of MRI and choline PET/CT resulted in a higher detection rate for LR versus choline PET/CT alone (34.2% vs 18.4%, $p = 0.04$). No significant differences were observed between 18F-CH PET/CT imaging and mpMRI imaging in terms of their detection rates for LR, LNR and BM, which were, respectively, as follows: 18.4% vs 31.6% ($p = 0.12$), 31.6% vs 26.3% ($p = 0.50$), and 7.9% vs 10.5% ($p = 1.00$) (Table 2). Distance metastases were detected by 18F-CH PET/CT in 5 patients (3 patients with mediastinal lymph node metastases, 1 with a supraclavicular nodal metastasis, and 1 with retroperitoneal metastases). Overall, the radiological findings of both tests disagreed in 10 cases.

The initially planned salvage treatment was modified in 22 patients (57.8%) due to mpMRI and/or 18F-CH PET/CT findings (Table 3).

Clinical variables associated with the radiological findings
The 21 patients with a positive mpMRI had significantly higher PSA values prior to imaging than patients with a negative mpMRI (Table 4). Patients with a positive mpMRI had a significantly higher median PSA at biochemical failure compared to patients with negative mpMRI findings (0.9 [1.2] ng/mL versus 0.4 [0.1] ng/mL, $p = 0.005$). PSA values were significantly associated with a positive mpMRI (odds ratio [OR]: 30.9; 95% confidence interval [CI]: 1.5–635.8) (Table 5).

The 20 patients with a positive 18F-CH PET/CT presented significantly higher PSA values prior to imaging than patients with a negative PET/CT (Table 4). Additionally, the Gleason score and subsequent PET/CT findings were significantly associated: of the 10 patients with a Gleason score >7, nine (90%) had a positive PET/CT; however, of the 28 patients with a Gleason score ≤7, only 11 (39.3%) had a positive PET/CT. Consequently, Gleason score > 7 was significantly associated with a positive PET/CT (OR: 13.9; 95% CI: 1.5–125.6) (Table 5).

LR occurred in 13 patients. Additional file 1 shows the distribution of clinical variables in this subgroup. On the multivariate analysis, a significant association was found between PSADT (OR: 1.3; 95% CI: 1.0–1.7), T stage (OR:

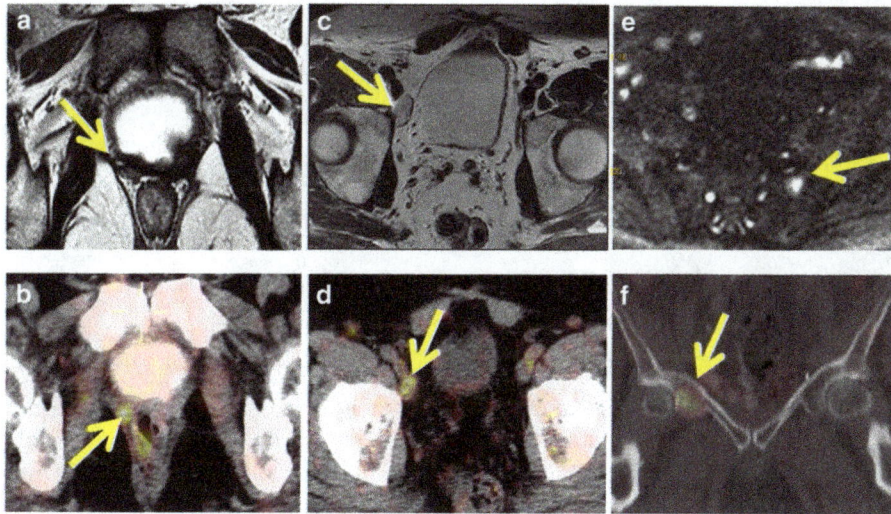

Fig. 1 Representative images of different pelvic tumor recurrences detected by mpMRI and 18F-CH PET/CT (*arrows*). **a** Local recurrence in axial T2-weighted MRI and **b** local recurrence in 18F-CH PET/CT. **c** Right external iliac lymph node detected by axial T2-weighted MRI. **d** 18F-CH PET/CT image at corresponding level demonstrates choline-avid right external iliac lymph node. **e** Axial Diffusion Weighted Imaging (DWI) of bone metastases in left sacrum (*arrow*) and; **f** 18F-CH PET/CT shows a hypermetabolic bone metastases in right acetabulum

21.1;95% CI:1.6–272.1), and the presence of LR (Additional file 2).

A total of 12 patients presented LNR. In patients with a Gleason score > 7, six of 10 patients (60%) developed a LNR versus only six of the 28 patients (21.4%) with a Gleason score ≤7, a significant difference ($p = 0.04$). PSA values (first PSA after surgery, PSA at biochemical failure, and nadir PSA after RP) were all significantly higher in patients who developed LNR. PSADT, the time elapsed from RP to first biochemical recurrence, and time elapsed from surgery to MRI and PET-CT, were all significantly shorter in patients who developed LNR (see Additional file 3). The univariate analysis showed a

significant association between Gleason score (OR: 5.5; 95% CI: 1.2–26.0), PSADT (OR: 0.74; 95% CI: 0.56–0.97) and the presence of LNR (see Additional file 4). On the multivariate analysis, no associations were observed between any of the clinical variables and LNR.

Discussion

To our knowledge, this is the first study to compare 3T-mpMRI without endorectal coil to 18F-CH PET/CT to determine their relative capacity to detect pelvic tumor recurrences following RP. Although the detection rate of LR, LNR and BM was similar in both imaging techniques, the combination of mpMRI and

Table 2 Comparison of the detection rate of mpMRI versus 18F-Choline PET/TC versus Both tests in the diagnosis of tumor recurrences in patients with biochemical relapse following radical prostactectomy. The right panel shows a Venn's Diagram of the distribution of the most frequent recurrences of these patients: LR and LNR

	Both tests (%)	PET/CT (%)	mpMRI (%)
LR	13/38 (34,2)	**7/38 (18,4) ***	12/38 (31,6)
Pelvic LNR	12/38 (31,6)	12/38 (31,6)	10/38 (26,3)
Pelvic BM	4/38 (10,5)	3/38 (7,9)	4/38 (10,5)
Global	25/38 (65,8)	20/38 (52,6)	21/38 (55,3)

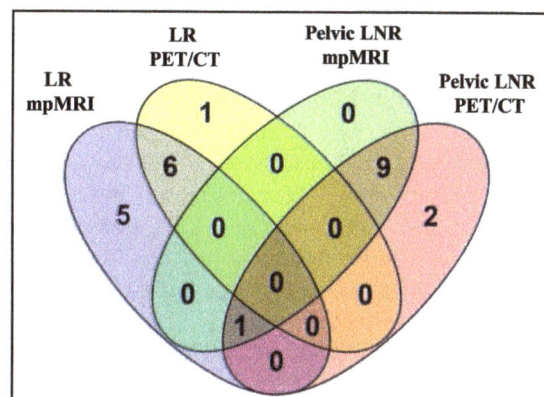

LR local recurrence, *LNR* lymph node recurrence, *BM* bone metastases
Statistically significant value, *$p < 0.05$ vs. Both test are in bold

Table 3 Modification of salvage treatment after radiological findings of mpMRI and/or 18F-CH PET/CT

N	Initial treatment	Salvage treatment, initially planned BEFORE imaging	Radiological findings of mpMRI and/or 18F-CH PET/CT	Salvage treatment, planned AFTER imaging
8	Radical prostatectomy	RT on prostate bed	LR	Boost on tumor bed
1	Radical prostatectomy	RT on prostate bed	Pelvic LNR + one pelvic BM	RT on pelvis (including LNR and pelvic BM with SIB) + ADT
1	Radical prostatectomy and ADT	RT on prostate bed	LR+ One pelvic BM	RT on bed + BM + ADT
8	Radical prostatectomy	RT on prostate bed	Pelvic LNR	RT on pelvis (including LNR with SIB) + ADT
1	Radical prostatectomy and adjuvant radiotherapy	ADT	Pelvic and retroperitoneal LNR + one pelvic BM	SBRT on affected node and BM + ADT
3	Radical prostatectomy and ADT	RT on prostate bed	LR + Pelvic LNR	RT on pelvis (including LR and LNR with SIB) + ADT

18F-CH PET/CT was superior to PET/CT alone in the detection of LR.

Few studies have compared mpMRI to choline PET/CT in the context of biochemical relapse after RP. Kitajima et al. retrospectively compared 11C-choline PET/CT to 1.5T and 3T mpMRI with endorectal coil to detect pelvic recurrences after RP in 115 PCa patients [8]. In that study, mpMR imaging with endorectal coil was superior to PET/CT in the detection of LR, but PET/CT was superior for detecting LNR; both were equally excellent for pelvic BM []. Panebianco et al. compared 3T MRI with endorectal coil to 18F-CH PET/CT in 84 patients with PCa recurrence [7], finding a diagnostic accuracy of MRI for LR higher than that of PET/CT.

In recent years, a new generation of targeted tracers for PET imaging, primarily PSMA, has shown promising results, with a better detection rate than MRI or choline imaging, even in patients with low PSA levels (≤ 0.5 ng/mL) [3]. However, we are still awaiting the results of validation studies currently in progress [16].

We found that, the tumor detection rate in our patient cohort was high: nearly two-thirds for combined MRI and PET/CT versus approximately half for both MRI and PET/CT alone. In addition, the combination of the imaging techniques versus choline PET/CT alone achieved a significantly higher detection rate for LR. It is worth highlighting the increasing clinical and diagnostic role of the integrated PET/MRI scanner, an advanced technique that combines the anatomical and functional information provided by MRI with the higher specificity of PET [17]. This hybrid PET-MRI system has shown promising results in terms of tumor detection compared to MRI or PET alone [17]. For this reason, the high detection rate for MRI and choline PET/CT allows us to define the site of recurrence, assess for metastatic disease, and personalize salvage therapy. Thus, the use of combined data in our study had an important impact on salvage RT treatment decisions, leading us to change the therapeutic approach in nearly 60% of cases.

Salvage RT is the primary treatment option in patients who suffer a relapse after RP. Although the most common approach is to irradiate the surgical bed (even when there is no radiological or histological evidence of disease), various questions remain unresolved with regard to optimal target volume definition and RT doses [16]. Of the 38 patients in our study, 13 (34.2%) developed LR. In 8 of these patients, we were able to escalate the RT dose to 76 Gy at the recurrence site. This is important because the dose needed to achieve biochemical control can vary depending on whether the recurrence is micro- or macroscopic [18]. Moreover, when the imaging studies show no evidence of recurrence, radiation oncologists define the prostate bed and clinical target volume (CTV) blindly, based on recommendations published in clinical guidelines [19]. However, in some cases, following these guidelines can result in the tumor being excluded from the CTV [20]. Similarly, the decision to irradiate the prostate bed or the whole pelvis will depend on the localization of the recurrence, which can be local or loco-regional.

Although metastatic PCa has traditionally been treated with ADT alone, the recent increase of metastases-directed therapy in oligometastatic patients, has made it even more important to accurate detect the presence of LNR and BM after RP in order to properly manage these patients [21]. In our study, oligometastatic lesions (bone and/or lymph nodes) were detected outside of the prostate bed in nearly 37% of patients. In these cases, the initial salvage RT plan to the prostate bed would have been completely ineffective. For this reason, the definitive treatment included metastases-directed therapy with RT and ADT. Although it is true that the optimal therapy in patients with nodal or pelvic bone involvement remains unclear, a recent review of studies that assessed surgical and RT treatment of oligometastatic PCa concluded that, in general, both of these treatment approaches can achieve good outcomes in terms of disease control and increased survival, with only limited toxicity [21].

In terms of the association between clinical variables and the findings of the imaging tests, several points are worth highlighting. Patients with positive MRI and PET/CT findings had PSA values that were significantly

Table 4 Comparison of the clinical variables of patients with positive and negative mpMRI and 18F-CH PET/CT

	mpMRI			18F-CH PET/CT		
	Positive n = 21	Negative/Uncertain n = 17	P value	Positive n = 20	Negative/Uncertain n = 18	P value
Age, years	63,2 ± 7,2	62,5 ± 7,4	0,767	63,4 ± 7,6	62,4 ± 6,8	0,703
Preoperative PSA, ng/mL	7,7 [14,0]	7,0 [8,4]	0,453	7,4 [9,1]	7,5 [12,1]	0,65
Pathologic T stage (%)						
T2	11 (44,0)	14 (56,0)	0,086	11 (44,0)	14 (56,0)	0,182
T3	10 (76,9)	3 (23,1)		9 (69,2)	4 (30,8)	
Pathologic N stage, n (%)						
N0	9 (56,3)	7 (43,8)	0,917	10 (62,5)	6 (37,5)	0,299
Nx	12 (54,5)	10 (45,5)		10 (45,5)	12 (54,5)	
Pathologic Gleason score, n (%)						
≤7	13 (46,4)	15 (53,6)	0,136	11 (39,3)	17 (60,7)	**0,009**
>7	8 (80,0)	2 (20,0)		9 (90,0)	1 (10,0)	
Positive surgical margin, n (%)						
Yes	8 (50,0)	8 (50,0)	0,578	6 (37,5)	10 (62,5)	0,111
No	13 (59,1)	9 (40,9)		14 (63,6)	8 (36,4)	
Perineural Invasion, n (%)						
Yes	10 (58,8)	7 (41,2)	0,691	9 (52,9)	8 (47,1)	0,973
No	11 (52,4)	10 (47,6)		11 (52,4)	10 (47,6)	
Lymphatic vessel invasion, n (%)						
Yes	2 (50,0)	2 (50,0)	1,000	2 (50,0)	2 (50,0)	1,000
No	19 (55,9)	15 (44,1)		18 (52,9)	16 (47,1)	
PSA levels, ng/mL						
Post radical prostatectomy	0,2 [1,4]	0,0 [0,1]	**0,006**	0,2 [1,3]	0,0 [0,1]	**0,007**
On day of biochemical failure	0,9 [1,2]	0,4 [0,1]	**0,005**	0,7 [1,1]	0,4 [0,1]	**0,009**
On day of CH PET/CT and mpMRI	2,0 [1,9]	0,4 [1,0]	**0,024**	2,0 [1,7]	0,4 [0,7]	**0,019**
Lowest PSA level after surgery	0,2 [1,4]	0,0 [0,1]	**0,012**	0,2 [1,2]	0,0 [0,1]	**0,003**
Treatment before mpMRI/18F-CH PET, n (%)						
Radical prostatectomy only	14 (51,9)	13 (48,1)	0,508	15 (55,6)	12 (44,4)	0,572
Prostatectomy and HT or RT	7 (63,6)	4 (36,4)		5 (45,5)	6 (54,5)	
Time from prostatectomy, months						
To first PSA recurrence	5,0 [36,0]	16,0 [18,5]	0,075	5,5 [21,0]	16,5 [25,0]	0,079
To mpMRI/PET/CT	31,0 [55,5]	27,0 [44,5]	0,596	10,5 [36,0]	32,0 [48,0]	0,187
PSA doubling time, months	4,0 [9,5]	5,8 [8,5]	0,634	3,1 [5,3]	8,5 [9,5]	0,135

Mean ± standard deviation; Median [interquartile range]
Statistically significant value, $p < 0.05$ are in bold

greater than those observed in patients with negative findings on the imaging tests. In fact, although we only found an association between PSA values at the time of biochemical failure and MRI positivity, many studies have reported an association between PSA and choline PET/CT [22]. Thus, after RP, the optimal PSA cut-off level for choline PET/CT analysis seems to be between 1 and 2 ng/mL [23], while for MRI, the corresponding value appears to range from 0.3 to 0.54 ng/mL [5]. In addition to the PSA value, several studies have reported

that PSA kinetics (PSADT, PSA velocity) are strong predictors for positive PET and MRI findings, even in patients with low PSA values [4, 5, 23]. We found that PSADT was significantly associated with the type of pelvic recurrence: patients with a higher PSADT had an increased probability of local recurrence. Hernández et al. demonstrated a significantly shorter PSADT in patients with LNR [5]. In the other hand, the Gleason score should be considered when evaluating the utility of 18F-CH PET/CT as it has been related to the PET/CT

Table 5 Univariate analysis of the clinic characteristics associated to the positivity of mpMRI and 18F-CH PET/CT

	mpMRI		18F-CH PET/CT	
	OR (95% CI)	p value	OR (95% CI)	p value
Age, years	1.01 (0.93–1.10)	0.759	1.02 (0.93–1.12)	0.694
Preoperative PSA, ng/mL	1.05 (0.95–1.15)	0.344	0.98 (0.89–1.07)	0.630
Pathologic T stage, T3	4.24 (0.94–19.26)	0.061	2.86 (0.69–11.82)	0.146
Pathologic N stage, Nx	0.93 (0.26–3.41)	0.917	0.50 (0.13–1.86)	0.301
Pathologic Gleason score, > 7	4.62 (0.83–25.73)	0.081	13.91 (1.54–125.63)	**0.019**
Positive surgical margin	0.69 (0.19–2.53)	0.578	0.34 (0.09–1.30)	0.116
Perineural Invasion	1.30 (0.36–4.72)	0.691	1.02 (0.28–3.68)	0.973
PSA levels, ng/mL				
Post radical prostatectomy	20.66 (0.45–964.07	0.121	2.17 (0.71–6.63)	0.172
On day of biochemical failure	30.90 (1.50–635.84)	**0.026**	2.48 (0.76–8.15)	0.135
On day of MRI-PET/CT	1.62 (0.88–2.98)	0.122	1.64 (0.90–2.99)	0.110
Lowest PSA level after surgery	16.77 (0.530–531.40)	0.110	2.03 (0.72–5.69)	0.180
Treatment before mpMRI/choline PET/CT				
Radical prostatectomy and hormonotherapy or radiotherapy	1.63 (0.38–6.87)	0.509	0.67 (0.16–2.73)	0.573
Time from prostatectomy				
To first PSA recurrence	0.99 (0.95–1.03)	0.568	0.98 (0.94–1.01)	0.217
To MRI-PET/CT	1.00 (0.98–1.02)	0.807	0.99 (0.97–1.01)	0.203
PSA doubling time, months	1.02 (0.92–1.12)	0.772	0.94 (0.85–1.05)	0.271

Statistically significant value, $p < 0.05$ are in bold

positivity [24]. T staging was also significantly associated with LR: patients with extracapsular involvement (T3) had an increased probability of developing LR, a finding that is congruent with the beneficial effect of adjuvant RT in the patient subgroup with extracapsular invasion or seminal vesicle involvement [23]. In short, all of these variables should be taken into account when re-staging patients who develop biochemical recurrence after RP in order to select the most appropriate salvage therapy.

Our study has several limitations. First, this was a retrospective analysis with a small sample size. Second, there was some patient selection bias, as evidenced by the fact that most patients who underwent mpMRI and 18F-CH PET/CT had positive radiological findings. This can be attributed to various factors, as follows: pre-imaging PSA values were relatively high in the entire cohort, the time to biochemical failure was short, and the PSADT values low. All of these clinical characteristics are indicative of highly aggressive disease with a high probability of tumor recurrence that are detectable on both imaging tests. Third, the specific choline PET/CT protocol and the radiotracer used in this study could have influenced the quality of the images and thus their interpretation. However, a recent metanalysis concluded that (11) C-choline and 18F-CH and the different acquisition protocols had no significant impact on the detection rate [25]. Fourth, the MRI and PET images were

acquired in separate imaging sessions and this may have affected the detection rate compared to the hybrid PET-MRI system, as mentioned before. Fifth, we did not use endorectal coil and this may have influenced the reliability of the MRI images [26]. Nevertheless, in patients with tumor recurrence after RP, the tumor detection rate using a 3T MRI seems not to be influenced by the type of coil [4]. Lastly, in our study 4 patients received ADT before MRI and PET/CT, which could have a limited uptake on the choline PET/CT and caused morphological changes and alterations in the parameters of the DWI and DCE on the MRI [27, 28]. However, data from our study and others [7] show that this does not directly influence the comparative analysis. In fact, in three of these four patients the recurrence was identified by both imaging techniques.

The strength of the study is the blinded evaluation of all images at the same institution by two different experts (an uro-radiologist and a nuclear medicine specialist). In addition, this is the first study to compare 3T mpMRI without endorectal coil to 18F-CH PET/CT in this context.

Conclusion

Multiparametric MRI and 18F-CH PET/CT yield similar detection rates for LR, LNR and pelvic BM. The combination of both imaging techniques provides a better

LR detection rate after RP versus choline PET/CT alone. The initially planned salvage treatment was modified in 57.8% of patients due to both imaging techniques findings. In addition to PSA values, Gleason score, T stage, and PSADT may provide valuable data to identify those patients that are most likely to benefit from undergoing both imaging procedures.

Abbreviations

18F-CH PET/CT: 18-fluorocholine positron emission tomography/computed tomography; ADC: Apparent diffusion coefficient; ADT: Androgen-deprivation therapy; BM: Bone metastases; DCE: Dynamic contrast enhanced; DWI: Diffusion weighted imaging; EAU: European Association of Urology; IQR: Interquartile range; ITP: Instituto Tecnológico PET; LNR: Lymph node recurrence; LR: Local recurrences; mpMRI: Multiparametric magnetic resonance imaging; PSADT: PSA doubling time; RP: Radical prostatectomy; RT: Radiotherapy; SBRT: Stereotactic fractioned body radiotherapy; SD: Standard deviation; SIB: Simultaneous integrated boost; SUVmax: Maximum standardized uptake value

Acknowledgments

We wish to thank all the members of the Clinical Radiology, Nuclear Medicine, Urology and Pathology Departments as well as MRI and PET/CT technicians of the Hospital Universitario Quiron Madrid for their invaluable collaboration in this study. We would like to thank Bradley Londres for his assistance in editing and improving the English text.

Funding

There was no funding for this work.

Authors' contributions

FC designed the project, collected and analyzed data, and drafted the manuscript; EDC, AAD, FJM, MR, AM contributed to project design and revised the drafted manuscript; DSR edited tables and figures and revised the manuscript; IT collected and analyzed data; KO revised and helped to translate the manuscript; MM revised the manuscript; LC revised the manuscript. All authors read and approved the final manuscript.

Competing interests

The authors declare that they have no competing interests.

Author details

[1]Department of Radiation Oncology, Hospital Universitario Quiron Madrid, Calle Diego de Velazquez, 1, 28223, Pozuelo de Alarcón, Madrid, Spain. [2]Department of Radiology, Hospital Universitario Quiron, Madrid, Spain. [3]Department of Nuclear Medicine, Hospital Universitario Quiron, Madrid, Spain. [4]School of Doctoral Studies and Research, Universidad Europea de Madrid, Madrid, Spain. [5]Clinical Department, School of Biomedical Sciences, Universidad Europea de Madrid, Madrid, Spain. [6]Hospital Universitario Quiron, Madrid, Spain. [7]Department of Radiation Oncology, Hospital Universitario La Princesa, Madrid, Spain.

References

1. Alfarone A, Panebianco V, Schillaci O, et al. Comparative analysis of multiparametric magnetic resonance and PET-CT in the management of local recurrence after radical prostatectomy for prostate cancer. Crit Rev Oncol Hematol. 2012;84(1):109–21.
2. Schiavina R, Ceci F, Borghesi M, et al. The dilemma of localizing disease relapse after radical treatment for prostate cancer: which is the value of the actual imaging techniques? Curr Radiopharm. 2013;6(2):92–5.
3. Kratochwil C, Afshar-Oromieh A, Kopka K, Haberkorn U, Giesel FL. Current status of prostate-specific membrane antigen targeting in nuclear medicine: clinical translation of chelator containing prostate-specific membrane antigen ligands into diagnostics and therapy for prostate cancer. Semin Nucl Med. 2016;46(5):405–18.

4. Couñago F, del Cerro E, Recio M, et al. Role of 3T multiparametric magnetic resonance imaging without endorectal coil in the detection of local recurrent prostate cancer after radical prostatectomy: the radiation oncology point of view. Scand J Urol. 2015;49(5):360–5.
5. Hernandez D, Salas D, Giménez D, et al. Pelvic MRI findings in relapsed prostate cancer after radical prostatectomy. Radiat Oncol. 2015;10:262.
6. Castellucci P, Ceci F, Graziani T, et al. Early biochemical relapse after radical prostatectomy: which prostate cancer patients may benefit from a restaging 11C-Choline PET/CT scan before salvage radiation therapy? J Nucl Med. 2014;55(9):1424–9.
7. Panebianco V, Sciarra A, Lisi D, et al. Prostate cancer: 1HMRS-DCEMR at 3T versus [(18)F]choline PET/CT in the detection of local prostate cancer recurrence in men with biochemical progression after radical retropubic prostatectomy (RRP). Eur J Radiol. 2012;81(4):700–8.
8. Kitajima K, Murphy RC, Nathan MA, et al. Detection of recurrent prostate cancer after radical prostatectomy: comparison of 11C-choline PET/CT with pelvic multiparametric MR imaging with endorectal coil. J Nucl Med. 2014;55(2):223–32.
9. Budiharto T, Joniau S, Lerut E, et al. Prospective evaluation of 11C-choline positron emission tomography/computed tomography and diffusion-weighted magnetic resonance imaging for the nodal staging of prostate cancer with a high risk of lymph node metastases. Eur Urol. 2011;60(1):125–30.
10. Heck MM, Souvatzoglou M, Retz M, et al. Prospective comparison of computed tomography, diffusion-weighted magnetic resonance imaging and [11C]choline positron emission tomography/computed tomography for preoperative lymph node staging in prostate cancer patients. Eur J Nucl Med Mol Imaging. 2014;41(4):694–701.
11. Pinaquy JB, De Clermont-Galleran H, Pasticier G, et al. Comparative effectiveness of [(18) F]-fluorocholine PET-CT and pelvic MRI with diffusion-weighted imaging for staging in patients with high-risk prostate cancer. Prostate. 2015;75(3):323–31.
12. Shen G, Deng H, Hu S, Jia Z. Comparison of choline-PET/CT, MRI, SPECT, and bone scintigraphy in the diagnosis of bone metastases in patients with prostate cancer: a meta-analysis. Skeletal Radiol. 2014;43(11):1503–13.
13. Couñago F, Del Cerro E, Díaz-Gavela AA, et al. Tumor staging using 3.0 T multiparametric MRI in prostate cancer: impact on treatment decisions for radical radiotherapy. Springerplus. 2015;4:789.
14. Couñago F, Recio M, Del Cerro E, et al. Role of 3.0 T multiparametric MRI in local staging in prostate cancer and clinical implications for radiation oncology. Clin Transl Oncol. 2014;16(11):993–9.
15. Oliveros JC. Venny. An interactive tool for comparing lists with Venn's diagrams. (2007–2015). http://bioinfogp.cnb.csic.es/tools/venny/index.html.
16. Amzalag G, Rager O, Tabouret-Viaud C, et al. Target definition in salvage radiotherapy for recurrent prostate cancer: the role of advanced molecular imaging. Front Oncol. 2016;6:73.
17. Lindenberg L, Ahlman M, Turkbey B, Mena E, Choyke P. Evaluation of prostate cancer with PET/MRI. J Nucl Med. 2016;57 Suppl 3:111S–6.
18. Dirix P, van Walle L, Deckers F, et al. Proposal for magnetic resonance imaging-guided salvage radiotherapy for prostate cancer. Acta Oncol. 2016;1–6. [Epub ahead of print].
19. Poortmans P, Bossi A, Vandeputte K, et al. Guidelines for target volume definition in post-operative radiotherapy for prostate cancer, on behalf of the EORTC Radiation Oncologuy Group. Radiother Oncol. 2007;84(2):121–7.
20. Wang L, Kudchadker R, Choi S, et al. Local recurrence map to guide target volume delineation after radical prostatectomy. Pract Rad Oncol. 2014;4:e239–46.
21. Van Poppel H, De Meerleer G, Joniau S. Oligometastatic prostate cancer: metastases-directed therapy? Arab J Urol. 2016;14(3):179–82.
22. Mapelli P, Incerti E, Ceci F, Castellucci P, Fanti S, Picchio M. 11C- or 18F-choline PET/CT for imaging evaluation of biochemical recurrence of prostate cancer. J Nucl Med. 2016;57 Suppl 3:43S–8.
23. Mottet N, Bellmunt J, Briers E, et al. Prostate cancer. European Association of Urology (EAU) guidelines. 2016. https://uroweb.org/guideline/prostate-cancer/
.
24. Rodado-Marina S, Coronado-Poggio M, García-Vicente AM. Clinical utility of (18) F-fluorocholine positron-emission tomography/computed tomography (PET/CT) in biochemical relapse of prostate cancer after radical treatment: results of a multicentre study. BJU Int. 2015;115(6):874–83.
25. von Eyben FE, Kairemo K. Acquisition with (11C)-choline and (18)F-fluorocholine PET/CT for patients with biochemical recurrence of prostate cancer: a systematic review and meta-analysis. Ann Nucl Med. 2016;30(6):385–92.
26. Barentsz OJ, Richenberg J, Clements R, Choyke P, et al. Esur prostate MR guidelines 2012. Eur Radiol. 2012;22:746 57.

2

Added value of diffusion-weighted imaging in hepatic tumors and its impact on patient management

Jana Taron[1], Jonas Johannink[2], Michael Bitzer[3], Konstantin Nikolaou[1], Mike Notohamiprodjo[1*] and Rüdiger Hoffmann[1]

Abstract

Background: To investigate the added diagnostic value of diffusion-weighted imaging (DWI) of the liver and its impact on therapy decisions in patients with hepatic malignancy.

Methods: Interdisciplinary gastrointestinal tumorboard cases concerning patients with hepatic malignancies discussed between 11/2015 and 06/2016 were included in this retrospective, single-center study. Two radiologists independently reviewed the respective liver MR-examination first without, then with DWI. The readers were blinded regarding number, position and size of hepatic malignancies. Cases in which DWI revealed additional findings concerning the hepatic tumor status as compared to conventional sequences alone were presented to experienced members of the interdisciplinary tumor board. In this retrospective setting changes in treatment decisions based on these additional findings in the DWI sequences were recorded.

Results: A total of 87 patients were included. DWI revealed additional findings in 12 patients (13,8%). These new findings had a direct effect on the therapy in 8 patients (9,2%): In 6 patients (6,9%) the surgical/interventional treatment was adapted ($n = 5$: extended resection, $n = 1$: with transarterial chemoembolization of a single hepatocellular carcinoma only detectable in DWI); 2 patients (2,3%) received systemic therapy ($n = 1$: neo-adjuvant, $n = 1$: palliative) based on the additional findings in DWI. In 4 patients (4.6%) additional DWI findings did not affect the therapeutic decision.

Conclusions: DWI is a relevant diagnostic tool in oncologic imaging of the liver. By providing further information regarding tumor load in hepatic malignancies it can lead to a significant change in treatment.

Keywords: Diffusion-weighted imaging, MRI, Additional value, Abdominal imaging, Liver tumors, Oncology

Background

Over the past two decades diffusion-weighted imaging (DWI) has evolved from being limited to intracranial implementations to an established technique in abdominal magnetic resonance imaging (MRI). Through a series of advances in acquisition techniques, sequence design and hardware, to overcome sensitivity to susceptibility and gross motion, DWI can now be readily integrated into clinical protocols, leading to its widespread use and acceptance [1–3]. Based on the principle of quantifying the degree of free or rather limited Brownian motion of protons [4], DWI inherits the property of detecting diffusion restriction in areas with high cellularity (i.e. malignancies) and cell membrane density. This ability to gather information on changes of diffusion on a cellular level explains its great importance to oncologic imaging [1], where it is used for the detection and characterization of a lesion as well as monitoring and predicting therapeutic response [1, 5–7]. For the management of oncologic patients, particularly with regard to potential surgical options, it is of major importance to reliably detect or rule out metastatic involvement. In abdominal imaging, the liver is of particular interest as it is

* Correspondence: Mike.Notohamiprodjo@uni-tuebingen.de
[1]Department of Diagnostic and Interventional Radiology, University Hospital of Tuebingen, Hoppe-Seyler-Str. 3, 72076 Tuebingen, Germany
Full list of author information is available at the end of the article

a common site for metastatic lesions as well as primary malignancies [8, 9].

Several studies have assessed the diagnostic accuracy of DWI for the detection of intrahepatic lesions. However to our knowledge, a study evaluating the impact and added value of diffusion-weighted imaging on therapeutic decision making and, thus, its direct impact on patient care has not yet been performed. As DWI has become an integral part of our daily imaging routine and a reliable diagnostic tool, this subject appears to be of major importance. Thus, aim of our investigation was to quantify the additional information gained through the performance of DWI in oncologic imaging of the liver and evaluate its clinical impact on patient management and therapeutic options.

Methods

Patient cohort

This retrospective single-center study was approved by the local institutional review board and written-informed consent was waived. We included all patients with primary hepatic tumors or hepatic metastases, who were referred to our interdisciplinary gastrointestinal tumor board between November 2015 and June 2016. Inclusion criteria was an existing on-site MRI examination (1.5 or 3 T, MAGNETOM Aera/Avanto/Skyra Siemens Healthcare GmbH, Erlangen, Germany) of the abdomen or the liver at the date of tumor board inclusion.

MR imaging protocol

Institutional standard imaging protocols consisted of the following sequences (acquired in the same order as listed): coronal T2-weighted half acquisition single shot turbo spin echo (HASTE), axial T2-weighted turbo spin echo sequence (TSE) and spectral fat saturation pulse (SPIR) for fat suppression, axial T1 in- and opposed-phase, axial echo planar imaging (EPI) for diffusion-weighted imaging with b-values of 0, 400 and 800 s/mm^2 and dynamic axial T1-weighted volumetric interpolated breath-hold examination (VIBE) sequence with fat saturation using the Dixon technique [10] after intravenous injection of 0.1 mmol of gadobutrol (Gadovist, Bayer HealthCare, Leverkusen, Germany) per kg body weight or 0.025 mmol of gadoxetate disodium (Primovist, Bayer HealthCare) per kg body weight. The intravenous application of contrast medium in patients with highly impaired renal function was spared.

Image Reading.

Evaluated was the current MRI examination at the date of tumor board inclusion. The MR images were reviewed by two independent and blinded radiologists (R.H. and J.T.; with 6 and 4 year of experience in abdominal MR-

imaging). First, the readers reviewed the conventional sequences excluding DWI regarding tumor localization, size and number. Thereafter, reading was repeated using conventional sequences including DWI. Deviations between both reading sessions (with and without DWI) were noted and the corresponding cases were reassessed in a consensus reading.

In a next step, cases with additional findings as agreed upon in the consensus reading were presented (using the available clinical data and liver MRI) to members of the institution's gastrointestinal tumor board consisting of an abdominal surgeon, a radiologist and a gastrointestinal oncologist (J.J., M.N., M.B.), who were not involved in initial board meeting and, thus, blinded to the actual therapeutic decision. The cases were re-discussed in this simulated setting of the repeated tumor board and hypothetical changes in treatment based on these additional findings in the DWI sequences were recorded and classified as: (a) Change in surgical/interventional procedure, (b) change in systemic treatment, (c) no change in treatment.

Finally, follow-up examinations and clinical reports were examined with respect to the additionally found lesions. If available, these lesions were matched to pathology reports, otherwise appearance and characteristics in the follow-up images served as validation.

Comprehensive data analysis was performed using Microsoft Excel (2007).

Results

A total of 87 patients (62 male, mean age 70.5 ± 10.5) were included in this study; in 57 patients MRI was performed using gadobutrol, 30 patients received gadoxetate disodium. Patient characteristics were the following: 43 patients presented hepatic metastases ($n = 26$ colorectal carcinomas, $n = 5$ neuroendocrine tumors (NET), $n = 3$ breast carcinomas, n = 1 bronchial carcinoma n = 1 melanoma, n = 1 oesophageal carcinoma, $n = 4$ pancreatic carcinoma, n = 1 ovarian carcinoma, n = 1 urothelial carcinoma), 35 patients hepatocellular carcinomas (HCC), 6 patients cholangiocarcinomas (CC) and 3 patients HCC-CC mixed-type carcinoma.

In 12/87 patients (13.8%) DWI revealed additional lesions as compared to reading the conventional MRI protocol alone. In the simulated tumor board setting the members agreed on a change in therapy in 8 of these cases (9.2%). Changes in management were as follows: In 6 patients (6.9%) the surgical treatment or interventional treatment was adapted with an extended resection in 5 cases ($n = 2$ NET, $n = 1$ colorectal carcinoma, n = 1 oesophageal carcinoma, n = 1 pancreatic carcinoma) and a transarterial chemoembolization in one case in which HCC was only identified in DWI; 2 patients (2,3%) received systemic therapy ($n = 1$ neo-adjuvant systemic therapy in a patient with colorectal cancer, n = 1 palliative systemic therapy in a patient with pancreatic cancer). (Figures 1, 2, 3 and 4).

In the other 4 cases ($n = 4.6\%$) additional findings did not affect the therapeutic decision due to multiple lesions (detectable in morphological sequences) which already indicated a palliative regimen ($n = 2$ colorectal cancer, n = 1 bronchial carcinoma, n = 1 CC).

Mean follow-up period of the 12 patients with additionally found lesions was 10.5 months [1; 24]. In two cases, the malignant entity of the additional found lesions by DWI could not be definitely confirmed. In both cases (n = 2 colorectal carcinoma) the lesions appeared cystic without progression in long-term follow-up of 17 and 28 months, respectively. A definite differentiation between benign hepatic cyst and cystic residuum was not possible in both cases. The simulated tumor board had decided on 'no effect on therapy' based on the additional findings in these two patients due to the presence of multiple intra- and extrahepatic lesions as described above. Regarding the other 10/12 cases, follow-up or histopathology confirmed the malignancy of the additionally found lesions. In these cases 6 patients presented progressive disease ($n = 1$ bronchial carcinoma, n = 1 CC, n = 1 neuroendocrine tumor n = 1 colorectal carcinoma, n = 1 oesophageal carcinoma, n = 1 pancreatic cancer, n = 1 bronchial carcinoma), 2 patients presented regressive disease under chemotherapy (n = 1 pancreatic cancer, n = neuroendocrine tumor), 1 patient presented a relapse of hepatic metastases of colorectal cancer, 1 patient was tumor-free after transarterial chemoembolization of HCC during our follow-up period.

Discussion

The results of our evaluation show that in about 14% of all patients with hepatic tumor lesions referred to our interdisciplinary tumor board additional suspicious hepatic lesions, which might have otherwise gone undetected, could be identified with diffusion-weighted imaging and, thus, be considered in decisions on individual therapeutic management.

This is especially relevant as the liver is a prevalent location in metastatic disease [9]. Additionally, the number of primary hepatic malignancies is steadily increasing, drawing a focus on HCC and CC- the two most common primary hepatic neoplasms [11–14]. In this context it is crucial to diagnose hepatic involvement for correct patient care in terms of systemic therapy or potential surgical/interventional options.

According to recent literature, the additional information gained by diffusion-weighting is thought to have a direct impact on surgical decisions as well as follow-up after an operational procedure [8, 9], a statement we can now corroborate with our results. While DWI revealed additional lesions in 13.8% of the patients, these findings changed surgical management in 9.2% and or indicated the need for a systemic/palliative therapy in 2.3%.

Previous studies have assessed the role of diffusion-weighted imaging in standard imaging protocols which generally consist of a T2-weighted as well as a T1-weighted in- and opposed phase sequence and a series of contrast enhanced images [8, 15]. In this context, DWI was found to be of higher sensitivity than T2-weighted images in detection of focal liver lesions, and a combination of a diffusion-weighted sequence plus contrast-enhanced series was described to deliver the highest sensitivity for the discovery of suspicious lesions [9, 16]. Colagrande et al. obtained similar results in their recently published study evaluating the value of DWI in contrast-enhanced scans in hepatic metastases of colorectal cancer. They found an improvement on diagnostic accuracy in non-contrast-enhanced examinations due to DWI as well as an increase in specificity in contrast-enhanced images [17].

Metastatic lesions were by far the most common entity in our patient collective and our results match the experience of the above mentioned studies. In our study 11 out of the 12 patients with additional lesions suffered from metastatic diseases. Furthermore, 7 out of the 8 patients with changes in therapy presented with hepatic metastases. This brings us to the assumption that especially in hepatic metastatic disease DWI has an

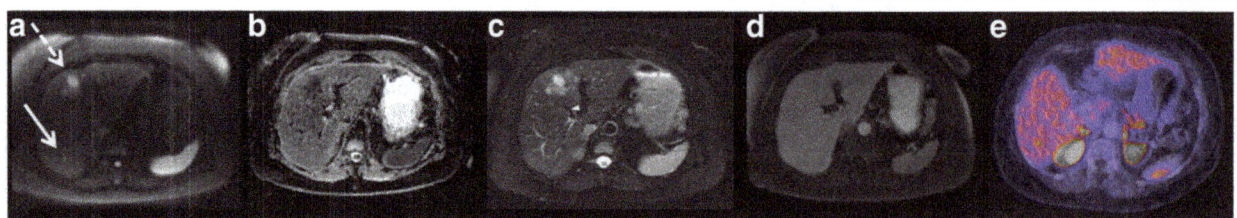

Fig. 1 55 year old female patient with hepatic metastases (dashed arrow) of a neuroendocrine tumor. Hepatic lesion (white arrow) was only detected in DWI. The simulated tumorboard decided on change in surgical procedure due to this additionally found lesion. **a**. Diffusion-weighted sequene (b-value 800). **b**. Corresponding ADC map. **c**. T2-weighted sequence. **d**. T1-weighted post-contrast scan. **e**. Corresponding PET-CT of hepatic lesion

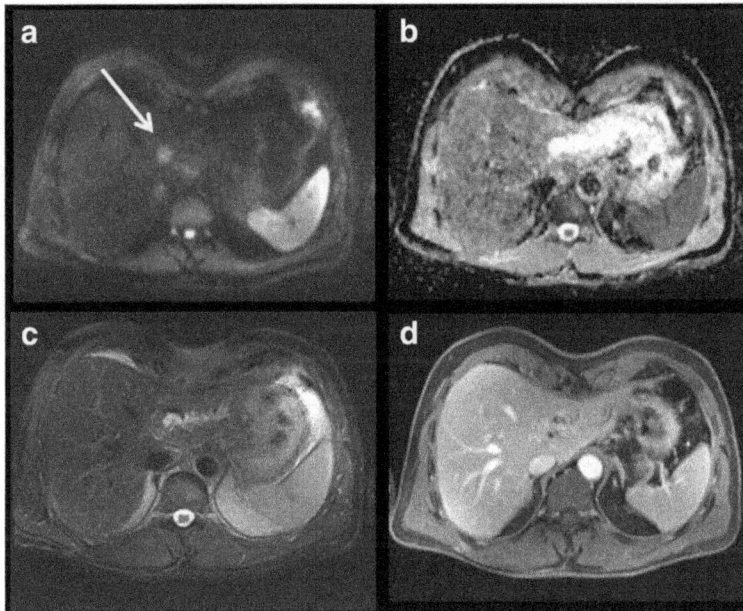

Fig. 2 48 year old male patient with hepatic metastases of a pancreatic carcinoma. Additional lesion in Counaud Segment II (white arrow). The simulated tumorboard decided on change in surgical procedure. **a**. Diffusion-weighted image (b-value 800). **b**. Corresponding ADC map. **c**. T2-weighted sequence. **d**. T1-weighted post-contrast scan

enormous impact on diagnostic imaging from which patients will largely benefit.

Although DWI has already proven to be exceptionally useful in the diagnosis of malignancies [18], its benefits seem to focus on metastases rather than HCC [19]. The detection of HCC in DWI has previously been discussed contradictorily [20, 21]. While larger HCCs usually present typical enhancement characteristics, this behavior alters with decreasing lesion size making it difficult to detect these smaller HCC foci. It is hypothesized that in early tumor development neovascularization might be too

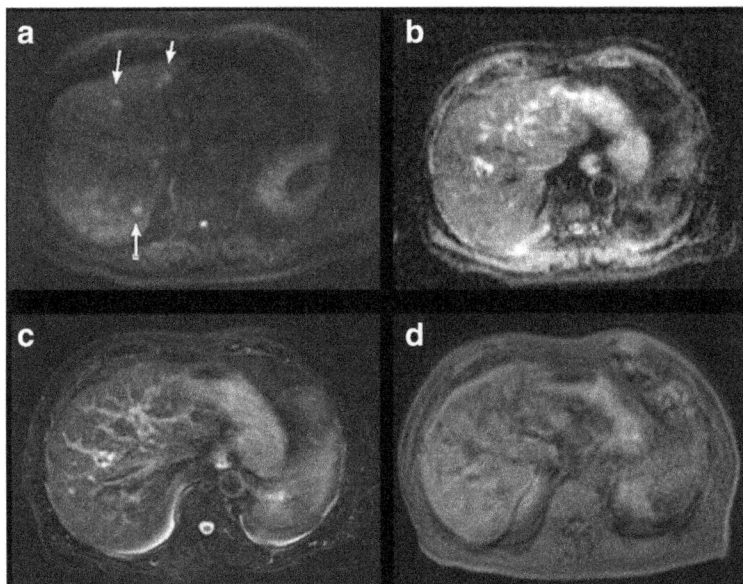

Fig. 3 80 year-old male patient with hepatic metastases of a pancreatic carcinoma. Imaging was performed without the intravenous application of contrast material due to highly elevated retention parameters. Motion artifacts due to difficulty in breathing with impairment in image quality. Hepatic lesions were only visible in diffusion-weighted sequences (white arrows). The simulated tumorboard decided on palliative regimen. **a**. Diffusion-weighted image (b-value 800). **b**. Corresponding ADC map. **c**. T2-weighted sequence. **d**. T1-weighted sequence

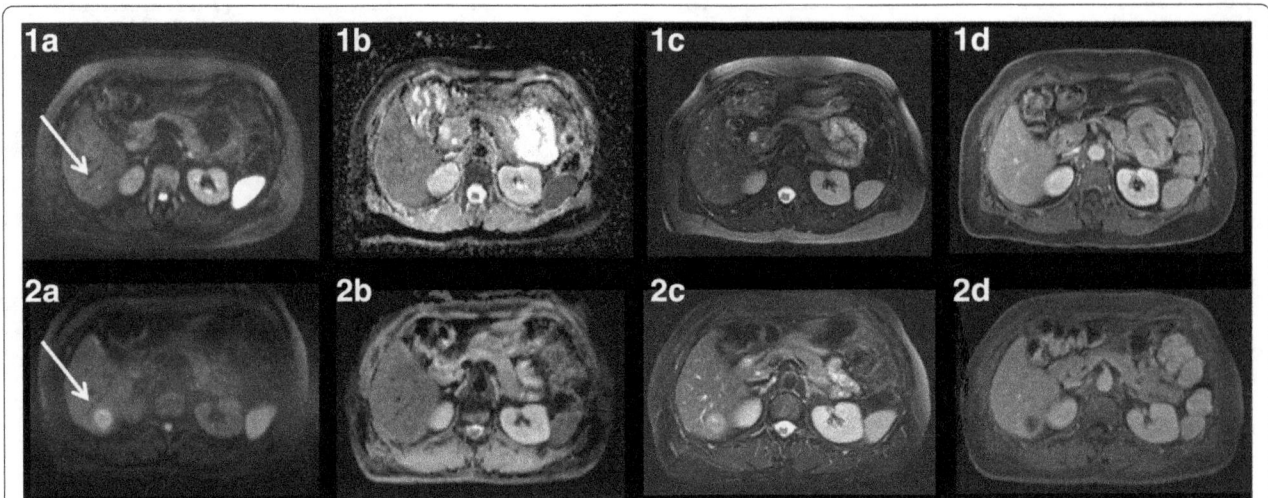

Fig. 4 51 year old female patient with hepatic metastases of a neuroendocrine tumor which was only detectable in DWI (white arrow). The simulated tumorboard decided on neoadjuvant chemotherapy. 1) Image series at baseline, 2) Image series after neoadjuvant chemotherapy with progressive disease. **a**. Diffusion-weighted image (b-value 800). **b**. Corresponding ADC map. **c**. T2-weighted sequence. **d**. T1-weighted post-contrast scan

faint to be sufficiently recorded by plain or contrast-enhanced images [8, 22]. However, by providing additional information on cell density DWI might be a further puzzle piece on the way to diagnosis [22, 23]. In our study 35 patients presented the diagnosis of a HCC, out of which DWI revealed additional information in one case. Even though there might be restrictions in detecting some cases of HCC in diffusion-weighted images, it needs to be stressed that in this specific example the HCC would have gone undetected without the additional diffusion-weighted sequence.

DWI has also been reported to increase diagnostic sensitivity in the diagnosis of CC [14, 24]. A study performed by Lee et al. revealed that the intensity of diffusion restriction can be used to establish a treatment regimen and improve the outcome of patients with intrahepatic cholangiocarcinoma [25]. Furthermore, DWI may be used in the differential diagnosis of benign strictures and the periductal infiltrating cholangiocarcinoma [14, 26]. Again, DWI in combination with standard abdominal imaging was described to lead to superior diagnosticswhen compared to MRI without an additional diffusion-weighted sequence [26]. With CC-patients being the minority in our collective, a conclusion cannot be made in this context.

Further, with DWI being a non-contrast-enhanced application it plays a special role in the diagnostic performance of patients with impaired renal function [2, 5, 27]. In our experience patients with elevated retention parameters usually present in a critical condition with limited tolerance to lengthy examinations - in these cases DWI is especially relevant as most diffusion-weighted

images are performed in free-breathing in a rather short period of time, which naturally plays in favor of limiting artifacts and scan time [2, 3]. The possibility of gaining additional information in an otherwise diagnostically limited image series is a major benefit we noticed in our retrospective evaluation.

There are limitations to this retrospective study. Firstly, imaging was performed with both, scanners of 1.5 and 3 T field strength, which might have affected image quality to a certain extent. Nevertheless, our study protocol was intended to resemble an everyday clinical setting where different scanners (i.e. different magnetic field strengths) are in use and patients are scheduled according to availability. Secondly, for the additionally detected lesions there was no established gold-standard and histological validation was not available for all lesions. In two cases without histopathological evaluation, confirmation of malignancy was not possible on the basis of the follow-up imaging. Therefore, false-positive results of DWI cannot be excluded in these two cases. Also, as above discussed, detection of HCC in diffusion-weighted images can be limited. Further, detailed information on the diagnostic value of DWI in single entities (such as specific metastases, HCC and CC) cannot be made due to small number of cases, so that larger multi-center studies are necessary. Another limitation is the fact that only patients with known hepatic malignancies were included in this evaluation which likely overinflates the rate of patients with additional findings in DWI when compared to a cohort of patients without suspected lesions or with proven extrahepatic malignancies (with a subsequently lower prevalence of liver lesions at all).

Conclusions

In conclusion, DWI is an important diagnostic tool in oncologic imaging of the liver. In comparison to conventional sequences, DWI reveals further information regarding the tumor load in patients with known hepatic malignancy influencing the therapeutic regimen.

Abbreviations

CC: Cholangiocarcinoma; DWI: Diffusion-weighted imaging; EPI: Echo planar imaging; HASTE: Half acquisition single shot turbo spin echo; HCC: Hepatocellular carcinoma; MRI: Magnetic resonance imaging; NET: Neuroendocrine tumor; TSW: Turbo spin echo sequence; VIBE: Volumetric interpolated breath-hold examination

Funding

Nothing to declare.

Authors' contributions

JT, RH and MN analyzed and interpreted the patient data regarding the added value of DWI. JJ and MB were experienced members of the interdisciplinary tumor board and provided information on treatment options. KN was a major contributor in writing the manuscript. All authors read and approved the final manuscript.

Competing interests

The authors declare that they have no competing interests.

Author details

[1]Department of Diagnostic and Interventional Radiology, University Hospital of Tuebingen, Hoppe-Seyler-Str. 3, 72076 Tuebingen, Germany. [2]Department of Visceral Surgery, University Hospital of Tuebingen, Tuebingen, Germany. [3]Department of Internal Medicine, University Hospital of Tuebingen, Tuebingen, Germany.

References

1. Koh D-M, Collins DJ. Diffusion-weighted MRI in the body: applications and challenges in oncology. Am J Roentgenol. 2007;188:1622–35. https://doi.org/10.2214/AJR.06.1403.
2. Taouli B, Beer AJ, Chenevert T, Collins D, Lehman C, Matos C, et al. Diffusion-weighted imaging outside the brain: consensus statement from an ISMRM-sponsored workshop. J Magn Reson Imaging. 2016;44:521–40. https://doi.org/10.1002/jmri.25196.
3. Taouli B, Koh D-M, Diffusion-weighted MR. Imaging of the liver. Radiology. 2009;254:47–66. https://doi.org/10.1148/radiol.09090021.
4. Stejskal EO, Tanner JE. Spin Diffusion Measurements: Spin echoes in the presence of a time-dependent field gradient. J Chem Phys. 1965;42:288–92. https://doi.org/10.1063/1.1695690.
5. Bharwani N, Koh DM. Diffusion-weighted imaging of the liver: an update. Cancer Imaging. 2013;13:171–85. https://doi.org/10.1102/1470-7330.2013.0019.
6. Padhani AR, Koh DM. Diffusion MR imaging for monitoring of treatment response. Magn Reson Imaging Clin N Am. 2011;19:181–209. https://doi.org/10.1016/j.mric.2010.10.004.
7. Bains LJ, Zweifel M, Thoeny HC. Therapy response with diffusion MRI: an update. Cancer Imaging. 2012;12:395–402. https://doi.org/10.1102/1470-7330.2012.9047.
8. van den Bos IC, Hussain SM, Dwarkasing RS, Hop WCJ, Zondervan PE, de Man RA, et al. MR imaging of hepatocellular carcinoma: relationship between lesion size and imaging findings, including signal intensity and dynamic enhancement patterns. J Magn Reson Imaging. 2007;26:1548–55. https://doi.org/10.1002/jmri.21046
9. Parikh T, Drew SJ, Lee VS, Wong S, Hecht EM, Babb JS, et al. Focal liver lesion detection and characterization with diffusion-weighted MR imaging: comparison with standard breath-hold T2-weighted imaging. Radiology. 2008;246:812–22. https://doi.org/10.1148/radiol.2463070432.
10. Dixon WT. Simple proton spectroscopic imaging. Radiology. 1984;153:189–94. https://doi.org/10.1148/radiology.153.1.6089263.
11. Jang KM, Kim SH, Min JH, Lee SJ, Kang TW, Lim S, et al. Value of diffusion-weighted MRI for differentiating malignant from benign intraductal papillary mucinous neoplasms of the pancreas. Am J Roentgenol. 2014;203:992–1000. https://doi.org/10.2214/AJR.13.11980.
12. Elbarbary AA, Saleh Elahwal HM, Elashwah ME. Role of diffusion weighted magnetic resonance imaging in evaluation of hepatic focal lesions. The Egyptian Journal of Radiology and Nuclear Medicine. 2015;46:325–34. https://doi.org/10.1016/j.ejrnm.2014.12.006.
13. Yang JD, Roberts LR. Hepatocellular carcinoma: a global view. Nat Rev Gastroenterol Hepatol. 2010;7:448–58. https://doi.org/10.1038/nrgastro.2010.100
14. Fábrega-Foster K, Ghasabeh MA, Pawlik TM, Kamel IR. Multimodality imaging of intrahepatic cholangiocarcinoma. Hepatobiliary Surg Nutr. 2017; 6:67–78. https://doi.org/10.21037/hbsn.2016.12.10.
15. Shinmura R, Matsui O, Kobayashi S, Terayama N, Sanada J, Ueda K, et al. Cirrhotic nodules: association between MR imaging signal intensity and intranodular blood supply. Radiology. 2005;237:512–9. https://doi.org/10.1148/radiol.2372041389.
16. Hardie AD, Naik M, Hecht EM, Chandarana H, Mannelli L, Babb JS, et al. Diagnosis of liver metastases: value of diffusion-weighted MRI compared with gadolinium-enhanced MRI. Eur Radiol. 2010;20:1431–41. https://doi.org/10.1007/s00330-009-1695-9.
17. Colagrande S, Castellani A, Nardi C, Lorini C, Calistri L, Filippone A. The role of diffusion-weighted imaging in the detection of hepatic metastases from colorectal cancer: a comparison with unenhanced and Gd-EOB-DTPA enhanced MRI. Eur J Radiol. 2016;85:1027–34. https://doi.org/10.1016/j.ejrad.2016.02.011.
18. Taouli B. Diffusion-weighted MR imaging for liver lesion characterization: a critical look. Radiology. 2012;262:378–80. https://doi.org/10.1148/radiol.11112417.
19. Kanematsu M, Goshima S, Watanabe H, Kondo H, Kawada H, Noda Y, et al. Detection and characterization of focal hepatic lesions with diffusion-weighted MR imaging: a pictorial review. Abdom Imaging. 2013;38:297–308. https://doi.org/10.1007/s00261-012-9940-0.
20. Park M-S, Kim S, Patel J, Hajdu CH, Do G, RK ML, et al. Hepatocellular carcinoma: detection with diffusion-weighted versus contrast-enhanced magnetic resonance imaging in pretransplant patients. Hepatology. 2012;56: 140–8. https://doi.org/10.1002/hep.25681.
21. Shankar S, Kalra N, Bhatia A, Srinivasan R, Singh P, Dhiman RK, et al. Role of diffusion weighted imaging (DWI) for hepatocellular carcinoma (HCC) detection and its grading on 3T MRI: a prospective study. J Clin Exp Hepatol. 2016;6:303–10. https://doi.org/10.1016/j.jceh.2016.08.012.
22. Vandecaveye V, De Keyzer F, Verslype C, Op de Beeck K, Komuta M, Topal B, et al. Diffusion-weighted MRI provides additional value to conventional dynamic contrast-enhanced MRI for detection of hepatocellular carcinoma. Eur Radiol. 2009;19:2456–66. https://doi.org/10.1007/s00330-009-1431-5.
23. Delso G, Fürst S, Jakoby B, Ladebeck R, Ganter C, Nekolla SG, et al. Performance measurements of the siemens mMR integrated whole-body PET/MR scanner. J Nucl Med. 2011;52:1914–22. https://doi.org/10.2967/jnumed.111.092726.
24. Park HJ, Kim YK, Park MJ, Lee WJ. Small intrahepatic mass-forming cholangiocarcinoma: target sign on diffusion-weighted imaging for differentiation from hepatocellular carcinoma. Abdom Imaging. 2013;38: 793–801. https://doi.org/10.1007/s00261-012-9943-x.
25. Lee J, Kim SH, Kang TW, Song KD, Choi D, Jang KT. Mass-forming intrahepatic cholangiocarcinoma: diffusion-weighted imaging as a preoperative prognostic marker. Radiology. 2016;281:119–28. https://doi.org/10.1148/radiol.2016151781.
26. Park HJ, Kim SH, Jang KM, Choi S-y, Lee SJ, Choi D. The role of diffusion-weighted MR imaging for differentiating benign from malignant bile duct strictures. Eur Radiol. 2014;24:947–58. https://doi.org/10.1007/s00330-014-3097-x.
27. Padhani AR, Koh D-M, Collins DJ. Whole-body diffusion-weighted MR imaging in cancer: current status and research directions. Radiology. 2011; 261:700–18. https://doi.org/10.1148/radiol.11110474.

3

Imaging of hepatocellular carcinoma and image guided therapies - how we do it

Jonathon Willatt*⊙, Julie A. Ruma, Shadi F. Azar, Nara L. Dasika and F. Syed

Abstract

Treatment options for hepatocellular carcinoma have evolved over recent years. Interventional radiologists and surgeons can offer curative treatments for early stage tumours, and locoregional therapies can be provided resulting in longer survival times. Early diagnosis with screening ultrasound is the key. CT and MRI are used to characterize lesions and determine the extent of tumour burden. Imaging techniques are discussed in this article as the correct imaging protocols are essential to optimise successful detection and characterisation. After treatment it is important to establish regular imaging follow up with CT or MRI as local residual disease can be easily treated, and recurrence elsewhere in the liver is common.

Background

Hepatocellular carcinoma (HCC) is the most common liver cancer and the fifth most common cancer worldwide. It results in between 250,000 and 1 million deaths globally per annum [1]. The number of deaths per year in HCC is close to that of the incidence throughout the world, which emphasizes the high case fatality rate of this aggressive cancer [1].

80% of HCC cases are associated with chronic hepatitis B and C virus infections [2]. Alcoholic liver disease is a risk factor in younger age groups, and the combination of alcoholic liver disease and viral hepatitis substantially increases the risk for the development of cirrhosis and HCC. The obesity epidemic has resulted in a growing population of patients with non-alcoholic fatty liver disease, cirrhosis and HCC [3].

In the United States, HCC, with its link to the hepatitis C epidemic, represents the fastest growing cause of cancer mortality overall and the second fastest growing cause of cancer deaths among women [4].

Surveillance

The AASLD (American Association for the Study of Liver Diseases) recommends screening for the following high-risk groups: Asian male hepatitis B carriers over age 40, Asian female hepatitis B carriers over age 50, hepatitis B carriers with a family history of HCC, Africans and

African Americans with hepatitis B, cirrhotic hepatitis B carriers, individuals with hepatitis C cirrhosis, individuals with stage 4 primary biliary cirrhosis, individuals with genetic hemochromatosis and cirrhosis, individuals with alpha 1-antitypsin deficiency and cirrhosis, individuals with cirrhosis from other etiologies [5].

We scan patients with cirrhosis from any etiology every 6 months with ultrasound [5, 6]. Ultrasonography remains the primary imaging modality of choice for HCC surveillance. It is more cost-effective than CT and MRI, and more widely available. A meta-analysis reported a sensitivity of 94% in detecting lesions and a specificity of >90% [7], although the figures were less favourable for lesions measuring less than 2 cm. The sensitivity for early HCC is 63%. Although our liver clinic routinely uses alpha-fetoprotein as an adjunct to imaging screening, it is acknowledged that it is neither sensitive nor specific for early diagnosis of HCC [8].

Once a nodule is detected, further follow-up depends on the size of the lesion(s), with both the American Association of the Society of Liver Diseases (AASLD) and the European Association for the Study of the Liver, European Organisation for Research and Treatment of Cancer (EASL–EORTC) using a threshold for further management of 1 cm. For nodules measuring less than 1 cm, the patient returns for a repeat ultrasound at 3 or 4 months. For nodules greater than 1 cm, the patient undergoes a dynamic contrast enhanced computed tomography (CT) or magnetic resonance imaging (MRI). The diagnosis of HCC is then determined by imaging characteristics.

* Correspondence: jwillatt@med.umich.edu
Veterans Administration, University of Michigan, Ann Arbor, MI, USA

CT or MRI

Unlike most other cancers, HCC can be diagnosed on imaging studies only without tissue sampling confirmation. Currently, all major consensus groups support the diagnosis of HCC with contrast-enhanced multiphasic CT, or with MRI using an extracellular contrast agent [5, 6]. Studies have shown a similar or slightly better diagnostic performance of dynamic MR imaging compared with multiphasic CT [9, 10] although the difference in sensitivities is small [11–13].

The decision to perform one over the other may depend on institutional preferences, individual patient needs, and availability. Advantages of CT over MRI include lower cost, increased availability, and faster scan times. Faster scan times in particular can be an advantage in the context of a cirrhotic population with multiple morbidities and difficulty in cooperating with the breath hold requirements of MRI. Advantages of MRI include the capacity to evaluate a greater variety of tissue properties including fat content, restriction of diffusion, or T2-weighted increased signal, all of which may help in lesion detection and characterization. Lack of ionizing radiation may also be a consideration in younger patients.

Ultrasound technique

We use a standard diagnostic 3–5 Mhz linear curved array probe to evaluate the liver. Subcostal real time imaging is performed of the left lobe, followed by intercostal and subcostal views of the right lobe. Both transverse and longitudinal projections are performed. Ask the patient to adopt a left lateral decubitus position for visualization of the right lobe after initially imaging in the supine position.

Initially information on the echogenicity and coarseness of the liver echotexture is assessed, as well as smoothness or nodularity of the liver surface. Then we look for focal lesions. Comparison with prior studies is essential to assess for stability or change in small hypoechoic or hyperechoic nodules. Once a new nodule or a change in a nodule is identified the patient goes on to CT or MRI, often on the same day.

We look at the hepatic vasculature. Although we do not do a full Doppler evaluation of the liver, we always look at the portal vein for direction of flow with both colour and spectral techniques and for any filling defects suggestive of tumor or bland thrombus.

An interval increase in the degree of splenomegaly can indicate a worsening of portal hypertension, so we measure the spleen as a final component of the study (Table 1).

MRI technique

We perform MRI of the liver at 1.5-T field strength, although a 3.0-T field strength can also be used [14]. A phased-array coil is routinely employed. Our protocol for imaging the cirrhotic liver includes T1-weighted gradient-recalled echo (GRE) in-phase and opposed-phase sequences, a moderately T2-weighted FSE sequence with an echo time of 80–90 msec, diffusion weighted imaging (DWI) and multiphase T1-weighted dynamic gadolinium-enhanced sequences.

A heavily T2-weighted sequence (echo time, ≥120 msec) can help to distinguish between cystic and solid lesions and a fast sequence, such as single-shot FSE (or half-Fourier acquisition turbo spin-echo—half-Fourier rapid acquisition with relaxation enhancement), is used for this purpose.

The sequences used can vary according to vendor and personal preferences. To improve image quality, sequences should be performed during suspended respiration or should be respiratory averaged (some T2-weighted sequences). Suspending respiration at end expiration produces more consistent breath holding compared with end inspiration but is more difficult for patients [15]. GRE sequences are widely used for T1-weighted imaging. Using a dual gradient-echo sequence that allows simultaneous acquisition of the earliest opposed-phase and in-phase images minimizes misregistration and improves the characterization of focal lesions and diffuse liver disease [16]. The acquisition of the earliest opposed-phase echo (2.2 msec at 1.5-T and 1.15 msec at 3-T imaging) followed by the subsequent

Table 1 Summary of imaging techniques for ultrasound, MRI and CT

Ultrasound liver	MRI liver	CT liver
3–5 MHz Curvilinear Probe	Sequences	Non contrast phase
Transverse and longitudinal imaging, to include supine and left lateral decubitus positions	Cor T2-w Single Shot Fast Spin Echo +/–Fat Saturation (FS)	IV Contrast: Iohexol 100 mL
Doppler evaluation of the portal vein	Ax T2-w Fast Spin Echo FS	Bolus tracking for arterial phase (average 30 s)
Spleen measurement	Ax Diffusion Weighted Imaging	Venous phase 65 s
	Ax dual gradient echo	Delayed phase 240 s
	Ax 3D Spoiled Gradient Echo FS pre and post dynamic contrast enhancement (and coronal reconstruction in venous phase)	Single breath for each phase
	Ax 2D Spoiled Gradient Echo FS post contrast delayed phase	Injection rate min 4 ml/s
	10 ml Gadavist	Slice thickness 3 mm no overlap
	Subtraction imaging provided	Coronal reconstructions in venous phases provided.
		Subtraction imaging optional

in-phase echo enables the distinction between signal intensity loss caused by the presence of lipid seen on opposed-phase images and signal intensity loss due to susceptibility artifact from hepatic iron deposition, which is exaggerated on the longer of the two echoes (usually in phase).

Three-dimensional gadolinium-enhanced GRE sequences are preferred to two-dimensional GRE sequences because of the thinner sections obtained, which improve lesion detection and permit multiplanar image reconstructions for presurgical planning [17]. Section thickness should not exceed 4 mm for three-dimensional sequences and 6 mm for two-dimensional sequences. Contrast agent bolus timing is strongly recommended, based on our experience and review of the literature [18], to ensure the consistent capturing of the arterial-dominant phase; fixed delay is not a reliable method in this patient population. Options include use of a test bolus and various automated detection methods [19]. Hypervascular HCC is most conspicuous in the late arterial phase and can be missed if the arterial-dominant phase images are acquired early [20]. A timing bolus is not essential if rapid multiphase arterial imaging is performed. To improve lesion characterization—for example, to detect washout or delayed contrast material retention of hemangioma and cholangiocarcinoma—multiphase dynamic gadolinium-enhanced imaging should include three contrast-enhanced phases or more. We routinely acquire four sets of images after gadolinium-based contrast material injection in the arterial-dominant (automated timing, usually 20–35 s), venous (60–90 s), interstitial (120–150 s), and delayed (5 min) phases of hepatic enhancement. The highest spatial resolution should be used without compromising signal intensity, taking into account patients' breath-holding capacity. Parallel imaging techniques can be applied to improve spatial resolution and/or reduce acquisition time. However, these techniques should be implemented with care, because they can result in image artifacts and reduced lesion conspicuity [21].

We find ourselves frequently dependent on subtraction imaging because of the intrinsic high signal demonstrated by nodules in the cirrhotic liver, including regenerative, dysplastic and malignant nodules. Intrinsic high signal can also be demonstrated in successfully treated HCC [22]. Unenhanced images can be subtracted from arterial-phase gadolinium-enhanced images to assess for arterial enhancement in nodules [23]. Subtraction can be performed if the unenhanced and gadolinium-enhanced imaging sequences are identical, if the imager is not retuned between acquisitions, and if there are no image rescaling issues. Acquiring the unenhanced and gadolinium-enhanced images in a single series rather than in separate series minimizes these differences and is possible with most systems. Patients

should be instructed to hold their breath in a similar fashion during all sequences to minimize misregistration artifacts, which appear as a bright line at the edge of organs owing to incomplete overlap. At this point the ability of the MR radiographer or technician to coach the patient is crucial. Consistent breath holds are important in many MR sequences because of the lengths of the scans, but for subtraction imaging it is impossible to overemphasise the absolute requirement for good breath holds. If the patient, despite careful coaching, is unable to hold his/her breath, then CT, despite the change in modality, may be the better form of imaging.

Diffusion weighted imaging increases the detection rate of HCC, particularly for small tumours [24–26]. B-values typically used include one in the low range (0–50 s/mm2) and one in the intermediate-to-high range (400–800 s/mm2). We find that the DWI sequence frequently helps us to lean in favour or against small arterial enhancing lesions with equivocal washout as HCC, as well as assisting us in bringing our attention to small lesions which are inconspicuous on contrast-enhanced sequences [27]. Tumors can be obscured on DWI because of the increased DWI signal in fibrotic liver parenchyma and subsequent decreased lesion to liver contrast [28]. In addition, DWI signal may be seen with other hepatic malignancies, such as metastases and intrahepatic cholangiocarcinomas [28–30].

Both extracellular and hepatobiliary agents can be used for imaging of the liver. We favour the use of the more expensive hepatobiliary agents only in specific cases where key decisions are to be made with regard to transplant or locoregional treatment. Indeed, hepatobiliary agents can present radiologists with greater diagnostic conundrums in contrast to more clarity.

Extracellular gadolinium-based contrast agents (for example, gadopentetate dimeglumine (Gd-DTPA), Magnevist®, Bayer HealthCare), distribute from the vascular space into the interstitial compartment. The standard dose is 0.1 mmol/kg typically injected intravenously at a rate of 2 mL/s followed by a normal saline "flush" of 20 to 50 mL.

Hepatobiliary agents distribute into the interstitial space, but, importantly for hepatic imaging, are also taken up by hepatocytes with subsequent biliary excretion. Multihance, Bracco Diagnostics, Princeton, NJ, USA) was the first to be approved. Approximately 95% of this agent is excreted by the kidney, but 3 to 5% is taken up by the normal hepatocytes and excreted into the biliary tract. Gadoxetate Disodium (U.S: Eovist, Europe: Primovist, Bayer Healthcare Pharmaceuticals, Wayne, NJ, USA) has approximately 50:50 excretion between renal (glomerular filtration) and hepatocyte uptake/biliary excretion. This can therefore be used for the early dynamic imaging phase in the liver, as above, followed by a 20 min T1-weighted imaging phase where the liver is of higher signal intensity and non-hepatocyte containing masses will be of low signal intensity. Hepatocyte-specific contrast agents have been shown in many studies to increase lesion sensitivity for HCC by capitalizing on evidence that poorly differentiated HCCs do not contain functioning hepatocytes and bile ducts, and therefore demonstrate hypointense signal relative to the surrounding liver parenchyma [30, 31]. Combining contrast-enhanced MRI features and hepatobiliary phase imaging has demonstrated sensitivities and specificities of greater than 90% [31].

Potential pitfalls that apply specifically to Eovist/Primovist include transient marked motion on arterial phase images, inability to assess washout after the portal venous phase due to early parenchymal enhancement, difficulty identifying "capsule appearance" due to hepatic parenchymal enhancement, and difficulty identifying venous tumor invasion due to more rapid venous clearance and decreased vein to liver contrast [32, 33].

The use of hepatobiliary agents for the diagnosis of HCC is in transition. Some major HCC imaging guidelines do not mention this class contrast agents [5, 6, 34], while other societies or organizations recommend their use [35]. It remains unclear whether hepatobiliary phase contrast hypoenhancement [32] will be more widely incorporated in comparison with conventional extracellular contrast agent imaging characteristics for the diagnosis of HCC (Table 1).

CT technique

Multidetector CT (MDCT) allows fast, high-quality, thin-section imaging and permits 3D reconstruction with better spatial resolution than that of MRI. Fast injection rates (4–8 ml/s) provide more reliable enhancement during the hepatic arterial phase and increase the sensitivity of CT to liver lesions. Studies have demonstrated hypervascular components in 81–89% of HCCs [36]. For patients with contraindications to MRI CT serves as an adequate alternative.

CT imaging technique is based on the same principles as dynamic contrast MRI, using arterial enhancement, delayed washout, and a delayed enhancing pseudocapsule as the pillars of diagnosis. The precontrast images serve as a baseline to gauge subsequent enhancement. Following the injection of 100 ml of Omnipaque 350 (Iohexol) we use a bolus tracking system (threshold attenuation in the aorta 150 HU) to initiate arterial phase breathhold imaging through the liver. Subsequent series of images are taken at 65 s and 240 s to provide venous and delayed phase imaging Subtraction images (postcontrast minus precontrast) may be helpful for detection of enhancement and evaluation of its degree [37] (Table 1).

Diagnosis of HCC and report writing

The hallmark feature of HCC on both CT and MRI is late arterial enhancement with washout relative to the liver parenchyma during the venous or delayed phases (3–5 min post injection) (Fig. 1). This pattern of enhancement has been shown to demonstrate high specificity and positive predictive value [38–40] making it the noninvasive standard for HCC diagnosis [5, 6, 35, 41–44].

In addition to the enhancement pattern, additional features of HCC have been described which are also specific for HCC including capsular enhancement [30, 45, 46]. Capsular enhancement (Fig. 2) is defined as a persistent peripheral enhancing rim seen on venous and delayed phases.

More specific to MRI, a diagnosis of HCC is often attributed to a lesion showing only arterial enhancement or only washout and pseudocapsule formation, if the lesion also demonstrates increased signal intensity on T2-weighted mages [47, 48] or if the lesion restricts

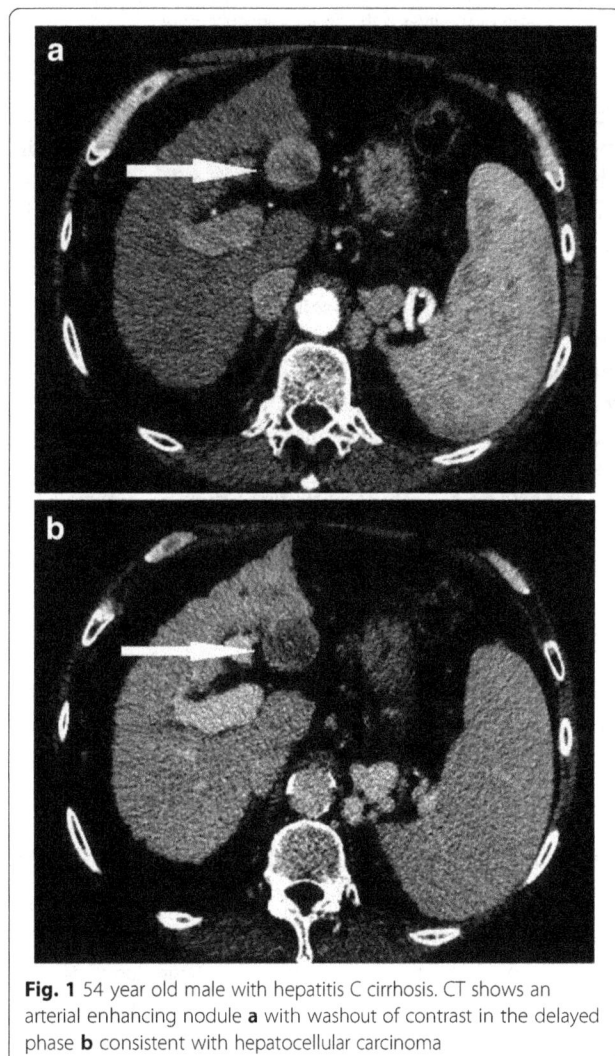

Fig. 1 54 year old male with hepatitis C cirrhosis. CT shows an arterial enhancing nodule **a** with washout of contrast in the delayed phase **b** consistent with hepatocellular carcinoma

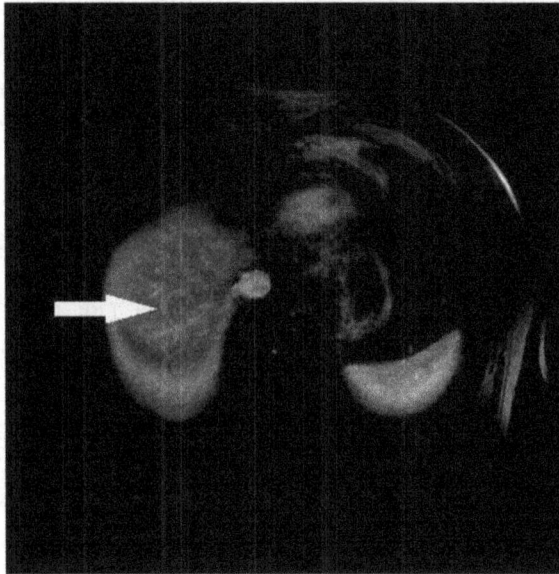

Fig. 2 67 year old male with alchohol liver disease and cirrhosis. Venous phase MRI with gadolinium demonstrates an HCC nodule at the dome of the liver with capsular enhancement

Fig. 3 71 year old male with hepatitis C cirrhosis. Signal drop out on opposed phase imaging (**b**) in comparison with in phase imaging (**a**). The findings represent intracellular lipid in an HCC tumour

diffusion [25, 27, 49], although some caution should be applied to both of these adjuncts as they can result in false positive interpretations [50] (Table 2).

Intracellular lipid detected within a nodule on dual-echo in and opposed phase T1-weighted MRI is an additional finding which has been shown to be reasonably specific for HCC. This can be a useful addition to the toolbox when looking at a lesion with non-specific enhancement characteristics as intracellular lipid is very rare in a regenerative or dysplastic nodules [51] (Fig. 3).

In the event of uncertainty a consensus opinion is reached from the available liver imaging specialists in the department. Lesions with focal hepatic arterial enhancement, but without washout, capsule enhancement, or abnormal increased T2 signal, are considered dysplastic nodules (if clearly a defined nodule) or non-specific hypervascular lesions (if nonmarginated and subcapsular).

We review prior imaging and clinical information for all patients. An understanding of the treatment options for HCC under the current guidelines is essential. We structure the conclusions of our reports so that the multidisciplinary liver group can make informed decisions in the context of the options available.

Reports indicate the size (largest axial or coronal section diameter), number, and location of HCC lesions. The Couinaud classification is used for anatomic reference [52]. Although the system was designed for surgical planning it is universally accepted, simple, and more concise than the descriptive terms for the segmental anatomy. The coronal measurement is frequently omitted in reports but is important because it affects the treatment stratification, both for transplant evaluation and for determination of the type of locoregional therapy to be used.

Table 2 MRI major and ancillary features for the diagnosis of HCC

HCC: major feature s	HCC: ancillary features
Arterial phase enhancement	T2-w hyperintensity
Delayed phase "washout"	Restriction of diffusion
Threshold growth	Intra-lesional fat
Delayed enhancing capsule	

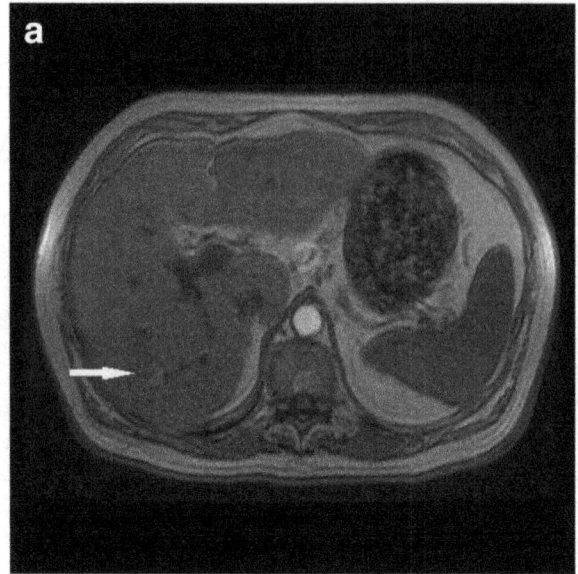

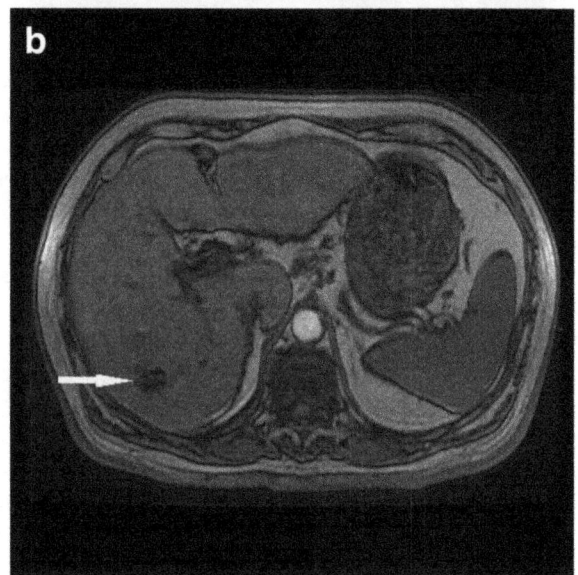

We number the tumors from 1 to 4. If there are more than 4 lesions then we determine whether there is unilobar or bilobar disease and describe how many lesions there are in each lobe, again numbering them so that they can be easily detected. We believe in the importance of providing series and image numbers for each lesion up to 4 lesions so that if the reporting radiologist is not present at the multidisciplinary meeting, or if surgeons or liver specialists are looking at the images, they can find the lesions quickly and not become confused by other confounding imaging findings.

For each lesion the T1-weighted, T2-weighted, diffusion weighted and contrast enhanced characteristics are always described. If there are ancillary findings, for example signal dropout on opposed phase imaging in contrast with in phase imaging, then we add those as well. Although we do not strictly apply a LIRADS (Liver Imaging Reporting and Data System) number to each lesion, we report findings in the context of the LIRADS criteria as these are the current most comprehensive guidelines used to stratify the risk malignancy in the context of cirrhosis and HCC [53]. LIRADS is a useful system to use when there is not close communication in a multidisciplinary setting. It is easily accessible online and the system is helpful for those cases where there is some uncertainty.

For specific examples which are not clearly covered by guidelines, our experiences are that small nodule-like arterial enhancing lesions which do not show associated washout, but which increase in conspicuity over time, merit close attention on follow up imaging as these often develop ancillary features of washout, pseudocapsule or restricted diffusion over time. Small foci of restricted diffusion or high T2-weighted signal with arterial enhancement often turn out to be HCC, whereas small foci or restricted diffusion without arterial enhancement, and without other ancillary features, are very common, and are almost always not related to cancer.

A review for extrahepatic disease is essential as metastatic disease changes all of the treatment pathways. The lungs should be imaged once HCC is diagnosed. Metastatic disease is seen in multiple locations but portal lymph nodes, peritoneum, adrenal glands and bones are the more frequent locations.

Selection and staging

Once a patient is diagnosed with HCC, a multidisciplinary approach is adopted to determine optimal therapy and further management. Our group includes transplant surgeons, hepatologists, oncologists, radiation oncologists, and cross-sectional and interventional radiologistsWe prepare the cases for presentation each week.

Although several staging schema have been developed, none have been universally adopted. A few main factors have been identified as influential in the prognosis of

patients with HCC. These include liver function, tumor size and number, tumor extent, including vascular invasion and extrahepatic spread, evidence of portal hypertension, and clinical performance status. Tumor proximity to large vessels and main bile ducts can also be pertinent with regard to ablative therapies, and is worth mentioning if these treatments are likely to be considered.

CT and MRI are useful in identifying tumor extent and extrahepatic spread. They also provide secondary evidence of portal hypertension, including the presence of splenomegaly and portosystemic collaterals. Imaging of the chest is also recommended as part of the initial work up, given that lung and bone are common sites for HCC metastasis. A bone scan can also be performed if there is a suspicion for osseous metastasis, or if the patient is being considered for liver transplantation.

The Barcelona Clinic Liver Cancer (BCLC) system links the staging of HCC in patients with cirrhosis with treatment options, making it the most commonly adopted staging system [5, 6].

The BCLC system identifies those patients with early stage HCC who may benefit from curative therapies (stage 0 and A), those at intermediate (stage B) or advanced (stage C) stages who may benefit from palliative treatments, and those who are most suitable for best supportive care (stage D). Curative treatment options, including transplantation, resection, and ablation for patients with early stage disease depends on local factors, patient specific issues, and patient preference. Palliative, non-curative treatment options include transcatheter arterial chemoembolization (TACE) for stage B disease, radioembolisation, and sorafenib for advanced stage C disease. TACE is also increasingly used as a "bridge" to transplant, and in some cases to downstage patients so that they can become candidates for a transplant list [54, 55].

In equivocal cases where the diagnosis of HCC is uncertain in small lesions, a reasonable approach is to wait 3 months and image again [56, 57].

Post therapy imaging

Because many patients with HCC do not meet criteria for transplantation or surgery, a large proportion of patients receive locoregional therapy or systemic therapy and therefore require post-therapy imaging to evaluate for initial response and recurrent disease. No established guidelines for ideal surveillance time intervals exist. Recurrence is 6.5 times more likely to occur in the first year after therapy than in the second year, so most guidelines suggest 3 monthly interval imaging in the first year after treatment [58]. We follow up with imaging at 3 month intervals for one year followed by 6 month intervals for 2 years, and then we return to ultrasound screening. It is important to use the same modality for each follow up as comparison between CT and MRI can

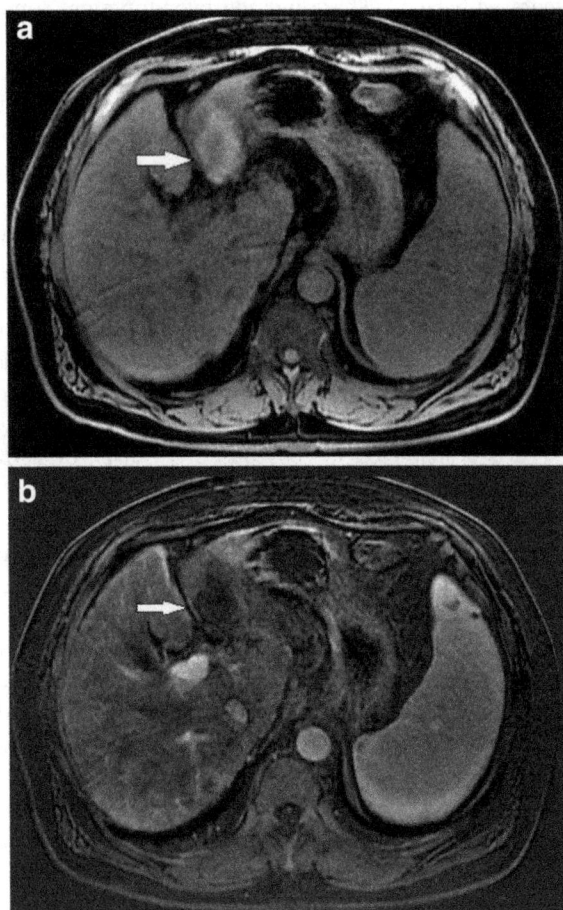

Fig. 4 66 year old female with hepatitis C cirrhosis post microwave ablation of HCC Precontrast image post microwave ablation (**a**) show a cavity with intrinsic high signal on T1 weighted imaging. A subtraction image (**b**) removes the high signal resulting in no evidence of enhancement

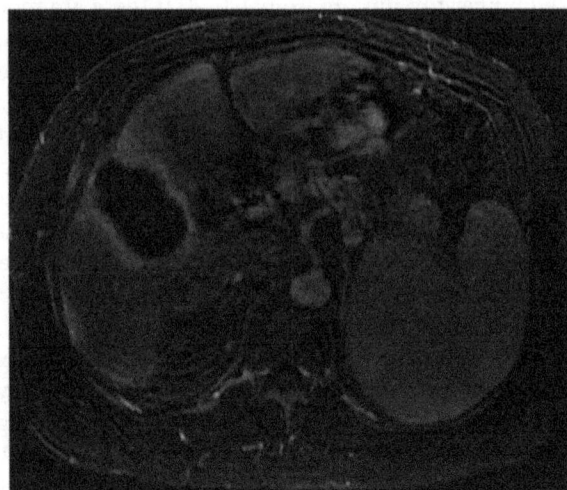

Fig. 5 63 year old male with cirrhosis and HCC treated with microwave ablation. A thin rim of enhancement post ablation, consistent with hyperemia adjacent to the ablation zone, is a normal finding and does not represent recurrent tumour

be challenging. We generally use MRI for follow up as the imaging findings can be more difficult to interpret following treatment and the subtraction images can be really useful (Fig. 4).

Several systems have been developed to objectively evaluate the response of HCC to locoregional therapy. Some of these are based on tumor size, such as the WHO (World Health Organisation) and RECIST (Response Evaluation Criteria in Solid Tumours) criteria [59, 60],

while others, such as EASL, AASLD, and mRECIST, are based on the assessment of residual enhancing HCC [61, 62]. mRECIST, or modified RECIST, therefore does not evaluate tumour bulk itself, as does RECIST, as this may not change after treatment, or may even increase, but assesses the volume of residual functional tumour or arterial enhancing tissue [63]. Studies have shown that the mRECIST and EASL enhancement-based protocols correlate more accurately with residual disease burden and with survival after therapy than the size-based protocols for patients treated with ablation, radioembolization and TACE [63–67]. At our multidisciplinary meetings we use a combination of mRECIST and EASL criteria to quantify residual or recurrent tumour, along with informed discussion from the team members (Table 3).

Prior to reporting we make sure we have established the procedures performed or therapies used, as lack of awareness of these can lead to embarrassing errors in reporting. Regardless of the therapy performed, treated tumor should demonstrate an absence of enhancement. A thin rim of enhancement can be seen as a normal finding after ablation and TACE due to adjacent hyperemia and fibrosis (Fig. 5). However, residual or

Table 3 Summary of mRECIST and EASL responses

	mRECIST	EASL
Complete Response	Disappearance of any intratumoral arterial enhancement in all target lesions (up to 2 measurable liver lesions)	Disappearance of any intratumoral arterial enhancement in all measurable arterial enhancing liver lesions
Partial Response	Decrease >30% in the sum of longest diameters of viable target lesions	Decrease >50% in the sum of the product of bidimensional diameters of viable target lesions
Progressive Disease	Increase >20% in the sum of longest diameters of viable target lesions	Increase >25% in the sum of the diameters of viable target lesions
Stable Disease	None of the above	None of the above

recurrent disease presents as thick or nodular peripheral arterial enhancement [65, 68, 69] (Fig. 6). Post-ablation changes are similar regardless of what type of ablation is performed. The ablation zone should be larger than the original tumor by between 5 and 10 mm. If it is not, then careful attention to subtle enhancing lesions is needed. Ablation zones can decrease in size with time. An ablation zone can demonstrate high signal intensity on pre-contrast T1-weighted images as a result of coagulative necrosis, making evaluation for arterial enhancement difficult in the absence of subtraction imaging. Subtractions should therefore be routinely included within the MRI protocol [22].

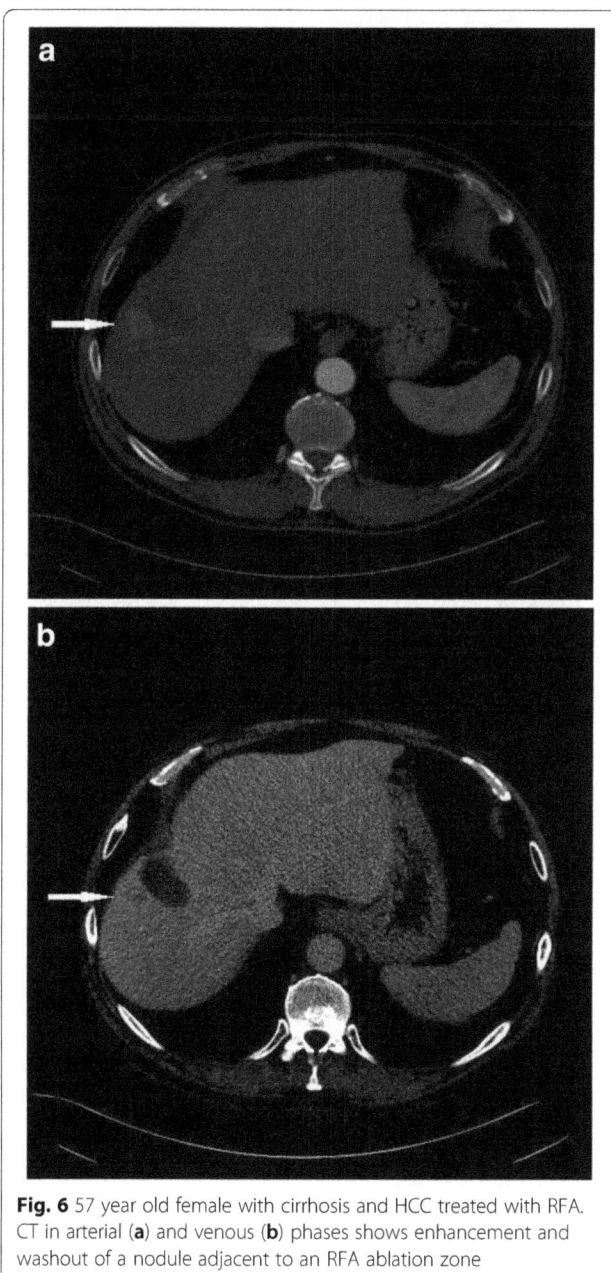

Fig. 6 57 year old female with cirrhosis and HCC treated with RFA. CT in arterial (**a**) and venous (**b**) phases shows enhancement and washout of a nodule adjacent to an RFA ablation zone

Conclusions

The accepted modality for hepatocellular carcinoma screening is ultrasound. Once HCC is suspected then CT or MRI may be used to confirm the diagnosis and establish the tumor burden for staging purposes. The BCLC classification system is the most frequently used for treatment planning. However, multidisciplinary meeting and planning is essential to ensure that the correct pathways are adopted within the context of each institution. Following surgical, locoregional, chemotherapeutic or radiotherapeutic treatment, follow up imaging and regular multidisciplinary discussion is adopted.

Abbreviations
AASLD: American Association for the Study of Liver Diseases; BCLC: Barcelona Clinic Liver Cancer; CT: Computed tomography; DWI: Diffusion weighted imaging; EASL–EORTC: European Association for the Study of the Liver, European Organisation for Research and Treatment of Cancer; FSE: Half-Fourier acquisition turbo spin-echo; Gd: Gadolinium; GRE: Gradient echo; HCC: Hepatocellular carcinoma; LIRADS: Liver Image and Reporting Data System; MDCT: Multidetector computed tomography; mRECIST: modified Response Evaluation Criteria in Solid Tumours; MRI: Magnetic resonance imaging; RECIST: Response Evaluation Criteria in Solid Tumours; TACE: Transcatheter arterial chemoembolization; WHO: World Health Organisation

Acknowledgements
Not applicable.

Funding
Not applicable.

Authors' contributions
JW was primary author and prepared the manuscript for publication. JR drafted the original manuscript. SA reviewed and helped edit the manuscript and provided help with images. ND reviewed, provided expert opinion and edits on treatments for HCC, and helped edit the manuscript. FS reviewed and helped edit the manuscript as an independent reviewer of the structure and content of the article. All authors read and approved the final manuscript.

Competing interests
The authors declare that they have no competing interests.

References
1. Torre LA, Bray F, Siegel RL, Ferlay J, Lortet-Tieulent J, Jemal A. Global cancer statistics, 2012. CA Cancer J Clin. 2015;65(2):87–108.
2. Perz JF, Armstrong GL, Farrington LA, Hutin YJ, Bell BP. The contributions of hepatitis B virus and hepatitis C virus infections to cirrhosis and primary liver cancer worldwide. J Hepatol. 2006;45(4):529–38.
3. Bugianesi E. EASL-EASD-EASO Clinical Practice Guidelines for the management of non-alcoholic fatty liver disease: disease mongering or call to action? Diabetologia. 2016;59(6):1145–7.
4. Seeff LB. Introduction: The burden of hepatocellular carcinoma. Gastroenterology. 2004;127(5 Suppl 1):S1–4.
5. Bruix J, Sherman M. Management of hepatocellular carcinoma: an update. Hepatology. 2011;53(3):1020–2.

6. EASL-EORTC clinical practice guidelines: management of hepatocellular carcinoma. J Hepatol. 2012;56(4):908–43.

7. Singal A, Volk ML, Waljee A, et al. Meta-analysis: surveillance with ultrasound for early-stage hepatocellular carcinoma in patients with cirrhosis. Aliment Pharmacol Ther. 2009;30(1):37–47.

8. Lok AS, Sterling RK, Everhart JE, et al. Des-gamma-carboxy prothrombin and alpha-fetoprotein as biomarkers for the early detection of hepatocellular carcinoma. Gastroenterology. 2010;138(2):493–502.

9. Choi TW, Lee JM, Kim JH, Yu MH, Han JK, Choi BI. Comparison of multidetector CT and gadobutrol-enhanced MR imaging for evaluation of small, solid pancreatic lesions. Korean J Radiol. 2016;17(4):509–21.

10. Guo J, Seo Y, Ren S, et al. Diagnostic performance of contrast-enhanced multidetector computed tomography and gadoxetic acid disodium-enhanced magnetic resonance imaging in detecting hepatocellular carcinoma: direct comparison and a meta-analysis. Abdom Radiol. 2016;41(10):1960–72.

11. Burrel M, Llovet JM, Ayuso C, et al. MRI angiography is superior to helical CT for detection of HCC prior to liver transplantation: an explant correlation. Hepatology. 2003;38(4):1034–42.

12. Kim YK, Kim CS, Chung GH, et al. Comparison of gadobenate dimeglumine-enhanced dynamic MRI and 16-MDCT for the detection of hepatocellular carcinoma. AJR Am J Roentgenol. 2006;186(1):149–57.

13. Lim JH, Kim CK, Lee WJ, et al. Detection of hepatocellular carcinomas and dysplastic nodules in cirrhotic livers: accuracy of helical CT in transplant patients. AJR Am J Roentgenol. 2000;175(3):693–8.

14. Hussain SM, Wielopolski PA, Martin DR. Abdominal magnetic resonance imaging at 3.0 T: problem or a promise for the future? Top Magn Reson Imaging. 2005;16(4):325–35.

15. Kimura T, Hirokawa Y, Murakami Y, et al. Reproducibility of organ position using voluntary breath-hold method with spirometer for extracranial stereotactic radiotherapy. Int J Radiat Oncol Biol Phys. 2004;60(4):1307–13.

16. Merkle EM, Nelson RC. Dual gradient-echo in-phase and opposed-phase hepatic MR imaging: a useful tool for evaluating more than fatty infiltration or fatty sparing. Radiographics. 2006;26(5):1409–18.

17. Lee VS, Lavelle MT, Rofsky NM, et al. Hepatic MR imaging with a dynamic contrast-enhanced isotropic volumetric interpolated breath-hold examination: feasibility, reproducibility, and technical quality. Radiology. 2000;215(2):365–72.

18. Sharma P, Kitajima HD, Kalb B, Martin DR. Gadolinium-enhanced imaging of liver tumors and manifestations of hepatitis: pharmacodynamic and technical considerations. Top Magn Reson Imaging. 2009;20(2):71–8.

19. Hussain HK, Londy FJ, Francis IR, et al. Hepatic arterial phase MR imaging with automated bolus-detection three-dimensional fast gradient-recalled-echo sequence: comparison with test-bolus method. Radiology. 2003;226(2):558–66.

20. Mori K, Yoshioka H, Takahashi N, et al. Triple arterial phase dynamic MRI with sensitivity encoding for hypervascular hepatocellular carcinoma: comparison of the diagnostic accuracy among the early, middle, late, and whole triple arterial phase imaging. AJR Am J Roentgenol. 2005;184(1):63–9.

21. Vogt FM, Antoch G, Hunold P, et al. Parallel acquisition techniques for accelerated volumetric interpolated breath-hold examination magnetic resonance imaging of the upper abdomen: assessment of image quality and lesion conspicuity. J Magn Reson Imaging. 2005;21(4):376–82.

22. Winters SD, Jackson S, Armstrong GA, Birchall IW, Lee KH, Low G. Value of subtraction MRI in assessing treatment response following image-guided loco-regional therapies for hepatocellular carcinoma. Clin Radiol. 2012;67(7):649–55.

23. Yu JS, Kim YH, Rofsky NM. Dynamic subtraction magnetic resonance imaging of cirrhotic liver: assessment of high signal intensity lesions on nonenhanced T1-weighted images. J Comput Assist Tomogr. 2005;29(1):51–8.

24. Park MS, Kim S, Patel J, et al. Hepatocellular carcinoma: detection with diffusion-weighted versus contrast-enhanced magnetic resonance imaging in pretransplant patients. Hepatology. 2012;56(1):140–8.

25. Xu PJ, Yan FH, Wang JH, Shan Y, Ji Y, Chen CZ. Contribution of diffusion-weighted magnetic resonance imaging in the characterization of hepatocellular carcinomas and dysplastic nodules in cirrhotic liver. J Comput Assist Tomogr. 2010;34(4):506–12.

26. Le Moigne F, Durieux M, Bancel B, et al. Impact of diffusion-weighted MR imaging on the characterization of small hepatocellular carcinoma in the cirrhotic liver. Magn Reson Imaging. 2012;30(5):656–65.

27. Wu LM, Xu JR, Lu Q, Hua J, Chen J, Hu J. A pooled analysis of diffusion-weighted imaging in the diagnosis of hepatocellular carcinoma in chronic liver diseases. J Gastroenterol Hepatol. 2013;28(2):227–34.

28. Park MJ, Kim YK, Lee MW, et al. Small hepatocellular carcinomas: improved sensitivity by combining gadoxetic acid-enhanced and diffusion-weighted MR imaging patterns. Radiology. 2012;264(3):761–70.

29. Miller FH, Hammond N, Siddiqi AJ, et al. Utility of diffusion-weighted MRI in distinguishing benign and malignant hepatic lesions. J Magn Reson Imaging. 2010;32(1):138–47.

30. Rhee H, Kim MJ, Park MS, Kim KA. Differentiation of early hepatocellular carcinoma from benign hepatocellular nodules on gadoxetic acid-enhanced MRI. Br J Radiol. 2012;85(1018):e837–44.

31. Liu X, Zou L, Liu F, Zhou Y, Song B. Gadoxetic acid disodium-enhanced magnetic resonance imaging for the detection of hepatocellular carcinoma: a meta-analysis. PLoS One. 2013;8(8):e70896.

32. Motosugi U, Bannas P, Sano K, Reeder SB. Hepatobiliary MR contrast agents in hypovascular hepatocellular carcinoma. J Magn Reson Imaging. 2015;41(2):251–65.

33. Hope TA, Fowler KJ, Sirlin CB, et al. Hepatobiliary agents and their role in LI-RADS. Abdom Imaging. 2015;40(3):613–25.

34. Wald C, Russo MW, Heimbach JK, Hussain HK, Pomfret EA, Bruix J. New OPTN/UNOS policy for liver transplant allocation: standardization of liver imaging, diagnosis, classification, and reporting of hepatocellular carcinoma. Radiology. 2013;266(2):376–82.

35. Kudo M, Izumi N, Kokudo N, et al. Management of hepatocellular carcinoma in Japan: consensus-based clinical practice guidelines proposed by the Japan Society of Hepatology (JSH) 2010 updated version. Dig Dis. 2011;29(3):339–64.

36. Murakami T, Kim T, Takamura M, et al. Hypervascular hepatocellular carcinoma: detection with double arterial phase multi-detector row helical CT. Radiology. 2001;218(3):763–7.

37. Miraglia R, Pietrosi G, Maruzzelli L, et al. Predictive factors of tumor response to trans-catheter treatment in cirrhotic patients with hepatocellular carcinoma: a multivariate analysis of pre-treatment findings. World J Gastroenterol. 2007;13(45):6022–6.

38. Forner A, Vilana R, Ayuso C, et al. Diagnosis of hepatic nodules 20 mm or smaller in cirrhosis: Prospective validation of the noninvasive diagnostic criteria for hepatocellular carcinoma. Hepatology. 2008;47(1):97–104.

39. Kim SE, Lee HC, Shim JH, et al. Noninvasive diagnostic criteria for hepatocellular carcinoma in hepatic masses >2 cm in a hepatitis B virus-endemic area. Liver Int. 2011;31(10):1468–76.

40. Leoni S, Piscaglia F, Golfieri R, et al. The impact of vascular and nonvascular findings on the noninvasive diagnosis of small hepatocellular carcinoma based on the EASL and AASLD criteria. Am J Gastroenterol. 2010;105(3):599–609.

41. Benson 3rd AB, Abrams TA, Ben-Josef E, et al. NCCN clinical practice guidelines in oncology: hepatobiliary cancers. J Natl Compr Canc Netw. 2009;7(4):350–91.

42. Omata M, Lesmana LA, Tateishi R, et al. Asian Pacific Association for the Study of the Liver consensus recommendations on hepatocellular carcinoma. Hepatol Int. 2010;4(2):439–74.

43. Verslype C, Rosmorduc O, Rougier P. Hepatocellular carcinoma: ESMO-ESDO Clinical Practice Guidelines for diagnosis, treatment and follow-up. Ann Oncol. 2012;23 Suppl 7:vii41–8.

44. Santillan CS, Tang A, Cruite I, Shah A, Sirlin CB. Understanding LI-RADS: a primer for practical use. Magn Reson Imaging Clin N Am. 2014;22(3):337–52.

45. Khan AS, Hussain HK, Johnson TD, Weadock WJ, Pelletier SJ, Marrero JA. Value of delayed hypointensity and delayed enhancing rim in magnetic resonance imaging diagnosis of small hepatocellular carcinoma in the cirrhotic liver. J Magn Reson Imaging. 2010;32(2):360–6.

46. Cruite I, Santillan C, Mamidipalli A, Shah A, Tang A, Sirlin CB. Liver imaging reporting and data system: review of ancillary imaging features. Semin Roentgenol. 2016;51(4):301–7.

47. Coenegrachts K, Delanote J, Ter Beek L, et al. Improved focal liver lesion detection: comparison of single-shot diffusion-weighted echoplanar and single-shot T2 weighted turbo spin echo techniques. Br J Radiol. 2007;80(955):524–31.

48. Parikh T, Drew SJ, Lee VS, et al. Focal liver lesion detection and characterization with diffusion-weighted MR imaging: comparison with standard breath-hold T2-weighted imaging. Radiology. 2008;246(3):812–22.

49. Piana G, Trinquart L, Meskine N, Barrau V, Beers BV, Vilgrain V. New MR imaging criteria with a diffusion-weighted sequence for the diagnosis of hepatocellular carcinoma in chronic liver diseases. J Hepatol. 2011;55(1):126–32.

50. Hicks RM, Yee J, Ohliger MA, et al. Comparison of diffusion-weighted imaging and T2-weighted single shot fast spin-echo: Implications for LI-RADS characterization of hepatocellular carcinoma. Magn Reson Imaging. 2016;34(7):915–21.

51. Sano K, Ichikawa T, Motosugi U, et al. Imaging study of early hepatocellular carcinoma: usefulness of gadoxetic acid-enhanced MR imaging. Radiology. 2011;261(3):834–44.

52. Couinaud C. Liver lobes and segments: notes on the anatomical architecture and surgery of the liver. Presse Med. 1954;62(33):709–12.

53. ACo. R. Liver imaging reporting and data system version. American College of Radiology: https://nrdr.acr.org/lirads/. Accessed 10 Dec 2016.

54. Prasad MA, Kulik LM. The role of bridge therapy prior to orthotopic liver transplantation. J Natl Compr Canc Netw. 2014;12(8):1183–90. quiz 91.

55. San Miguel C, Muffak K, Triguero J, et al. Role of transarterial chemoembolization to downstage hepatocellular carcinoma within the Milan criteria. Transplant Proc. 2015;47(9):2631–3.

56. An C, Choi YA, Choi D, et al. Growth rate of early-stage hepatocellular carcinoma in patients with chronic liver disease. Clin Mol Hepatol. 2015;21(3):279–86.

57. Jha RC, Zanello PA, Nguyen XM, et al. Small hepatocellular carcinoma: MRI findings for predicting tumor growth rates. Acad Radiol. 2014;21(11):1455–64.

58. Boas FE, Do B, Louie JD, et al. Optimal imaging surveillance schedules after liver-directed therapy for hepatocellular carcinoma. J Vasc Interv Radiol. 2015;26(1):69–73.

59. Bogaerts J, Ford R, Sargent D, et al. Individual patient data analysis to assess modifications to the RECIST criteria. Eur J Cancer. 2009;45(2):248–60.

60. Miller AB, Hoogstraten B, Staquet M, Winkler A. Reporting results of cancer treatment. Cancer. 1981;47(1):207–14.

61. Lencioni R. New data supporting modified RECIST (mRECIST) for Hepatocellular Carcinoma. Clin Cancer Res. 2013;19(6):1312–4.

62. Lencioni R, Llovet JM. Modified RECIST (mRECIST) assessment for hepatocellular carcinoma. Semin Liver Dis. 2010;30(1):52–60.

63. Gillmore R, Stuart S, Kirkwood A, et al. EASL and mRECIST responses are independent prognostic factors for survival in hepatocellular cancer patients treated with transarterial embolization. J Hepatol. 2011;55(6):1309–16.

64. Bargellini I, Bozzi E, Campani D, et al. Modified RECIST to assess tumor response after transarterial chemoembolization of hepatocellular carcinoma: CT-pathologic correlation in 178 liver explants. Eur J Radiol. 2013;82(5):e212–8.

65. Forner A, Ayuso C, Varela M, et al. Evaluation of tumor response after locoregional therapies in hepatocellular carcinoma: are response evaluation criteria in solid tumors reliable? Cancer. 2009;115(3):616–23.

66. Riaz A, Memon K, Miller FH, et al. Role of the EASL, RECIST, and WHO response guidelines alone or in combination for hepatocellular carcinoma: radiologic-pathologic correlation. J Hepatol. 2011;54(4):695–704.

67. Yeo DM, Choi JI, Lee YJ, Park MY, Chun HJ, Lee HG. Comparison of RECIST, mRECIST, and choi criteria for early response evaluation of hepatocellular carcinoma after transarterial chemoembolization using drug-eluting beads. J Comput Assist Tomogr. 2014;38(3):391–7.

68. Kloeckner R, Otto G, Biesterfeld S, Oberholzer K, Dueber C, Pitton MB. MDCT versus MRI assessment of tumor response after transarterial chemoembolization for the treatment of hepatocellular carcinoma. Cardiovasc Intervent Radiol. 2010;33(3):532–40.

69. Sainani NI, Gervais DA, Mueller PR, Arellano RS. Imaging after percutaneous radiofrequency ablation of hepatic tumors: part 2, abnormal findings. AJR Am J Roentgenol. 2013;200(1):194–204.

4

Review of radiological classifications of pancreatic cancer with peripancreatic vessel invasion: are new grading criteria required?

Y. N. Shen[1,2], X. L. Bai[1,2], G. G. Li[1,2] and T. B. Liang[1,2*]

Abstract

Pancreatic cancer is mainly diagnosed at an advanced stage when adjacent vessel invasion is present; however, radical resection is potentially curative for selected patients with adjacent vessel invasion. Therefore, accurately judging the resectability of patients with adjacent vessel invasion represents a crucially important step in diagnosis and treatment. Currently, decisions regarding resectability are based on imaging studies, commonly contrast computed tomography (CT). Several radiological classifications have been published for vascular infiltration in pancreatic cancer. However, radiologists always formulate these CT grading systems according to their own experience, resulting in different judgment methods and parameters. And it is controversial in evaluating performance and clinical application. Besides, the conventional CT grading systems mainly focus on the evaluation of vessel invasion so as to less on the outcome of patient evaluation. In this review, we summarize the mainstream CT grading systems for vascular invasion in pancreatic cancer, with the aim of improving the clinical value of CT grading systems for predicting resectability and survival.

Keywords: Pancreatic cancer, Vessel invasion, Computed tomography criterion, Resectability, Review

Background

Pancreatic cancer is a highly lethal disease with high morbidity and a dismal prognosis [1, 2]. The 5-years survival rates for white and black American patients with pancreatic cancer are 8 and 7%, respectively, and the overall survival rate for all races is only 8% [2]. Approximately 90% of patients diagnosed with pancreatic cancer ultimately die of the disease [3]. Patients who do not have specific symptoms in the early stages are frequently diagnosed at an advanced stage, for which surgical therapy is usually not possible. Only 20% of patients with pancreatic cancer are eligible for one-stage resection [4]; however, 14–30% of these cases will be found to be unsuitable for resection during surgery [5]. Therefore, the ability to accurately judge the resectability of pancreatic cancer represents a

crucially important step in diagnosis and treatment, and could help to more accurately determine appropriate therapeutic approaches and predict the prognosis of individual patients. Moreover, once a patient is confirmed as unsuitable for surgery, palliative or neoadjuvant radiochemotherapy can be given in a timelier manner.

Computed tomography (CT) currently plays an important role in the diagnosis and stage evaluation of pancreatic cancer [6]. Preoperative CT evaluation of peripancreatic vascular infiltration in pancreatic cancer is an essential parameter used to assess whether resection can be performed. Several researchers [7–13] have assessed vascular involvement in pancreatic cancer and established a series of preoperative CT criteria to enable more accurate and reliable assessment. However, differences in imaging practices and interpretation [6], local experience and even the ethnicity of the patients have contributed to variations in these criteria, which are also limited by the technology and resources available. The clinical application of these criteria is also affected by their low accuracy. Therefore, it is imperative to

* Correspondence: liangtingbo@zju.edu.cn
[1]Department of Hepatobiliary and Pancreatic Surgery, Second Affiliated Hospital of Zhejiang University School of Medicine, Zhejiang University, Jiefang Road, Shangcheng District, Hangzhou, China
[2]Zhejiang Provincial Key Laboratory of Pancreatic Disease, Hangzhou, China

Table 1 Loyer's Criteria [7]

Type	Imaging features
A	Fat plane separates tumor and/or normal pancreatic parenchyma from adjacent vessels.
B	Normal parenchyma separates hypodense tumor from adjacent vessels.
C	Hypodense tumor is inseparable from adjacent vessels, points of contact form a convexity against vessels.
D	Hypodense tumor is inseparable from adjacent vessels, points of contact form a concavity against or partially encircle vessels.
E	Hypodense tumor encircles adjacent vessels, no fat plane is identifiable between tumor and vessels.
F	Tumor occludes vessels.

establish widely-accepted criteria for vascular involvement in pancreatic cancer with higher precision and clinical value. Though the National Comprehensive Cancer Network (NCCN) established definitions for borderline resectable pancreatic cancer in 2014 [14] in which imaging features provide an important reference, we hold the opinion that the problems described above still persist. This review aimed to systematically summarize the mainstream CT criteria for peripancreatic vascular infiltration in pancreatic cancer published in recent few decades to provide a more comprehensive reference for radiologists and surgeons. Moreover, this information could contribute to the design and establishment of improved CT imaging criteria for vascular involvement in pancreatic cancer.

Characteristics of existing criteria for vascular involvement in pancreatic cancer

Loyer's criteria (1996)

Loyer et al. [7] suggested CT criteria for vascular infiltration in pancreatic carcinoma in 1996 (Table 1). These criteria could be divided into six types (Type A – F) [7]: in Type A, a fat plane separates the tumor from adjacent vessels; Type

B: normal pancreatic parenchyma separates the tumor from adjacent vessels; Type C: hypodense tumor not separated from vessels, and the points of contact form a convexity against the vessels; Type D: hypodense tumor not separated from vessels, and the points of contact form a concavity against or partially encircle the vessels; Type E: hypodense tumor encircled by adjacent vessels, while the fat plane between the tumor and blood vessels cannot be identified; and Type F: a tumor occluding the vessel (Fig. 1).

For Type A/B pancreatic cancer, the resectable rate reached 100% (22/22). However, one patient with Type B accepted venous resection as normal pancreatic tissue was present within the tumor and around the portal vein, resulting in a resection rate without venous resection of 95% for Type A/B (21/22). For Type C, the resectable rate was 89% (8/9), and 55% for resection without venous resection. For Type D, the resectable rate was 47% (7/15), but only 7% for resection without venous resection (1/15).

Loyer's criteria [7] were the first attempt to stratify patients with vascular invasion to distinguish clearly unresectable cases from potentially resectable cases [15]. The researchers calculated the resection rate for the included patients, which had a certain clinical significance. However, this method is complex and relatively subjective, and failed to provide definite definitions of resectable and unresectable tumors [15]. Moreover, Loyer et al. only paid attention to imaging features, and did not consider intraoperative and pathological findings, since a pathologist was not asked to prepare histologic sections of the vascular wall in the early cases [7]. This may have limited the accuracy of this system. In addition, arterial and venous infiltrations were not differentiated. There is another limitation as well: Type C is described as a hypodense tumor with a point of contact forming a convexity against the vessel. However, if a tumor, which is densely fibrotic, simply impinges the venous wall, thus having a convex border or point of contact with the vein, it would be

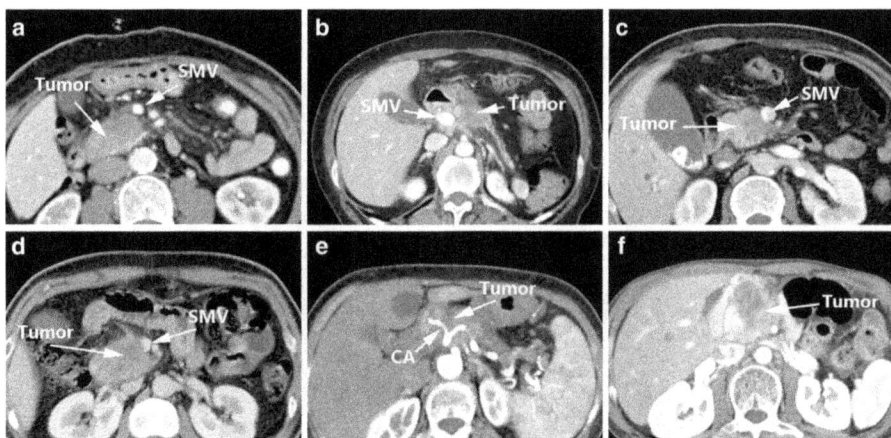

Fig. 1 Loyer's Criteria: Type A (**a**), Type B (**b**), Type C (**c**), Type D (**d**), Type E (**e**), Type F (**f**)

Table 2 Lu's Criteria [12]

Grade	Imaging features
0	No contiguity of tumor to vessel.
1	Tumor contiguous to less than one-quarter circumference.
2	Between one-quarter and one-half circumference.
3	Between one-half and three-quarters circumference.
4	Greater than three-quarters circumferential involvement or any vessel constriction.

classified as type C. However, this imaging finding was later-on called to be a "tear-drop deformity", which is actually highly suggestive of venous wall invasion.

Lu's criteria (1997)

In 1997, Lu et al. [12] assessed 25 patients who underwent surgery for pancreatic adenocarcinoma and designed classification criteria for tumor resectability (Table 2). Imaging features of peripancreatic vessels were the main assessment for this criteria, and were classified into five grades: Grade 0: the tumor does not touch adjacent vessels; Grade 1: less than one quarter of the tumor circumference contacts vessels; Grade 2: one quarter to half of the tumor circumference contacts vessels; Grade 3: half to three quarters of the tumor circumference contacts vessels; Grade 4: over three quarters of the tumor circumference contacts vessels, or any vascular constriction (Fig. 2). When combined with intra-operative assessment, the higher the grade, the lower the resectability rate.

Lu's criteria [12] considered a vessel circumferential involvement of 1/2 (180°) as the threshold of whether the tumor was resectable, which resulted in a sensitivity and specificity of 84 and 98%, respectively, and a positive predictive value (PPV) and negative predictive value (NPV) for unresectability of 95 and 93% (Table 7). These criteria were subsequently recognized and used by many

scholars [16–18]. However, Lu's criteria only focused on circumferential involvement, and ignored other important parameters like the length of tumor contact and stenosis, which could explain their relatively low sensitivity (84%). In addition, Valls et al. [15] stated that the main limitations of Lu's criteria [12] were that only 11 patients were eventually resectable, and most of the surgical correlations were based on venous vessels.

Li's criteria (2005)

Li et al. reported sequential studies [8, 9] in 2005 and 2006 and designed a set of criteria for arterial and venous invasion in pancreatic cancer according to imaging features and intra-operative findings (Table 3). The criteria could be divided into four signs: Sign A: arteries embedded within the tumor or blocked veins; Sign B: circumferential involvement greater than 180°; Sign C: irregular vessel walls; and Sign D: vessel caliber stenosis. Then two criteria were recommended. Criteria of arterial invasion: presence of sign A, or combination of sign B with either sign C and/or D. Criteria of venous invasion: presence of one of the following signs: sign A, sign B, sign C, sign D and sign E (teardrop SMV) (Fig. 3).

The heterogeneity of Li's criteria [8, 9] is acceptable, but this system had a low sensitivity when used for assessment of artery and venous involvement. Therefore, the researchers realized specific assessments are needed for arterial and venous invasion (Nakayama et al. [19] expressed a similar opinion in 2001). In their recommended criteria, Li et al. [8, 9] stated artery invasion may meet Sign A or Sign B combined with either Sign C or Sign D, and venous invasion may meet Sign A, Sign B, Sign C, Sign D or Sign E (teardrop shape performance of the superior mesenteric vein). The sensitivity of these arterial and venous assessments for vessel invasion reached 79% (23/29) and 92% (45/49), respectively

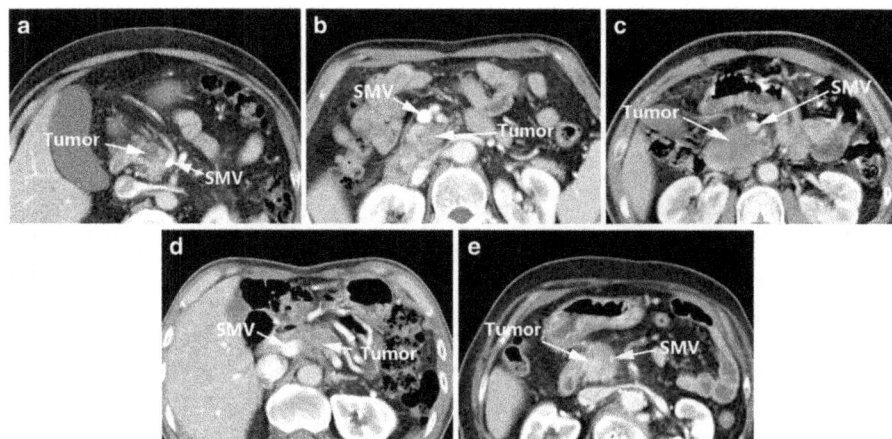

Fig. 2 Lu's Criteria: Grade 0 (**a**), Grade 1 (**b**), Grade 2 (**c**), Grade 3 (**d**), Grade 4 (**e**)

Table 3 Li's Criteria [8, 9]

Sign	Imaging features
A	Arterial embedment in tumor or venous obliteration.
B	Tumor surrounding 1/2 circumference of the vessel.
C	Vessel wall irregularity.
D	Vessel caliber stenosis.

Recommended criteria
Criteria of arterial invasion: presence of sign A, or combination of sign B with either sign C and/or D
Criteria of venous invasion: presence of one of the following signs: sign A, sign B, sign C, sign D and sign E (teardrop SMV)

(Table 7). The researchers considered that venous and arterial invasion present different CT signs of invasion, because the venous wall is thinner and weaker than the muscular arterial wall. When veins are surrounded or infiltrated by tumor, the wall tends to be irregular and the calibre becomes narrowed. At the same time, tumor often penetrates the venous wall and forms thrombus since the flow rate in veins becomes slow, causing venous occlusion finally [8].

Klauss's criteria (2008)

In 2008, Klauss et al. [13] proposed a new preoperative CT system to assess the resectability of pancreatic cancer (Table 4) based on the relation of peripancreatic vessels to the tumor, and verified the results using intraoperative findings and postoperative pathological reports. In this system, artery and venous assessments are separate (Fig. 4). Compared to the previous versions described above, Klauss's criteria include more assessment items and more detail. For example, the venous assessment includes assessment of the length of tumor contact, circumferential involvement and other abnormalities; the length of tumor contact and circumferential involvement are recorded to an accuracy of mm and degrees. The length of tumor contact and circumferential involvement assessment was also added for the artery assessment. Furthermore, this system provides a corresponding score for each assessment item, and the total score is calculated by adding the score for each item after the assessment. Generally, the total score was used to judge the resectability of the tumor and assess peripancreatic vessel invasion. Finally, 11 points was selected as the cut-off point for

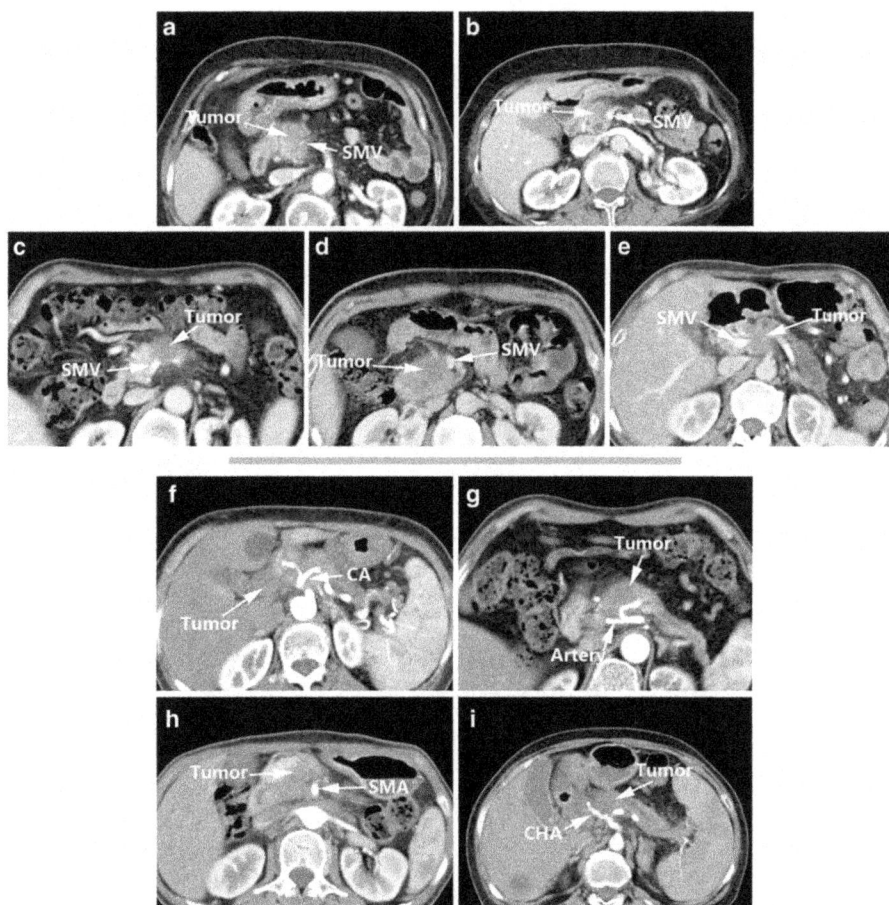

Fig. 3 Li's Criteria (vein): Sign A (**a**), Sign B (**b**), Sign C (**c**), Sign D (**d**), Sign E (**e**); Li's Criteria (artery): Sign A (**f**), Sign B (**g**), Sign C (**h**), Sign D (**i**)

Table 4 Klauss's Criteria [13]

Length of tumor contact (mm)	Circumferential Involvement (°)	Other abnormalities	Score
Veins			
0	0		1
< 5	1–45		2
5–10	46–90		3
11–20	91–180	Flattened	4
21–40	181–270	Long-segment contour deformity	5
> 40	> 270	Obliteration or severe contour deformity	6
Total score			Σ
Arteries			
0	No		1
< 5	In Places		2
5–10	Continuously < 45		3
11–20	45–180		4
21–40	181–270		5
> 40	270 to complete obliteration		6
Total score			Σ

evidence of vessel invasion. That is to say, the vessel was invaded by the tumor in case of the total score of single vessel was equivalent with or higher than 11 points.

One major limitation of Klauss' Score is the fact that this very meticulous scoring system was developed with the same patient cohort, which was then also used to validate the score. For such an advanced scoring system

a separate validation cohort would have been reliable. Based on their criteria, Klauss et al. [13] verified whether the superior mesenteric vein (SMV), superior mesenteric artery (SMA), splenic vein and portal vein (PV) or celiac trunks were involved in each patient. The sensitivity of this method for vessel invasion reached 66.7 to 100% (Table 7). Among the 28 patients, the sensitivity and specificity of the tumor resectability assessment reached 95.5% (21/22) and 100% (6/6), respectively [13]. Compared to other related systems or criteria, Klauss's criteria have a higher sensitivity and specificity and warrant increased use in the clinic. However, Klauss et al. [13] stated their criteria also had a number of limitations, including the fact benign tumors would also lead to vessel compression and could lead to diagnostic errors.

Marinelli's criteria (2014)

The assessment system designed by Marinelli et al. [10] (Table 5) was mainly designed to assess peripancreatic venous invasion such as portal vein (PV) and superior mesenteric vein (SMV), with the aim of selecting the appropriate therapeutic approach after accurate preoperative assessment to improve the treatment and prognosis of patients with borderline resectable disease. Compared to other criteria, the design of this system is more complicated. The items assessed are: tumor contact with vessel, length of tumor contact, circumferential involvement and stenosis. It is noteworthy that the tumor contact with vessel criterion employed the system included in Loyer's criteria [7]. However, interestingly Marinelli et al. [10] combined Loyer's Grade A and Grade B in their system. Marinelli et al. maintained there is no significant difference between these two grades in terms of surgical outcome, since both

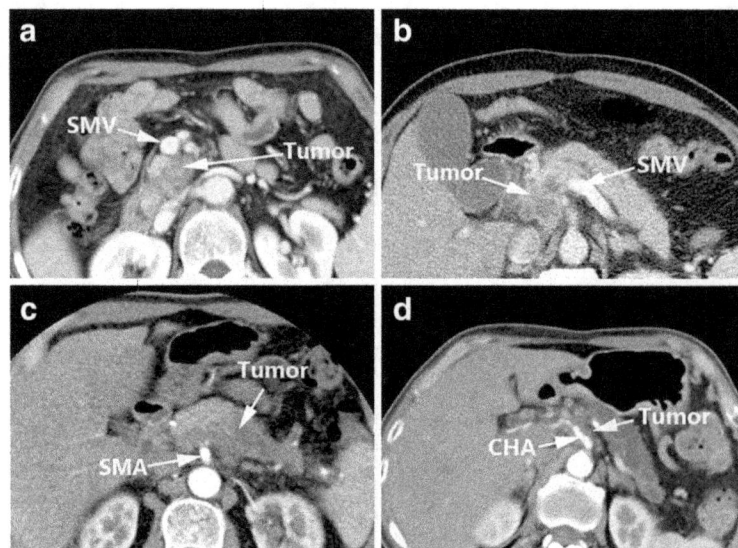

Fig. 4 Klauss's Criteria (vein): Score < 11 (**a**), Score > 11 (**b**); Klauss's Criteria (artery): Score < 11 (**c**), Score > 11 (**d**)

Table 5 Marinelli's Criteria [10]

Grade (likelihood of vascular invasion)	Tumor contact with vessel[a]	Length of tumor contact with vessel (mm)	Circumferential vein involvement (°)	Stenosis
1	Grade A–B	= 0 mm	= 0°	No stenosis
2	Grade C	< 5 mm	= 0°–90°	No stenosis
3	Grade C–D	> 5 mm	= 0°–90°	Flattened
4	Grade D	> 5 mm	>90° < 180° >180°	Occlusion thrombus
	Grade E/F	-		-

Grade 1, Definite absence of invasion; Grade 2, Probable absence of invasion; Grade 3, Probable presence of invasion; Grade 4, Definite presence of invasion
[a]Grades A–F, according to Loyer's Criteria [8]:
Grade A: fat plane visible between tumour and vessels
Grade B: normal pancreatic tissue between tumour and vessels
Grade C: tumour adjacent to vessel with a convex contour towards vessels
Grade D: tumour adjacent to vessel with a concave contour towards vessels
Grade E: circumferential involvement of vessels
Grade F: vascular occlusion

are clearly resectable [10]. The "length of tumor contact" was classified as 0 mm, < 5 mm and > 5 mm; "circumferential involvement" as 0°, 0° to 90°, 90° to 180°, and > 180°, respectively. Four grades were defined in Marinelli's criteria [10]: Grade 1, definite absence of invasion; Grade 2, probable absence of invasion; Grade 3, probable presence of invasion; and Grade 4, definite presence of invasion. In Grade 1, the tumor contacts with vessels of Grade A–B, and length of tumor contact is 0 mm with circumferential involvement of 0 and no stenosis. In Grade 2, the tumor contacts with vessels of Grade C, with a length of tumor contact < 5 mm, circumferential involvement is 0°–90° and no stenosis. There are two kinds of situations in Grade 3, the tumor contacts with vessels of Grade C, with a length of tumor contact > 5 mm, circumferential involvement is

0°–90° or flattened vessels. Another situation is circumferential involvement is 0–90° with flattened vessels, Grade D tumor vessel contact. Grade 4 includes three scenarios: grade E or F tumor vessel contact and circumferential involvement > 180°; narrowing of vessels; or Grade D tumor contact, contact length > 5 mm and circumferential involvement of 90° to 180° (Fig. 5).

The advantage of Marinelli's score over Klauss' criteria [13] is the fact that Marinelli's scoring system refers to actual clinical situations instead of adding score numbers. Marinelli et al. [10] verified their standard in 56 patients with pancreatic cancer and obtained sensitivity and specificity values for PV invasion of 80 and 100%, respectively. The PPV and NPV were 80 and 96%. For the SMV, the sensitivity and specificity of this method reached 100 and 94%, and the PPV and NPV were 75 and 100% (Table 7). The innovation in this method was that the researchers analyzed the prognosis of the patients by grade. For the PV infiltration score, the survival time was inversely proportional to grade, though the trend was not significant ($P = 0.106$). Additionally, the researchers proposed that both the PV and SMV infiltration scores were associated with metastatic disease and the resection margins status [10].

Teramura's criteria (2016)

Teramura et al. [11] assessed whether pathological PV invasion (pPV) in pancreatic cancer could be accurately identified by preoperative CT in order to select patients who could benefit from surgery. The researchers established a CT diagnostic standard according to the degree of vascular invasion, intra-operative findings and pathology results (Table 6). The classification method for this criteria is similar to Loyer's criteria [7] and is divided into five types (Type

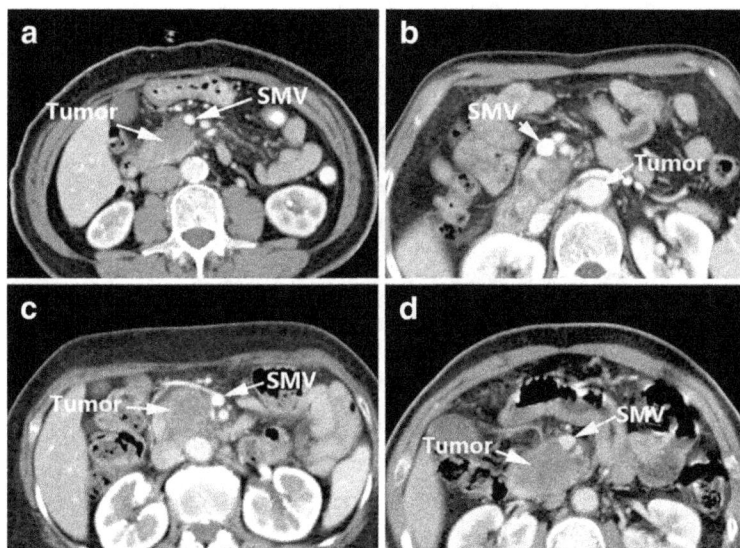

Fig. 5 Marinelli's Criteria: Grade 1 (**a**), Grade 2 (**b**), Grade 3 (**c**), Grade 4 (**d**)

Table 6 Teramura's Criteria [11]

Type	Diagnosis	CT findings	
0	Negative	Negative	c vessels.
1		Soft tissue density	Soft tissue density between tumor and portal vein.
2	Positive	Contact	Tumor is inseparable from adjacent vessels, and points of contact from a convexity against the vessels.
3		Stenosis	Deformation, narrowing or stenosis on portal vein.
4		Obstruction	Portal vein is completely obstructed by tumor.

0 – 4): In Type 0, a fat plane separates the tumor and (or) normal pancreatic tissues from adjacent vessels; in Type 1, soft tissue density exists between the tumor and vessels; in Type 2, the tumor cannot be separated from the adjacent vessels and the points of contact from a convexity against the vessels; in Type 3, the PV is deformed, narrowed or exhibits stenosis; and in Type 4, the PV is completely blocked by the tumor (Fig. 6).

Teramura et al. [11] demonstrated that the prognosis of Type 0 vs. Type 3/4 was significantly different ($P = 0.02$), but not for Types 0 vs. 1/2 and Types 1/2 vs. 3/4 ($P = 0.30$ and $P = 0.10$, respectively). The 5-years survival rates for Type 0, 1/2 and 3/4 were 23.1, 11.4 and 3.2%, respectively. Although a significant difference in 5-years survival was not observed between Type 1/2 and Type 3/4, a higher percentage of patients with Type 1/2 than Type 3/4 survived for 36 months (10/35 vs. 1/32). Therefore, this method was feasible to assess whether patients are suitable for pancreaticoduodenectomy with PV resection via preoperative CT [11]. However, while the sensitivity and NPV were 97.6 and 97.5%, respectively, the specificity was only 60% and the PPV was 61.2% (Table 7).

Clinical significance

With respect to resectability, patients with Type A and B vascular involvement according to Loyer's criteria [7] are suggested to undergo pancreatic resection, while Type E and F are considered inoperable. In their study, one case of Type E/F underwent surgery with vessel resection, though a positive margin was detected in the pathological examination. Resection was recommended for Type C, but the tumor may or may not attach to the vessel wall. A detailed plan of the surgical approach should be made before pancreatic resection in cases of Type D. It is important to note that venous resection should not be attempted if the surgeon lacks relevant experience. In addition, Loyer's [7] study did not provide a definite definition of resectable and unresectable, as previously discussed. Teramura et al. [11] mainly focused on the relationship between prognosis and vascular invasion. They reported patients with "stenosis", "obstruction", or a Klauss score [13] ≥ 11 are likely to have a poor prognosis, even with portal vein reconstruction (PVR) [11], and recommended resectability should be assessed from the perspective of prognosis. According to the aforementioned data, Lu et al. [12] used one-half of the circumference of the vessel as the threshold; resection should be recommended if the value was higher. Furthermore, Li et al. [8, 9] and Hough et al. [20] found that a tear drop appearance of the SMV can be a contraindication for resection. However, unambiguous definitions of resectable tumors were not provided in the criteria by Klauss [13] and Marinelli [10].

In recent years, these rigid concepts of vascular invasion (meaning non-resectability) have been somehow overruled by the concept of "borderline resectable", which has been adopted by many cancer centers and institutions. According to the NCCN guidelines (Version 1.2017), the "borderline resectable" could be defined as several resectability statuses as follows:

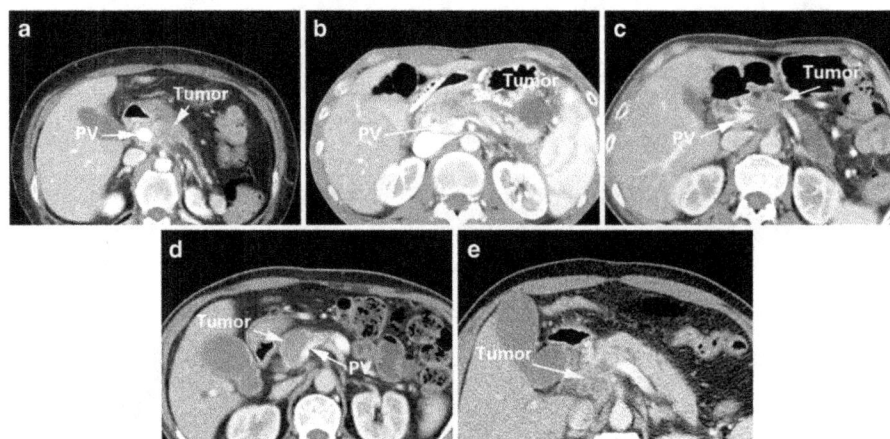

Fig. 6 Teramura's Criteria: Type 0 (**a**), Type 1 (**b**), Type 2 (**c**), Type 3 (**d**), Type 4 (**e**)

Table 7 Sensitivity and specificity of each criteria for vessel invasion in pancreatic cancer

Criteria	Vessel	Sensitivity (%)	Specificity (%)	PPV (%)	NPV (%)
Loyer et al. (n = 56)	NA	NA	NA	NA	NA
Lu et al. (n = 25)	Vein/ Artery	84	98	95	93
Li et al. (n = 54)	Vein	92	100	NA	NA
	Artery	79	99	NA	NA
Klauss et al. (n = 28)	SMV	100	95.8	80	100
	Splenic vein	66.7	100	100	96.2
	PV	100	96.2	66.7	100
	Celiac trunk	100	100	100	96.4
	SMA	100	100	100	96.4
Marinelli et al. (n = 56)	PV	80	100	80	96
	SMV	96	94	75	100
Teramura et al. (n = 107)	PV/SMV	97.6	60	61.2	97.5

PV portal vein, *SMV* superior mesenteric vein, *SMA* superior mesenteric artery, *NA* not available, *PPV* positive predictive value, *NPV* negative predictive value

1. Venous
   - Solid tumor contact with SMV or PV of > 180°, contact of < = 180° with contour irregularity of the vein or thrombosis of the vein but with suitable vessel proximal and distal to the site of involvement allowing for safe and complete resection and vein reconstruction;
   - Solid tumor contact with the inferior vena cava (IVC).
2. Arterial
   2.1 Pancreatic head/uncinate process:
   - Solid tumor contact with common hepatic artery (CHA) without extension to celiac axis or hepatic artery bifurcation allowing for safe and complete resection and reconstruction;
   - Solid tumor contact with the superior mesenteric artery (SMA) of < = 180°;
   - Solid tumor contact with variant arterial anatomy (ex: accessory right hepatic artery, replaced right hepatic artery, replaced CHA, and the origin of replaced or accessory artery) and the presence and degree of tumor contact should be noted if present as it may affect surgical planning.
   2.2 Pancreatic body/tail:
   - Solid tumor contact with the celiac axis (CA) of < = 180°;
   - Solid tumor contact with the CA of > 180° without involvement of the aorta and with

intact and uninvolved gastroduodenal artery thereby permitting a modified Appleby procedure.

Interestingly, Teramura et al. [11] doubted the definition of "borderline" pancreatic head cancer established in the newest NCCN guidelines, and pointed out that circumferential contact of the PV did not have high diagnostic value and may even affect assessment of the resectability of "borderline" pancreatic head cancer.

Other studies also considered prognosis. Nakao et al. [21] showed the imaging features of PV correlated with long-term survival; survival was poorer for patients with bilateral narrowing or stenosis/obstruction with collaterals than patients with unilateral narrowing [21]. Moreover, they also suggested that radiographic classification of PV invasion was more appropriate than pathological classification [21]. A similar report by Chun et al. [22] showed patients with bilateral narrowing were less likely to benefit from preoperative treatment.

Another useful feature of these criteria [7–13] summarized by us is the prediction of vascular invasion. Some researchers previously believed perivascular changes were not specific for pancreatic carcinoma [23–25]. However, Megibow maintained that patients with pathological confirmed ductal adenocarcinoma are likely to have tumor infiltration if perivascular changes can be observed on CT [26]; this supposition was supported by Loyer [7]. In the study by Zeman et al. [27], vascular invasion could be identified if the caliber was irregular, circumferential involvement > 180°, or vessel thrombosis was present. In the study by Furukawa et al. [28], vascular invasion is classified as positive if circumferential involvement is more than 90°. Klauss et al. [13] considered it was difficult to assess vascular invasion as the contact between the vessels and tumor does not always indicate whether the vessels have been truly infiltrated; Teramura et al. [11] expressed a similar view. In research published in 2012, Nakao et al. [21] found imaging classifications of PV invasion correlated with the pathological grade of invasion.

Conclusions

From the information above, we can conclude that the previous studies suggesting criteria for assessing the resectability of pancreatic cancer via CT are basically consistent, and while some criteria are suitable for clinical practice (for example, the sensitivity and specificity of the Klauss's criteria [13] reach 95.5 and 100%, respectively), they also remain controversial. In most studies, the length of tumor contact, circumferential involvement, stenosis and other imaging findings are taken as reference items. However, in the latest study, Teramura et al. [11] reported circumferential involvement had low diagnostic value and they removed this feature from their criteria. In addition, scoring systems with a high reference value like Klauss's criteria also have limitations. For instance, it is difficult to distinguish whether vessels are oppressed by a benign or malignant tumor on CT.

In conclusion, we hold the opinion that the current criteria [7–13] have superior clinical value to previous systems, The scoring system, especially from Klauss' and Marinelli's, is worthy of being applied to the clinical practice. However, the criteria above still remain controversial, especially with respect to the lack of the prognostic criteria. We believe that with continuous developments in CT technology and accumulation of experience by radiologists, more improved and accurate criteria will be established.

Abbreviations

CA: Celiac axis; CHA: Hepatic artery; CT: Computed tomography; NCCN: National comprehensive cancer network; NPV: Negative predictive value; PPV: Positive predictive value; PV: Portal vein; SMA: Superior mesenteric artery; SMV: Superior mesenteric vein

Acknowledgements
Not applicable.

Funding
This study is supported by National High Technology Research and Development Program of China (No. SS2015AA020405), Training Program of the Key Program of the National Natural Science Foundation of China (No. 91442115), National Natural Science Foundation of China (No.81672337), Key Program of the National Natural Science Foundation of China (No. 81530079), Key research and development Project of Zhejiang Province (No. 2015C03044), Zhejiang Provincial Program for the Cultivation of High-level Innovative Health talents, Zhejiang Provincial Key Innovation Team of Pancreatic Cancer Diagnosis & Treatment (No.2013TD06).

Authors' contributions
All the authors contributed equally to this work. All authors read and approved the final manuscript.

Competing interests
The authors who have taken part in this study declared that they do not have any conflict of interest with respect to this manuscript.

References
1. Kamisawa T, Wood LD, Itoi T, Takaori K. Pancreatic cancer. Lancet. 2016; 388(10039):73–85.
2. Siegel RL, Miller KD, Jemal A. Cancer statistics, 2016. CA Cancer J Clin. 2016; 66(1):7–30.
3. Ryan DP, Hong TS, Bardeesy N. Pancreatic adenocarcinoma. N Engl J Med. 2014;371(22):2140–1.
4. Gillen S, Schuster T, Meyer ZBC, Friess H, Kleeff J. Preoperative/neoadjuvant therapy in pancreatic cancer: a systematic review and meta-analysis of response and resection percentages. PLoS Med. 2010;7(4):e1000267.
5. White R, Winston C, Gonen M, et al. Current utility of staging laparoscopy for pancreatic and peripancreatic neoplasms. J Am Coll Surg. 2008;206(3):445–50.
6. Pietryga JA, Morgan DE. Imaging preoperatively for pancreatic adenocarcinoma. J Gastrointest Oncol. 2015;6(4):343–57.
7. Loyer EM, David CL, Dubrow RA, Evans DB, Charnsangavej C. Vascular involvement in pancreatic adenocarcinoma: reassessment by thin-section CT. Abdom Imaging. 1996;21(3):202–6.
8. Li H, Zeng MS, Zhou KR, Jin DY, Lou WH. Pancreatic adenocarcinoma: the different CT criteria for peripancreatic major arterial and venous invasion. J Comput Assist Tomogr. 2005;29(2):170–5.
9. Li H, Zeng MS, Zhou KR, Jin DY, Lou WH. Pancreatic adenocarcinoma: signs of vascular invasion determined by multi-detector row CT. Br J Radiol. 2006; 79(947):880–7.
10. Marinelli T, Filippone A, Tavano F, et al. A tumour score with multidetector spiral CT for venous infiltration in pancreatic cancer: influence on borderline resectable. Radiol Med. 2014;119(5):334–42.
11. Teramura K, Noji T, Nakamura T, et al. Preoperative diagnosis of portal vein invasion in pancreatic head cancer: appropriate indications for concomitant portal vein resection. J Hepatobiliary Pancreat Sci. 2016;23(10): 643-9.
12. Lu DS, Reber HA, Krasny RM, Kadell BM, Sayre J. Local staging of pancreatic cancer: criteria for unresectability of major vessels as revealed by pancreatic-phase, thin-section helical CT. AJR Am J Roentgenol. 1997;168(6):1439–43.
13. Klauss M, Mohr A, von Tengg-Koblig H, et al. A new invasion score for determining the resectability of pancreatic carcinomas with contrast-enhanced multidetector computed tomography. Pancreatology. 2008;8(2):204–10.
14. Tempero MA, Malafa MP, Behrman SW, et al. Pancreatic adenocarcinoma, version 2.2014: featured updates to the NCCN guidelines. J Natl Compr Canc Netw. 2014;12(8):1083–93.
15. Valls C, Andía E, Sanchez A, et al. Dual-phase helical CT of pancreatic adenocarcinoma: assessment of resectability before surgery. AJR Am J Roentgenol. 2002;178(4):821–6.
16. Horton KM, Fishman EK. Multidetector CT angiography of pancreatic carcinoma: part 2, evaluation of venous involvement. AJR Am J Roentgenol. 2002;178(4):833–6.
17. Lepanto L, Arzoumanian Y, Gianfelice D, et al. Helical CT with CT angiography in assessing periampullary neoplasms: identification of vascular invasion. Radiology. 2002;222(2):347–52.
18. O'Malley ME, Boland GW, Wood BJ, Fernandez-del CC, Warshaw AL, Mueller PR. Adenocarcinoma of the head of the pancreas: determination of surgical unresectability with thin-section pancreatic-phase helical CT. AJR Am J Roentgenol. 1999;173(6):1513–8.
19. Nakayama Y, Yamashita Y, Kadota M, et al. Vascular encasement by pancreatic cancer: correlation of CT findings with surgical and pathologic results. J Comput Assist Tomogr. 2001;25(3):337–42.
20. Hough TJ, Raptopoulos V, Siewert B, Matthews JB. Teardrop superior mesenteric vein: CT sign for unresectable carcinoma of the pancreas. AJR Am J Roentgenol. 1999;173(6):1509–12.
21. Nakao A, Kanzaki A, Fujii T, et al. Correlation between radiographic classification and pathological grade of portal vein wall invasion in pancreatic head cancer. Ann Surg. 2012;255(1):103–8.
22. Chun YS, Milestone BN, Watson JC, et al. Defining venous involvement in borderline resectable pancreatic cancer. Ann Surg Oncol. 2010;17(11):2832–8.
23. Schulte SJ, Baron RL, Freeny PC, Patten RM, Gorell HA, Maclin ML. Root of the superior mesenteric artery in pancreatitis and pancreatic carcinoma: evaluation with CT. Radiology. 1991;180(3):659–62.
24. Luetmer PH, Stephens DH, Fischer AP. Obliteration of periarterial retropancreatic fat on CT in pancreatitis: an exception to the rule. AJR Am J Roentgenol. 1989;153(1):63–4.
25. Baker ME, Cohan RH, Nadel SN, Leder RA, Dunnick NR. Obliteration of the fat surrounding the celiac axis and superior mesenteric artery is not a specific CT finding of carcinoma of the pancreas. AJR Am J Roentgenol. 1990;155(5):991–4.
26. Megibow AJ. Pancreatic adenocarcinoma: designing the examination to evaluate the clinical questions. Radiology. 1992;183(2):297–303.
27. Zeman RK, Cooper C, Zeiberg AS, et al. TNM staging of pancreatic carcinoma using helical CT. AJR Am J Roentgenol. 1997;169(2):459–64.
28. Furukawa H, Kosuge T, Mukai K, et al. Helical computed tomography in the diagnosis of portal vein invasion by pancreatic head carcinoma: usefulness for selecting surgical procedures and predicting the outcome. Arch Surg. 1998;133(1):61–5.

5

Portal vein embolization with n-butyl-cyanoacrylate through an ipsilateral approach before major hepatectomy: single center analysis of 50 consecutive patients

José Hugo Mendes Luz[1*], Paula Mendes Luz[2], Tiago Bilhim[3], Henrique Salas Martin[1], Hugo Rodrigues Gouveia[1], Élia Coimbra[3], Filipe Veloso Gomes[3], Roberto Romulo Souza[1], Igor Murad Faria[1] and Tiago Nepomuceno de Miranda[1]

Abstract

Purpose: To evaluate the efficacy of portal vein embolization (PVE) with n-Butyl-cyanoacrylate (NBCA) through an ipsilateral approach before major hepatectomy. Secondary end-points were PVE safety, liver resection and patient outcome.

Methods: Over a 5-year period 50 non-cirrhotic consecutive patients were included with primary or secondary liver cancer treatable by hepatectomy with a liver remnant (FLR) volume less than 25% or less than 40% in diseased livers.

Results: There were 37 men and 13 women with a mean age of 57 years. Colorectal liver metastases were the most frequent tumor and patients were previously exposed to chemotherapy. FLR increased from 422 ml to 629 ml ($P < 0.001$) after PVE, corresponding to anincrease of 52%. The FLR ratio increased from 29.6% to 42.3% ($P < 0.001$). Kinetic growth rate was 2.98%/week. A negative association was observed between increase in the FLR and FLR ratio and FLR volume before PVE ($P = 0.002$). In 31 patients hepatectomy was accomplished and only one patient presented with liver insufficiency within 30 days after surgery.

Conclusions: PVE with NBCA through an ipsilateral puncture is effective before major hepatectomy. Meticulous attention is needed especially near the end of the embolization procedure to avoid complications.

Keywords: Portal vein, Embolization, Future liver remnant, Extended hepatectomy, Hepatic insufficiency

Background

More than 30 years after its first publication, portal vein embolization (PVE) is still abundantly used to successfully promote hepatic hypertrophy before major hepatectomies [1]. Hepatic resection is currently the cornerstonein the curative treatment of primary liver malignancies such as cholangiocarcinoma, hepatocellular carcinoma and metastasis from colorectal cancer and other primary origins [2].

To allow hepatic resection most hepatobiliary services admit a future liver remnant (FLR) of at least 25% in healthy livers [3]. For diseased livers, as in heavily chemotherapy treated patients [4, 5]or in hepatic cirrhosis candidates [6], larger FLR of 35% to 40% are required. Embolization of the aimed portal vein territory will diverge all blood flow containing trophic and growth factors to the FLR, inducing hypertrophy and permitting the prearranged future surgery [7]. As with PVE, liver surgery greatly evolved over the years allowing more patients to undergo this potentially curative treatment [8, 9]. Systemic chemotherapy additionally played an important role downsizing tumors and converting previously unresectable patients

* Correspondence: jluz@inca.gov.br; jhugoluz@gmail.com
[1]Department of Interventional Radiology, Radiology Division, National Cancer Institute, INCA, Praça Cruz Vermelha 23, Centro, Rio de Janeiro CEP 20230-130, Brazil
Full list of author information is available at the end of the article

into surgical candidates [10]. PVE has been shown to besafe and effective in promoting FLR growth [3, 11] and is currently adopted in the preoperative scenario in many hepatobiliary units worldwide [12].

A myriad of technical approaches and different embolic materials have been proposed [13]. To date, n-butyl-cyanoacrylate (NBCA) has been used for PVE and some publications have suggested that it may be more efficient than other embolic agents [14]. PVE with NBCA has been widely adopted throughout the last 3 decades. However, the percutaneous access has been nearly exclusively through the FLR as originally described in France [4, 15].Nevertheless, access to the portal vein is usually through the diseased liver that is going to be surgically removed (ipsilateral side) when using other embolic agents, such as particle embolics and coils [16–20]. Furthermore, in situations that PVE with NBCA was attempted through the ipsilateral side authors have done it with the aid of either amplatzer plugs [21, 22] or occlusion balloons [23] in order to minimize the risk of NBCA reflux to FLR. We conducted the present study to assessthe efficacy and safety of PVE solely with NBCA through an ipsilateral approach.

Methods

Patients

Over a 5-year period 50 consecutive patients with primary and secondary liver cancer referred for PVE before major hepatectomy were assessed for analysis. Inclusion criteria were: patients with primary and secondary liver cancer treatable by hepatectomy with a proportion of FLR volume to the total functional liver volume (TFLV) less than 25% orless than 40% in patients with previous chemotherapy or hepatic cirrhosis. Exclusion criteria were: extensive ipsilateral tumor precluding safe access to the portal vein, unmanageable coagulopathy, extensive extra-hepatic disease, liver abscess or infection. PVE indications and details, including embolization of segment IV, were discussed and decided previously in the weekly multidisciplinary liver tumor board meeting. All patients gave their written informed consent to be submitted to PVE. The ethics committee of the Brazilian's National Cancer Institute (INCA) approved the study protocol (Approval #67703317.1.0000.5274). The clinical and imaging records from these sequential patients were retrospectively gathered from the hospital archive and liver volumetric data was generated as stated in the liver volume section.

Study endpoints

Primary endpoint was to evaluate the efficacy of PVE with the NBCA through an ipsilateral approach. Secondary end-points were accomplishment of liver surgery, patient out-come after hepatectomy and safety of the proposed PVE technique. Efficacy was measured according to FLR volume changes, growth rate and kinetic growth rate and was obtained from 37 out of the 50 patients due to unavailable full imaging follow-up data (pre or post-PVE complete set of imaging studies) in 13 patients. All other analysis refers to the total study population (50 patients).

Portal vein Embolization

On the day of PVE patients were assigned to a hospital bed with an anticipated 24 h hospitalization. Patients were kept on intravenously conscious sedation (n = 33) or general anesthesia (n = 17) depending on patient collaboration and anesthesiologist preference. Except for the side which we decided to puncture the liver, our PVE technique was accomplished similarly as reported elsewhere [4, 15]. In brief, a non-FLR portal branch was punctured through ultrasound guidance always avoiding tumor transgression. A 6-F vascular sheath (Terumo, Tokyo, Japan) was placed in the portal vein branch accessed and a subtraction acquisition was performed through a 5F pigtail angiographic catheter (Cook Medical, Bloomington, IN). Selective catheterization of each second-order portal vein branches was achieved with 5F Simmons 1 or 2 catheters (Cook Medical) in the first 30 patients. Coaxial microcatheters (2.8-F Progreat, Terumo) were additionally used in the last 20 patients. Small boluses of n-butyl-cyanocrylate (NBCA - Hystoacryl˚, Trudell Medical International, London, Canada) with iodized oil (Lipiodol˚ Guerbet, France) in a ratio that varied from1-to-3 to 1-to-5 depending on the specific portal vein branch flow, flushed with 5% dextrose, was used for embolization. Segment IV embolization was also completed with glue (n = 6) except in technically defiant or very small branches in which polyvinyl alcohol microparticles (100-300 μm Beadblock, Biocompatibles, Farnham, UK) were used (n = 4) as suggested in previous publications [24]. A post-embolization direct portography was obtained and the glue cast image was recorded. Liver parenchymal tract occlusion was performed with the NBCA lipiodol mixture. Intravenous prophylactic antibiotics were administered at the moment of PVE. After hospital discharge patients were kept on oral analgesics as needed.

Liver volumetry

A 3.0 mmor less slice thickness CT was obtained during the arterial and portal phases with a 16-detector row multislice CT scanner (Phillips, The Netherlands). On individual slices the whole liver, the tumor and the FLR (accordingly to previously surgical planning) were delineated with a handheld cursor using a freely downloadable open-source image analysis software package, OsiriX˚. This open-source PAC software system was agreed to be used since it has been reported and validated for liver volumetric assessment elsewhere [25]. Once all of the regions of interest were selected within one series, the volumetric calculations were obtained using OsiriX* by multiplying surface and slice thickness and then adding up individual slice volumes [25]. TFLV comprehended the total hepatic volume subtracted by the tumor volume. FLR was defined as the portion of the liver that would remain after the proposed hepatectomy. The ratio between the FLR and the TFLV was calculated and defined as the FLR/TFLV ratio. The increase in the FLR after PVE was also quantified and calculated by the formula ((FLR post PVE - FLR pre PVE) ÷ FLR pre PVE) as suggested in guidelines [26]. Additionally, the kinetic growth rate (KGR), defined as the increase in the FLR/TFLV ratio divided by the length of time (in weeks) was calculated [27].

Complications and patient outcome

Pain during and after PVE was assessed with 10-point pain scales. Complications were obtained from the clinical, imaging and laboratory data files and from PVE reports. Complications were classified as suggested in previous publications [15, 28]. Major complications were defined as events that promoted significant morbidity raising the level of medical treatments, or that prolonged hospitalization or provoked hospital re-admissions. Events that did not promote longer hospitalization or did not require specific treatment were considered as incidental findings (e.g., migration of minimal NBCA fragments in the FLR) [15]. Liver enzymes and liver function were assessed before PVE, before surgery and in the immediate postoperative scenario. Patients' charts were scrutinized for submission to surgery, reasons for precluding surgery, surgical complications, intensive care unit admissions, transfusions, length of hospital permanence and death. For all 50 patients included in this study, medical reports were analyzed to the most updated available information up to December 2016 or death. The mean follow-up time was 23.5 months (range 1-60, SD 19.22).

Statistical analysis

Descriptive statistics including mean, standard deviation and range were calculated for numerical variables while absolute numbers and percentages were calculated for categorical variables. Comparison of TFLV and FLR volumes before and after PVE were performed by either paired t-test or paired Wilcoxon rank-sum test, as appropriate. Linear regression models were used to test the association between FLR volume before PVE and FLR volume increase after PVE and between FLR/TFLV ratio before PVE and FLR volume increase after PVE. The association between the use of microcatheter and the occurrence of complications was tested using Fisher's exact test and Chi-squared test.

Results

There were 37(74%) men and 13(26%) women with a mean age of 57 years ±15 (range, 5–80 years). Colorectal liver metastases were the most frequent tumor (Table 1). All patients with colorectal cancer had been previously exposed to systemic chemotherapy. No patients presented with liver cirrhosis, including the ones with hepatocellular carcinoma. Four patients showed biliary obstruction at presentation and were percutaneously drained before (n = 3) or at the moment (n = 1) of PVE.In 49 (98%) patients the ipsilateral approach was performed while in 1 patient both ipsilateral and contra-lateralside punctures were performed. Mean pain score during and after the procedure was 2.5 ±2.5 points. Mean hospital stay was 1.1 days. Thirty-eight (76%) patients had a right PVE,10 (20%) patients had a right PVE plus segment IV and 2 patients underwent PVE of segments VI and VII (4%), (Fig. 1).

PVE was technically successful in 49 (98%) patients. Assisted secondary technical success was obtained in all 50 patients. PVE was technically incomplete in 1 patient as it was necessary to repeat the procedure to achieve full occlusion of an anterior sectorial branch that was overlooked. Segment IV embolizations were carried out by the ipsilateral approach in all but one patient. This patient was submitted to a second PVE to occlude segment IV branches as decided in the tumor board meeting a few days after the completion of the first PVE procedure. Since all right portal vein branches were already occluded we were obligated to perform segment IV embolization through the contralateral approach. In this case it was necessary to puncture the FLR, which occurred uneventfully.

Regarding biliary obstruction; in 3 patients we obtained a significant reduction of bilirubin levels after

Table 1 Patients' characteristics

Number of patients	50
Age, mean (SD)	56.5(15.1)
Male patients, N (%)	37 (74)
Tumor, N (%)	
Cholangiocarcinoma	7 (14)
Colorectal	36 (72)
HCC	3 (6)
Hepatoblastoma	2 (4)
Metastases Wilms Tumor	1 (2)
Retroperitoneal Leiomyiosarcoma	1 (2)
Chemotherapy, N (%)	39 (78)
Biliary drainage, N (%)	4 (8)
Arterial embolization, N (%)	3 (6)
Ablation before PVE, N (%)	4 (8)

SD Standard Deviation

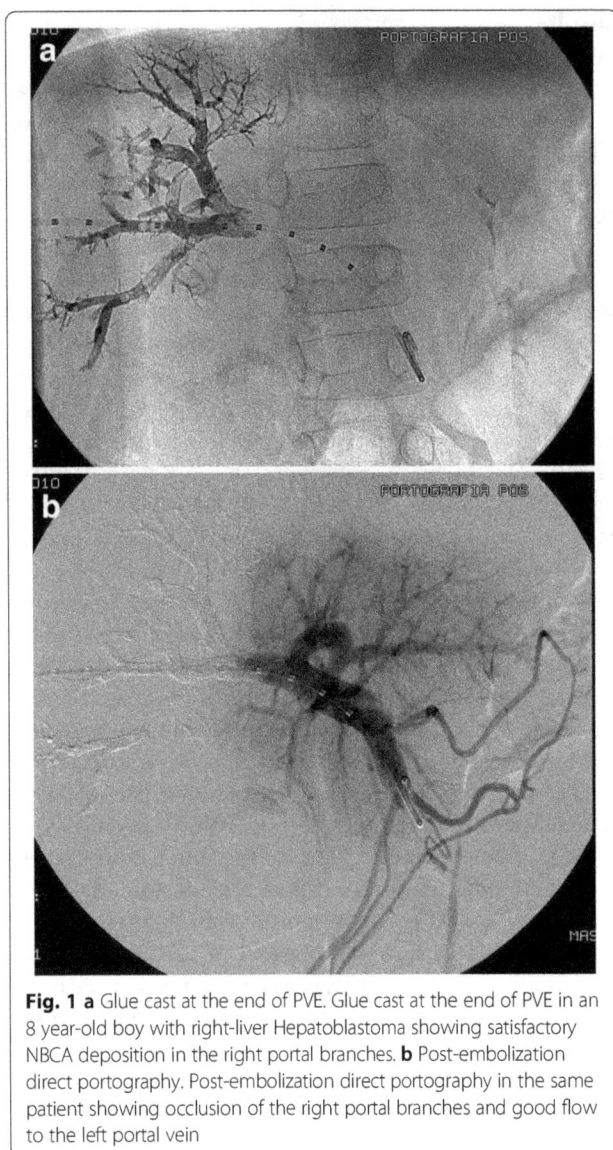

Fig. 1 a Glue cast at the end of PVE. Glue cast at the end of PVE in an 8 year-old boy with right-liver Hepatoblastoma showing satisfactory NBCA deposition in the right portal branches. **b** Post-embolization direct portography. Post-embolization direct portography in the same patient showing occlusion of the right portal branches and good flow to the left portal vein

Table 2 Liver volumetry before and after PVE

PVE segments, N (%)	
Right plus IV PVE	10 (20)
Right PVE	38 (76)
Segments VI and VII	2 (4)
PVE approach, N (%)	
Ipsilateral	49 (98)
Ipsi and Contra-lateral	1 (2)
Microcathether, N (%)	20 (40)
Glue: Lipidol ratio (range)	1-3 to 1-4
Before PVE[a]	
Total functional liver volume, mL, mean (SD)	1473.57 (432.78)
Future liver remnant, mL, mean (SD)	421.95 (132.54)
After PVE[a]	
Total functional liver volume, mL, mean (SD)	1531.24 (459.77)
Future liver remnant, mL, mean (SD)	628.97 (191.64)
FLR increase[a], %	51.67 (21.81)
FLR ratio increase[a], %	12.73 (4.8)
Kinetic growth rate[a], %/week	2.98 (1.29)

[a]Data available for 37 patients
SD Standard Deviation

and 3). The FLR/TFLV ratio increased from 29.6% ± 8.3% to 42.3% ± 9.8% ($P < 0.001$). Kinetic growth rate was 2.98%/week ± 1.29%/week. The TFLV slightly increased from 1474 ± 433 to 1531 ± 460 after PVE did not reach statistical significance ($P = 0.070$). Laboratory values showed no significant changes of measured parameters at 4–5 weeks after PVE when compared with measurements before PVE (Table 2).

Association of factors with FRL increase after PVE

A negative association was observed between FLR volume and increase in the FLR after PVE (Beta = −0.06, $P = 0.017$, Fig. 4 top) and between the FLR/TFLV ratio before PVE and the increase in the FLR after PVE (Beta = −1.29, $P = 0.002$, Fig. 4 bottom).

Complications

Of the 50 patients submitted to 52 PVE procedures three experienced major complications (5.7%): significant migration of NBCA fragments to the FLR ($n = 1$), a subcapsular biloma ($n = 1$) and FLR portal vein stenosis due to NBCA fragment dislodgment associated with cholangitis ($n = 1$) and. The latter patient was a 74 year-old male patient with cholangiocarcinoma submitted to percutaneous biliary drainage and PVE at the same time. During catheter manipulation there was glue dislodgment to the main left portal vein creating a stenosis. This patient showed the lowest rate of FLR increase in our study (20%). He was re-admitted to the hospital

drainage, before performing PVE. In 1 patient the biliary drainage was accomplished at the same moment of PVE. For this patient we performed PVE followed by biliary drainage at the same procedure. This tactic was implemented to try to optimize the time gap between PVE and surgery, as it is suggested in some publications [29]. Currently we first obtain an adequate biliary decompression with undoubtful evidence of declining levels of bilirubin before we proceed to PVE in such subset of patients [30].

Volumetric liver results and laboratory values

CT assessments were performed on average 15 (range 1–22) days before PVE. Imaging interval from the day of PVE to the post procedure volumetric CT was 32.7 ±14.5 days. FLR increased froma mean value of 422 ml ±133 to 629 ml ±192 ($P < 0.001$) after PVE, corresponding to a mean FLR increase of 52%±22% (Table 2, Figs. 2

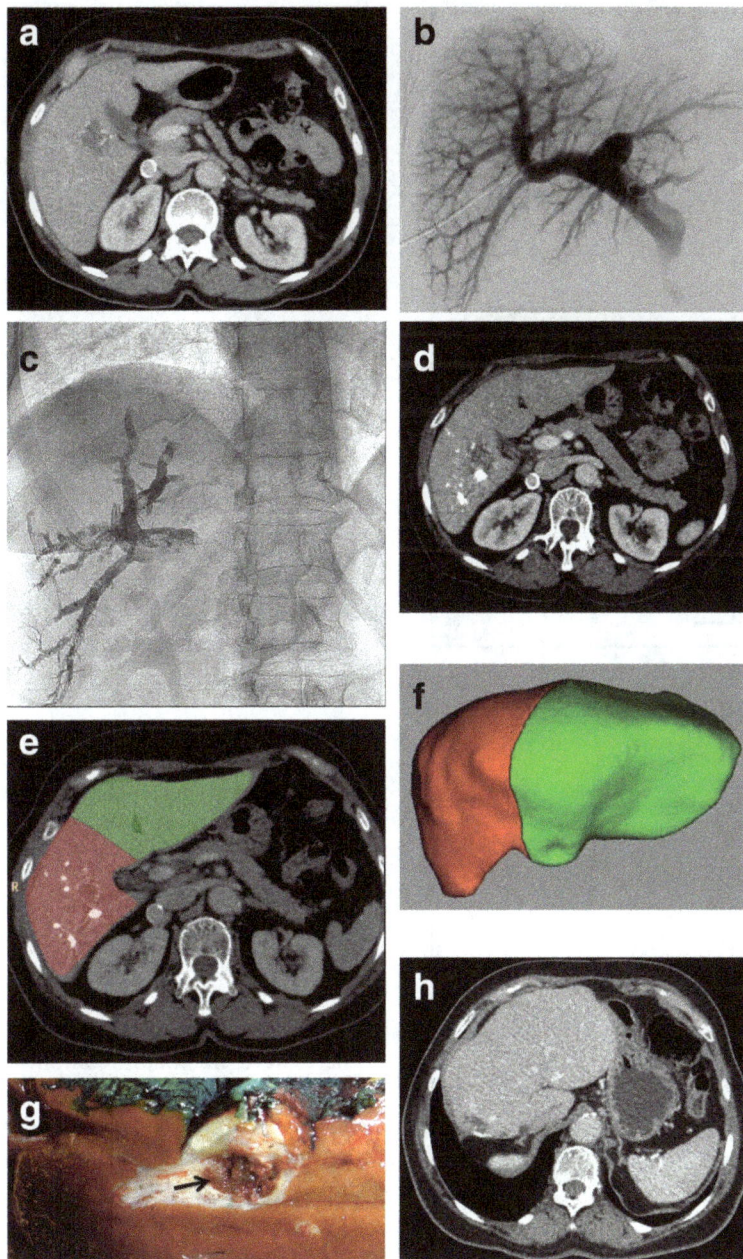

Fig. 2 a Computed tomography before PVE. A contrasted portal phase computed tomography before PVE in a 67 year-old female with colorectal cancer and liver metastasis. **b** Direct portography. Direct portography depicting normal portal vein anatomy during PVE. **c** Glue cast. Glue cast in the right portal branches at the end of PVE showing satisfactory distribution of the NBCA-lipiodol mixture. **d** Computed tomography 30 days after PVE. Portal venous phase computed tomography 30 days after PVE showing an important hypertrophy of the left liver. **e** and **f** Computed tomography volumetry after PVE. Computed tomography volumetry yielded a FLR increase of 44% and a FLR/TFLV ratio expansion from 34% to 47% after 30 days. **g** Liver specimen after right hepatectomy. Liver specimen after right hepatectomy showing glue in a right portal vein branch from the previous portal vein embolization. **h** 3-year post-operative computed tomography. Post-operative portal venous phase computed tomography 3 years after PVE with a good remnant liver volume

25 days after PVE with cholangitis and deceased 7 days afterwards due to refractory sepsis. Solely in this patient the complication precluded liver surgery (Fig. 5a and b).

Nine patients presented incidental findings or adverse events: 5 cases of very mild and minimal NBCA migration to the non-embolized liver, 1 case of small NBCA fragment migration to the right hepatic vein and 3 cases of nauseas and vomiting. All these patients with minute fragments of glue in the FLR or in the right hepatic vein presented satisfactory hypertrophy levels

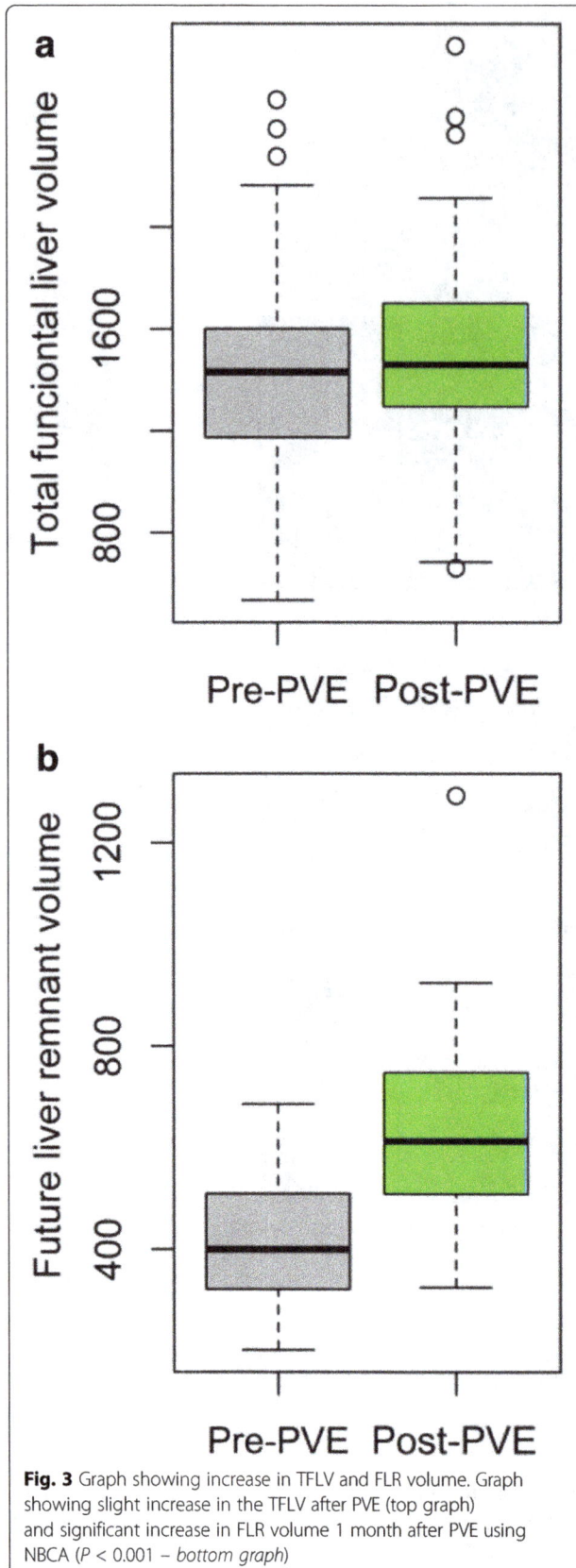

Fig. 3 Graph showing increase in TFLV and FLR volume. Graph showing slight increase in the TFLV after PVE (top graph) and significant increase in FLR volume 1 month after PVE using NBCA ($P < 0.001$ – *bottom graph*)

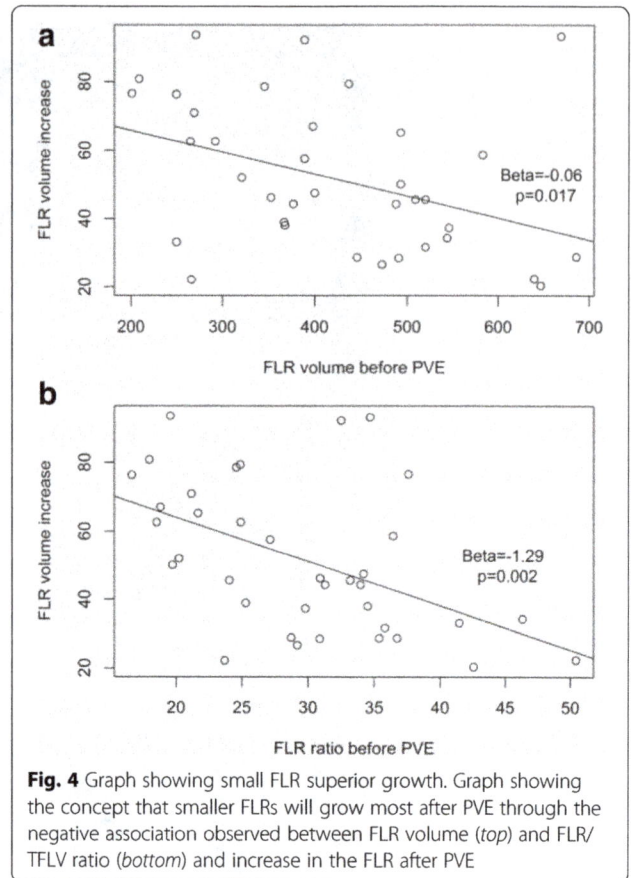

Fig. 4 Graph showing small FLR superior growth. Graph showing the concept that smaller FLRs will grow most after PVE through the negative association observed between FLR volume (*top*) and FLR/TFLV ratio (*bottom*) and increase in the FLR after PVE

probably secondary to their very small size and non-occlusive arrangement [15].

Complications and the use of microcatheters
There were no major complications, regarding NBCA, in patients where PVE was achieved with a microcatheter. Moreover incidental findings and adverse events were much more common in patients that a microcatheter was not used ($n = 7$) than in patients in whom it was adopted ($n = 2$). This analysis did not reach statistical significance ($p = 0.189$).

Surgical outcomes
Thirty-four patients were taken to the operating room although 3 patients presented intraoperative disease progression that prohibited liver resection. Thirty-onepatients eventually were submitted to hepatic surgery (62%). The executed liver resection procedures were as follows: right hepatectomy in 19 patients, right hepatectomy extended to segment IV in 8 patients, right hepatectomy extended to segment IV with resection of the caudate lobe and left portal vein reconstruction in 1 patient, resection of segments VI and VII in 2 patients and Associating Liver Partition and Portal vein Ligation for Staged hepatectomy (ALPPS) in 1 patient. Post hepatectomy complications

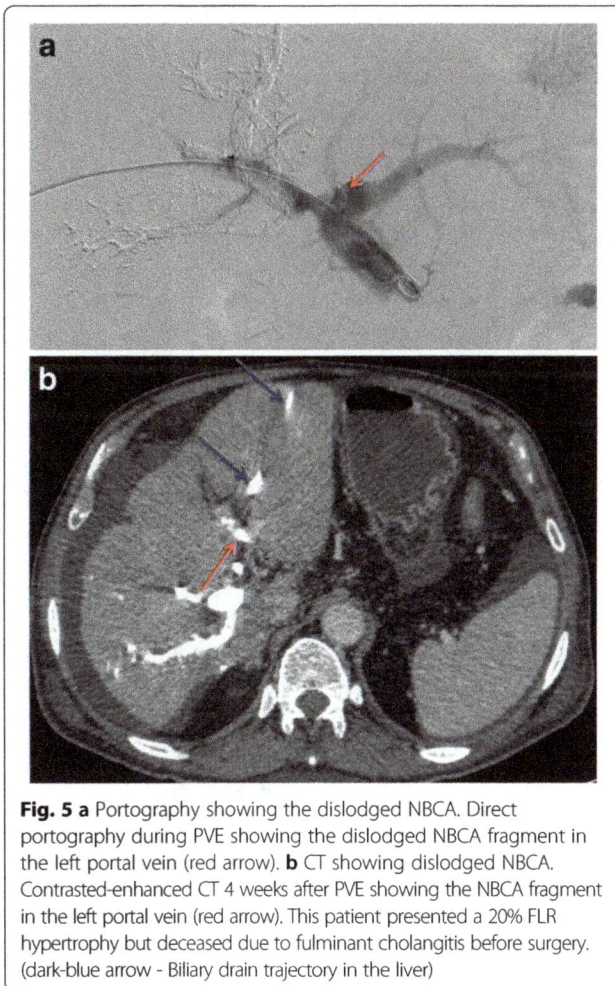

Fig. 5 a Portography showing the dislodged NBCA. Direct portography during PVE showing the dislodged NBCA fragment in the left portal vein (red arrow). **b** CT showing dislodged NBCA. Contrasted-enhanced CT 4 weeks after PVE showing the NBCA fragment in the left portal vein (red arrow). This patient presented a 20% FLR hypertrophy but deceased due to fulminant cholangitis before surgery. (dark-blue arrow - Biliary drain trajectory in the liver)

comprised bile leak or fistula or biloma ($n = 3$), pneumonia ($n = 1$), intraoperative hepatic bleeding (n = 3), sepsis (n = 1), subcapsular abscess (n = 1) and liver insufficiency (n = 1). Hospital stay was 9.97 days on average (range 3 to 56 days). Three patients needed blood transfusion. Thirteen patients eventually died (four patientswithin 30 days of hepatectomy - three from liver hemorrhage and one from a severe pneumonia). Sixteen patients were not taken to surgery due to disease progression ($n = 14$), cholangitis, liver insufficiency and death (n = 1) and uncontrolled comorbidities (n = 1).

Discussion

Liver surgery has certainly evolved in the last decades [5, 10] and for patients with less than adequate FLR volume before hepatic resections PVE is the procedure of choice in most hepatobiliary treatment centers [31]. Different PVE techniques and approaches have been described and numerous embolization materials have been tested to stimulate remnant liver growth [3, 13, 32]. Analyses of the induced hypertrophy of PVE with NBCA using

animaland afterwards human subjects showed its greater capacity compared to that of PVE with other embolic materials [14, 32] that might be related to the provoked periportal inflammatory response [4, 32]. Patients in the present study presented a substantial degree of FLR hypertrophy and increase in the FLR/TFLV ratio in accordance with previously published data including studies that compared NBCA glue with microparticles and coils [14, 22, 33]. The mean absolute FLR volume increase of 52% and the FLR/TFLV ratio expansion of 12% are superior to the published hypertrophy results in studies using other embolic agents than NBCA [14, 21, 34, 35]. Previously reported figures for PVE using NBCA, polyvinyl alcohol particles (PVA) plus coils/vascular plugs, gelatin sponge, PVA alone and fibrin glue are in the range of 47%-79%, 24%-54%, 17%-37%, 24%-32% and 27%-31% of FLR volume increase respectively [4, 24, 36, 37].

Another important and very discussed technical point in PVE is which side should be elected for the puncture, the contralateral, achieved through an access of the FLR's peripheral portal branch, or the ipsilateral, attained by the puncture of the portal vein that will be removed in the near future hepatectomy. In the contralateral approach, developed in France [15, 38, 39], there is a potentially easier catheterization of the right portal subdivisions and the possibility to use smaller catheters [15] with the drawbackof potential harm to the FLR's portal vein. The ipsilateral approach, in contrast, avoids puncture of the FLR but has a trickier catheterization [40]. In a systematic review that included studies from 1990 to 2011 [33], the ipsilateral approach accounted for 55% ($n = 963$) of all PVE procedures but in only 3% (28 procedures) the glue-lipiodol mixture (without coils nor particles nor amplatzer plug) was adopted as their sole embolic material. Moreover, the authors from this systematic review argued that it would be hard to manipulate glue from the ipsilateral side. Albeit we agree that PVE with glue requires extra caution, is a technically demanding procedure [24], and has a steep learning curve, the present study suggests that it can be performed through an ipsilateral approach. To our knowledge, this is one of the largest PVE series employing solely NBCA-lipiodol mixture as the embolic material through an ipsilateral approach.

These results show that the initial FLR volume and FLR/TFLV ratio were predictive factors for FLR hypertrophy after PVE, indicating that patients with lesser FLR volume or minor FLR/TFLV ratios at presentation will be the ones we can expect the greatest FLR enlargement. This association has been previously described in a study analyzing predictors of hypertrophy of the FLR after PVE in a non-cirrhotic population [24]. In cirrhotic patients with primary liver tumors this analysis was also performed and likewise similar results were shown [41,

42]. This correlation was also demonstrated in the surgical series that scrutinized liver regeneration and influencing factors. The general conclusion is that liver regeneration rate after resection is proportional to the volume of hepatic parenchyma removed at surgery whether or not liver dysfunction is present [43, 44]. As far as expectations and indications go for PVE these findings have direct influence in its daily practice. Since the degree of hypertrophy is inversely associated with the initial FRL volume, one should reaffirm PVE indication even for very small FLR volumes [24].

Of all complications associated with PVE recorded in our sample, only one precluded future liver surgery. This latter patient presented a stenosis of the left portal vein through the dislodgment of a glue fragment ensued near the completion of PVE and deceased 32 days after that from cholangitis and liver insufficiency. In this case we could have tried to pull the NBCA fragment back into the right portal vein as shown elsewhere [45], even though at that moment we did not have the appropriated material. While it is not stated in PVE guidelines or quality improvement statements [26] we currently maintain adequate retrieval materials such as snares and angioplasty balloons at our interventional radiology department, principally when dealing with embolic materials such as glue. It is also advisable to get satisfactory bilirubin clearance before PVE instead of performing both percutaneous biliary drainage and PVE procedures at the same time [29] as recommended in guidelines [26]. Particular attention should be devoted to avoid FLR glue migration since it can preclude liver surgery. When comparing complication rates between the groups with and without additional use of microcatheters there were no cases of major NBCA migration or dislodgment with its use and it was suggested that glue migration might be avoided with this coaxial technique. This difference did not reach statistical significance probably due to the small sample size. Additionally, the interpretation of this finding also suffers from the allocation of the use of the microcatheter, which was not random. We believe the use of microcatheters associated with the administration of small glue aliquots (e.g. 0.3 mL) in between abundant flushing with dextran or glucose 5% [26], is highly advisable when performing PVE with NBCA through an ipsilateral approach. Technical advises have been systematically addressed in the PVE NBCA publications, alerting for the extra care towards the end of the procedure where most of the targeted portal branches are already occluded, the few branches left usually demonstrate slow flow and complications, particularly embolic material reflux to the left portal vein, might occur [15].

The technical success rate (98%) and the clinical success rate of PVE (96%) in the present study were high and in accordance with the previous reported results [33]. Two patients (4%) presented insufficient hypertrophy after PVE and one of them could not be submitted to the planned surgery because of the associated development cholangitis and liver insufficiency. The other patient had a FLR before PVE which accounted for 17% of the TFLV and despite the significant hypertrophy of 76% and an increase to 30% in the FLR/TFLV ratio the liver surgeon decided to perform an ALPPS procedure to amplify FLR growth. The ALPPS was performed in May 2014 and this patient is currently on follow-up with no evidence of cancer related disease. In this series thirty-one patients (62%) were submitted to liver resections. One patient presented signs of liver failure within 30 days from hepatectomy with posterior convalescence. Out of the 31 patients submitted to liver surgery 18 (58%) are alive with no signs of hepatic insufficiency. Our 62% liver resection rate is below the usual published statistics for PVE in which approximately 70% to 80% of the originally planned liver resections after PVE are performed [33, 46]. In our group the vast majority of patients were not taken to liver resection after PVE due to disease progression. While this is the most frequent cause of not performing hepatectomies after PVE [33, 47], some of our cohort patients also suffered from inadequate long waiting periods for surgery after PVE due to local institutional impairments which might influence disease progression. Besides that, during PVE-induced liver regeneration, disease progression may be secondary to undetectable pre-existing tumor growth, and PVE may, consequently, perform as a surrogate marker of cancer biology, removing patients that are not suitable for surgery [46]. Notwithstanding tumor progression, FLR growth following PVE would have been sufficient to permit the planned hepatic resection in all but one of these patients.

This study has limitations. This was a retrospective study occurring over a period of five years and as such it is plausible that the improved patient selection for PVE and radiologists' experience gained over the years could result in better outcomes. The data collection and extraction relied primarily on medical charts. The small sample hindered us from exploring other factors that might be linked to greater FLR increase. A strength of this study was the relative homogeneous patient population conceded only by non-cirrhotic patients which otherwise could have confused our hypertrophy results because of cirrhosis regeneration recognized variances [48]. Furthermore, even though NBCA is one of the main embolic agents used worldwide for PVE and it is suggested that it induces the highest FLR growth, its administration has been reported almost exclusively from the contralateral side. This study was able to show that it is possible to use NBCA for PVE without approaching the FLR.

Conclusions

This study suggests that PVE with NBCA through an ipsilateral puncture is an effective procedure to permit major hepatectomies in patients with a small FLR. Meticulous attention is needed especially near the end of the embolization procedure to avoid complications.

Abbreviations

ALPPS: Associating Liver Partition and Portal vein Ligation for Staged hepatectomy; CT: Computed tomography; FLR: Future liver remnant; KGR: Kineticgrowthrate; NBCA: n-butyl-cyanoacrylate; PVE: Portal vein embolization; TFLV: Total functional liver volume

Acknowledgments

We acknowledge the liver surgeons, Dr. Gustavo Stoduto, Dr. Rinaldo Gonçalves, Dr. Mauro Monteiro, Dr. Eduardo Linhares, Dr. Rafael Albagli, Dr. Marcus Valdão, Dr. André Maciel, Dr. Leonaldson Castro, Dr. Sergio Bertholace, Dr. Carlos Eduardo Santos,Dr. Marcelo Enne, among others, with the scientific insights during the elaboration of the manuscript.

Funding

This work was supported by the Brazilian National Cancer Institute (INCA 31770814.7.000.5274) but with no specific funding.

Meetings

Part of this work was shown as an oral presentation at the annual European Congress of Radiology (ECR) of the European Society of Radiology, March 1–5, 2017, in Vienna, Austria.

Authors' contributions

JHML Interventional Radiologist. Contributed to the conception and design of this work. Performed part of the interventional procedures. He is a contributor responsible for the overall content as guarantor. Reviewed the manuscript. Approved the final version to be published. Agreed to be accountable to all aspects of this work. PML Contributed in the analyses and interpretation of data. Reviewed the manuscript. She is a contributor responsible for the overall content as guarantor. Approved the final version to be published. Agreed to be accountable to all aspects of this work. TB Interventional Radiologist. Contributed to the design of the manuscript. Reviewed the manuscript. Approved the final version to be published. Agreed to be accountable to all aspects of this work. HSM Interventional Radiologist. Contributed to the conception and design of this work. Established the ideal technique for PVE. Performed part of the interventional procedures. Reviewed the manuscript. Approved the final version to be published. Agreed to be accountable to all aspects of this work. HRG Interventional Radiologist. Contributed to the conception and design of this work. Established the ideal technique for PVE. Performed part of the interventional procedures. Reviewed the manuscript. Approved the final version to be published. Agreed to be accountable to all aspects of this work. EC Interventional Radiologist. Contributed to the design of the manuscript. Reviewed the manuscript. Approved the final version to be published. Agreed to be accountable to all aspects of this work. FVG Interventional Radiologist. Contributed to the design of the manuscript. Reviewed the manuscript. Approved the final version to be published. Agreed to be accountable to all aspects of this work. IFM Interventional Radiology fellow. Contributed in the analyses and interpretation of data. Reviewed the manuscript. Approved the final version to be published. Agreed to be accountable to all aspects of this work. RRS Interventional Radiology fellow. Contributed in the analyses and interpretation of data. Reviewed the manuscript. Approved the final version to be published. Agreed to be accountable to all aspects of this work. TNdM Interventional Radiology fellow. Contributed in the analyses and interpretation of data. Reviewed the manuscript. Approved the final version to be published. Agreed to be accountable to all aspects of this work.

Competing interests

The authors declare that they have no competing interests.

Author details

[1]Department of Interventional Radiology, Radiology Division, National Cancer Institute, INCA, Praça Cruz Vermelha 23, Centro, Rio de Janeiro CEP 20230-130, Brazil. [2]National Institute of Infectious Disease EvandroChagas, Oswaldo Cruz Foundation, Rio de Janeiro, Brazil. [3]Department of Interventional Radiology, Centro Hepato-Bilio-Pancreático e de Transplantação.Hospital Curry Cabral, CHLC, Lisbon, Portugal.

References

1. Kinoshita H, Sakai K, Hirohashi K, Igawa S, Yamasaki O, Kubo S. Preoperative portal vein embolization for hepatocellular carcinoma. World J Surg. 1986;10(5):803–8.
2. Aoki T, Kubota K. Preoperative portal vein embolization for hepatocellular carcinoma: consensus and controversy. World J Hepatol. 2016;8(9):439–45.
3. Abdalla EK, Hicks ME, Vauthey JN. Portal vein embolization: rationale, technique and future prospects. Br J Surg. 2001;88(2):165–75.
4. de Baere T, Roche A, Elias D, Lasser P, Lagrange C, Bousson V. Preoperative portal vein embolization for extension of hepatectomy indications. Hepatology. 1996;24(6):1386–91.
5. Azoulay D, Castaing D, Smail A, Adam R, Cailliez V, Laurent A, Lemoine A, Bismuth H. Resection of nonresectable liver metastases from colorectal cancer after percutaneous portal vein embolization. Ann Surg. 2000;231(4):480–6.
6. Kubota K, Makuuchi M, Kusaka K, Kobayashi T, Miki K, Hasegawa K, Harihara Y, Takayama T. Measurement of liver volume and hepatic functional reserve as a guide to decision-making in resectional surgery for hepatic tumors. Hepatology. 1997;26(5):1176–81.
7. Starzl TE, Francavilla A, Halgrimson CG, Francavilla FR, Porter KA, Brown TH, Putnam CW. The origin, hormonal nature, and action of hepatotrophic substances in portal venous blood. Surg Gynecol Obstet. 1973;137(2):179–99.
8. Jaeck D, Bachellier P, Guiguet M, Boudjema K, Vaillant JC, Balladur P, Nordlinger B. Long-term survival following resection of colorectal hepatic metastases. Association Française de Chirurgie. Br J Surg. 1997; 84(7):977–80.
9. Jaeck D, Oussoultzoglou E, Rosso E, Greget M, Weber JC, Bachellier P. A two-stage hepatectomy procedure combined with portal vein embolization to achieve curative resection for initially unresectable multiple and bilobar colorectal liver metastases. Ann Surg. 2004;240(6): 1037–49. discussion 1049-51
10. Adam R, Delvart V, Pascal G, Valeanu A, Castaing D, Azoulay D, Giacchetti S, Paule B, Kunstlinger F, Ghémard O, Levi F, Bismuth H. Rescue surgery for unresectable colorectal liver metastases downstaged by chemotherapy: a model to predict long-term survival. Ann Surg. 2004;240(4):644–57. discussion 657-8
11. May BJ, Talenfeld AD, Madoff DC. Update on portal vein embolization: evidence-based outcomes, controversies, and novel strategies. J Vasc Interv Radiol. 2013;24(2):241–54.
12. Madoff DC, Abdalla EK, Vauthey JN. Portal vein embolization in preparation for major hepatic resection: evolution of a new standard of care. J Vasc Interv Radiol. 2005;16(6):779–90.
13. de Baere T, Denys A, Madoff DC. Preoperative portal vein embolization: indications and technical considerations. Tech Vasc Interv Radiol. 2007;10(1):67–78.
14. Guiu B, Bize P, Gunthern D, Demartines N, Halkic N, Denys A. Portal vein embolization before right hepatectomy: improved results using n-butyl-cyanoacrylate compared to microparticles plus coils. Cardiovasc Intervent Radiol. 2013;36(5):1306–12.
15. Di Stefano DR, de Baere T, Denys A, Hakime A, Gorin G, Gillet M, Saric J, Trillaud H, Petit P, Bartoli JM, Elias D, Delpero JR. Preoperative percutaneous portal vein embolization: evaluation of adverse events in 188 patients. Radiology. 2005;234(2):625–30.

16. Madoff DC, Abdalla EK, Gupta S, Wu TT, Morris JS, Denys A, Wallace MJ, Morello FA, Ahrar K, Murthy R, Lunagomez S, Hicks ME, Vauthey JN. Transhepatic ipsilateral right portal vein embolization extended to segment IV: improving hypertrophy and resection outcomes with spherical particles and coils. J Vasc Interv Radiol. 2005;16(2 Pt 1):215–25.

17. Madoff DC, Hicks ME, Abdalla EK, Morris JS, Vauthey JN. Portal vein embolization with polyvinyl alcohol particles and coils in preparation for major liver resection for hepatobiliary malignancy: safety and effectiveness–study in 26 patients. Radiology. 2003;227(1):251–60.

18. Nagino M, Kamiya J, Nishio H, Ebata T, Arai T, Nimura Y. Two hundred forty consecutive portal vein embolizations before extended hepatectomy for biliary cancer: surgical outcome and long-term follow-up. Ann Surg. 2006; 243(3):364–72.

19. Hong YK, Choi SB, Lee KH, Park SW, Park YN, Choi JS, Lee WJ, Chung JB, Kim KS. The efficacy of portal vein embolization prior to right extended hemihepatectomy for hilar cholangiocellular carcinoma: a retrospective cohort study. Eur J Surg Oncol. 2011;37(3):237–44.

20. Mise Y, Passot G, Wang X, Chen HC, Wei S, Brudvik KW, Aloia TA, Conrad C, Huang SY, Vauthey JN. A Nomogram to predict hypertrophy of liver segments 2 and 3 after right portal vein Embolization. J Gastrointest Surg. 2016;20(7):1317–23.

21. Libicher M, Herbrik M, Stippel D, Poggenborg J, Bovenschulte H, Schwabe H. Portal vein embolization using the amplatzer vascular plug II: preliminary results. Rofo. 2010;182(6):501–6.

22. Jaberi A, Toor SS, Rajan DK, Mironov O, Kachura JR, Cleary SP, Smoot R, Tremblay St-Germain A, Tan K. Comparison of clinical outcomes following glue versus polyvinyl alcohol portal vein Embolization for hypertrophy of the future liver remnant prior to right hepatectomy. J Vasc Interv Radiol. 2016;27(12):1897–905. e1

23. Nagino M, Nimura Y, Kamiya J, Kondo S, Kanai M. Selective percutaneous transhepatic embolization of the portal vein in preparation for extensive liver resection: the ipsilateral approach. Radiology. 1996;200(2):559–63.

24. de Baere T, Teriitehau C, Deschamps F, Catherine L, Rao P, Hakime A, Auperin A, Goere D, Elias D, Hechelhammer L. Predictive factors for hypertrophy of the future remnant liver after selective portal vein embolization. Ann Surg Oncol. 2010;17(8):2081–9.

25. van der Vorst JR, van Dam RM, van Stiphout RS, van den Broek MA, Hollander IH, Kessels AG, Dejong CH. Virtual liver resection and volumetric analysis of the future liver remnant using open source image processing software. World J Surg. 2010;34(10):2426–33.

26. Denys A, Bize P, Demartines N, Deschamps F, De Baere T, Europe, C. a. I. R. S. o. Quality improvement for portal vein embolization. Cardiovasc Intervent Radiol. 2010;33(3):452–6.

27. Shindoh J, Truty MJ, Aloia TA, Curley SA, Zimmitti G, Huang SY, Mahvash A, Gupta S, Wallace MJ, Vauthey JN. Kinetic growth rate after portal vein embolization predicts posthepatectomy outcomes: toward zero liver-related mortality in patients with colorectal liver metastases and small future liver remnant. J Am Coll Surg. 2013;216(2):201–9.

28. Goldberg SN, Grassi CJ, Cardella JF, Charboneau JW, Dodd GD, Dupuy DE, Gervais D, Gillams AR, Kane RA, Lee FT, Livraghi T, McGahan J, Phillips DA, Rhim H, Silverman SG, Committee, S. o. I. R. T. A, Ablation, I. W. G. o. I.-G. T. Image-guided tumor ablation: standardization of terminology and reporting criteria. Radiology. 2005;235(3):728–39.

29. Guiu B, Bize P, Demartines N, Lesurtel M, Denys A. Simultaneous biliary drainage and portal vein embolization before extended hepatectomy for hilar cholangiocarcinoma: preliminary experience. Cardiovasc Intervent Radiol. 2014;37(3):698–704.

30. Lee EC, Park SJ, Han SS, Park HM, Lee SD, Kim SH, Lee IJ, Kim HB. Mortality after portal vein embolization: two case reports. Medicine (Baltimore). 2017;96(6):e5446.

31. Adams RB, Haller DG, Roh MS. Improving resectability of hepatic colorectal metastases: expert consensus statement by Abdalla et al. Ann Surg Oncol. 2006;13(10):1281–3.

32. de Baere T, Denys A, Paradis V. Comparison of four embolic materials for portal vein embolization: experimental study in pigs. Eur Radiol. 2009;19(6):1435–42.

33. van Lienden KP, van den Esschert JW, de Graaf W, Bipat S, Lameris JS, van Gulik TM, van Delden OM. Portal vein embolization before liver resection: a systematic review. Cardiovasc Intervent Radiol. 2013;36(1):25–34.

34. Covey AM, Brown KT, Jarnagin WR, Brody LA, Schwartz L, Tuorto S, Sofocleous CT, D'Angelica M, Getrajdman GI, DeMatteo R, Kemeny NE, Fong Y. Combined portal vein embolization and neoadjuvant chemotherapy as a treatment strategy for resectable hepatic colorectal metastases. Ann Surg. 2008;247(3):451–5.

35. van den Esschert JW, de Graaf W, van Lienden KP, Busch OR, Heger M, van Delden OM, Gouma DJ, Bennink RJ, Laméris JS, van Gulik TM. Volumetric and functional recovery of the remnant liver after major liver resection with prior portal vein embolization : recovery after PVE and liver resection. J Gastrointest Surg. 2009;13(8):1464–9.

36. Giraudo G, Greget M, Oussoultzoglou E, Rosso E, Bachellier P, Jaeck D. Preoperative contralateral portal vein embolization before major hepatic resection is a safe and efficient procedure: a large single institution experience. Surgery. 2008;143(4):476–82.

37. Covey AM, Tuorto S, Brody LA, Sofocleous CT, Schubert J, von Tengg-Kobligk H, Getrajdman GI, Schwartz LH, Fong Y, Brown KT. Safety and efficacy of preoperative portal vein embolization with polyvinyl alcohol in 58 patients with liver metastases. AJR Am J Roentgenol. 2005;185(6):1620–6.

38. de Baere T, Roche A, Vavasseur D, Therasse E, Indushekar S, Elias D, Bognel C. Portal vein embolization: utility for inducing left hepatic lobe hypertrophy before surgery. Radiology. 1993;188(1):73–7.

39. Azoulay D, Castaing D, Krissat J, Smail A, Hargreaves GM, Lemoine A, Emile JF, Bismuth H. Percutaneous portal vein embolization increases the feasibility and safety of major liver resection for hepatocellular carcinoma in injured liver. Ann Surg. 2000;232(5):665–72.

40. Denys A, Prior J, Bize P, Duran R, De Baere T, Halkic N, Demartines N. Portal vein embolization: what do we know? Cardiovasc Intervent Radiol. 2012; 35(5):999–1008.

41. Imamura H, Shimada R, Kubota M, Matsuyama Y, Nakayama A, Miyagawa S, Makuuchi M, Kawasaki S. Preoperative portal vein embolization: an audit of 84 patients. Hepatology. 1999;29(4):1099–105.

42. Denys A, Lacombe C, Schneider F, Madoff DC, Doenz F, Qanadli SD, Halkic N, Sauvanet A, Vilgrain V, Schnyder P. Portal vein embolization with N-butyl cyanoacrylate before partial hepatectomy in patients with hepatocellular carcinoma and underlying cirrhosis or advanced fibrosis. J Vasc Interv Radiol. 2005;16(12):1667–74.

43. Tani M, Tomiya T, Yamada S, Hayashi S, Yahata K, Tamura Y, Akiyama M, Kawai S, Masaki N, Fujiwara K. Regulating factors of liver regeneration after hepatectomy. Cancer Chemother Pharmacol. 1994; 33(Suppl):S29–32.

44. Nagino M, Ando M, Kamiya J, Uesaka K, Sano T, Nimura Y. Liver regeneration after major hepatectomy for biliary cancer. Br J Surg. 2001;88(8):1084–91.

45. Dobrocky T, Kettenbach J, Lopez-Benitez R, Kara L. Disastrous portal vein Embolization turned into a successful intervention. Cardiovasc Intervent Radiol. 2015;38(5):1365–8.

46. Ironside N, Bell R, Bartlett A, McCall J, Powell J, Pandanaboyana S. Systematic review of perioperative and survival outcomes of liver resections with and without preoperative portal vein embolization for colorectal metastases. HPB (Oxford). 2017;19(7):559–66.

47. Pamecha V, Glantzounis G, Davies N, Fusai G, Sharma D, Davidson B. Long-term survival and disease recurrence following portal vein embolisation prior to major hepatectomy for colorectal metastases. Ann Surg Oncol. 2009;16(5):1202–7.

48. Yamanaka N, Okamoto E, Kawamura E, Kato T, Oriyama T, Fujimoto J, Furukawa K, Tanaka T, Tomoda F, Tanaka W. Dynamics of normal and injured human liver regeneration after hepatectomy as assessed on the basis of computed tomography and liver function. Hepatology. 1993;18(1):79–85.

6

Assessment and diagnostic accuracy of lymph node status to predict stage III colon cancer using computed tomography

Erik Rollvén[1*], Mirna Abraham-Nordling[2], Torbjörn Holm[2] and Lennart Blomqvist[1]

Abstract

Background: To study different imaging criteria for prediction of lymph node metastases (Stage III disease) in colon cancer using CT.

Methods: In a retrospective setting, 483 consecutive patients with histology proven colon cancer underwent elective primary resection during 2008–2011, a cohort of 119 patients were included. Contrast enhanced CT examinations, in portal-venous phase, were reviewed with assessment of the number of lymph nodes, their anatomical distribution, size, size ratio, internal heterogeneity, presence of irregular outer border and attenuation values. Sensitivity, specificity, PPV and NPV for each studied criteria for prediction of stage III disease was calculated.

Results: According to histopathology 80 patients were stage I-II and 39 were stage III. Of the studied CT-criteria for lymph node metastases per patient, internal heterogeneity in at least one lymph node resulted in the best performance with sensitivity, specificity, PPV and NPV of 79, 84, 70 and 89%, Odds ratio (OR) 20. Presence of irregular outer border resulted in a sensitivity, specificity, PPV and NPV of 59, 81, 61 and 82%, OR 6.2. If both internal heterogeneity and/or irregular outer border was used as a criterion this resulted in a sensitivity, specificity, PPV and NPV of 85, 75, 62 and 91%, OR 16.5. None of the size criteria used were predictive for stage III disease.

Conclusions: When performing preoperative CT in patients with colon cancer, the imaging criteria that allow best prediction of stage III disease on CT are either presence of at least one lymph node with internal heterogeneity or internal heterogeneity and/or irregular outer border. These criteria have to be validated in a prospective study.

Keywords: Colon cancer, Computed tomography, Staging, Stage III, Lymph nodes

Background

Colon cancer is the third most common malignancy in the western world. In Sweden the incidence is increasing with an aging population while the mortality is slowly decreasing [1].

The treatment is surgical removal of the tumour containing segment of the bowel together with local and regional lymph nodes. In addition, adjuvant chemotherapy is standard treatment for patients with stage III disease and in some patients with stage II disease, depending on presence of additional histological risk factors.

Well-known important prognostic factors in colon cancer are tumour stage (T), extramural vascular invasion (EMVI) and lymph node involvement (N) [2]. Even the total number of harvested lymph nodes at surgery and lymph node ratio (the ratio between lymph node metastases and examined lymph nodes, LNR) assessed by the pathologist has a prognostic importance [3–5].

A complete preoperative evaluation of patients with colon cancer includes staging of the primary tumour and evaluation of distant metastases in the liver and lungs with computed tomography (CT). In recent years, some studies advocate and support the use of CT also for local staging of colon cancer including treatment planning and selection of patients for neoadjuvant treatment [6–8]. If selection of patients for neoadjuvant treatment is being used routinely

* Correspondence: erik.rollven@ki.se
[1]Department of Molecular Medicine and Surgery, Karolinska Institutet, Department of Radiology, Karolinska University Hospital, Solna SE - 171 76, Stockholm, Sweden
Full list of author information is available at the end of the article

in the clinic, pretreatment knowledge of regional lymph node involvement will be even more important.

To date, there are no validated imaging criteria for the assessment of lymph node metastases in colon cancer. Previous studies have applied different criteria based on either size and/or morphology. Lymph node size >1 cm, short-long axis diameter ratio, internal heterogeneity (IH), irregular outer border (IOB), attenuation values >100 Hounsfield units (HU) and cluster of three or more normal sized lymph nodes, or any combination of the above, have all been used as a single criterion or combined criteria [6, 9–14]. In a systematic review by Leufkens et al. including 753 patients with colon cancer in altogether 11 studies a sample sized weighted sensitivity and specificity of CT for N-staging of 76 and 55% was reported [15]. Most of the studies included were performed with older CT-technology that is no longer used and that does not allow true multiplanar assessment. Furthermore, the studies did not consider the distribution and location of lymph nodes within the colonic mesentery adjacent to the cancer as a potential marker of lymph node involvement.

Today, when CT scanners are configured with multiple rows of detectors, multiplanar assessment can be performed allowing for more detailed assessment of size and morphology of pathological lesions [16].

The aim of this study was to assess whether the number of lymph nodes, their anatomical distribution, size, size ratio, internal heterogeneity, irregular outer border and attenuation values on preoperative CT, either alone or in combination, were predictive for stage III disease.

Methods

From the Swedish colorectal cancer registry (SCRCR), 483 consecutive patients having a histology proven colon cancer and operated between the years 2008 and 2011 and examined with abdominal CT (64 detector CT-scanner) before surgery at our institution were included. A cohort of 119 patients was determined, after the following patients were excluded: insufficient CT examination (no iv contrast, CT-Colonography, no 64-slice) including examination performed outside the University hospital ($n = 80$), patients having emergency colonic surgery ($n = 78$), patients with T4 tumours ($n = 68$), metastatic disease ($n = 67$), no detectable tumour on the preoperative CT ($n = 18$), co-malignant disease ($n = 15$), CT examination >60 days prior to surgery ($n = 13$), patients with neo-adjuvant chemotherapy ($n = 11$), previous colon cancer surgery ($n = 9$), CT after treatment with colon stenting ($n = 3$) and perforated tumour or abscess ($n = 2$).

In the remaining cohort with histologically proven colon cancer there were 63 women and 56 men with a median age of 69 (range 32–91 years).

Most of the tumours were located in the sigmoid colon (Table 1). The majority of the tumors were classified on

Table 1 Demographics table of 119 patients/tumours

Characteristics	Number (%)
Sex (female/male)	63/56
Age (median)	69 (32–91)
Histopathological evaluation	
Tumour localization	
Caecum	23 (19%)
Ascending colon	22 (18%)
Hepatic flexure	8 (7%)
Transverse colon	11 (9%)
Splenic flexure	4 (3%)
Descending colon	6 (5%)
Sigmoid colon	45 (38%)
Tumor Stage	
T1	10 (8%)
T2	16 (13%)
T3	93 (78%)
Positive lymph node status	
T1 tumours	2/10 (20%)
T2 tumours	2/16 (12%)
T3 tumours	35/93 (38%)
Stage	
Stage I	22 (18%)
Stage II	58 (49%)
Stage III	39 (33%)
Lymph nodes, total number	
Harvested lymph nodes PAD	2542
Positive lymph nodes PAD	123
CT evaluation	
Detected lymph nodes ≥4 mm/tot	442/1312 (34%)
Region 1	261/835 (31%)
Region 2	161/389 (41%)
Region 3	20/88 (23%)

histopathology as T3 tumours (Table 1). Thirty-nine out of 119 patients had lymph node positive (stage III) disease (28 patients N1 and 11 patients N2) (Table 1). The median age for patients with stage I-II disease was 70 years, and the median age for patients with stage III disease was 63 years.

All patients had preoperative investigations with CT of the abdomen with intravenous contrast (0.5 mg Iodine/kg) in portal-venous phase (delay 90 s) on one of four different 64 slice CT scanners (Lightspeed VCT, General Electric, Milwaukee, USA). All examinations were performed at 120 kV and with tube current modulation. For abdomen the median dose length product (DLP) was 583 mGy-cm (range 393 to 878 mGy-cm). Median pitch factor was 1.375 (range 0.516 to 1.50). Medium noise index was 30 (range 26 to 42). The variation in both pitch factor and noise index are due to differences in the four CT scanners that were used. In 56 CT examinations arterial phase imaging of the abdomen at the tumour location and liver was also performed. After the examination, reformatted images in axial, coronal and sagittal planes with 5 mm thickness (increment 2.5 mm) were routinely generated together with the original (thin slices) 0.625 mm images.

CT evaluation

All CT examinations were retrospectively reviewed by one radiologist (E.R.) with more than 15 years of experience in cross sectional imaging of colorectal cancer and blinded for the histology and surgical reports. Examinations were assessed according to a dedicated evaluation proforma.

All measurements and assessments were performed on a Sectra Workstation IDS7 (version 15.1.14.41) using the 5 mm reformatted images with 2.5 mm increment. The original thin slices (0.625 mm) were used for detection of small lymph nodes (≤4 mm).

Anatomical distribution

The colonic mesentery, 5 cm oral and aboral from the tumour site, was divided in three anatomical regions (region 1–3), as a modified variant of the guidelines of the Japanese Society for Cancer in the Colon and Rectum [17]. Region 1 was defined as the region most adjacent to the tumour (+/–5 cm) and 3 cm proximal along the vessels to the branch artery divides covering the pericolonic and marginal lymph nodes. Region 3 was defined as the most proximal part of the mesentery including the undivided mesenteric artery from the aorta (proximal lymph nodes). Region 2 was defined as the region between region 1 and 3 (Fig. 1).

Number, size and size-ratio of lymph nodes

All lymph nodes ≥2 mm in size were separately registered in total and in each anatomical region. For lymph nodes ≥4 mm in shortest diameter, the short axis and the long axis were also separately measured and the ratio between the short and long axis diameter was calculated. The size ratio (ratio between two orthogonal (short/long) axis diameters) was used to test whether a more rounded shape was predictive for metastasis. A >0.8 ratio between diameter was used as cut off point according to a previous study [18]. The presence of a cluster (within a range of the lymph node diameter) of three or more lymph nodes was also separately noted in every region.

Internal heterogeneity and irregular outer borders

As possible morphological predictors of metastases, the internal heterogeneity (IH, mixed attenuation within the

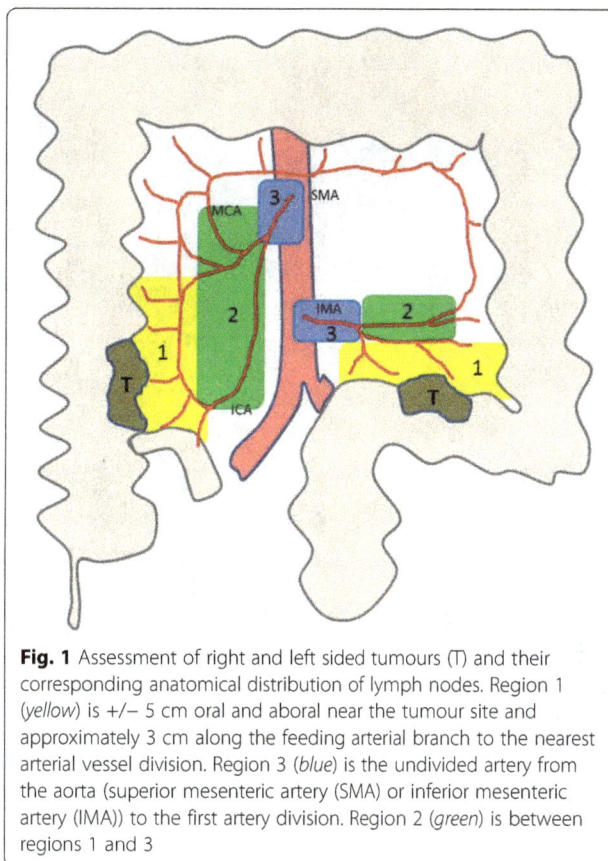

Fig. 1 Assessment of right and left sided tumours (T) and their corresponding anatomical distribution of lymph nodes. Region 1 (*yellow*) is +/– 5 cm oral and aboral near the tumour site and approximately 3 cm along the feeding arterial branch to the nearest arterial vessel division. Region 3 (*blue*) is the undivided artery from the aorta (superior mesenteric artery (SMA) or inferior mesenteric artery (IMA)) to the first artery division. Region 2 (*green*) is between regions 1 and 3

lymph node) as well as the irregular outer border (IOB, indistinct demarcation of the lymph node) were evaluated both on reformatted and thin sections (Figs. 2 and 3).

Attenuation values

Attenuation measurements of each lymph node in the portal venous phase and, when available, in the arterial phase were also performed. All density measurements (using HU) were performed by placing as large a region of interest (ROI) as possible (>2 mm^2) on the lymph node in the portal venous phase and in the arterial phase when available. Attenuation values of ≥50 and ≥100 HU in the portal venous phase were separately noted as well as ratio portal venous/arterial phase. Inhomogeneous contrast enhancement as indicative for tumour involvement was separated from either presence of a fatty lymph node hilum or a contrast filled vessel in the vicinity of a lymph node.

Surgery

All patients in the study were operated in an elective setting and according to colorectal surgery praxis. The resection of colon cancer was made by clear lateral margins, resection of the loco-regional lymph node bearing mesentery.

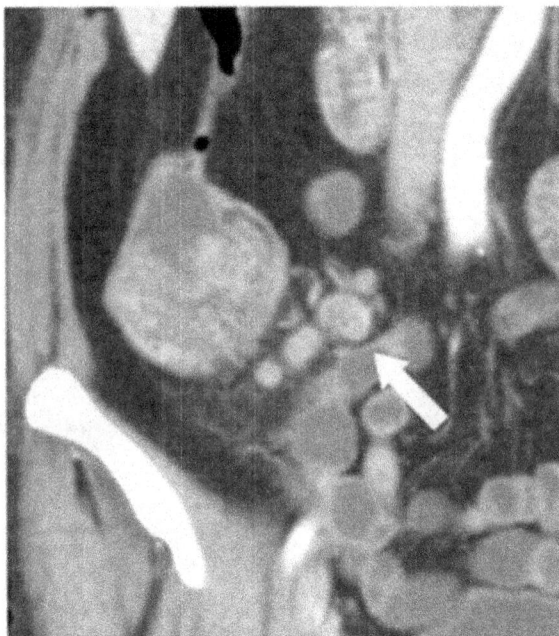

Fig. 2 Coronal reformation (5 mm section post iv contrast portal phase) CT image illustrating the apperance of 10 × 15 mm lymph node (*white arrow*) in region 1 with internal heterogeneity thus well defined borders in a patient with pT3 tumour in the ascending colon. At histopathology, 4 metastatic lymph nodes out of 43 were harvested

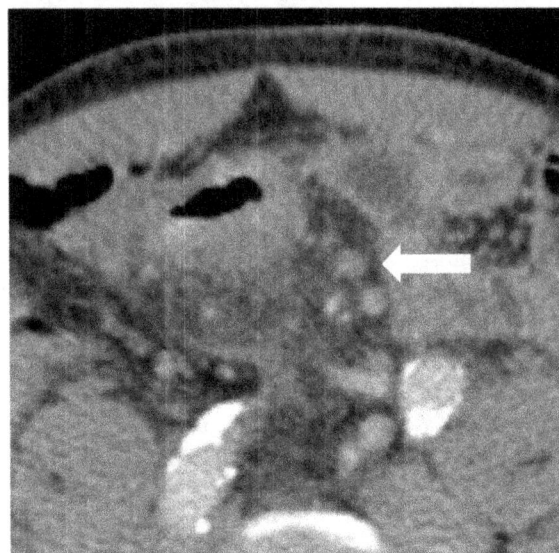

Fig. 3 Transaxial reformation (5 mm section post iv contrast portal phase) CT image illustrating the apperance of a 7 × 7 mm mesocolic lymph node (*white arrow*) in region 2 with irregular outer border and internal heterogeneity in a patient with a pT3 tumour in the sigmoid colon with 1 metastatic lymph nodes out of 16 harvested at histopathology

Histopathology

Histopathology was performed according to standard procedures at the university hospital pathology department by a specialized GI pathologist (initially using TNM version 6 and later TNM version 7) [19, 20]. From the pathologists' original report the T- and N-stage, the total number of harvested and metastatic lymph nodes served as reference standard.

Statistics

Data were evaluated using statistical analysis software SPSS, IBM. Descriptive statistics were applied to the different lymph node characteristics calculating sensitivity, specificity, PPV, NPV and Odds ratio for the prediction of stage III disease. Mann–Whitney U test were used to test significance which was set to $p \leq 0.05$. Univariate and multiple logistic regression analyses were performed for categorical data. Receiver operating characteristics (ROC) and area under the curve (AUC) were used to compare the optimal lymph node size criterion.

Results
Patients and histopathology

The median time interval between pre-operative CT examination and surgery was 28 days (range 4 – 59 days), mean 29 days (standard deviation 13 days).

A total of 2542 lymph nodes were harvested (median 19 lymph nodes/patient, range 4–69) and of those 123 were assessed as metastases (median, 2 lymph nodes/patient, range 1–10). The change from TNM 6 to TNM 7 did not affect the result.

CT evaluation

Number, anatomical distribution, size and size-ratio of lymph nodes

At CT, most of the lymph nodes were located in region 1. Region 2 had higher proportion of lymph nodes ≥4 mm (41%) compared to the other regions (Table 1). The mean number of lymph nodes found was 7.2 for pT1 tumours, 8.6 for pT2 tumours and 11.8 for pT3 tumours (not shown in Table).

Evaluation of lymph nodes

Using size thresholds of ≥4, 5, 6, 7, 8 and 10 mm as criteria for lymph node metastases, the results are presented as a ROC-curve in Fig. 4.

Size ratio with a cutoff point of 0.8 had an overall sensitivity and specificity of 85 and 30% (Table 2). If divided into the three anatomical regions, the sensitivity and specificity were as follows: region 1, 80 and 35%; region 2, 54 and 74% and region 3, 5 and 94%, respectively.

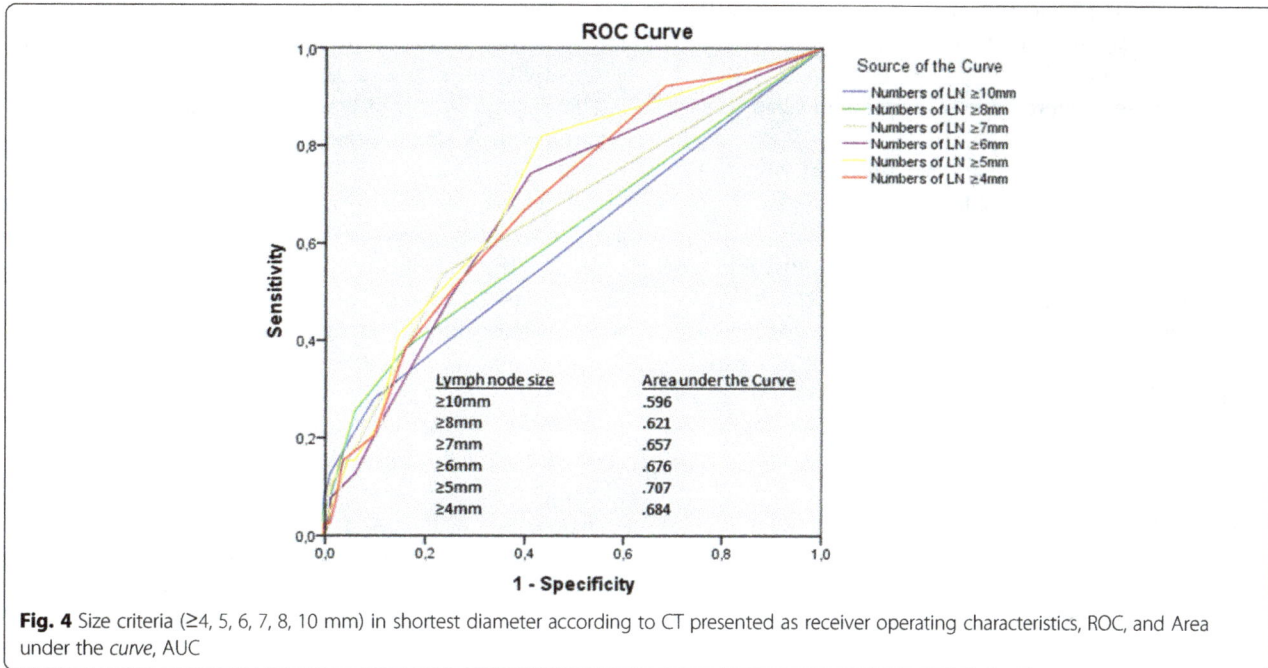

Fig. 4 Size criteria (≥4, 5, 6, 7, 8, 10 mm) in shortest diameter according to CT presented as receiver operating characteristics, ROC, and Area under the *curve*, AUC

Internal heterogeneity and irregular outer border

Forty-four out of 119 patients had at least one (range 1–6) lymph node with internal heterogeneity according to CT and a total number of 94 lymph nodes with this morphological feature were detected. Compared to histopathology, the sensitivity and specificity for predicting stage III disease with this criterion was 79 and 84%, respectively, $p \leq < .001$, OR = 20 (Table 2). If divided by anatomical region, the sensitivity and specificity were as follows: region 1, 64 and 91%; region 2, 51 and 92% and region 3, 3 and 97%, respectively.

Thirty-eight patients had at least one (range 1–8) lymph node with an irregular outer border.

Compared to histopathology, lymph nodes with an irregular outer border showed sensitivity and specificity for prediction of stage III disease of 59 and 81%, respectively, $p \leq < .001$, OR = 6.3 (Table 2). If divided by anatomical region, the sensitivity and specificity were as follows: region 1, 49 and 89%; region 2, 33 and 91%, and region 3, 0 and 99%, respectively.

In patients with at least one lymph node with internal heterogeneity *and* a lymph node with an irregular outer border, regardless of location, the sensitivity and specificity for stage III disease was 54 and 90%, respectively.

Patients with any lymph node showing internal heterogeneity and/or irregular outer borders, meaning that either one of the criteria were present or both in combination, showed an overall sensitivity and specificity for stage III disease of 85 and 75%, respectively, $p \leq < .001$, OR = 16.5 (Table 2).

Contrast enhancement

The overall sensitivity and specificity prediction of stage III disease for lymph nodes having a HU value ≥50 or ≥100

Table 2 Sensitivity, specificity, PPV and NPV (%) for the different CT characteristics of lymph nodes > 4 mm in shortest diameter

Variables	Number	Sensitivity	Specificity	PPV	NPV	OR	p-value
Size ≥5 mm	287	90	31	39	86	1.33	0.002
Size ≥10 mm	29	28	90	58	72	2.67	0.009
Ratio cut off 0.8	244	85	30	37	80	2.36	0.090
Internal heterogeneity (IH)	94	79	84	70	89	20.0	<0.001
Irregular outer border (IOB)	73	59	81	61	82	6.23	<0.001
IH and/or IOB	67	85	75	62	91	16.5	<0.001
HU ≥50	396	95	20	37	89	4.63	0.049
HU ≥100	81	44	68	40	71	1.60	0.239
Cluster of three	14	13	89	36	68	1.16	0.803

Note: *HU* Hounsfield units, *OR* Odds ratio

post contrast in portal venous phase were, 95 and 20%, and 44 and 68%, respectively (Table 2).

Cluster of three or more normal shaped and sized lymph nodes

This criterion resulted in an overall sensitivity of 13% and a specificity of 89% (Table 2).

Combination of different variables using multivariate logistic regression analyses

The strongest predictor for stage III disease in our study was internal heterogeneity. No other variable contributed significantly when the variable internal heterogeneity was included in the multivariate regression model (Fig. 5).

Discussion

To our knowledge, this report is the first to study previously reported criteria for lymph node metastases on CT separately or in comparison as a predictor for stage III disease in colon.

Of all the studied imaging criteria in this study, morphological criteria was superior to size criteria. Internal heterogeneity and irregular outer borders were the two variables that display best, both alone or combined, with reasonable sensitivity and specificity. The combination of internal heterogeneity and/or irregular outer borders still resulted in a moderate sensitivity of 85% and specificity of 75%. The strongest predictor in our study for stage III disease was internal heterogeneity both alone or combined with other variables (Fig. 5). Our results using CT are inferior, but for sensitivity comparable with previous work by Brown et al., which used morphological predictors for mesorectal lymph node status in magnetic

resonance imaging (MRI) of rectal cancer where mixed signal intensity or irregular border resulted in a sensitivity of 85% and specificity of 97% [21].

The majority (64%) of lymph nodes that were detected, regardless of N-stage, were located in region 1, but presence of lymph nodes in this region were not predictive for nodal disease (stage III) ($p = 0.182$). In region 2 there was a slightly higher proportion of lymph nodes in favour of stage III (160 out of 471 lymph nodes (34%)) vs stage II (229 out of 841 lymph nodes (27%)) ($p = 0.006$). In the whole cohort, only 39 patients had lymph nodes in region 3, and there was no difference between the two groups regardless of T-stage. The high specificity in region 3 for the criteria internal homogeneity, irregular outer border and size ratio cut off <0.8 is due to a very limited number of lymph nodes fulfilling those criteria.

In a study, with 106 patients and up to date computed tomography technique using >1 cm and/or cluster of ≥3 lymph nodes as criteria for nodal disease resulted in a sensitivity of 71% and specificity of 41% [22]. In the present study, only 19 patients had lymph nodes ≥10 mm and only 14 patients had lymph nodes in a cluster of three, thus reducing the impact of these criteria for prediction of stage III.

Regarding lymph node size, lymph nodes >5 mm and/or irregular outer border were considered positive for nodal disease in the study by Dighe et al. with sensitivity and specificity of 64 and 53%, respectively [8]. In our study, this criterion showed a similar sensitivity of 56% but a higher specificity of 84%. We have no explanation for this difference.

Size criteria alone can really be questioned and not supported by our study. It has been reported that up to 70% of lymph nodes with metastases in colorectal cancer

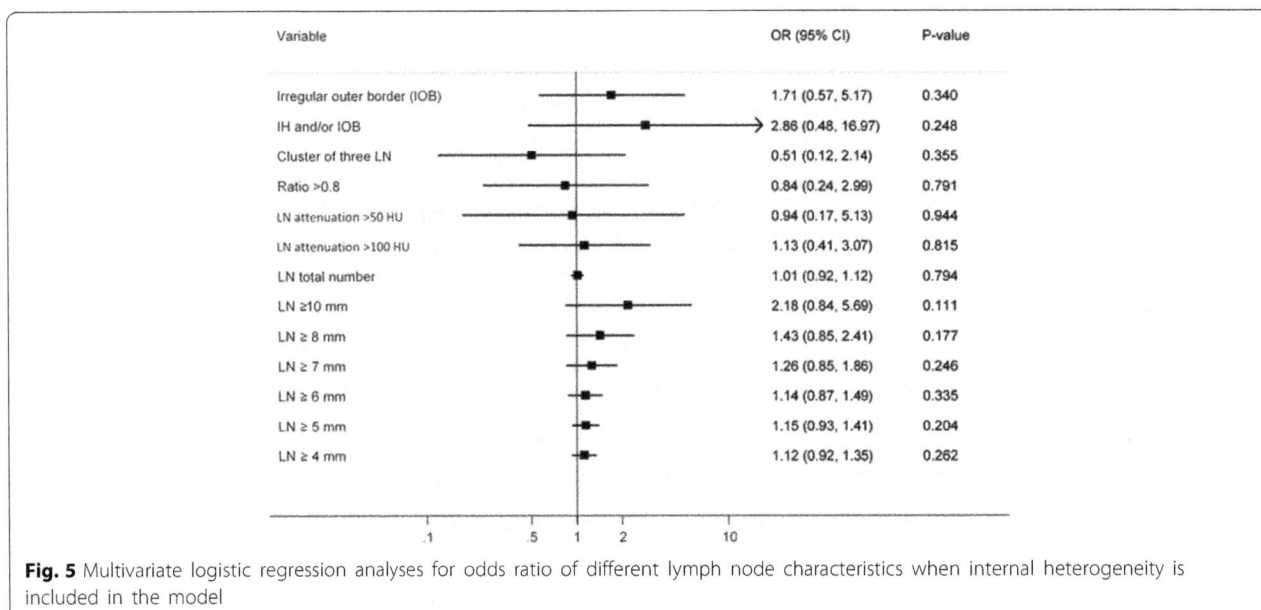

Variable		OR (95% CI)	P-value
Irregular outer border (IOB)		1.71 (0.57, 5.17)	0.340
IH and/or IOB		2.86 (0.48, 16.97)	0.248
Cluster of three LN		0.51 (0.12, 2.14)	0.355
Ratio >0.8		0.84 (0.24, 2.99)	0.791
LN attenuation >50 HU		0.94 (0.17, 5.13)	0.944
LN attenuation >100 HU		1.13 (0.41, 3.07)	0.815
LN total number		1.01 (0.92, 1.12)	0.794
LN ≥10 mm		2.18 (0.84, 5.69)	0.111
LN ≥ 8 mm		1.43 (0.85, 2.41)	0.177
LN ≥ 7 mm		1.26 (0.85, 1.86)	0.246
LN ≥ 6 mm		1.14 (0.87, 1.49)	0.335
LN ≥ 5 mm		1.15 (0.93, 1.41)	0.204
LN ≥ 4 mm		1.12 (0.92, 1.35)	0.262

Fig. 5 Multivariate logistic regression analyses for odds ratio of different lymph node characteristics when internal heterogeneity is included in the model

are ≤5 mm in diameter [23]. The majority of the detected lymph nodes (*n* = 870, 66%) in our study were <4 mm and thus could not be further assessed because of their small size and uncertainty in characterization using CT.

In the study of Kwak et al., a combination of criteria regarding assessment of lymph node metastases, including a cluster of more than three nodes along the loco-regional vascular pedicle, spiculated and indistinct node borders, and a mottled heterogeneous pattern were all integrated in the assessment and together with the size threshold of ≥10 mm reporting a sensitivity and specificity of 87 and 29%, respectively, with CT alone [24]. The specificity was surprisingly low maybe due to the large threshold size. The results with positron emission tomography/computed tomography (PET/CT), with a slightly different setting of defined criteria, did not markedly improve the overall results with a sensitivity and specificity of 66 and 60%, respectively.

Other studies using fluoro-2-deoxy-D-glucose-PET (FDG-PET) reported low sensitivities (29–37%) but higher specificity (87%) for nodal staging, suggesting that PET/CT is of limited additional value in detecting metastatic regional lymph nodes surrounding the primary tumour due to high false negative rate [25, 26]. Some authors argues that routine use of PET/CT can alter or change the management in stage III patients (6.5%) and stage IV patients (12.7%) while other authors claim that it does not [27, 28].

Regarding contrast enhancement/attenuation features, this does not seem to increase diagnostic accuracy. Arterial or portal venous phase attenuation post contrast was not predictive for stage III disease in this study. The differences in attenuation between arterial and portal-venous phase was not predictive for stage III disease.

Furthermore, regarding lymph node size ratio, Kanamoto et al. reported both high sensitivity and specificity of 87 and 80%, respectively, using the criteria of cutoff point of 0.8 or greater in short/long axis diameter ratio measured in the axial plane of the CT images [18]. In this current study the reformatted images were used to measure the true short and long axis and found similar sensitivity (85%) for this criterion but much lower specificity (30%) due to a high rate of false positive findings (70%). Benign lymph nodes can be either oval or rounded, which is a limitation using this criterion.

The use of CT assessed lymph node status alone as predictor of prognosis is still premature. If selection for neoadjuvant chemotherapy was made by the best combination of criteria (heterogeneity and/or irregular border) in this study, 6 patients out of 39 (15%) would potentially be undertreated and 20 patients out of 80 (25%) overtreated. This emphasizes the need to decide on such treatment based on other prognostic factors or use them in combination with the assessed lymph node status.

The strength of this study, beside the use of several imaging criteria for lymph node metastases, is the homogenous patient cohort; all examined with 64-multidetector CT and all having primary surgery allowing histopathology of the resected specimen as reference.

Limitations of the study were the retrospective setting. The assessment by only one observer could reduce the robustness and reproducibility of the imaging criteria. These criteria must be validated in a multi reader setting. There were also a limited number of patients with some of the criteria. Furthermore, the histopathological tissues were not reevaluated and there was no possibility to match individual lymph nodes between imaging and histopathology. Another possible limitation was that we also excluded T4 tumours in the study. We argue that the high rate of lymph node metastases in this group of patients (around 37%) is likely to bias the radiologist when looking on CT and assessing the lymph nodes. No texture analysis software was available at the time of the study. We believe that texture analysis may have a role in the context of characterizing regional lymph nodes on CT in colon cancer although the approach in this setting is rather unexplored and may be subjected to a separate study.

Conclusion

Various imaging criteria for lymph node metastases on CT have been used in previous literature. The results of the present study do not support use of any the commonly used criteria for lymph node metastases. When performing preoperative CT in patients with colon cancer, the imaging criteria that allow the best prediction of stage III disease are either the presence of at least one lymph node with internal heterogeneity or the presence of at least one lymph node with internal heterogeneity and/or irregular outer border. These criteria have to be validated in prospective studies.

Acknowledgements
No acknowledgements.

Funding
Financial support was provided through the regional agreement on medical training and clinical research (ALF) between the Stockholm County Council and Karolinska Institutet.

Authors' contributions
Study concepts and design: ER, MA-N, TH, LB. Performing study: ER, LB. Evaluating exams: ER, LB. Collection of data: ER. Analysis of data: ER, MA-N, TH, LB. Manuscript preparation: ER, LB. Manuscript reviewing and editing: ER, MA-N, TH, LB. All authors read and approved the final manuscript.

Competing interests
The authors declare that they have no competing interests.

Author details

[1]Department of Molecular Medicine and Surgery, Karolinska Institutet, Department of Radiology, Karolinska University Hospital, Solna SE - 171 76, Stockholm, Sweden. [2]Department of Molecular Medicine and Surgery, Karolinska Institutet, Center for Digestive Diseases, Karolinska University Hospital, Stockholm, Sweden.

References

1. Swedish Colorectal Cancer Study Group. National Colon Cancer Report. 2011. http://www.cancercentrum.se/sv/Kvalitetsregister/-Kolorektalcancer/ Rapporter. ISBN 000-91-89048-46-6.
2. Dighe S, Swift I, Brown G. CT staging of colon cancer. Clin Radiol. 2008;63: 1372–9.
3. Derwinger K, Carlsson G, Gustavsson B. A study of lymph node ratio as a prognostic marker in colon cancer. Eur J Surg Oncol. 2008;34:771–5.
4. Ceelen W, Van Nieuwenhove Y, Pattyn P. Prognostic value of the lymph node ratio in stage III colorectal cancer: a systematic review. Ann Surg Oncol. 2010;17:2847–55.
5. Chang YJ, Chang YJ, Chen LJ, Chung KP, Lai MS. Evaluation of lymph nodes in patients with colon cancer undergoing colon resection: a population-based study. World J Surg. 2012;36:1906–14.
6. Smith NJ, Bees N, Barbachano Y, Norman AR, Swift RI, Brown G. Preoperative computed tomography staging of nonmetastatic colon cancer predicts outcome: implications for clinical trials. Br J Cancer. 2007;96:1030–6.
7. Huh JW, Jeong YY, Kim HR, Kim YJ. Prognostic value of preoperative radiological staging assessed by computed tomography in patients with nonmetastatic colon cancer. Ann Oncol. 2012;23:1198–206.
8. Dighe S, Swift I, Magill L, Handley K, Gray R, Quirke P, et al. Accuracy of radiological staging in identifying high-risk colon cancer patients suitable for neoadjuvant chemotherapy: a multicentre experience. Colorectal Dis. 2012;14:438–44.
9. Acunas B, Rozanes I, Acunas G, Celik L, Sayi I, Gokmen E. Preoperative CT staging of colon carcinoma (excluding the recto-sigmoid region). Eur J Radiol. 1990;11:150–3.
10. Burton S, Brown G, Bees N, Norman A, Biedrzycki O, Arnaout A, et al. Accuracy of CT prediction of poor prognostic features in colonic cancer. Br J Radiol. 2008;81:10–9.
11. Zbar AP, Rambarat C, Shenoy RK. Routine preoperative abdominal computed tomography in colon cancer: a utility study. Tech Coloproctol. 2007;11:105–9.
12. Harvey CJ, Amin Z, Hare CM, Gillams AR, Novelli MR, Boulos PB, et al. Helical CT pneumocolon to assess colonic tumors: radiologic-pathologic correlation. AJR Am J Roentgenol. 1998;170:1439–43.
13. Gazelle GS, Gaa J, Saini S, Shellito P. Staging of colon carcinoma using water enema CT. J Comput Assist Tomogr. 1995;19:87–91.
14. Hundt W, Braunschweig R, Reiser M. Evaluation of spiral CT in staging of colon and rectum carcinoma. Eur Radiol. 1999;9:78–84.
15. Leufkens AM, van den Bosch MA, van Leeuwen MS, Siersema PD. Diagnostic accuracy of computed tomography for colon cancer staging: a systematic review. Scand J Gastroenterol. 2011;46:887–94.
16. Anderson EM, Betts M, Slater A. The value of true axial imaging for CT staging of colonic cancer. Eur Radiol. 2011;21:1286–92.
17. Watanabe T, Itabashi M, Shimada Y, Tanaka S, Ito Y, Ajioka Y, et al. Japanese society for cancer of the colon and rectum (JSCCR) guidelines 2010 for the treatment of colorectal cancer. Int J Clin Oncol. 2012;17:1–29.
18. Kanamoto T, Matsuki M, Okuda J, Inada Y, Tatsugami F, Tanikake M, et al. Preoperative evaluation of local invasion and metastatic lymph nodes of colorectal cancer and mesenteric vascular variations using multidetector-row computed tomography before laparoscopic surgery. J Comput Assist Tomogr. 2007;31:831–9.
19. Sobin LH. TNM, sixth edition: new developments in general concepts and rules. Semin Surg Oncol. 2003;21:19–22.
20. Sobin LH, Compton CC. TNM seventh edition: what's new, what's changed: communication from the International Union against cancer and the American Joint Committee on cancer. Cancer. 2010;116:5336–9.
21. Brown G, Richards CJ, Bourne MW, Newcombe RG, Radcliffe AG, Dallimore NS, et al. Morphologic predictors of lymph node status in rectal cancer with use of high-spatial-resolution MR imaging with histopathologic comparison. Radiology. 2003;227:371–7.
22. de Vries FE, da Costa DW, van der Mooren K, van Dorp TA, Vrouenraets BC. The value of pre-operative computed tomography scanning for the assessment of lymph node status in patients with colon cancer. Eur J Surg Oncol. 2014;40:1777–81.
23. Rodriguez-Bigas MA, Maamoun S, Weber TK, Penetrante RB, Blumenson LE, Petrelli NJ. Clinical significance of colorectal cancer: metastases in lymph nodes < 5 mm in size. Ann Surg Oncol. 1996;3:124–30.
24. Kwak JY, Kim JS, Kim HJ, Ha HK, Yu CS, Kim JC. Diagnostic value of FDG-PET/CT for lymph node metastasis of colorectal cancer. World J Surg. 2012; 36:1898–905.
25. Abdel-Nabi H, Doerr RJ, Lamonica DM, Cronin VR, Galantowicz PJ, Carbone GM, et al. Staging of primary colorectal carcinomas with fluorine-18 fluorodeoxyglucose whole-body PET: correlation with histopathologic and CT findings. Radiology. 1998;206:755–60.
26. Furukawa H, Ikuma H, Seki A, Yokoe K, Yuen S, Aramaki T, et al. Positron emission tomography scanning is not superior to whole body multidetector helical computed tomography in the preoperative staging of colorectal cancer. Gut. 2006;55:1007–11.
27. Lee JH, Lee MR. Positron emission tomography/computed tomography in the staging of colon cancer. Ann Coloproctol. 2014;30:23–7.
28. Cipe G, Ergul N, Hasbahceci M, Firat D, Bozkurt S, Memmi N, et al. Routine use of positron-emission tomography/computed tomography for staging of primary colorectal cancer: does it affect clinical management? World J Surg Oncol. 2013;11:49.

7

MRI features of combined hepatocellular-cholangiocarcinoma versus mass forming intrahepatic cholangiocarcinoma

Jennifer Sammon[1], Sandra Fischer[2], Ravi Menezes[1], Hooman Hosseini-Nik[1], Sara Lewis[3], Bachir Taouli[3] and Kartik Jhaveri[1*]

Abstract

Background: Combined hepatocellular-cholangiocarcinoma (cHCC-CC) is a rare primary liver tumor, which has overlapping imaging features with mass forming intra-hepatic cholangiocarcinoma (ICC) and hepatocellular carcinoma (HCC). Previous studies reported imaging features more closely resemble ICC and the aim of our study was to examine the differential MRI features of cHCC-CC and ICC with emphasis on enhancement pattern observations of gadolinium enhanced MRI.

Methods: Institutional review board approval with consent waiver was obtained for this retrospective bi-centric study. Thirty-three patients with pathologically proven cHCC-CC and thirty-eight patients with pathologically proven ICC, who had pre-operative MRI, were identified. MRI images were analyzed for tumor location and size, T1 and T2 signal characteristics, the presence/absence of: cirrhosis, intra-lesional fat, hemorrhage/hemosiderin, scar, capsular retraction, tumor thrombus, biliary dilatation, degree of arterial enhancement, enhancement pattern, pseudocapsule and washout. Associations between MRI features and tumor type were examined using the Fisher's exact and chi-square tests.

Results: Strong arterial phase enhancement and the presence of: washout, washout and progression, intra-lesional fat and hemorrhage were all strongly associated with cHCC-CC ($P < 0.001$). While cHCC-CC had a varied enhancement pattern, the two most common enhancement patterns were peripheral persistent ($n = 6$) and heterogeneous hyperenhancement with washout ($n = 6$), compared to ICC where the most common enhancement patterns were peripheral hypoenhancement with progression ($n = 18$) followed by heterogeneous hypoenhancement with progression ($n = 14$) ($P < 0.001$).

Conclusion: The cHCC-CC enhancement pattern seems to more closely resemble HCC with the degree of arterial hyperenhancement and the presence of washout being valuable in differentiating cHCC-CC from ICC. However the presence of washout and progression, in the same lesion or a predominantly peripheral /rim hyperenhancing mass were also seen as important features that should alert the radiologist to the possibility of a cHCC-CC.

Keywords: Combined hepatocellular-cholangiocarcinoma, Intrahepatic cholangiocarcinoma, Biphenotypic tumor, Liver MRI, Primary liver tumor

* Correspondence: kartik.jhaveri@uhn.ca
[1]Toronto Joint Department of Medical Imaging, University Health Network, Sinai Health System and Women's College Hospitals, University of Toronto, Toronto, Canada
Full list of author information is available at the end of the article

Background

Combined hepatocellular-cholangiocarcinoma (cHCC-CC) is a rare primary liver tumor that expresses both biliary and hepatocellular markers on immunohistochemistry. The WHO reclassified cHCC-CC in 2010 into two subgroups: cHCC-CC classical type and cHCC-CC with stem cell features. These tumors must show unequivocal hepatocellular (HCC) and cholangiocarcinoma (ICC) components which have transition zones, thus differentiating cHCC-CC from collision tumors [1].

As cHCC-CC is a rare tumor, only a few studies have looked at prognosis and management of this tumor, with complete tumor resection and lymph node clearance having the best prognosis. Survival rates post resection appear to be worse than HCC and similar to ICC [2–7], with several studies reporting 5-year survival rates of 16–41.1% for cHCC-CC post-transplant compared to near 70% for HCC patients [8–11]. There are no accepted transplant criteria for cHCC-CC to date, with previous studies reporting poor outcome post liver transplant for patients with presumed HCC who were found to have cHCC-CC on the explant pathology. As patients can proceed to transplant without histology, pre-operative diagnosis of cHCC-CC is important, but remains challenging, as there is both clinical and radiological overlap in these tumors. cHCC-CC can occur in patients with risk factors for HCC and in patients with risk factors for ICC and due to the heterogeneity of the tumor, cHCC-CC can have overlapping imaging features with HCC and ICC. Tumor markers cannot be relied upon to differentiate, as only just over half of patients in one study had elevated Alpha-fetoprotein (AFP) and/or carbohydrate antigen 19.9 (CA19.9) [1].

Previous studies report imaging features of cHCC-CC appear to more closely resemble ICC and metastasis rather than HCC [12–18] and to the best of our knowledge there are only a few studies that have attempted to investigate the MRI features of cHCC-CC [12–15]. We performed a step-wise systematic evaluation of MRI examinations of pathologically proven cHCC-CC versus ICC. The aim of our study was to examine the differential MRI features of cHCC-CC and ICC with emphasis on enhancement pattern observations of gadolinium enhanced MRI.

Methods

Patients

Institutional review board approval with consent waiver was obtained for this retrospective bi-centric study. Pathology databases at both centers were searched for consecutive cHCC-CC/biphenotypic tumors between January 2005 and December 2014 and these results were cross-referenced with radiology databases, excluding any patients who did not have preoperative MRI. Over the same period the pathology and radiology databases were searched for ICC cases.

The patient demographics of the two groups are summarized in Table 1. Thirty-three patients who had pathologically proven cHCC-CC and MRI at baseline were identified. Within this cohort, 25 of the patients were male and 8 were female. The mean age was 59.5 years with an age range of 36–82. Twenty-five patients had chronic liver disease: 16 patients had hepatitis B, 9 patients had hepatitis C, 3 patients had a history of alcohol abuse, 1 patient had hemochromatosis, 1 patient had non-alcoholic steatohepatitis and 1 patient had primary biliary cirrhosis. Two of the patients with histories of alcohol excess were also hepatitis C positive and 1 patient had both hepatitis B and hepatitis C positive serology. Twenty-three (69.7%) of the patients had cirrhosis on imaging, defined as lobar redistribution (hypertrophy of the caudate and left lateral segments, with atrophy of the right lobe and left medial segments) and/or nodular hepatic contour.

AFP was recorded for 29 patients pre-treatment and 8 patients had an AFP > 100 ng/ml, with 5 patients in the cohort having an AFP > 400 ng/ml (range < 5–353,014). Only 7 patients had CA19.9 recorded pre-treatment and 4 of those had elevated CA19.9 (> 37 U/ml), with only one greater than twice the normal limit at 125 U/ml. The remaining patients with a positive CA19.9 ranged from 38 to 49 U/ml.

Forty consecutive patients with pathologically proven ICC with MRI at baseline were identified. Two patients were excluded; one as they did not have dynamic contrast enhanced imaging and the other, as the quality of the study was deemed non-diagnostic. Within this cohort there were a similar amount of male and female patients with 20 males and 18 females. The mean age was 61, with an age range of 32–86. Ten patients had risk factors for liver disease, 7 had hepatitis B and 3 had hepatitis C.

AFP was recorded in 24 patients pre-treatment and no patient had an elevated AFP. CA19.9 was recorded in 26 patients pre-treatment and the median CA19.9 was

Table 1 Patient demographics

Parameter	cHCC-CC	Cholangiocarcinoma
Mean age (range)	59.5 (36–82)	61 (32–86)
Sex (M:F)	25:8	20:18
Median AFP (range)	23.5 ng/ml (< 5–353,014)	2 ng/ml (< 5–15)
Median Ca19.9 (range)	25 U/ml (< 1–49)	16.5 U/ml (< 1–129,207)
Hepatitis B	16	7
Hepatitis C	9	3

16.5 U/ml (range < 1–129,207). Seven patients had a CA19.9 > 37 U/ml.

Image acquisition

MRI examinations were performed at 1.5 T or 3 T ($n = 63$ at 1.5 T and $n = 8$ at 3 T) using a phased array torso coil. MRI protocol included: T2 single shot turbo spin echo with TE 180, axial T2 turbo spin echo with TE 90, axial T1 volumetric interpolated breath-hold (VIBE) opposed-in phase sequences, axial diffusion weighted imaging and axial T1 VIBE pre-contrast and dynamic post-contrast images (Table 2). The majority of the patients (22 cHCC-CC and 38 ICC) received routine extracellular gadolinium based contrast agent gadobutrol (Gadovist, Bayer Healthcare, Berlin, Germany) at a dose of 0.1 mmol/kg at 1 ml/s. Eleven cases in the cHCC-CC group and 3 cases in the ICC group had imaging with hepatocyte specific contrast agent gadoxetic acid (Primovist, Bayer AG, Germany) at a dose of 0.025 mmol/kg at 1 ml/s. At our institution, the primary contrast agent for initial liver imaging is an extracellular based gadolinium contrast agent, and as this is a retrospective study, only the extracellular phases of contrast imaging were analyzed.

Image analysis

Two abdominal radiologists (one abdominal imaging fellow and one faculty with 15 years subspecialty MRI experience) retrospectively reviewed the studies in consensus. Images were reviewed on a picture archive communication system. The following characteristics were evaluated: tumor location and size, T1 and T2 signal characteristics, the presence/absence of: cirrhosis on imaging, intra-lesional fat, hemorrhage/hemosiderin, scar, capsular retraction, tumor thrombus, biliary dilatation, degree of arterial enhancement, enhancement pattern on arterial portal-venous and delayed (5 min) phases, pseudocapsule and washout. T2 intermediate signal intensity was defined as the same signal intensity as the spleen and T2 hyperintense lesions were defined as being of higher signal intensity than the spleen. Capsular retraction was recorded for peripheral tumors, which we defined as being within 1 cm of the liver capsule. The degree of arterial enhancement was defined as being strong if any part of the lesion showed similar enhancement to the aorta, mild to moderate if the enhancement was less than the aorta and absent if there was no arterial enhancement. For the overall enhancement pattern, lesions were characterized as being associated with washout even if there was an area of progressive enhancement in the same lesion as our main aim of this study was comparing cHCC-CC to ICC. Lesions with both washout and progression were captured separately. Lesions were defined as having peripheral enhancement patterns, rather than heterogeneous enhancement patterns, if there was peripheral (< 1 cm depth) enhancement on the arterial or venous phase (in lesions that were hypoenhancing on arterial phase). If there was any central enhancement these lesions were characterized as a heterogeneous enhancement pattern. Evidence of cirrhosis included a lobulated/nodular contour and/or volume redistribution to the left lobe and caudate.

Statistical analysis

Descriptive statistics (frequencies, percentage, mean) were used to summarize demographics, clinical history and MRI features, by tumor type. Associations between MRI features and tumor type were examined using the Fisher's exact and chi-square tests. All tests were two

Table 2 MRI parameters

Image sequence	TR (ms)	TE (ms)	NEX	FOV (mm)	ST (mm)	Gap (mm)	Matrix (phase × frequency)
Pre-contrast imaging:							
Axial T2 HASTE SPAIR	1600	90	1	360	5	1	259 × 320
Axial T2 HASTE SPAIR	1600	180	1	360	5	1	259 × 320
Axial T1 VIBE opp/in	4.43	1.39–2.49	1	360	3	0	218 × 320
ep2d diff b100,600	7600	66	6	380	5	0	156 × 192
T1 VIBE axial SPAIR	4.19	1.47	1	300	3	0	195 × 320
Post-contrast imaging:							
T1 VIBE axial SPAIR dynamic: arterial (care bolus trigger), venous (45–60 s) and interstitial phase (90–120 s)	4.19	1.47	1	300	3	0	195 × 320
T1 VIBE axial SPAIR 5-min delay	4.19	1.47	1	300	3	0	195 × 320
[a]Post-contrast Primovist:							
T1 VIBE axial SPAIR 20 min	4.37	1.47	1	300	4	0	195 × 320
T1 VIBE axial SPAIR 20 min	4.19	1.47	1	300	1.5	0	202 × 320

[a]If hepatocyte specific contrast agent (gadoxetic acid) used

sided, and $p < 0.05$ was considered an indicator of a statistically significant association. Statistical analyses were performed using SPSS software (version 20.0, IBM).

Results

The MRI features of cHCC-CC and ICC are summarized in Table 3. On T1 the majority of the lesions were homogenously hypointense in the cHCC-CC and ICC groups, 23/33 and 30/38 respectively. On T2, the majority of the cHCC-CC group (23/33), had a homogenous intermediate/hyperintense appearance. In the ICC group, 14/38 had heterogeneous signal intensity on T2, 12/38 had homogenous intermediate/hyperintense appearance and peripheral hyperintensity with a central hypointense region was seen in 9/38.

Two patients in the cHCC-CC group had intra-lesional fat and 4 patients in the cHCC-CC group had intra-lesional hemorrhage. No patient in the ICC cohort had intra-lesional fat. One patient in the ICC cohort had evidence of intra-lesional hemorrhage, however this patient had a percutaneous biopsy three days prior to the MRI. Excluding the post biopsy patient in the ICC group, both intra-lesional fat and intra-lesional hemorrhage are highly specific (100%) for cHCC-CC versus ICC, although they have poor sensitivities (6% {95% CI: -2 to 14%} and 12% {95% CI: 1–23%} respectively).

In the cases of peripherally located tumors, 13/21 in the ICC group showed capsular retraction compared to 3/23 in the cHCC-CC group ($P < 0.001$).

The presence of biliary dilatation associated with the mass was seen in 5 of the cHCC-CC group and 23 of the ICC group, P-value of less than 0.001. Portal vein tumor thrombus was seen in 3 of the cHCC-CC group compared to 0 in the ICC group.

The enhancement characteristics of cHCC-CC and ICC are summarized in Table 4. Arterial enhancement was seen in 90.9% ($n = 30$) of the cHCC-CC group compared to 57.9% ($n = 22$) of the ICC group. The degree of arterial enhancement in 15 patients in the cHCC-CC group was similar to the degree of enhancement of the aorta (strong) and in the remaining 15 patients it was less intense (mild to moderate) than the aorta, compared to 1 and 22, respectively in the ICC group ($P < 0.001$; strong arterial enhancement). Peripheral rim enhancement on the arterial phase was seen in 14 cases in both the cHCC-CC group and the ICC group.

With regards to the overall enhancement characteristics of the lesions, the most common enhancement patterns in the cHCC-CC group were peripheral persistent ($n = 6$) (Fig. 1) and heterogeneous hyperenhancement with washout ($n = 6$). The most common enhancement pattern in the ICC group was peripheral hypoenhancement with progression ($n = 18$) followed by heterogeneous hypoenhancement with progression ($n = 14$) (Fig. 2). Combining peripheral hypoenhancement with progression, heterogeneous hypoenhancement with progression and hypoenhancement versus the other subgroups, there was a statistically significant difference between the ICC and cHCC-CC groups. 79% of the patients who had either one of these three enhancement patterns had ICC and 89% of the patients in the other category had cHCC-CC ($P < 0.001$).

Progressive enhancement was seen in 13 of the cHCC-CC group and 33 of the ICC group ($P < 0.001$). Washout was seen in 13 of the cHCC-CC group and in 0 of the ICC group ($P < 0.001$), with a sensitivity of 39% (95% CI: 23–56%) and specificity of 100% in differentiating cHCC-CC from ICC. Both washout and progression were seen in the same tumor in 3 cases in the cHCC-CC group.

Table 3 MRI characteristics of cHCC-CC and ICC

Parameter	cHCC-CC	Cholangiocarcinoma	P-value
T1 WI			
Hypointense	23	30	0.37
Heterogeneous	9	5	0.136
Isointense/not seen	1	3	0.375
T2 WI			
Homogenously intermediate/hyperintense	23	12	0.001
Peripheral hyperintensity and central hypointensity	3	9	0.102
Heterogeneous	7	14	0.15
Isointense/not seen	0	3	0.99
Intralesional fat	2	0	0.124
Intralesional hemorrhage	4	1[a]	0.119
Capsular retraction[b]	3/23 (13%)	13/21 (62%)	< 0.001
Cirrhosis on imaging	23	0	< 0.001
Biliary dilatation	5	23	< 0.001
Tumor thrombus	3	0	0.058

[a]This patient had recently had a percutaneous biopsy
[b]Recorded for lesions within 1 cm of the liver capsule

Table 4 Enhancement characteristics of cHCC-CC and ICC

Parameter	Combined HCC/CC	Cholangiocarcinoma	P value
Degree of arterial enhancement	Strong: 15/33	Strong: 1/38	< 0.001
	Mild: 15/33	Mild: 22/38	0.295
	Hypo: 3/33	Hypo: 15/38	0.003
Peripheral rim arterial enhancement	14 (42%)	14 (37%)	0.631
Progression	13 (39%)	33 (87%)	< 0.001
Washout	13 (39%)	0	< 0.001
Washout and Progression	3 (9%)	0	0.058

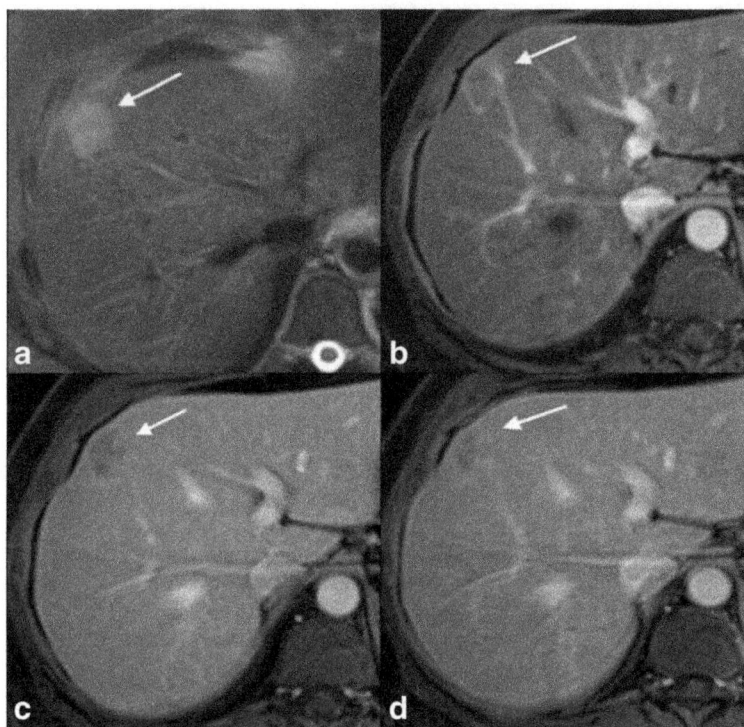

Fig. 1 Pathologically proven cHCC-CC with peripheral persistent enhancement: There is a T2 hyperintense (**a**) lesion in segment 8/4A of the liver, which demonstrates peripheral arterial hyperenhancement (**b**). The enhancement pattern remains peripheral on both the portal venous and delayed phases (**c** & **d**). This enhancement pattern (peripheral persistent) was one of the most common enhancement patterns of cHCC-CC seen in our cohort

Three patients in the cHCC-CC cohort also had a separate mass characteristic of HCC on their MRI. In two of these cases, the cHCC-CC tumors had similar imaging characteristics to the foci of HCC within the same liver, in that they demonstrated arterial hyperenhancement and washout. In one case, the cHCC-CC and HCC were both over 4 cm in diameter and in this case the cHCC-CC was relatively hypovascular compared to the HCC and it did not contain fat, unlike the HCC. The HCC demonstrated washout, but the cHCC-CC did not (Fig. 3). In two other cases, separate 1–2 cm foci of HCC were identified on the explanted liver, but not detected on pre-operative imaging.

Discussion

Few studies have been published evaluating the imaging features of cHCC-CC, with most of the earlier studies using the Allen and Lisa or Goodman classifications, which include collision tumors. As mentioned previously most studies report similar imaging characteristics to ICC [12–19]. However, the enhancement characteristics of cHCC-CC in our study appear to more closely resemble HCC rather than ICC, with 13/33 patients in the cHCC-CC cohort having a typical HCC enhancement

pattern (arterial enhancement and washout). This may be partly explained by the demographics of our population. In our study the prevalence of cirrhosis (69.7%) and positive hepatitis serology (hepatitis B: 48% and hepatitis C: 27%) in the cHCC-CC cohort is greater than previously reported North American studies [14, 20, 21], where patient demographics and the presence of chronic liver disease risk factors resembled those of ICC rather than HCC. However, some of the earlier studies of cHCC-CC are in Asian populations and these studies report demographics, risk factors and survival similar to HCC [1–3, 22–24]. One European study suggests that the risk factors of the cHCC-CC population lie in between the HCC and ICC groups, but continued to report a male predominance [25]. The differences in our group compared to previously published North American studies could be explained by the increasing Asian population in Canada, higher prevalence of chronic liver disease and increasing incidence of liver cancer [26].

There were also other features associated with HCC in the cHCC-CC group: $n = 2$ had intra-lesional fat and $n = 4$ had intra-lesional hemorrhage. While these features are highly specific in differentiating cHCC-CC from ICC, the low sensitivity does not help in differentiating cHCC-CC

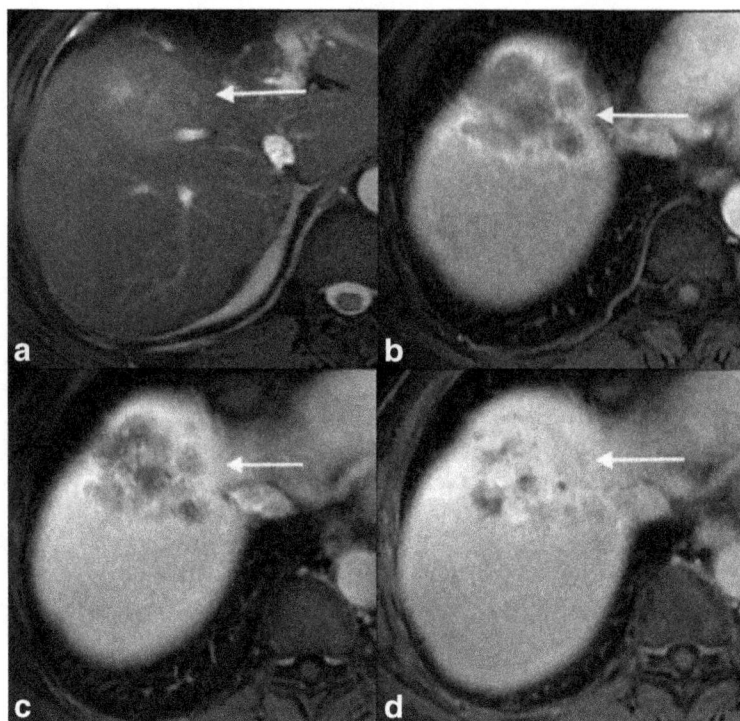

Fig. 2 Pathologically proven cHCC-CC with peripheral progressive enhancement: There is a large mass, which is predominantly intermediate signal on T2-WI (**a**) in segment 8 of the liver. This demonstrates peripheral arterial hyperenhancement (**b**), but then shows progressive enhancement on the portal venous and delayed phases (**c** & **d**) demonstrating enhancement pattern similar to that seen in mass forming ICC

from ICC. In 3 cases of cHCC-CC there was both washout and progression in the same lesion (Fig. 4), which does differentiate cHCC-CC from ICC, as washout is not seen in ICC. These features can be seen in scirrhous HCC, but this should alert the radiologist to the possibility of a cHCC-CC tumor and consideration for biopsy as the potential treatment options for these two tumors vary [27, 28].

Previous studies have reported that tumor markers can be helpful in raising the possibility of a cHCC-CC tumor, where both CA19.9 and AFP can be elevated [4, 14, 29, 30]. In our cHCC-CC cohort, AFP was recorded for 29 patients pre-treatment with 8 patients having an AFP > 100 ng/ml and 7 patients had CA19.9 recorded pre-treatment, with 4 of those patients having an elevated CA19.9. While the midrange elevation of AFP helps differentiate these tumors from ICC, there was only one patient who had a CA19.9 above twice the upper limit of normal. This could partially be due to limited sampling in these patients, as the presumptive diagnosis was HCC in the setting of cirrhosis and cHCC-CC was a post resection/explant or post biopsy diagnosis. With previous studies reporting low to mid-level elevation of CA19.9, it does raise an argument for routine CA19.9 testing in patients who have a liver mass as this would alert

the radiologist to the possible presence of a cHCC-CC tumor and prompt biopsy, to aid in a pre-treatment diagnosis.

Our study has several limitations, including that this is a retrospective study and the readers were aware the cohort comprised of cHCC-CC and ICC, even though specific pathological diagnosis was not known at the time of image review. Our study group is also small, with only 33 patients in the cHCC-CC group, however this is attributable to the rare nature of this tumor. Despite this, our population for MRI is larger than most other published studies. Another limitation is the absence of histological quantification of HCC and ICC components in the cHCC-CC tumors as not all cases went to resection.

Conclusion

Pre-operative imaging diagnosis of cHCC-CC tumors remains a challenge. In our study, cHCC-CC tumors displayed predominant arterial hyperenhancement pattern and the presence of washout, similar to HCC, perhaps due to a population with a high prevalence of HCC risk factors. We found that the presence of washout; washout and progression in the same lesion; intra-lesional fat and intra-lesional hemorrhage help differentiate cHCC-CC from ICC.

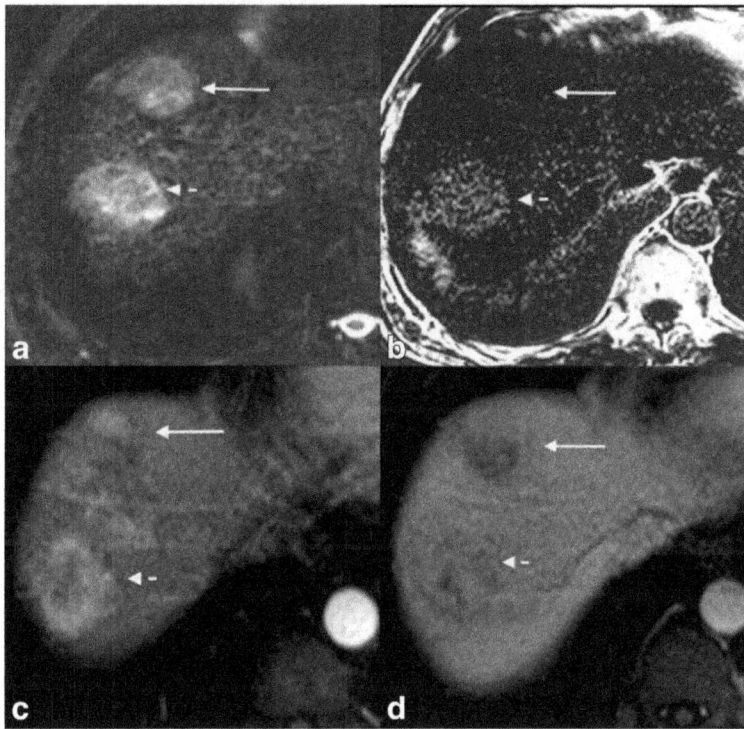

Fig. 3 cHCC-CC (long arrow) and HCC (short dashed arrow) in the same liver; show similar T2-WI imaging characteristics (**a**). However the HCC tumor shows intra-lesional fat on in-opposed phased subtraction image (**b**), arterial phase hyper enhancement (**c**) and washout (**d**) compared to the cHCC-CC tumor, which shows no internal fat (**b**) heterogeneous arterial enhancement (**c**) and no washout (**d**). The presence of two different enhancement patterns in similar sized lesions in the same liver should prompt biopsy to confirm that both are HCC as cHCC-CC can occur in the same liver as HCC given the overlap of risk factors

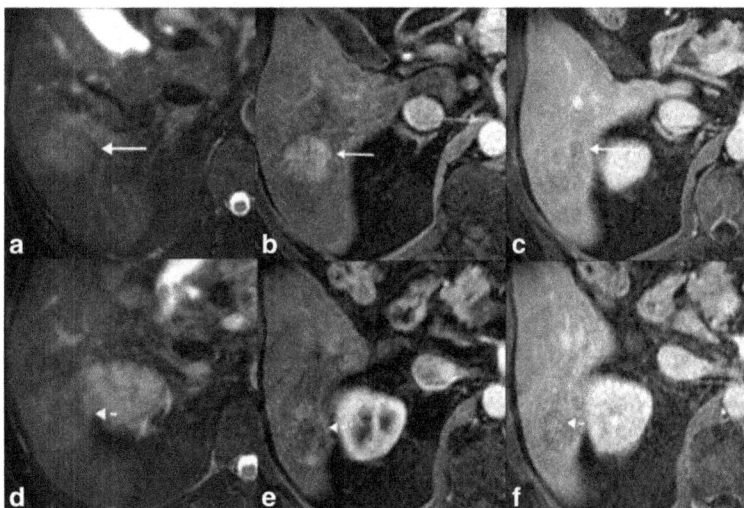

Fig. 4 Pathologically proven cHCC-CC tumor demonstrating both washout and progression: **a-c** is the superior aspect of the tumor and d-f is the more inferior aspect of the tumor. The superior portion of the tumor is T2 intermediate (**a**) and shows show arterial hyperenhancement and washout (**b**, **c**), typical of HCC. However the more inferior component of the tumor has some internal T2 hypointense components (**d**), and relatively hypovascular on the arterial phase (**e**) and shows some progression of enhancement on the delayed phase (**f**). The presence of washout and progression in the same lesion should alert the radiologist to the possibility of a cHCC-CC tumor

Abbreviations
AFP: Alpha-fetoprotein; CA19.9: Carbohydrate antigen 19.9; cHCC-CC: Combined hepatocellular-cholangiocarcinoma; HCC: Hepatocellular carcinoma; ICC: Intra-hepatic cholangiocarcinoma; MRI: Magnetic resonance imaging

Acknowledgements
N/A

Funding
No funding was provided for this study.

Authors' contributions
JS and KJ analyzed and interpreted the images. JS is the primary author. KJ and BT critically reviewed the paper and revised it. HH and SL performed the database search and literary review. HH and SL also contributed to the primary draft of the manuscript. SF did the pathology review and analysis. RM performed the statistical analysis. All authors read and approved the final manuscript.

Competing interests
The authors declare that they have no competing interests.

Author details
[1]Toronto Joint Department of Medical Imaging, University Health Network, Sinai Health System and Women's College Hospitals, University of Toronto, Toronto, Canada. [2]Department of Pathology, University Health Network, University of Toronto, Toronto, Canada. [3]Department of Radiology, Mount Sinai New York, New York, USA.

References
1. Yin X, Zhang B-H, Qiu S-J, Ren Z-G, Zhou J, Chen X-H, et al. Combined hepatocellular carcinoma and cholangiocarcinoma: clinical features, treatment modalities, and prognosis. Ann Surg Oncol. 2012;19(9):2869–76. http://www.springerlink.com/index/10.1245/s10434-012-2328-0.
2. Koh KC, Lee H, Choi MS, Lee JH, Paik SW, Yoo BC, et al. Clinicopathologic features and prognosis of combined hepatocellular cholangiocarcinoma. Am J Surg. 2005;189(1):120–5. http://linkinghub.elsevier.com/retrieve/pii/S0002961004004799.
3. Lee WS, Lee KW, Heo JS, Kim SJ, Choi SH, Kim YI, et al. Comparison of combined hepatocellular and cholangiocarcinoma with hepatocellular carcinoma and intrahepatic cholangiocarcinoma. Surg Today. 2006;36(10):892–7.
4. Kassahun WT, Hauss J. Management of combined hepatocellular and cholangiocarcinoma. Int J Clin Pract. 2008;62(8):1271–8. http://onlinelibrary.wiley.com/doi/10.1111/j.1742-1241.2007.01694.x/abstract.
5. Chi M, Mikhitarian K, Shi C, Goff LW. Management of combined hepatocellular-cholangiocarcinoma: a case report and literature review. Gastroint Cancer Res. 2012;5(6):199–202. http://www.pubmedcentral.nih.gov/articlerender.fcgi?artid=3533848&tool=pmcentrez&rendertype=abstract.
6. Zuo H-Q, Yan L-N, Zeng Y, Yang J-Y, Luo H-Z, Liu J-W, et al. Clinicopathological characteristics of 15 patients with combined hepatocellular carcinoma and cholangiocarcinoma. Hepatobiliary Pancreat Dis Int. 2007;6(2):161–5. http://www.ncbi.nlm.nih.gov/pubmed/17374575.
7. Lee J-H, Chung GE, Yu SJ, Hwang SY, Kim JS, Kim HY, et al. Long-term prognosis of combined hepatocellular and cholangiocarcinoma after curative resection comparison with hepatocellular carcinoma and cholangiocarcinoma. J Clin Gastroenterol. 2011;45(1):69–75. http://www.ncbi.nlm.nih.gov/pubmed/20142755.
8. Garancini M, Goffredo P, Pagni F, Romano F, Roman S, Sosa JA, et al. Combined hepatocellular-cholangiocarcinoma: a population-level analysis of an uncommon primary liver tumor. Liver Transpl. 2014;20(8):952–9. http://www.ncbi.nlm.nih.gov/pubmed/24777610.
9. Sapisochin G, Fidelman N, Roberts JP, Yao FY. Mixed hepatocellular cholangiocarcinoma and intrahepatic cholangiocarcinoma in patients undergoing transplantation for hepatocellular carcinoma. Liver Transpl. 2011;17(8):934–42. http://www.ncbi.nlm.nih.gov/pubmed/21438129.
10. Panjala C, Senecal DL, Bridges MD, Kim GP, Nakhleh RE, Nguyen JHH, et al. The diagnostic conundrum and liver transplantation outcome for combined hepatocellular-cholangiocarcinoma. Am J Transplant. 2010;10(5):1263–7. http://doi.wiley.com/10.1111/j.1600-6143.2010.03062.x.
11. Sapisochin G, de Lope CR, Gastaca M, de Urbina JO, López-Andujar R, Palacios F, et al. Intrahepatic cholangiocarcinoma or mixed hepatocellular-cholangiocarcinoma in patients undergoing liver transplantation: a Spanish matched cohort multicenter study. Ann Surg. 2014;259(5):944–52. http://www.ncbi.nlm.nih.gov/pubmed/24441817.
12. de Campos ROP, Semelka RC, Azevedo RM, Ramalho M, Heredia V, Armao DM, et al. Combined hepatocellular carcinoma-cholangiocarcinoma: report of MR appearance in eleven patients. J Magn Reson Imaging. 2012;36(5):1139–47. http://doi.wiley.com/10.1002/jmri.23754.
13. Hwang J, Kim YK, Park MJ, Lee MH, Kim SH, Lee WJ, et al. Differentiating combined hepatocellular and cholangiocarcinoma from mass-forming intrahepatic cholangiocarcinoma using gadoxetic acid-enhanced MRI. J Magn Reson Imaging. 2012;36(4):881–9.
14. Fowler KJ, Sheybani A, Parke R a., Doherty S, Brunt EM, Chapman WC, et al. Combined hepatocellular and cholangiocarcinoma (biphenotypic) tumors: imaging features and diagnostic accuracy of contrast-enhanced CT and MRI. Am J Roentgenol 2013;201(2):332–339.
15. Potretzke TA, Tan BR, Doyle MB, Brunt EM, Heiken JP, Fowler KJ. Imaging features of biphenotypic primary liver carcinoma (hepatocholangiocarcinoma) and the potential to mimic hepatocellular carcinoma: LI-RADS analysis of CT and MRI features in 61 cases. AJR Am J Roentgenol. 2016;207:1–7.
16. Akoi K, Takayasu K, Kawano T, Muramatsu Y, Moriyama N, Wakao F, et al. Combined hepatocellular carcinoma and cholangiocarcinoma: clinical features and computed tomographic findings. Hepatology. 1993;18(5):1090–5.
17. Jeon T, Kim S, Lee W, Lim H. The value of gadobenate dimeglumine-enhanced hepatobiliary-phase MR imaging for the differentiation of scirrhous hepatocellular carcinoma and cholangiocarcinoma with or without hepatocellular carcinoma. Abdom Imaging. 2010;35(3):337–45. http://resolver.scholarsportal.info/resolve/09428925/v35i0003/337_tvogdhcwowhcxml.
18. Wells ML, Venkatesh SK, Chandan VS, Fidler JL, Fletcher JG, Johnson GB, et al. Biphenotypic hepatic tumors : imaging findings and review of literature. Abdom Imaging. 2015;40(7):2293–305. https://doi.org/10.1007/s00261-015-0433-9.
19. Allen RA, Lisa JR. Combined liver cell and bile duct carcinoma. Am J Pathol. 1949;25:647–55.
20. Jarnagin WR, Weber S, Tickoo SK, Koea JB, Obiekwe S, Fong Y, et al. Combined hepatocellular and cholangiocarcinoma. Cancer. 2002;94(7):2040–6. http://doi.wiley.com/10.1002/cncr.10392.
21. Bhagat V, Javle M, Yu J, Agrawal A, Gibbs JF, Kuvshinoff B, et al. Combined hepatocholangiocarcinoma: case-series and review of literature. Int J Gastrointestinal Cancer. 2006;37(1):27–34.
22. Yano Y, Yamamoto J, Kosuge T, Sakamoto Y, Yamasaki S, Shimada K, et al. Combined hepatocellular and cholangiocarcinoma : a clinicopathologic study of 26 resected cases. Jpn J Clin Oncol. 2003;33(6):283–7.
23. Park HS, Bae JS, Jang KY, Lee JH, Yu HC, Jung JH, et al. Clinicopathologic study on combined hepatocellular carcinoma and cholangiocarcinoma: with emphasis on the intermediate cell morphology. J Korean Med Sci. 2011;26(8):1023. http://synapse.koreamed.org/DOIx.php?id=10.3346/jkms.2011.26.8.1023.
24. Lee SD, Park S-J, Han S-S, Kim SH, Kim Y-K, Lee S-A, et al. Clinicopathological features and prognosis of combined hepatocellular carcinoma and cholangiocarcinoma after surgery. Hepatobiliary Pancreat Dis Int. 2014;13(6):594–601. http://www.hbpdint.com/CN/abstract/abstract4238.shtml.

25. Cazals-hatem D, Rebouissou S, Bioulac-sage P, Bluteau O, Franco D, Belghiti J, et al. Clinical and molecular analysis of combined hepatocellular-cholangiocarcinomas. J Hepatol. 2004;41:292–8.

26. Jiang X, Pan SY, De Groh M, Liu S, Morrison H. Increasing incidence in liver cancer in Canada, 1972–2006: age-period-cohort analysis. J Gastrointest Oncol. 2011;2(4):223–31.

27. Kim SH, Lim HK, Lee WJ, Choi D, Park CK. Scirrhous hepatocellular carcinoma: comparison with usual hepatocellular carcinoma based on CT-pathologic features and long-term results after curative resection. Eur J Radiol. 2009;69(1):123–30. http://www.ejradiology.com/article/S0720048X07004676/fulltext.

28. Chung YE, Park M-S, Park YN, Lee H-J, Seok JY, Yu J-S, et al. Hepatocellular carcinoma variants: radiologic-pathologic correlation. AJR Am J Roentgenol. 2009;193(1):W7–13. http://www.ajronline.org/doi/full/10.2214/AJR.07.3947.

29. Maximin S, Ganeshan DM, Shanbhogue AK, Dighe MK, Yeh MM, Kolokythas O, et al. Current update on combined hepatocellular-cholangiocarcinoma. Eur J Radiol Open. 2014;1:40–8. http://linkinghub.elsevier.com/retrieve/pii/S2352047714000021.

30. O'Connor K, Walsh JC, Schaeffer DF. Combined hepatocellular-cholangiocarcinoma (cHCC-CC): a distinct entity. Ann Hepatol. 2014;13(3):317–22.

8

Incremental diagnostic utility of systematic double-bed SPECT/CT for bone scintigraphy in initial staging of cancer patients

Catherine Guezennec[*] ⓘ, Nathalie Keromnes, Philippe Robin, Ronan Abgral, David Bourhis, Solène Querellou, Romain de Laroche, Alexandra Le Duc-Pennec, Pierre-Yves Salaün and Pierre-Yves Le Roux

Abstract

Background: SPECT/CT has been shown to increase the diagnostic performance of bone scintigraphy for staging of malignancies. A systematic double-bed SPECT/CT of the trunk may allow further improvement. However, this would be balanced by higher dosimetry and longer acquisition time. The objective was to assess the incremental diagnostic utility of a systematic double-bed SPECT/CT acquisition for bone scintigraphy in initial staging of cancer patients, especially compared with the usual approach consisting in a whole body planar scan (WBS) plus one single-bed targeted SPECT/CT.

Methods: One hundred two consecutive patients referred for bone scintigraphy for initial staging of malignancy were analyzed. All patients underwent a double-bed SPECT/CT acquisition of the trunk. Images were interpreted by two nuclear medicine physicians in a 3-step procedure. Firstly, only WBS planar images were used; secondly, one additional single-bed SPECT/CT chosen based on planar images was used; finally, WBS planar and double-bed SPECT/CT images were interpreted. Lesions were classified as benign, equivocal or suspicious for metastasis. A per-lesion, per-anatomical region and per-patient analysis was performed.

Results: In a per-lesion analysis, the number of equivocal and suspicious lesions was 91 and 241 using WBS planar images, 17 and 259 using a single-bed SPECT/CT acquisition and 11 and 269 using double-bed SPECT/CT images, respectively. In a per-patient analysis, the diagnostic conclusion was negative, equivocal or suspicious for malignancy in 35, 53 and 14 patients using WB planar images, 77, 6 and 19 patients using an additional single-bed SPECT/CT and 76, 7 and 19 using double-bed SPECT/CT images, respectively.

Seventeen lesions unseen on WBS images were interpreted as suspicious ($n = 12$) or equivocal ($n = 5$) on double-bed SPECT/CT images. Six lesions unseen on "WBS + targeted single-bed SPECT/CT" were interpreted as suspicious on double-bed SPECT/CT, with no shift in the metastatic status of patients.

Conclusion: A systematic double-bed SPECT/CT acquisition has a limited incremental diagnostic value over an oriented single-bed SPECT/CT in terms of specificity and conclusiveness of bone scintigraphy in the initial staging of cancer patients. However, it slightly improved the sensitivity of the test by detecting unseen lesions on WBS, which may be of value for initial staging of cancer.

Keywords: Bone scintigraphy, SPECT/CT, Staging, Cancer, Bone metastasis

* Correspondence: catherine.guezennec@chu-brest.fr
Service de Médecine Nucléaire, EA3878 (GETBO) IFR 148, CHRU de Brest,
Brest, France

Background

Evaluating the metastatic status in cancer is of utmost importance in order to provide the best patient's management. Bone scintigraphy is currently a reference test in the initial staging of cancer, mainly prostate and breast cancers, to assess the presence of metastatic lesions. The accuracy of staging is a major challenge since the whole patient management may completely change, from a curative and local treatment for local diseases to a palliative treatment for metastatic patients in most cases [1–3].

Bone scintigraphy historically consists in a planar whole-body acquisition (whole-body scintigraphy -WBS), which is quickly acquired and has a large field of view. WBS has been proved to have a high sensitivity in detecting metastasis. However, the tracer uptake not being tumor-specific, its specificity is quite low [4–7]. Technologic innovation of these past 20 years has offered the opportunity to perform SPECT (single photon-emission computed tomography), then SPECT/CT, in addition to the WBS in clinical routine. SPECT has been shown to be more accurate than WBS to distinguish between malignant and benign lesions [8, 9]. SPECT/CT allows an even better characterization of equivocal uptakes on WBS by differentiating metastatic from benign lesions such as degenerative changes, fractures or other benign lesions [10, 11]. As a result, SPECT/CT has been shown to dramatically reduce the proportion of inconclusive results and increase the specificity of bone scintigraphy [5, 12–14]. Therefore, in most of nuclear medicine centers, the usual protocol for staging of bone metastases consists in a whole-body planar acquisition followed, if needed, by a targeted SPECT/CT to characterize suspicious or equivocal uptakes seen on WBS.

There is much less data on the usefulness of SPECT/CT to improve the sensitivity of the test. Some studies reported a slight increase of sensitivity which would be of interest in the setting of initial staging of malignancy [15]. Accordingly, although increasing the acquisition time and the effective dose, a systematic double-bed SPECT/CT of the trunk may be proposed to improve both specificity and conclusiveness but also sensitivity of bone scan in the initial staging of malignancy. Some studies have shown the diagnostic utility of a double-bed SPECT/CT as compared with WBS alone [15]. However, no study has yet compared the diagnostic performance of a systematic double-bed SPECT/CT of the trunk compared to the commonly used "WBS plus one single–bed targeted SPECT/CT" strategy.

The aim of this study was to assess the incremental diagnostic utility of a systematic double-bed SPECT/CT acquisition for bone scintigraphy in initial staging of cancer patients compared with the conventional "WBS plus single-bed targeted SPECT/CT" strategy.

Methods

Patients

Consecutive patients referred for bone scintigraphy for initial staging of biopsy proven malignancy to the nuclear medicine department of Brest University Hospital, France, from February to June 2014, were analyzed. Exclusion criteria included monoclonal gammapathy, patients under 18 years of age, technical issues not allowing a double–bed SPECT/CT acquisition, double-bed SPECT/CT acquisition not centered from the upper cervical spine to the proximal femora. The study was performed in accordance with the Declaration of Helsinki and was approved by the institutional ethics committee (Number 2015, CE26). All patients gave their informed consent.

Image acquisition

Bone scintigraphy systematically consisted in a planar whole-body scintigraphy (WBS) and a double-bed SPECT/CT from the cervical spine to the proximal femora. Images were acquired on Symbia Intevo 6 and Symbia T6 gamma-cameras (Siemens Healthcare, Erlangen, Germany). Both these hybrid systems incorporate a 6-slice X-ray CT scanner, and allow the acquisition of coregistered CT and SPECT images in one session. The acquisition was standard with low-energy high-resolution (LEHR) collimators, energy window 140 keV (+/- 7,5%), WBS was performed approximately 3 h after the intravenous injection of 9 MBq/kg of 99mTc-DPD (99mTc 3,3-diphosphono-1,2-propanedicarboxylic acid - Teceos®, IBA Molecular, Gif-sur-Yvette, France). Planar images were acquired with the following parameters: image matrix 256×1024, scanning speed 32 cm/min post-filtered with OncoFlash (Siemens Medical Solutions, USA). A double-bed SPECT/CT was acquired immediately after WBS from the upper cervical spine to the proximal femora. SPECT images were obtained with the following parameters: 10 secondes per step acquiring 120 projections with 180° rotation for each camera head, on a 128×128 pixel matrix. SPECT data were reconstructed using Flash 3D (Siemens) with ordered subset expectation maximization (OSEM) (8 iterations, 16 subsets and 10 mm Gaussian post filtering). CT imaging consisted in a low-dose technique with the following parameters: modulated tube current intensity (Care4D, 90mAs), 130 kV, total collimation 6x1mm, pitch 1, and was performed on the same anatomical region as the SPECT. The estimated irradiation dose received by the patients was simulated with the CT-Expo v2.1 package.

Image interpretation

Images were interpreted by two nuclear medicine physicians in a 3-step procedure and by consensus. Firstly, only WBS planar images were considered. Secondly, a single-bed SPECT/CT chosen based on planar images was used if WBS demonstrated any equivocal or suspicious uptake. Finally, WBS and double-bed SPECT/CT images were used for interpretation. A per-lesion, a per-anatomical region and a per-patient analysis were performed. Ten different regions were considered: cervical spine, thoracic spine, lumbar spine, pelvis, ribs, sternum, shoulders, skull, femora, other [15]. Each lesion was registered up to a maximum of 10 lesions per anatomical region. At each step, lesions, regions and diagnostic conclusions were classified using a 3-level scale, as negative for malignancy, equivocal or suspicious for metastasis [14].

Results

Patients' characteristics

Between February and June 2014, 104 consecutive patients referred for initial staging of malignancy underwent a planar whole body scintigraphy and a double-bed SPECT/CT of the trunk. Two patients could not be analyzed due to technical problems (one CT and one CT + SPECT lacking in the PACS system). One hundred and two patients were analyzed (male = 79, female = 23, mean age +/- SD = 68,7 +/- 11,5 years). The repartition of cancer was as follows: prostate $n = 67$, breast $n = 17$, lung $n = 6$, bladder $n = 6$, kidney $n = 4$, brain $n = 1$, ovary $n = 1$. The estimated effective dose received by the patients was 10,2 mSv with the double-bed SPECT/CT.

Whole body scintigraphy

Results of WBS interpretation are displayed in Table 1 and Fig. 1. Distribution of suspicious and equivocal regions is shown in Table 2. On WBS planar images, the

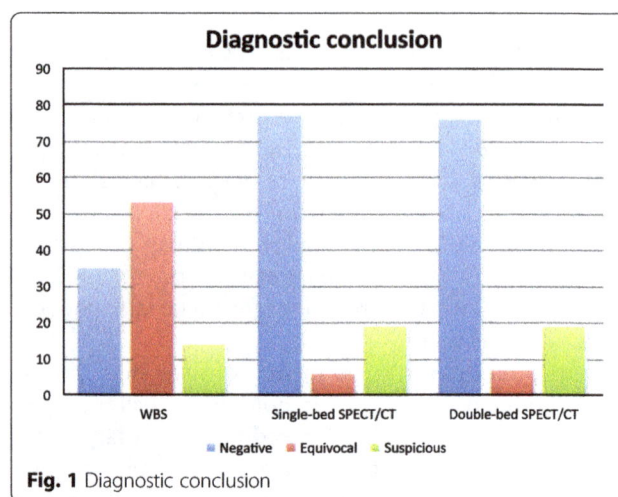

Fig. 1 Diagnostic conclusion

number of equivocal and suspicious lesions was 91 and 250, respectively. The diagnostic conclusion was negative, equivocal or suspicious for malignancy in 35 (34.3%), 53 (52%) and 14 (13.7%) patients, respectively.

WBS + targeted single-bed SPECT/CT strategy

With this strategy, the number of equivocal and suspicious lesions was 17 and 262, respectively; the diagnostic conclusion was negative, equivocal or suspicious for malignancy in 77 (75.5%), 6 (5.9%) and 19 (18.6%) patients, respectively (See Table 1 and Fig. 1).

Comparison between WBS and WBS + one single-bed SPECT/CT interpretations is shown in Table 3. Out of the 91 equivocal uptakes on WBS images, 65 (71.4%) were classified as benign and 13 (14.3%) as suspicious, while only 13 (14.3%) remained equivocal using one additional single-bed SPECT/CT acquisition. Similarly, out of the 53 equivocal diagnostic conclusions on WBS, 39

Table 1 Number and status of lesions, regions, and diagnostic conclusion for each modality

	WBS	Single-bed SPECT/CT	Double-bed SPECT/CT
Lesions			
Suspicious	250	262	265
Equivocal	91	17	18
Regions			
Suspicious	58	64	70
Equivocal	67	10	9
Benign	997	1048	1043
Diagnostic conclusion			
Suspicious	14	19	19
Equivocal	53	6	7
Negative	35	77	76

Table 2 Distribution of suspicious and equivocal regions between anatomical regions

Regions	WBS			Single SPECT/CT			Double-bed SPECT/CT		
	S	E	B	S	E	B	S	E	B
Cervical spine	3	1	98	3	1	98	5	0	97
Thoracic spine	7	11	84	9	2	91	10	1	91
Lumbar spine	7	16	79	8	1	93	8	1	93
Pelvis	9	18	75	8	2	92	10	2	90
Ribs	9	11	82	11	2	89	13	1	88
Sternum	4	2	96	4	0	98	3	1	98
Shoulders	4	2	96	6	0	96	6	1	95
Skull	5	0	97	5	0	97	5	0	97
Femora	6	5	91	7	1	94	7	1	94
Others	4	1	97	3	1	98	3	1	98

S suspicious, *E* equivocal, *B* benign

Table 3 Comparison between WBS and single-bed SPECT/CT

WBS	Single-bed SPECT/CT		
	Suspicious	Equivocal	Benign
Lesions			
Suspicious	243	0	7
Equivocal	13	13	65
Benign	6	4	
Regions			
Suspicious	53	0	5
Equivocal	9	9	49
Benign	2	1	994
Diagnostic conclusion			
Suspicious	11	0	3
Equivocal	8	6	39
Negative	0	0	35

Table 4 Comparison between WBS and double-bed SPECT/CT

WBS	Double-bed SPECT/CT		
	Suspicious	Equivocal	Benign
Lesions			
Suspicious	235	5	10
Equivocal	18	8	65
Benign	12	5	
Regions			
Suspicious	51	2	5
Equivocal	13	5	49
Benign	6	2	989
Diagnostic conclusion			
Suspicious	11	0	3
Equivocal	8	7	38
Negative	0	0	35

(73.6%) were re-classified as negative and 8 (15.1%) as suspicious.

Six lesions unseen on WBS images were interpreted as suspicious on SPECT/CT images. Four additional lesions unseen on WBS were classified as equivocal on SPECT/CT acquisition. None of these 10 new lesions induced a shift in the metastatic status of patients.

WBS + systematic double-bed SPECT/CT strategy

With this strategy, the number of equivocal and suspicious lesions was 18 and 265 respectively; the diagnostic conclusion was negative, equivocal or suspicious for malignancy in 76 (74.5%), 7 (6.9%) and 19 (18.6%) patients, respectively (See Table 1 and Fig. 1).

Comparison with WBS

Comparison between WBS and WBS + systematic double-bed SPECT/CT interpretation is shown in Table 4. Out of the 91 equivocal uptakes on WBS images, 65 (71.4%) were re-classified as benign and 18 (19.8%) as suspicious, while only 8 (8.8%) remained equivocal using a double-bed SPECT/CT acquisition. Similarly, out of the 53 equivocal diagnostic conclusions, 38 (71.7%) were re-classified as negative and 8 (15.1%) as suspicious.

Twelve lesions unseen on WBS images were interpreted as suspicious on double-bed SPECT/CT images. Five additional lesions unseen on WBS were classified as equivocal on double-bed SPECT/CT acquisition.

Comparison with WBS + single-bed SPECT/CT strategy

Comparison between "WBS + single-bed SPECT/CT" and "WBS + double-bed SPECT/CT" interpretation is shown in Table 5. Out of the 17 equivocal uptakes on WBS + single-bed SPECT/CT images, none was re-

classified as benign, 5 (29.4%) as suspicious, and 12 (70.6%) remained equivocal using a double-bed SPECT/CT acquisition. These lesions were found on patients already considered suspicious on both modalities. Out of the 262 suspicious uptakes on WBS + single-bed SPECT/CT, 5 (1.9%) were re-classified as equivocal and 3 (1.1%) as benign, while 254 (97%) remained suspicious.

Six lesions unseen by the "WBS + one single-bed SPECT/CT" strategy were interpreted as suspicious on double-bed SPECT/CT images, corresponding to 4 new suspicious regions. These new lesions did not induce a shift in the metastatic status of patients. The 4 suspicious regions concerned 3 (3%) patients. Two patients had lung cancers with diffuse bone metastases. The third one had prostate cancer with only one suspicious region

Table 5 Comparison between single-bed SPECT/CT and double-bed SPECT/CT

Single-bed SPECT/CT	Double-bed SPECT/CT		
	Suspicious	Equivocal	Benign
Lesions			
Suspicious	254	5	3
Equivocal	5	12	0
Benign	6	1	
Regions			
Suspicious	62	2	0
Equivocal	4	6	0
Benign	4	1	1043
Diagnostic conclusion			
Suspicious	19	0	0
Equivocal	0	6	0
Negative	0	1	76

(lumbar spine) on single-bed SPECT/CT and two more suspicious regions (ribs and shoulders) on double-bed SPECT/CT.

One additional lesion unseen on single-bed SPECT/CT was classified as equivocal on double-bed SPECT/CT acquisition. It induced a change in conclusion diagnostic in one patient with prostate cancer (1%) from benign to equivocal. WBS was interpreted as equivocal, with 2 equivocal lesions on the ribs. Based on single-bed SPECT/CT on the thorax, the 2 lesions on the ribs were re-classified as benign. On the double-bed SPECT/CT, 1 equivocal lesion was found in the iliac bone on the scan inducing an equivocal diagnostic conclusion. A guided biopsy of the equivocal lesion did not show malignancy (See Fig. 2). No patient had a change of diagnostic conclusion to suspicious for malignancy on double-bed SPECT/CT.

Discussion

We evaluated in this study the incremental diagnostic utility of a systematic double-bed SPECT/CT acquisition for the initial staging of cancer patients with bone scintigraphy. Consistent with previous data, adding SPECT/CT to WBS drastically reduced the number of equivocal lesions and diagnostic conclusions in favor of a higher specificity. However, comparing systematic double-bed SPECT/CT with single-bed SPECT/CT strategies, the incremental value was limited in terms of specificity and conclusiveness. On the other hand, a systematic double-bed SPECT/CT increased the sensitivity of bone scan, identifying unseen lesions and reclassifying regions considered benign on the WBS as suspicious on SPECT/CT, with a potential therapeutic impact on patient management.

Adding SPECT/CT to WBS drastically reduced the number of equivocal diagnostic conclusion in favor of a higher specificity of SPECT/CT compared to WBS alone. Indeed, out of the 53 patients with an "equivocal" diagnostic conclusion on WBS, only 7 patients' staging remained "equivocal" with double-bed SPECT/CT. In per-lesion analysis, 71.4% and 19.8% of equivocal uptake on WBS images were reclassified as benign and suspicious, respectively, while only 8.8% remained equivocal. This data is consistent with previous studies [5, 12–14]. In a study from Palmedo et al., 47.3%, 18.7% and 34% of lesions were considered benign, equivocal and suspicious on WBS, and 60.1%, 3.5% and 36.4% with a double-bed SPECT/CT, also showing a higher shift from equivocal to benign than to suspicious lesions [15]. In another publication from Heylar et al., out of equivocal lesions seen on WBS, 68% were reclassified as benign, 24% as suspicious and 8% remained equivocal [16]. Our data confirms the increase in specificity when adding SPECT/CT to WBS.

In terms of specificity and conclusiveness, the impact of a systematic double-bed SPECT/CT acquisition

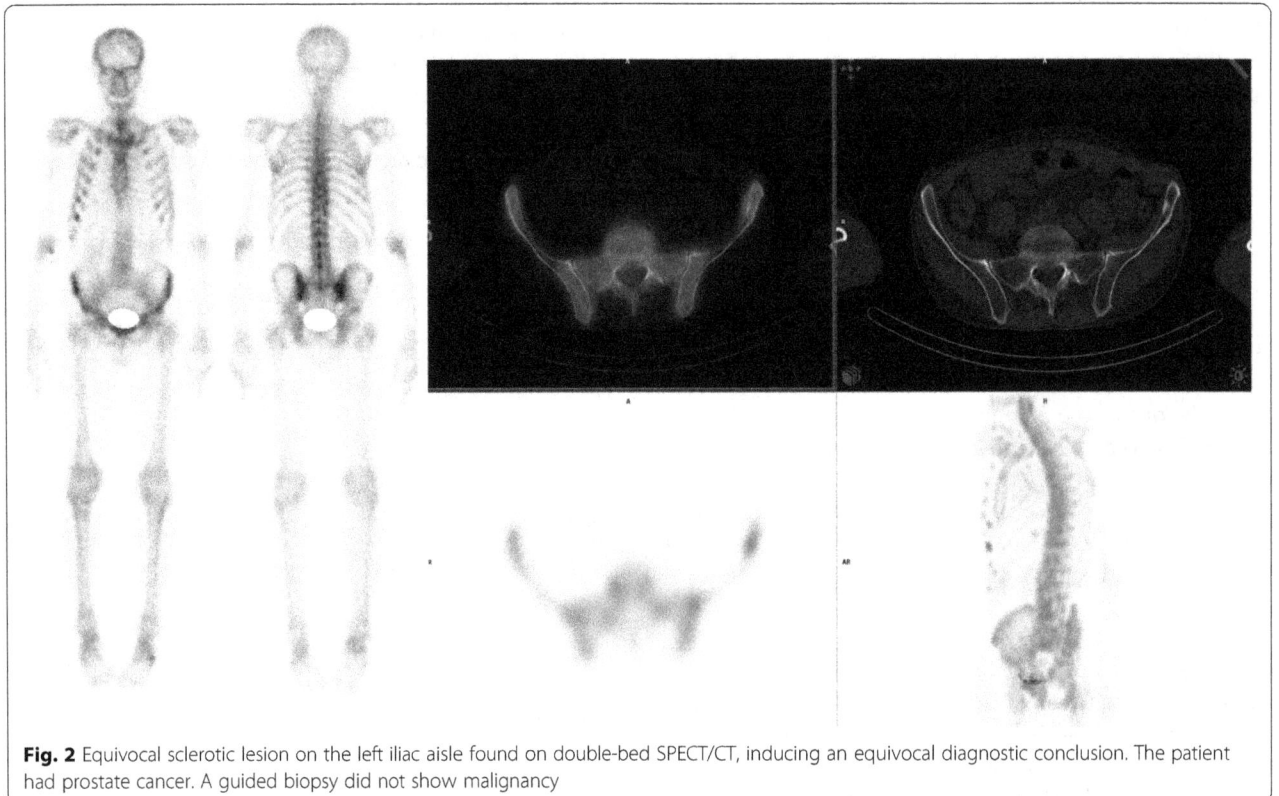

Fig. 2 Equivocal sclerotic lesion on the left iliac aisle found on double-bed SPECT/CT, inducing an equivocal diagnostic conclusion. The patient had prostate cancer. A guided biopsy did not show malignancy

compared to a single-bed SPECT/CT acquisition was limited. Indeed, there was no change in the proportion of equivocal and suspicious lesions (6.4% and 6.1%, respectively) or regions (93.6% and 93.9%, respectively). Nevertheless, the impact was not trivial as 5 equivocal lesions were re-classified as suspicious and conversely 5 suspicious lesions were downstaged as equivocal on double-bed SPECT/CT.

The ability of SPECT/CT to improve bone scan sensitivity is more controversial. Palmedo et al. reported in a large series a slight impact in breast cancer but not in prostate cancer [15]. In our study, we found an increase in sensitivity when adding a double-bed SPECT/CT. Overall, SPECT/CT detected 12 suspicious and 5 equivocal lesions unseen on WBS in 5 and 3 patients, respectively. Moreover there was also a slight increase in sensitivity when comparing WBS + single-bed SPECT/CT with WBS + double-bed SPECT/CT. Indeed, double-bed SPECT/CT detected 6 suspicious and 1 equivocal lesions in 4 and 1 patients respectively, when compared with single-bed SPECT/CT. The 6 suspicious lesions concerned 4 new suspicious regions in 3 (3%) patients. This increased sensitivity appears relevant in the setting of initial staging of cancer.

In our series, the impact on patient's management was however limited. There was only one change in diagnostic conclusion using the double-bed SPECT strategy as compared with the single-bed SPECT strategy. No patient was upstaged to suspicious for metastasis. The only change in diagnostic conclusion, from benign to equivocal, concerned a patient with prostate cancer. On double-bed SPECT/CT, there was a slight uptake in the iliac bone on an equivocal morphologic lesion. However, a guided biopsy did not show malignancy (Fig. 2). Three patients had the same diagnostic conclusion (evidence of bone metastases) but had additional lesions on double-bed SPECT/CT images not seen on WBS. Out of them, 2 had lung cancers with diffuse bone metastases, with no therapeutic consequences. The third one had prostate cancer with one isolated suspicious region (lumbar spine) on single-bed SPECT/CT and two additional suspicious regions (ribs and shoulders) on double-bed SPECT/CT. In this patient, this increase in sensitivity could potentially have a therapeutic impact, especially with the development of radiotherapy with curative aim for oligometastatic disease [17]. Oligometastatic disease concerns patients with 1 to 5 suspicious lesions [18]. In our study, we found no shift from oligometastatic to multi-metastatic status or from multi-metastatic to oligometatastic status. Indeed, amongst the patients with an oligometastatic status, when analyzing new suspicious lesions on double-bed SPECT/CT, 4 patients initially oligometastatic with respectively 1, 1, 1 and 4 suspicious lesions remained oligometastatic on double-bed SPECT/

CT with respectively 3 (2 new suspicious lesions overlooked on WBS + single-bed SPECT/CT), 2, 2 and 5 (1 equivocal lesion becoming suspicious for these last 3 patients). On the other hand, when analyzing the lesion shifts from suspicious to equivocal or benign, they all concerned the same patient who had prostate cancer with diffuse bone metastases. However, depending on the location of the metastasis or the symptoms associated with them, the increased sensitivity may also support a palliative treatment such as analgesic radiotherapy. Moreover this more precise characterization of the number and location of suspicious lesions on double-bed SPECT/CT may also better evaluate the therapeutic response to chemotherapy, hormonotherapy or internal radiotherapy treatment.

In terms of radiation exposure, a systematic double SPECT/CT acquisition induces an approximately 5 mSv increase of the effective dose. Indeed the estimated effective dose received by the patients was 10,2 mSv for a double-bed SPECT/CT versus 4,7 mSv for a single-bed SPECT/CT (abdomen). In addition, a systematic double-bed SPECT/CT is approximately 13 min longer compared to a single-bed SPECT/CT. These inconveniences appear acceptable in the setting of staging of cancer, if a double-bed SPECT/CT increases the sensitivity of the test and prevents further other irradiating examinations to specify undetermined lesions.

In these past 10 years, instrumentation of gamma cameras has evolved a lot, in terms of physics properties and reconstruction methods, resulting in an improved sensitivity. In our study, we used Flash 3D reconstruction method. In parallel, with the development of PET/CT, 18-F FNa PET/CT has been adopted in some centres as an alternative to bone scintigraphy in the detection of bone metastases, with a high sensitivity and specificity, and was showed to outperform SPECT/CT in several studies [5].

There are limitations in our study that deserve further discussion. Firstly, we included consecutive patients referred for initial staging of cancer whatever the type of cancer. The impact of a double-bed SPECT/CT may be different according to the primary. Nevertheless, this approach reflects the usual activity of a nuclear medicine department proposing the same protocol for all cancer patients. Secondly, the scale of our study was limited with a small number of patients. Larger studies including more patients would help further analyzing the impact on diagnostic conclusion of a systematic double SPECT/CT with an inter-observer reproducibility analysis. Thirdly, the targeted SPECT/CT strategy could also consist in a targeted double-bed SPECT/CT when needed, depending on the lesions seen on WBS. However, in our study, the main interest of a systematic double-bed SPECT/CT was to detect unseen lesions of

WBS. Acquiring single or double SPECT/CT acquisitions on the base of WBS interpretation would not increase the sensitivity of the test. Moreover, some studies proposed a multi-bed SPECT/CT [19]. In our study, the double-bed SPECT/CT was only performed from the cervical spine to proximal femora, and did not include the lower limbs and the skull. However, metastatic lesions of extremities were previously found to be very rare without an axial extension [15, 20, 21]. Finally, in our study, the scanning speed when acquiring WBS was 32 cm/min, quite fast when compared with previous studies. Yet, we used a post-treatment denoising step using a Pixon method, Oncoflash. This method produces an image equivalent to the one deriving from an acquisition half as fast, thus in our case at a scanning speed of 16 cm/min, which is average when compared with other studies [22].

Conclusions

A systematic double-bed SPECT/CT acquisition has a limited incremental diagnostic value over an oriented single-bed SPECT/CT in terms of specificity and conclusiveness of bone scintigraphy in the initial staging of cancer patients. However, it slightly improves the sensitivity of the test by detecting unseen lesions on WBS, which may be of value for initial staging of cancer.

Abbreviations
SPECT/CT: Single-Photon Emission Computed Tomography/Computed Tomography; WBS: Whole-body scintigraphy

Aknowledgements
Not applicable.

Funding
Not applicable.

Authors' contributions
CG, NK, PR, RA, SQ, PYS, PYLR contributed to designing the study. CG, DB, RDL contributed to managing imaging procedures. CG, NK contributed to interpreting images. CG, NK, PR, AP, PYS, PYLR contributed to analyzing the data. All authors contributed to writing the manuscript. All authors read and approved the final manuscript.

Authors' information
Not applicable.

Competing interests
The authors declare that they have no competing interests.

Endnotes
Not applicable.

References

1. Heidenreich A, Bastian PJ, Bellmunt J, Bolla M, Joniau S, van der Kwast T, et al. EAU guidelines on prostate cancer. part 1: screening, diagnosis, and local treatment with curative intent-update 2013. Eur Urol. 2014;65(1):124–37.
2. Heidenreich A, Bastian PJ, Bellmunt J, Bolla M, Joniau S, van der Kwast T, et al. EAU guidelines on prostate cancer. Part II: treatment of advanced, relapsing, and castration-resistant prostate cancer. Eur Urol. 2014;65(2):467–79.
3. Senkus E, Kyriakides S, Ohno S, Penault-Llorca F, Poortmans P, Rutgers E, et al. Primary breast cancer: ESMO clinical practice guidelines for diagnosis, treatment and follow-up. Ann Oncol Off J Eur Soc Med Oncol. 2015;26 Suppl 5:v8–v30.
4. Even-Sapir E, Metser U, Mishani E, Lievshitz G, Lerman H, Leibovitch I. The detection of bone metastases in patients with high-risk prostate cancer: 99mTc-MDP Planar bone scintigraphy, single- and multi-field-of-view SPECT, 18 F-fluoride PET, and 18 F-fluoride PET/CT. J Nucl Med Off Publ Soc Nucl Med. 2006;47(2):287–97.
5. Jambor I, Kuisma A, Ramadan S, Huovinen R, Sandell M, Kajander S, et al. Prospective evaluation of planar bone scintigraphy, SPECT, SPECT/CT, (18)F-NaF PET/CT and whole body 1.5 T MRI, including DWI, for the detection of bone metastases in high risk breast and prostate cancer patients: SKELETA clinical trial. Acta Oncol Stockh Swed. 2016;55(1):59–67.
6. Shen G, Deng H, Hu S, Jia Z. Comparison of choline-PET/CT, MRI, SPECT, and bone scintigraphy in the diagnosis of bone metastases in patients with prostate cancer: a meta-analysis. Skeletal Radiol. 2014;43(11):1503–13.
7. Thuraiaja R, McFarlane J, Traill Z, Persad R. State-of-the-art approaches to detecting early bone metastasis in prostate cancer. BJU Int. 2004;94(3):268–71.
8. Keidar Z, Israel O, Krausz Y. SPECT/CT in tumor imaging: technical aspects and clinical applications. Semin Nucl Med. 2003;33(3):205–18.
9. Schirrmeister H, Glatting G, Hetzel J, Nüssle K, Arslandemir C, Buck AK, et al. Prospective evaluation of the clinical value of planar bone scans, SPECT, and (18)F-labeled NaF PET in newly diagnosed lung cancer. J Nucl Med Off Publ Soc Nucl Med. 2001;42(12):1800–4.
10. Nozaki T, Yasuda K, Akashi T, Fuse H. Usefulness of single photon emission computed tomography imaging in the detection of lumbar vertebral metastases from prostate cancer. Int J Urol Off J Jpn Urol Assoc. 2008;15(6):516–9.
11. Even-Sapir E, Keidar Z, Bar-Shalom R. Hybrid imaging (SPECT/CT and PET/CT)–improving the diagnostic accuracy of functional/metabolic and anatomic imaging. Semin Nucl Med. 2009;39(4):264–75.
12. Utsunomiya D, Shiraishi S, Imuta M, Tomiguchi S, Kawanaka K, Morishita S, et al. Added value of SPECT/CT fusion in assessing suspected bone metastasis: comparison with scintigraphy alone and nonfused scintigraphy and CT. Radiology. 2006;238(1):264–71.
13. Strobel K, Burger C, Seifert B, Husarik DB, Soyka JD, Hany TF. Characterization of focal bone lesions in the axial skeleton: performance of planar bone scintigraphy compared with SPECT and SPECT fused with CT. AJR Am J Roentgenol. 2007;188(5):W467–74.
14. Römer W, Nömayr A, Uder M, Bautz W, Kuwert T. SPECT-guided CT for evaluating foci of increased bone metabolism classified as indeterminate on SPECT in cancer patients. J Nucl Med Off Publ Soc Nucl Med. 2006;47(7):1102–6.
15. Palmedo H, Marx C, Ebert A, Kreft B, Ko Y, Türler A, et al. Whole-body SPECT/CT for bone scintigraphy: diagnostic value and effect on patient management in oncological patients. Eur J Nucl Med Mol Imaging. 2014;41(1):59–67.
16. Helyar V, Mohan HK, Barwick T, Livieratos L, Gnanasegaran G, Clarke SEM, et al. The added value of multislice SPECT/CT in patients with equivocal bony metastasis from carcinoma of the prostate. Eur J Nucl Med Mol Imaging. 2010;37(4):706–13.
17. Palacios-Eito A, García-Cabezas S. Oligometastatic disease, the curative challenge in radiation oncology. World J Clin Oncol. 2015;6(4):30–4.
18. Palma DA, Salama JK, Lo SS, Senan S, Treasure T, Govindan R, et al. The oligometastatic state - separating truth from wishful thinking. Nat Rev Clin Oncol. 2014;11(9):549–57.
19. Giovanella L, Castellani M, Suriano S, Ruberto T, Ceriani L, Tagliabue L, et al. Multi-field-of-view SPECT is superior to whole-body scanning for assessing metastatic bone disease in patients with prostate cancer. Tumori. 2011;97(5):629–33.
20. Libson E, Bloom RA, Husband JE, Stoker DJ. Metastatic tumours of bones of the hand and foot. A comparative review and report of 43 additional cases. Skeletal Radiol. 1987;16(5):387–92.
21. Muller N, Didon-Poncelet A, Rust E. Evaluation de la stratégie optimale d'imagerie osseuse scintigraphique dans le bilan d'extension initial des patients avec un adénocarcinome prostatique à risque métastatique intermédiaire ou élevé. Médecine Nucl. 2016;40(4):315–28.
22. Wesolowski CA, Yahil A, Puetter RC, Babyn PS, Gilday DL, Khan MZ. Improved lesion detection from spatially adaptive, minimally complex, Pixon reconstruction of planar scintigraphic images. Comput Med Imaging Graph Off J Comput Med Imaging Soc. 2005;29(1):65–81.

9

Imaging features of fibrolamellar hepatocellular carcinoma in gadoxetic acid-enhanced MRI

Viktoria Palm[1], Ruofan Sheng[2], Philipp Mayer[1,3], Karl-Heinz Weiss[4,3], Christoph Springfeld[5,3], Arianeb Mehrabi[6,3], Thomas Longerich[7,3], Anne Katrin Berger[5], Hans-Ulrich Kauczor[1,3] and Tim Frederik Weber[1,3]*

Abstract

Background: Fibrolamellar hepatocellular carcinoma (FLC) is a rare malignancy occurring in young patients without cirrhosis. Objectives of our study were to analyze contrast material uptake in hepatobiliary phase imaging (HBP) in gadoxetic acid-enhanced liver MRI in patients with FLC and to characterize imaging features in sequence techniques other than HBP.

Methods: In this retrospective study on histology-proven FLC, contrast material uptake in HBP was quantitatively assessed by calculating the corrected FLC enhancement index (CEI) using mean signal intensities of FLC and lumbar muscle on pre-contrast imaging and HBP, respectively. Moreover, enhancement patterns in dynamic contrast-enhanced MRI and relative signal intensities compared with background liver parenchyma were determined by two radiologists in consensus for HBP, diffusion-weighted imaging using high b-values (DWI), and T2 and T1 weighted pre-contrast imaging.

Results: In 6 of 13 patients with FLC gadoxetic acid-enhanced liver MRI was available. The CEI suggested presence of HBP contrast material uptake in all FLCs. A mean CEI of 1.35 indicated FLC signal increase of 35% in HBP compared with pre-contrast imaging. All FLCs were hypointense in HBP compared with background liver parenchyma. Three of 6 FLCs had arterial hyperenhancement and venous wash-out. In DWI and T2 weighted imaging, 5 of 6 FLCs were hyperintense. In T1 weighted imaging, 5 of 6 FLCs were hypointense.

Conclusion: Hepatobiliary uptake of gadoxetic acid was quantitatively measurable in all FLCs investigated in our study. The observation of hypointensity of FLCs in HBP compared with background liver parenchyma emphasizes the role of gadoxetic acid-enhanced liver MRI for non-invasive diagnosis of FLC and its importance in the diagnostic work-up of indeterminate liver lesions.

Keywords: Diagnostic imaging, Magnetic resonance imaging, Liver neoplasms, Contrast media, Delayed diagnosis

Background

Fibrolamellar hepatocellular carcinoma (FLC) is a very rare form of primary hepatic cancer accounting for approximately 5% of all hepatocellular carcinomas (HCCs) [1]. FLCs are composed of well-differentiated neoplastic hepatocytes surrounded by fibrous bands often arranged in lamellar distribution [2]. The molecular basis for the difference between conventional HCC and FLC has recently been elucidated: a translocation resulting in a fusion transcript of the DNAJB1- and PRKACA-genes can be found in all patients with FLC, but not in other forms of liver cancer [3, 4]. Aside from these specific histologic and molecular properties, FLC has decisive clinical features that differ from conventional HCC: FLC develops preferably de novo in the non-cirrhotic liver of young patients without history of chronic liver disease.

From a radiologists' point of view, it is of utmost importance to distinguish FLC from focal nodular hyperplasia (FNH). FNH is a hepatic tumor that is observed in

* Correspondence: tim.weber@med.uni-heidelberg.de
[1]Department of Diagnostic and Interventional Radiology, Heidelberg University Hospital, INF 110, 69120 Heidelberg, Germany
[3]Liver Cancer Center Heidelberg, Heidelberg University Hospital, INF 224, 69120 Heidelberg, Germany
Full list of author information is available at the end of the article

young patients without chronic liver disease as well, but is always benign, has no potential for malignant transformation and requires no specific therapy. Radiologic discrimination between FLC and FNH can be challenging in magnetic resonance imaging (MRI) because FLC and FNH share important imaging features in pre-contrast and post-contrast scans using conventional extracellular gadolinium-based contrast agents [5–7]. Overlapping imaging features include the presence of a central scar and hypervascularity in arterial phase post-contrast scans. Considering MRI after injection of gadoxetic acid as a liver-specific contrast agent eliminated significantly via the biliary system (Primovist or Eovist; Bayer Vital, Leverkusen, Germany), it is well known that FNH typically shows enhancement during hepatobiliary phase imaging due to hepatocellular uptake of contrast material [8]. To our knowledge, there are incomplete data investigating the behavior of FLC on MRI using liver-specific contrast material.

Primary objective of this study was to investigate presence of enhancement of FLC in post-contrast hepatobiliary phase MRI. Secondary objectives of this study were to describe general imaging features of FLC including morphology and distribution, relative signal intensities in conventional sequence techniques other than post-contrast hepatobiliary phase MRI and presence of accompanying findings.

Methods
Study design and study population
This analysis was a retrospective single-center exploratory study on patients that have been identified by chart review of prospectively generated institutional research databases. Approval by the local institutional review board was available. Requirements for inclusion were (1) histology-proven FLC, (2) age ≥ 18 years, and (3) availability of gadoxetic acid-enhanced MRI. If patients had undergone local minimally invasive interventions (i.e. transarterial chemoembolisation [TACE]) prior to gadoxetic acid-enhanced MRI, only viable FLC components were considered. Clinical data were reported via an electronic medical record by the attending oncologists and medical staff. Information included time to FLC diagnosis, primary differential diagnoses on prior imaging studies other than gadoxetic acid-enhanced MRI, and clinical evidence of chronic liver disease. Time to FLC diagnosis was defined as the time period between initial evidence of a hepatic mass and histological diagnosis of malignancy.

Image analysis
The following sequence techniques covering the liver parenchyma were intended to be included: T2-weighted images without fat saturation (T2wi), pre-contrast T1-weighted images with and without fat-saturation (T1wi), high b-value diffusion weighted images (DWI), and hepatic

arterial phase (HAP), portal venous phase (PVP), and hepatobiliary phase (HBP) post-contrast T1-weighted images with fat saturation.

A consensus review of all images was performed by two radiologists. For each imaging sequence, the predominant signal intensities and their homogeneity were visually graded as hyperintense, hypointense, or isointense compared with background liver parenchyma. For quantitative assessment of FLC enhancement, the corrected enhancement index (CEI) was determined for each FLC according to an approach published by Watanabe et al. for hepatobiliary phase liver parenchyma enhancement using the following formula [9]:

$$\text{CEI} = (\text{SI liver HBP}/\text{SI muscle HBP})/(\text{SI liver PRE}/\text{SI muscle PRE}),$$

where "SI liver HBP" is the FLC signal intensity in HBP, "SI muscle HBP" is the lumbar muscle signal intensity in HBP, "SI liver PRE" is the FLC signal intensity in pre-contrast T1wi with fat saturation, and "SI muscle PRE" is the lumbar muscle signal intensity in pre-contrast T1wi with fat saturation. Signal intensities were assessed using region of interest (ROI) analyses. Ellipsoid ROIs were drawn on representative areas of viable FLC and lumbar muscle on the same slice. Liver and muscle ROIs, respectively, were equivalent concerning size and location for both pre-contrast imaging and HBP. Each measurement was performed three times, and the mean signal intensity was used for CEI calculation.

Predominant enhancement patterns from HAP to PV compared with background liver parenchyma were assigned to either APHE/WO pattern (arterial phase hyperenhancement followed by portal venous hypoenhancement), non-APHE/WO pattern.

Accompanying findings including presence of intralesional necrosis or hemorrhage, bile duct dilatation, bile duct tumor thrombosis, and portal vein tumor thrombosis were analyzed. Presence of intralesional necrosis or hemorrhage was only considered evaluable in patients that had no history of TACE.

Results
Patients
Of a total of 13 FLC patients, 6 patients were identified meeting our inclusion criteria. Clinical information on these 6 study patients is summarized in Table 1. Median age at FLC diagnosis was 37 years (range 18–65), and 3 patients were female. FLC diagnosis was delayed in 2 patients with time to FLC diagnosis of 10 months and 20 months, respectively. Delayed diagnosis was associated with advanced tumor stage and early death. These patients were primarily diagnosed with probable FNH at initial presentation at an

Table 1 Clinical information

	#1	#2	#3	#4	#5	#6
Age (years)	52	18	65	26	48	18
Sex	M	F	M	M	F	F
Tumor stage (initial)	pT2 pN0 cM0 (UICC II)	cT1 cN1 cM1 (UICC IVB)	cT1 cN0 cM0 (UICC I)	pT2 cN0 cM0 (UICC II)	cT3b cN0 cM0 (UICC IIIB)	pT3b pN1 cM0 (UICC IVA)
Time to diagnosis (months)	1	10	1	1	1	20
TACE prior to gadoxetic acid enhanced MRI	No	Yes	Yes	No	Yes	No
Treatment	Resection	Sorafenib	TACE, Sorafenib	Resection	Sorafenib	Resection
Survival times	PFS ongoing for 24 months	OS 2 months	OS 29 months	PFS ongoing for 46 months	Lost to follow-up	OS 7 months

TACE transarterial chemoembolisation, *MRI* magnetic resonance imaging, *PFS* progression free survival, *OS* overall survival

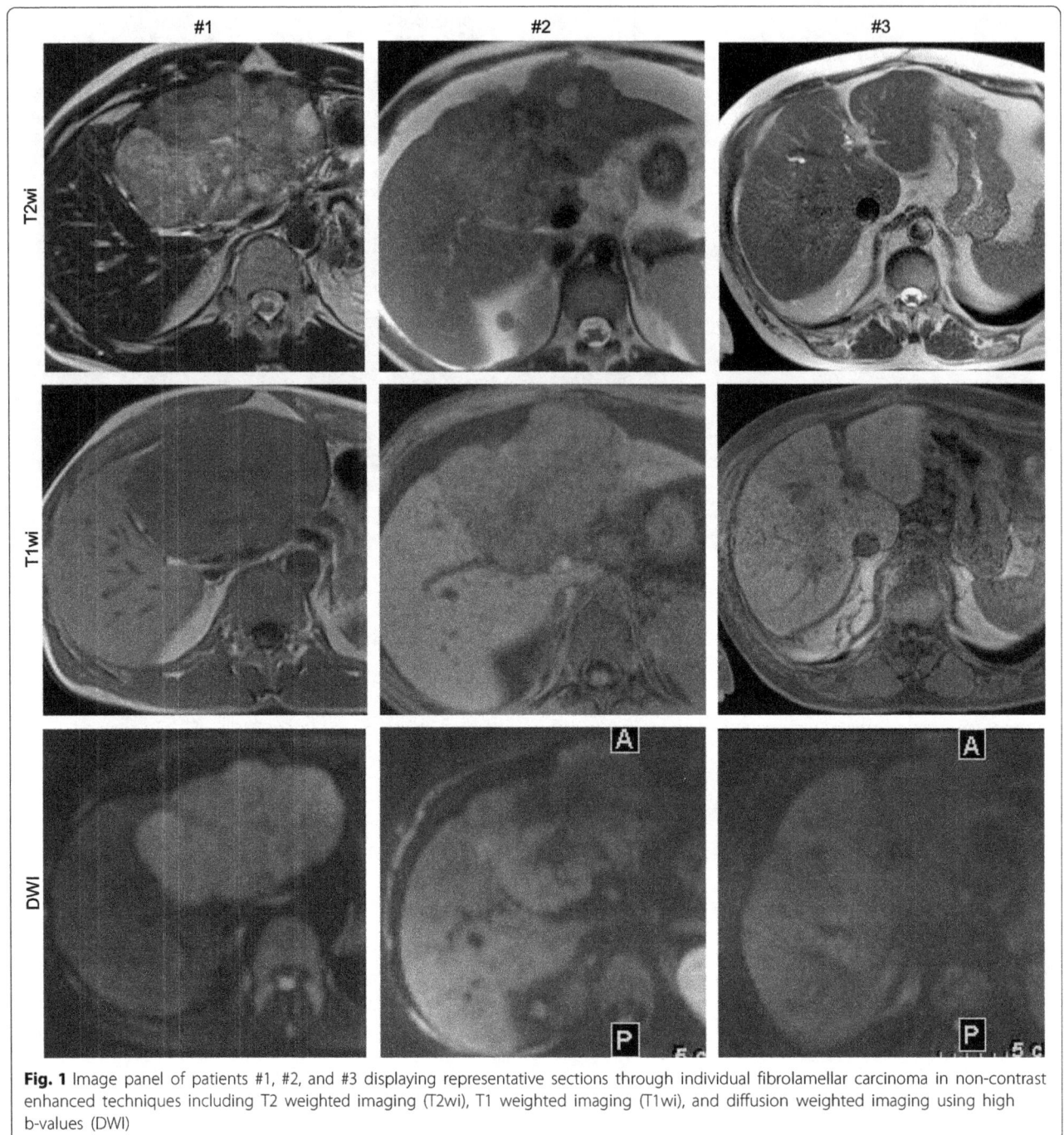

Fig. 1 Image panel of patients #1, #2, and #3 displaying representative sections through individual fibrolamellar carcinoma in non-contrast enhanced techniques including T2 weighted imaging (T2wi), T1 weighted imaging (T1wi), and diffusion weighted imaging using high b-values (DWI)

outside institution. One of these 2 patients presented initially in the early days of clinical introduction of gadoxetic acid. 3 patients had history of TACE with the last intervention 3, 8, and 12 months, respectively, prior to gadoxetic acid-enhanced MRI.

Imaging

Gadoxetic acid-enhanced MRI was performed between September 2007 and May 2016. All scanners were 1.5 T

devices (Siemens Magnetom Avanto or Siemens Magnetom Aera, Siemens Healthineers, Erlangen, Germany). Specific sequence parameters such as relaxation times and echo times differed between individual MRI protocols. General sequence design is summarized as follows: T2wi was half-Fourier acquisition single-shot turbo spin echo imaging in 5 of 6 examinations and turbo spin echo imaging in 1 examination. Slice thicknesses were 6 mm. T1wi without fat saturation was two-dimensional fast low angle shot imaging in all 6 examinations. Slice thicknesses were 6 mm. DWI was echo planar imaging in all 6 examinations. The highest available b-values were 800 s/mm^2 in 5 examinations, 600 s/mm^2 in 1 examination. Slice thicknesses were 6 mm. Pre- and post-contrast T1-weighted imaging with fat-saturation was three-dimensional fast low angle shot imaging in all 6 examinations. Slice thicknesses were 3 mm. HBP was acquired with a median delay after HAP of 18:06 min (range, 16:44–20:43 min). Details on contrast material injection were available for 3 patients. In 2 of these, contrast material was injected with a rate of 1 ml/s and in 1 with a rate of 2 ml/s. Contrast material injection was followed by a saline flush. The contrast material volume was weight dependent and was 10 ml at a maximum with 0.025 mmol/ml gadoxetic acid.

Lesion features

In 5 of 6 patients the FLC was unifocal. In 1 patient FLC was multifocal with disseminated confluent lesions within the whole liver. In this patient, only the predominant part

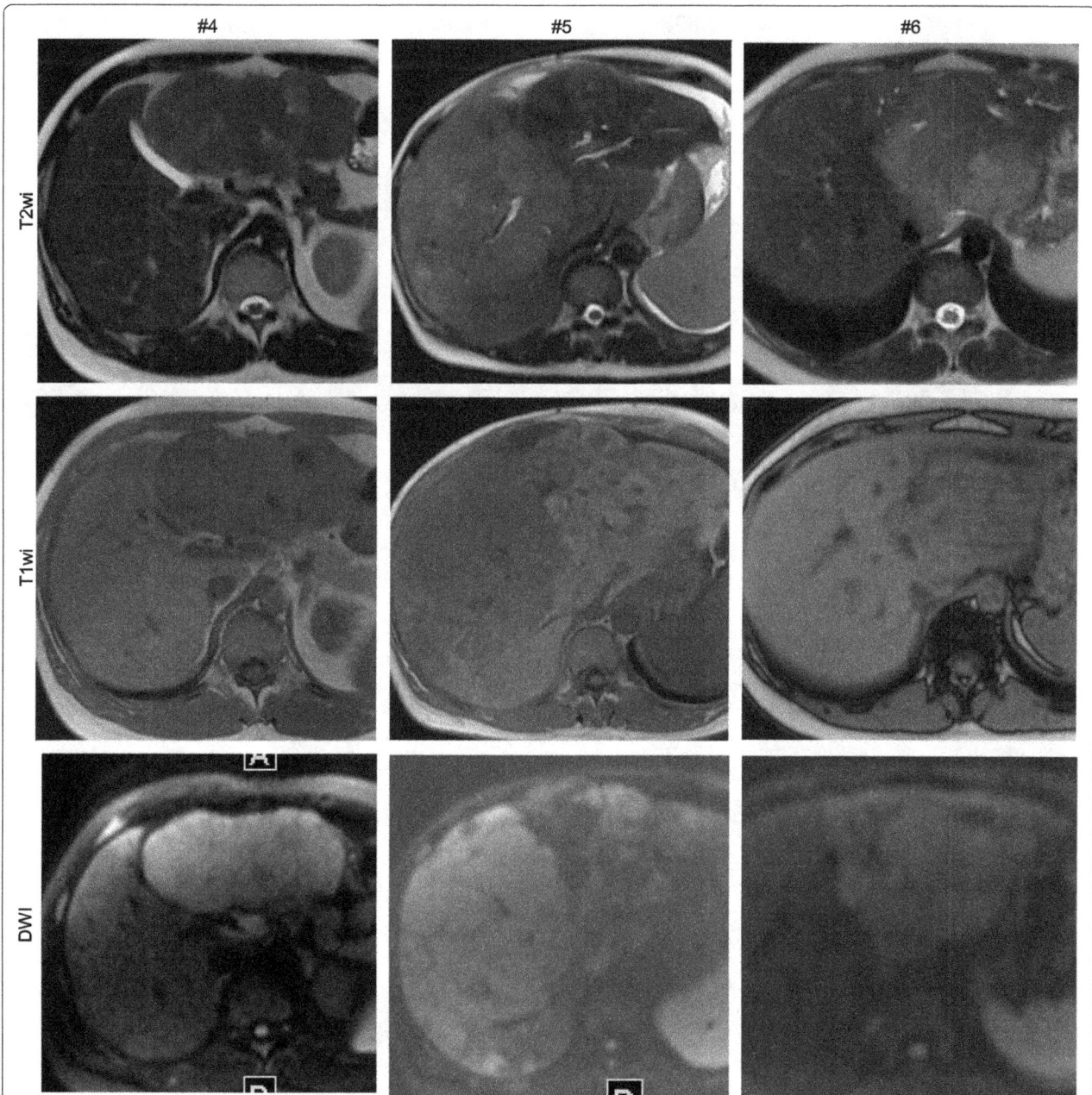

Fig. 2 Image panel of patients #4, #5, and #6 displaying representative sections through individual fibrolamellar carcinoma in non-contrast enhanced imaging techniques including T2 weighted imaging (T2wi), T1 weighted imaging (T1wi), and diffusion weighted imaging using high b-values (DWI)

of the lesion was evaluated. Thus, the evaluated FLCs had a median maximum diameter of 10.5 cm (range, 8.8–14.0). Panels of representative images of each FLC are shown in Figs. 1, 2, 3, and 4. Imaging features are summarized in Table 2.

In HBP, all FLCs were hypointense compared with background liver parenchyma. The CEI indicated presence of hepatobiliary contrast enhancement in all FLCs (Fig. 5). The mean CEI averaged over all FLCs was 1.35 indicating a FLC SI increase of 35% in HBP compared with pre-contrast T1wi normalized to muscle SI. Mean SI of FLCs and lumbar muscle and the CEI are shown in Table 3. In HAP, 5 FLCs had predominantly arterial hyperenhancement and 1 FLC had arterial hypoenhancement in lesion components considered viable. In PVP, 4 FLC were predominantly hypointense and 2 FLC was predominantly isointense in lesion components considered viable. The enhancement pattern was considered APHE/WO pattern in 3 FLCs.

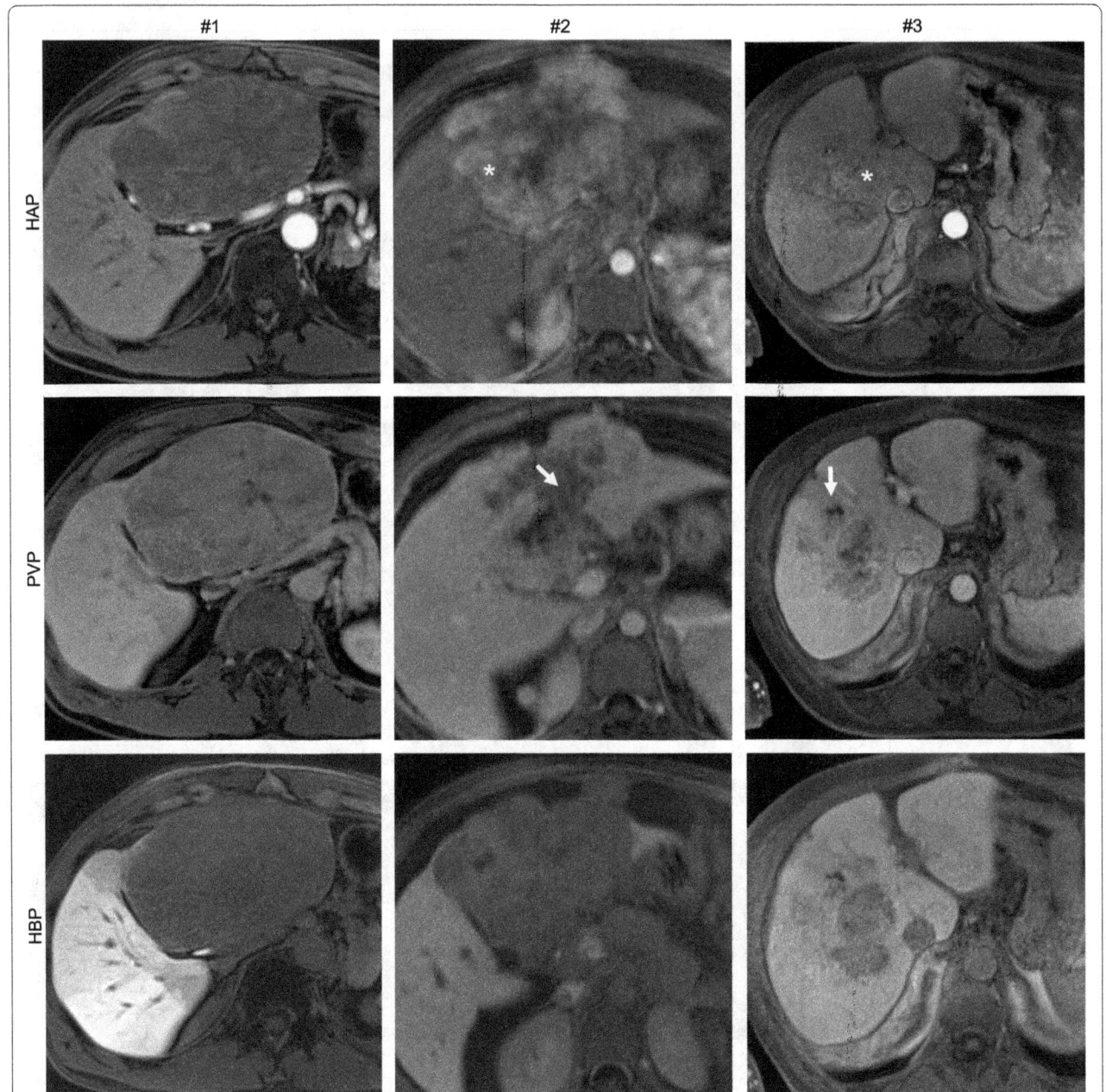

Fig. 3 Image panel of patients #1, #2, and #3 displaying representative sections through individual fibrolamellar carcinoma in contrast enhanced imaging techniques including hepatic arterial phase T1 weighted imaging (HAP), portal venous phase T1 weighted imaging (PVP), and hepatobiliary phase T1 weighted imaging (HBP). In patients with history of TACE prior to gadoxetic acid enhanced MRI (#2, #3) areas of non-viable tumor are indicated in the portal venous phase (arrows) and areas of viable tumor are indicated in the hepatic arterial phase (star)

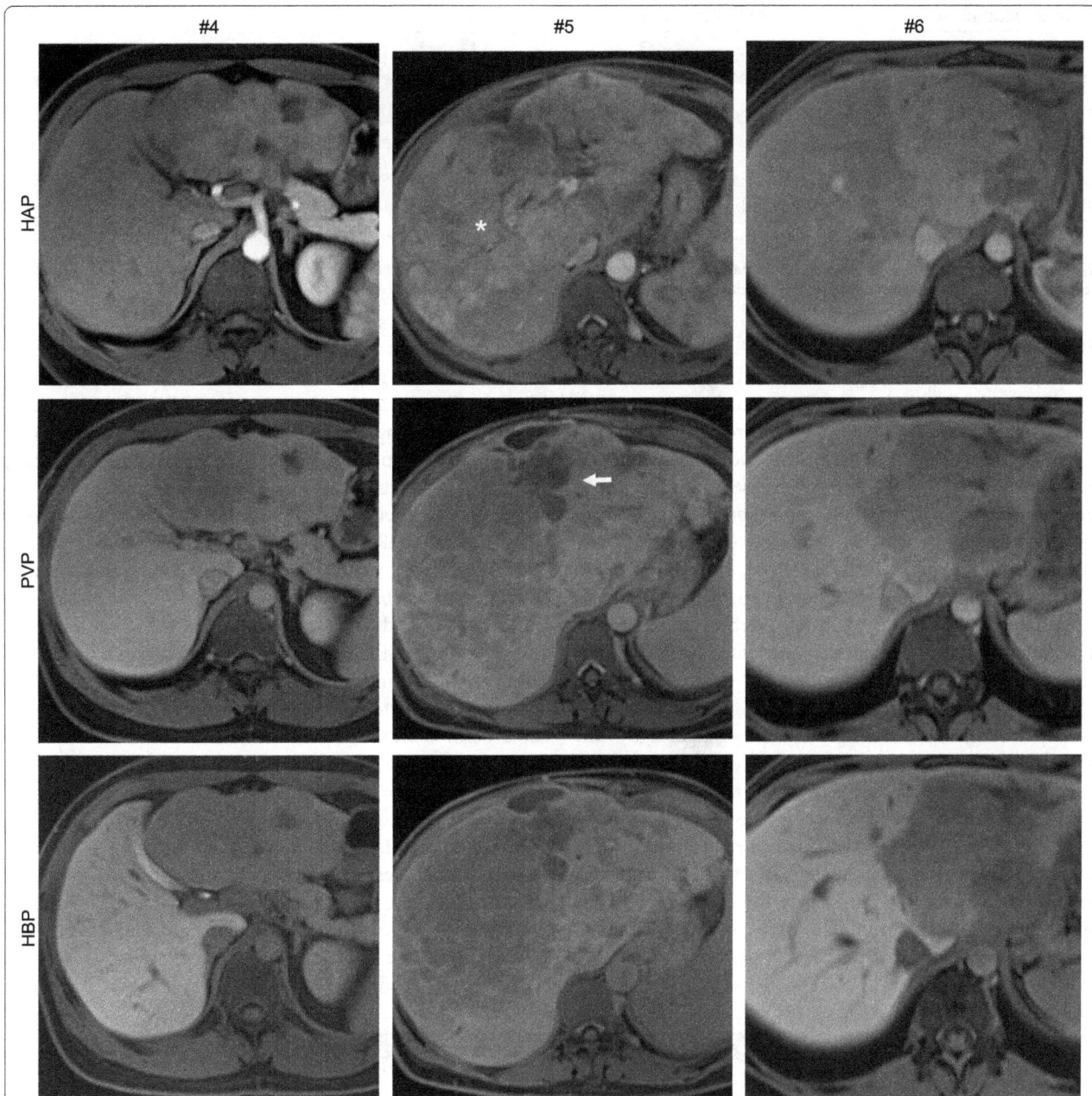

Fig. 4 Image panel of patients #1, #2, and #3 displaying representative sections through individual fibrolamellar carcinoma in contrast enhanced imaging techniques including hepatic arterial phase T1 weighted imaging (HAP), portal venous phase T1 weighted imaging (PVP), and hepatobiliary phase T1 weighted imaging (HBP). In patients with history of TACE prior to gadoxetic acid enhanced MRI (#5) areas of non-viable tumor are indicated in the portal venous phase (arrows) and areas of viable tumor are indicated in the hepatic arterial phase (star)

T1wi and T2wi were available in all patients. In T1wi, 5 FLCs were predominantly hypointense, and 1 FLC was predominantly isointense compared to background liver parenchyma. In T2wi, 5 FLCs were predominantly but heterogeneously hyperintense and 1 FLC was predominantly isointense compared to background liver parenchyma.

DWI and apparent diffusion coefficient (ADC) maps were available in all patients. In DWI with high b-value, 5 FLCs were predominantly hyperintense and 1 FLC was predominantly isointense compared to background liver parenchyma. In ADC map, 4 FLCs were predominantly hyperintense and 2 FLCs were predominantly isointense compared to background liver parenchyma.

Intrahepatic bile duct dilatation, bile duct tumor thrombosis, and portal vein thrombosis were present in 3, 1, and 1 patient, respectively. Intralesional necrosis and intralesional hemorrhage were present in 2 and 0 patients, respectively, of those patients without history of TACE.

Table 2 Predominant imaging features of fibrolamellar carcinomas

	#1	#2	#3	#4	#5	#6
T2wi	hyperintense	hyperintense	isointense	hyperintense	hyperintense	hyperintense
T1wi	hypointense	hypointense	hypointense	hypointense	hypointense	isointense
DWI	hyperintense	hyperintense	isointense	hyperintense	hyperintense	hyperintense
HAP	hypoenhanced	hyperenhanced	hyperenhanced	hyperenhanced	hyperenhanced	hyperenhanced
PVP	hypoenhanced	isoenhanced	hypoenhanced	isoenhanced	hypoenhanced	hypoenhanced
HBP	hypoenhanced	hypoenhanced	hypoenhanced	hypoenhanced	hypoenhanced	hypoenhanced

T2wi T2 weighted imaging, *T1wi* T1 pre contrast weighted imaging, *DWI* diffusion weighted imaging with high b-value, *HAP* hepatic arterial phase post contrast T1 weighted imaging, *PVP* portal venous phase post contrast T1 weighted imaging, *HBP* hepatobiliary phase post contrast T1 weighted imaging

Discussion

In the present analysis on gadoxetic acid-enhanced MRI of 6 patients with histology-proven FLC, contrast enhancement during HBP was present in all FLCs according to calculation of the corrected FLC enhancement index. At visual assessment, all FLCs were hypointense compared with background liver parenchyma. Important imaging features identified frequently in other sequence techniques include heterogeneous hyperintensity in T2wi, hyperintensity in DWI using high b-values, arterial phase hyperenhancement followed by venous wash-out after injection of contrast material, and presence of accompanying findings generally associated with malignancy.

FLC is an infrequent form of HCC mainly occurring equally in female and male patients of younger age without underlying liver disease. Only 20% of FLCs are found in cirrhotic livers [1]. Rarity of FLC and communalities of FLC with other liver lesions may be reasons for preference of benign differential diagnoses in conventional imaging studies and for delayed time to FLC diagnosis. In two of our patients, FLCs were mistaken for FNH at initial presentation. Prolonged time to FLC diagnoses was associated with poor outcome in these cases.

Among benign liver lesions that may be erroneously preferred over malignancy in patients without chronic liver disease, FNH is the most important misdiagnosis in cases of FLC. Mistaking FLC for FNH may have disastrous consequences on patient prognosis if tumor progression during the interval to FLC diagnosis leads to worsening of tumor stage and/or impossibility of curative resection. In patients diagnosed with FLC, positive lymph node status, distant metastatic disease and incomplete resection are associated with decreased survival [10, 11].

Both FLC and FNH are predominantly characterized by generally subtle deviations of signal intensities in pre-contrast T1wi and T2wi compared to background liver parenchyma, arterial hyperenhancement, and presence of a central scar. Imaging features that may favor FLC over FNH in MRI are greater heterogeneity of lesion texture of FLC including necrosis and hemorrhage, hypointensity of the central scar of FLC in T2wi, and portal venous hypoenhancement [12]. Calcifications are reported to be present in approximately 50% of FLCs and not in FNH but are depicted insufficiently in MRI [13]. These imaging features are, however, unreliable discriminators: E.g., the signal intensity of the central scar in

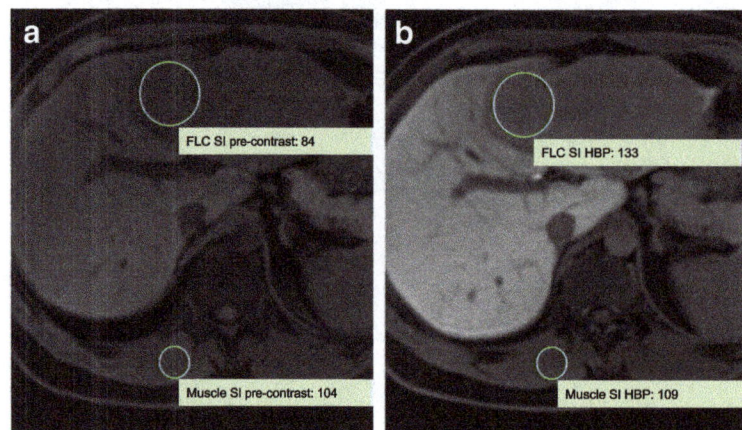

Fig. 5 Assessment of the corrected enhancement index (CEI) in patient #4. **a** shows the pre-contrast scan. **b** shows the hepatobiliary phase. CEI is 1.51 indicating a signal increase of 51% normalized to lumbar muscle signal intensity. FLC, fibrolamellar carcinoma; HBP, hepatobiliary phase; SI, signal intensity

Table 3 Signal intensity and signal intensity ratios

	#1	#2	#3	#4	#5	#6
SI liver PRE	146	114	131	84	96	145
SI muscle PRE	145	151	142	104	112	134
SI liver HBP	136	163	198	133	138	174
SI muscle HBP	99	149	158	109	125	141
CEI	1.38	1.45	1.36	1.50	1.30	1.13

SI signal intensity, *PRE* pre-contrast T1 weighted imaging, *HBP* hepatobiliary phase post-contrastT1 weighted imaging, *CEI* corrected enhancement index ([SI liver HBP /SI muscle HBP]/[SI liver PRE/SI muscle PRE])

T2wi has been shown to be variable [14]. We did not specifically analyze the presence of a central scar and its imaging features in this study, because TACE, which has been performed in 3 of our patients, was considered to affect central scar characterization within treated lesion components.

Gadoxetic acid is a liver-specific gadolinium-based contrast agent that was demonstrated to be of great value for HCC detection in the cirrhotic liver and FNH diagnosis in ambiguous liver lesions [15, 16]. FNHs are characterized by strong uptake of gadoxetic acid leading to iso- or hyperintensity in HBP. Conventional HCCs in the cirrhotic liver are typically hypointense in HBP compared to background liver parenchyma. However, approximately 10% of HCCs in the cirrhotic liver are reported to be not hypointense in HBP due to retained expression of the OATP8 receptor internalizing gadoxetic acid into the hepatocyte [17]. In the non-cirrhotic liver, 5 of 27 HCCs were not hypointense in HBP in a study by Kim et al. [18], but it was not reported if FLCs were included. Thus, precise data on signal behavior of FLC in gadoxetic acid-enhanced MRI are scarce.

In one case report of a pediatric FLC patient the tumor was considered to not show uptake of gadoxetic acid in HBP [19]. In a larger cohort of 37 FLCs only one gadoxetic acid-enhanced MRI was performed, and the tumor was uniformly hypointense in HBP compared with background liver parenchyma [14]. Apart from that, there are apparently only exemplary case presentations available in review articles on liver imaging showing hypointensity of FLC in HBP as well [20–22]. Interestingly, in one illustrative FLC case, uptake of gadoxetic acid in HBP with focal intralesional areas of isointensity was shown by Ringe et al. [22]. To our knowledge, quantitative data on uptake of gadoxetic acid of FLCs or conventional HCC in HBP have not been reported so far. Our case series shows that contrast material uptake may be generally measurable even in FLCs that are in total hypointense compared with background liver parenchyma. This suggests that OATP8 expression is reduced but probably generally present in FLCs.

Concerning DWI in FLC, published experience was very limited so far, but diffusion restriction was suggested to be the most salient finding [12]. The FLCs assessed in our study were qualitatively predominantly isointense ($n = 1$) or predominantly hyperintense ($n = 4$) in the ADC map compared to background liver parenchyma. As other groups have shown that the majority of FNHs are mildly hyperintense in DWI when using high b-values and that the ADC values of FNHs have substantial overlap with the ADC value of background liver parenchyma, we suppose that DWI may not be helpful for distinguishing FLC from FNH either [23, 24].

Limitations

This single-center study is limited by the small case number due to rarity of the tumor. However, to the best of our knowledge, so far no larger series on gadoxetic acid enhanced MRI of FLC has been reported. Moreover, in 3 of 6 patients TACE had been performed prior to acquisition of gadoxetic acid-enhanced MRI. To ensure a reasonably large study cohort, these patients were not excluded from analysis, but only FLC components were analyzed that progressed after TACE to address possible effects of TACE on lesion features. There was technical heterogeneity of MRI protocols, especially concerning DWI. Thus, ADC value calculation was not feasible. We did not carry out a comparative analysis between FLC and FNH. However, imaging features of FNH including DWI and HBP are well known and analysis of these was suggested not to enhance the data significantly.

Conclusion

A variable extent of hepatobiliary gadoxetic acid uptake is suggested to be generally present in FLCs. However, the observation of hypointensity of active FLC components in HBP of gadoxetic acid-enhanced liver MRI compared with background liver parenchyma underscores the role of gadoxetic acid for non-invasive diagnosis of FLC and its importance in the diagnostic work-up of indeterminate liver lesions including FNH.

Abbreviations

ADC: Apparent diffusion coefficient; APHE/WO: Arterial phase hyperenhancement followed by portal venous hypoenhancement; CEI: Corrected enhancement index; DWI: Diffusion weighted imaging; FLC: Fibrolamellar hepatocellular carcinoma; FNH: Focal nodular hyperplasia; HAP: Hepatic arterial phase; HBP: Hepatobiliary phase; HCC: Hepatocellular carcinoma; MRI: Magnetic resonance imaging; PVP: Portal venous phase; ROI: Region of interest; SI: Signal intensity; T1wi: T1-weighted imaging; T2wi: T2-weighted imaging; TACE: Transarterial chemoembolisation

Funding

Not applicable

Authors' contributions

VP: manuscript preparation, literature research. RS: data analysis, literature research, manuscript preparation. PM: data acquisition, manuscript editing. KHW: patient selection, database search, manuscript editing. CS: patient selection, database search, manuscript editing. AM: manuscript editing. TL: patient selection, database search, manuscript editing. AKB: collection of clinical data, manuscript editing. HUK: manuscript editing. TFW: study concept, data analysis, manuscript preparation. All authors read and approved the manuscript.

Competing interests

The authors declare that they have no competing interests.

Author details

[1]Department of Diagnostic and Interventional Radiology, Heidelberg University Hospital, INF 110, 69120 Heidelberg, Germany. [2]Department of Radiology, Zhongshan Hospital, Fudan University, 180 Fenglin Road, Shanghai 200032, China. [3]Liver Cancer Center Heidelberg, Heidelberg University Hospital, INF 224, 69120 Heidelberg, Germany. [4]Department of Gastroenterology, Infectious Diseases, Intoxication, Heidelberg University Hospital, INF 410, 69120 Heidelberg, Germany. [5]Department of Medical Oncology, National Center for Tumor Diseases (NCT), Heidelberg University Hospital, INF 460, 69120 Heidelberg, Germany. [6]Department of General, Visceral and Transplantation Surgery, Heidelberg University Hospital, INF 110, 69120 Heidelberg, Germany. [7]Division Translational Gastrointestinal Pathology, Institute of Pathology, Heidelberg University Hospital, INF 224, 69120 Heidelberg, Germany.

References

1. Torbenson M. Fibrolamellar carcinoma: 2012 update. Scientifica (Cairo). Hindawi. 2012;2012:743790–15.
2. Craig JR, Peters RL, Edmondson HA, Omata M. Fibrolamellar carcinoma of the liver: a tumor of adolescents and young adults with distinctive clinico-pathologic features. Cancer. 1980;46:372–9.
3. Honeyman JN, Simon EP, Robine N, Chiaroni-Clarke R, Darcy DG, Lim IIP, et al. Detection of a recurrent DNAJB1-PRKACA chimeric transcript in fibrolamellar hepatocellular carcinoma. Science. 2014;343:1010–4.
4. Graham RP, Jin L, Knutson DL, Kloft-Nelson SM, Greipp PT, Waldburger N, et al. DNAJB1-PRKACA is specific for fibrolamellar carcinoma. Mod Pathol. 2015; 28:822–9.
5. Corrigan K, Semelka RC. Dynamic contrast-enhanced MR imaging of fibrolamellar hepatocellular carcinoma. Abdom Imaging. 1995;20:122–5.
6. Ichikawa T, Federle MP, Grazioli L, Madariaga J, Nalesnik M, Marsh W. Fibrolamellar hepatocellular carcinoma: imaging and pathologic findings in 31 recent cases. Radiology. 1999;213:352–61.
7. Grazioli L, Morana G, Federle MP, Brancatelli G, Testoni M, Kirchin MA, et al. Focal nodular hyperplasia: morphologic and functional information from MR imaging with gadobenate dimeglumine. Radiology. 2001;221:731–9.
8. Husainy MA, Sayyed F, Peddu P. Typical and atypical benign liver lesions: a review. Clin Imaging. 2017;44:79–91.
9. Watanabe H, Kanematsu M, Goshima S, Kondo H, Onozuka M, Moriyama N, et al. Staging hepatic fibrosis: comparison of Gadoxetate disodium–enhanced and diffusion-weighted MR imaging—preliminary observations. Radiology. 2011;259:142–50.
10. Kaseb AO, Shama M, Sahin IH, Nooka A, Hassabo HM, Vauthey J-N, et al. Prognostic indicators and treatment outcome in 94 cases of fibrolamellar hepatocellular carcinoma. Oncology. 2013;85:197–203.
11. Darcy DG, Malek MM, Kobos R, Klimstra DS, DeMatteo R, La Quaglia MP. Prognostic factors in fibrolamellar hepatocellular carcinoma in young people. Journal of Pediatric Surgery Elsevier; 2015;50:153–156.
12. Ganeshan D, Szklaruk J, Kundra V, Kaseb A, Rashid A, Elsayes KM. Imaging features of fibrolamellar hepatocellular carcinoma. AJR Am J Roentgenol. 2014;202:544–52.
13. McLarney JK, Rucker PT, Bender GN, Goodman ZD, Kashitani N, Ros PR. Fibrolamellar carcinoma of the liver: radiologic-pathologic correlation. Radiographics. 1999;19:453–71.
14. Do RKG, McErlean A, Ang CS, DeMatteo RP, Abou-Alfa GK. CT and MRI of primary and metastatic fibrolamellar carcinoma: a case series of 37 patients. Br J Radiol. 2014;87:20140024.
15. Suh CH, Kim KW, Kim GY, Shin YM, Kim PN, Park SH. The diagnostic value of Gd-EOB-DTPA-MRI for the diagnosis of focal nodular hyperplasia: a systematic review and meta-analysis. Eur Radiol. 2015;25:950–60.
16. Liu X, Zou L, Liu F, Zhou Y, Song B. Gadoxetic acid disodium-enhanced magnetic resonance imaging for the detection of hepatocellular carcinoma: a meta-analysis. Ahn SH. PLoS One. 2013;8:e70896.
17. Kitao A, Matsui O, Yoneda N, Kozaka K, Kobayashi S, Koda W, et al. Hypervascular hepatocellular carcinoma: correlation between biologic features and signal intensity on gadoxetic acid-enhanced MR images. Radiology. 2012;265:780–9.
18. Kim R, Lee JM, Joo I, Lee DH, Woo S, Han JK, et al. Differentiation of lipid poor angiomyolipoma from hepatocellular carcinoma on gadoxetic acid-enhanced liver MR imaging. Abdom Imaging. 2015;40:531–41.
19. Matsuda M, Amemiya H, Kawaida H, Okamoto H, Hosomura N, Asakawa M, et al. Typical fibrolamellar hepatocellular carcinoma in a Japanese boy: report of a case. Surg Today. 2014;44:1359–66.
20. Bartolozzi C, Battaglia V, Bozzi E. HCC diagnosis with liver-specific MRI–close to histopathology. Dig Dis. 2009;27:125–30.
21. Ba-Ssalamah A, Uffmann M, Saini S, Bastati N, Herold C, Schima W. Clinical value of MRI liver-specific contrast agents: a tailored examination for a confident non-invasive diagnosis of focal liver lesions. Eur Radiol Springer-Verlag. 2009;19:342–57.
22. Ringe KI, Husarik DB, Sirlin CB, Merkle EM. Gadoxetate disodium-enhanced MRI of the liver: part 1, protocol optimization and lesion appearance in the noncirrhotic liver. AJR Am J Roentgenol. 2010;195:13–28.
23. Dohan A, Soyer P, Guerrache Y, Hoeffel C, Gavini J-P, Kaci R, et al. Focal nodular hyperplasia of the liver: diffusion-weighted magnetic resonance imaging characteristics using high b values. J Comput Assist Tomogr. 2014;38:96–104.
24. Donati F, Boraschi P, Gigoni R, Salemi S, Falaschi F, Bartolozzi C. Focal nodular hyperplasia of the liver: diffusion and perfusion MRI characteristics. Magn Reson Imaging. 2013;31:10–6.

10

Reproducibility and repeatability of same-day two sequential FDG PET/MR and PET/CT

David Groshar[1,2†], Hanna Bernstine[1,2†], Natalia Goldberg[1], Meital Nidam[1], Dan Stein[1], Ifat Abadi-Korek[1] and Liran Domachevsky[1*]

Abstract

Background: To determine PET/CT and PET/MR reproducibility and PET/MR repeatability of fluorine 18 fluorodeoxyglucose (FDG) uptake measurements in tumors in cancer patients.

Methods: This IRB approved prospective study was performed between October 2015 and February 2016 in consecutive patients who performed same day PET/CT and two sequential PET/MR. Thirty three patients with visible tumors ($N = 63$) were included. SUV for body weight (SUV) and lean body mass (SUL) were obtained. Volume of interest (VOI) with a threshold of 40% was used and SUV/L's, metabolic tumor volume (MTV) and tumor to liver ratio (T/L) were calculated. Measurements were plotted in a scattered diagram to visually identify correlation, a regression line was drawn and the equation of the line was calculated. Bland-Altman plots expressed as percentages were constructed to assess the agreement between measurements. The maximal clinically acceptable limits range was defined as ±30%.

Results: Lesional SUV's, SUL's and MTV corrected to body weight (BW) and lean body mass (LBM) demonstrated strong positive linear correlation between PET/CT and PET/MR and between two sequential PET/MR. The 95% limits of agreement ranged from -27.7 to 17.5 with a mean of -5.1 and -27.6 to 17.9 with a mean of -4.9 for SUVpeak and SULpeak, respectively for sequential PET/MR. Other PET metrics demonstrated limits range that is above ±30% between PET/CT and PET/MR and between two sequential PET/MR.

Conclusion: PET/MR SUV/L peak has a clinically acceptable repeatability performance and can be used to evaluate the response to treatment.

Keywords: PET/MR, SUV, Reproducibility, Repeatability, Reliability

Background

The introduction of hybrid PET/MR imaging offers a new modality that combines high soft-tissue contrast resolution of MR with metabolic imaging from PET within a single imaging session. This modality has shown promising results in oncological imaging and could be useful in the management of patients with cancer [1]. Quantitative or semi-quantitative imaging biomarkers such as fluorine 18 fluorodeoxyglucose (FDG) may predict response to therapy earlier compared to conventional

imaging as metabolic changes in tumors may precede changes in tumor size and texture and determine tissue viability [2].

FDG uptake can be assessed qualitatively as mild, moderate or intense compared to the background uptake in normal appearing tissues of which liver parenchyma is the most commonly used. However, quantitative or semi-quantitative PET metrics, rather than qualitative assessments, should be used in order to obtain comparable results both from sequential studies of a single patient and between different patient groups [3]. Indeed, SUV that is a semi quantitative measurement to evaluate FDG uptake in a tumor or organ by PET/CT has been successfully used in clinical studies in addition to visual assessments.

* Correspondence: liranura@gmail.com
†Equal contributors
[1]Department of Nuclear Medicine, Assuta Medical Center, 20 habarzel st., 6971028 Tel-Aviv, Israel
Full list of author information is available at the end of the article

The use of semi-quantitative measurements for patient follow-up or for comparison between different scanners relies on the high degree of repeatability and reproducibility, respectively. Knowledge of the expected range in reproducibility and repeatability is needed to determine what change in parameters between two examinations can be considered significant in an individual patient or between patient groups. Commercially available Dixon-based PET/MR attenuation correction (MRAC) differs from density-based PET/CT attenuation correction (CTAC) and has been shown to affect FDG uptake measurements in tumor lesions and in normal appearing structures [4]. Several studies have compared FDG PET images from PET/CT and PET/MR in clinical data [1, 5–13] and found similar diagnostic performance and detection rates, despite some differences in the semi-quantitative assessment of FDG uptake [14]. Unlike previous reports the test-retest repeatability in this study was performed on the same day and patients were randomized regarding the order of PET/CT and PET/MR studies. Same-day repeatability with studies performed in sequence enables evaluation of the PET/MR system reliability as variables related to the patient such as patient habitus or changes in tissues following therapy are similar, while randomization of patients obviates differences in biodistribution which still affect FDG uptake even with a modest temporal offset. The purpose of this observational prospective study is to determine PET/CT and PET/MR reproducibility and test-retest PET/MR repeatability of lesional FDG PET metrics obtained by PET/CT and by two sequential PET/MR examinations performed on the same day in patients with cancer.

Methods

This observational prospective study was approved by the institutional review board. Informed written consent was obtained from all patients participating in the study. Between October 2015 and February 2016, consecutive patients who performed PET/CT and two sequential non-enhanced whole-body PET/MR were enrolled. All patients had a biopsy-proven cancer (Table 1) and underwent PET/CT either for initial evaluation or for follow-up. Patients were randomized using a simple randomization to a group in which sequential PET/MR was performed first and to a second group in which PET/CT was performed first (Table 1). The sequential PET/MR studies were conducted in a row (i.e., immediately after the first PET/MR scan was ended the second PET/MR was started). Only patients with visible tumor based on PET/CT and PET/MR findings were included. A total of 33 out of 67 patients with 63 conspicuous tumor lesions (mean age 53.1 ± 12.1years, 19 females, mean age 52.4 ± 11.8 years and 14 males, mean age 54.1 ± 12.5 years) were included (Table 1).

Table 1 Patient characteristic

		Patients with visible lesions (N = 33)
Age (years)		53.1 ± 12.1 (28–75)
Gender	Female	n = 19, age 52.4 ± 11.8
	Male	n = 14, age 54.1 ± 12.5
MR first		16
CT first		17
Time to CT (minutes)		110 ± 32 (47–185)
Time to MR (minutes)		104 ± 36 (41–175)
Time to exam (minutes)		81 ± 22 (41–175)
Time between exams (minutes)		53 ± 17 (25–88)
Blood glucose levels (mg/dl)		95.47 ± 26.4 (69–203)
BMI		25.8 ± 5.1 (16.2–35.7)
Disease	Breast	12
	Lung	7
	Lymphoma	2
	Melanoma	1
	CRC	7
	Head and neck	3
	other	1
Number of lesions		
	1	13
	2	10
	3	10

PET/CT Protocol

PET/CT was performed using an integrated PET/CT scanner (GEMINI TF, PHILIPS Medical Systems, Cleveland, Ohio, USA). Intravenously FDG dose of 5.18MBq/kg (varied from 370 to 666 MBq) and 800–1000 mL of diluted iodinated contrast material was administered orally for bowel opacification. Contrast-enhanced 64-slice multi-detector CT was performed from skull base to mid-thigh with the arm-up position with tube voltage of 120 kVp, spiral CT at 0.8s per rotation with modulated 30–250 mAs, section thickness of 3.00 mm, and 3.00 mm interval with image reconstruction every 3.0 mm. Intravenous iodine contrast media (Omnipaque 300; iohexol 0.623 g/ml, GE Healthcare, USA; 1.5 cm3/kg) was administered in all examinations, except for patients with known iodine hypersensitivity or renal insufficiency. PET emission images were obtained with 2 min of acquisition per bed position with five to six bed positions from skull base to mid-thigh. PET data was reconstructed using 3D- ordered subset expectation maximization (OSEM), (3 iteration and 20 subsets,

4 mm Gaussian filter) on 144 matrix with CT-based attenuation correction.

PET/MR Protocol

FDG PET/MR was performed from skull base to mid-thigh with the arm-down position, on the Biograph mMR (Siemens AG, healthcare sector, Erlangen, Germany) simultaneous PET/MR system. Patients were positioned supine and multi-step/multi-bed scanning was performed in caudo-cranial direction with four bed positions. We used a 24 –channel spine RF coil integrated within the MR bed and 3 surface body coils (6 channel each) to cover the thorax, abdomen and pelvis. For the neck we used a 16-channel RF head/neck coil.

PET data was acquired in the list mode and reconstructed with 3D-OSEM, (3 iteration and 21 subsets, 4 mm Gaussian filter) on 172 matrix. Each bed position was started with coronal Dixon-based sequences for MR attenuation correction (MRAC) (breath holding) (19s). This was followed by axial T2 half-fourier acquisition single shot turbo spin echo (HASTE) (free breathing) (36s), coronal T2 HASTE with fat suppression (FS) (Inversion recovery (IR) –based) (44s) and axial T1 volumetric interpolated breath-hold examination (VIBE) Dixon (breath holding) (20s). PET data was acquired simultaneously with acquisition time of 5 min for each bed position. Similar parameters were used for the sequential PET/MR scan.

Image analysis

We used dedicated software (Syngo.via; Siemens AG, healthcare sector, Erlangen, Germany) for maximal, peak and mean SUV calculations normalized for body weight (SUV) and lean body mass (SUL).

SUV/Lmax is a single-pixel value of the maximal SUV/L within the sphere, whereas SUV/Lpeak is the mean SUV/L within a predetermined volume of interest (VOI) of 1ml around the voxel with the highest SUV/L in the sphere. SUV/Lmean is the average SUV/L value within the sphere.

Normalization for BW was performed using the patient weight in kg, measured before FDG injection and for LBM using the following formula:

$$LBM \text{ (female)} = (1.07 \text{ X BW}) \text{ (kg)}$$
$$- 148 [BW \text{ (kg)}/\text{body height (cm)}]^2$$

$$LBM \text{ (male)} = (1.1 \text{ X BW}) \text{ (kg)}$$
$$- 128 [BW \text{ (kg)}/\text{body height (cm)}]^2$$

Studies were searched for the presence of lesions by visual analysis. Characterization of lesions was performed based on increased FDG uptake compared to surrounding tissue and abnormal structure on CT and MR and was conducted by a dual board-certified in radiology and nuclear medicine physician (L.D., with 3 years of experience) and a board-certified nuclear medicine physician (H.B., with 9 years of PET/CT experience). However, measurements were only conducted by a board-certified nuclear medicine physician (H.B.). There was no lower or upper size limit for any visible lesion.

A spherical VOI was placed in the lesion and an iso-contour VOI with a threshold of 40% of SUV/Lmax corrected to LBM and BW was drawn in up to 3 distinct separated lesions (i.e., the largest lesions were selected) per each patient. In addition, a VOI with a diameter of 3 cm was drawn on the right lobe of the liver and tumor to liver ratio was determined. All VOI's were visually evaluated on axial, sagittal and coronal planes to be certain that the VOI is well located in the desired area.

Statistical analysis

Values are shown as mean ± SD from sequential PET/MR variables and from variables values from PET/MR and PET/CT. For PET/MR and PET/CT comparison, the average of the two PET/MR measurements was used. Measurements were plotted in a scattered diagram to visually identify correlation, a regression line was drawn and the equation of the line was calculated.

Bland-Altman plots were constructed for each PET metrics variable to assess the agreement between the measurements. The maximal clinically acceptable limits range was defined as ±30%, based on the PERCIST definition for partial response and progressive disease [15].

Statistical analysis was performed using SPSS (IBM version 21) and MedCalc (version 16.2.0).

Results

Lesional correlation and agreement between PET/CT and PET/MR

A mixed effects model that accounted for correlation of several lesional measurements within a patient showed no significant effect on the results. PET/CT and PET/MR SUV and SUL measurements of lesions, liver and tumor to liver ratio are shown in Table 2. Lesional SUV's and SUL's corrected to BW and LBM demonstrated strong positive linear correlation between PET/CT and PET/MR (Fig. 1).

The 95% limits of agreement and mean difference expressed as percentages for lesional SUV max, peak and mean corrected to BW and LBM were above the clinically acceptable range (Table 4).

Representative Bland-Altman plots for SUVpeak with y-axis values expressed as percentages showed 95% limits of agreement ranging from -27 to 54 with a mean of 13.8 and -27.3 to 54.7 with a mean of 13.7 corrected to BW and LBM, respectively (Fig. 1). Lesional MTV corrected to BW and LBM demonstrated strong linear

Table 2 PET/CT and PET/MR SUV and SUL measurements of tumor, liver and tumor to liver ratio (ratio)

	Tumor	Liver	Ratio
SUV max			
PET/CT	10.54 ± 5.41	2.74 ± 0.57	4.97 ± 2.91
PET/MR	10.02 ± 5.23	2.30 ± 0.69	4.76 ± 3.18
SUV mean			
PET/CT	6.11 ± 3.13	2.17 ± 0.41	3.01 ± 1.81
PET/MR	5.66 ± 2.84	1.80 ± 0.36	3.24 ± 1.69
SUV peak			
PET/CT	8.14 ± 4.32	2.66 ± 0.41	3.21 ± 1.92
PET/MR	7.25 ± 3.95	2.01 ± 0.39	3.75 ± 2.21
SUL max			
PET/CT	7.81 ± 3.97	2.28 ± 0.31	3.58 ± 2.04
PET/MR	7.42 ± 3.85	1.64 ± 0.29	4.74 ± 2.78
SUL mean			
PET/CT	4.5 ± 2.27	1.56 ± 0.25	3.08 ± 1.84
PET/MR	4.17 ± 2.09	1.30 ± 0.24	3.35 ± 1.85
SUL peak			
PET/CT	6.01 ± 3.1	1.92 ± 0.25	3.28 ± 1.94
PET/MR	5.35 ± 2.88	1.46 ± 0.26	3.79 ± 2.23

correlation between PET/CT and PET/MR (Fig. 2). Bland-Altman plots for MTV with y-axis values expressed as percentages showed 95% limits of agreement ranging from -41.7 to 96.2 with a mean of 27.3 and -43.4 to 88 with a mean of 22.3 corrected to BW and LBM, respectively (Fig. 2).

Lesional correlation and agreement between two sequential PET/MR

Two sequential PET/MR SUV and SUL measurements of lesions, liver and tumor to liver ratio are shown in Table 3. Lesional SUV's and SUL's corrected to BW and LBM demonstrated strong positive linear correlation between two sequential PET/MR (Fig. 3). The 95% limits of agreement and mean difference expressed as percentages for lesional SUVpeak corrected to BW and LBM were below the clinically acceptable range of ±30%, but was larger for SUVmax and mean (Table 4). Representative Bland-Altman plots for SUVpeak with y-axis values expressed as percentages showed 95% limits of agreement ranging from -27.7 to 17.5 with a mean of -5.1 and -27.6 to 17.9 with a mean of -4.9 corrected to BW and LBM, respectively (Fig. 3). Lesional MTV corrected to BW and LBM demonstrated strong linear correlation between two sequential PET/MR (Fig. 4). Bland-Altman plots for MTV with y-axis values expressed as percentages showed 95% limits of agreement ranging from -42.8 to 59.1 with a mean of 8.1 and -44.3 to 59.9 with a mean of 7.8 corrected to BW and LBM, respectively (Fig. 4). After exclusion of tumors with

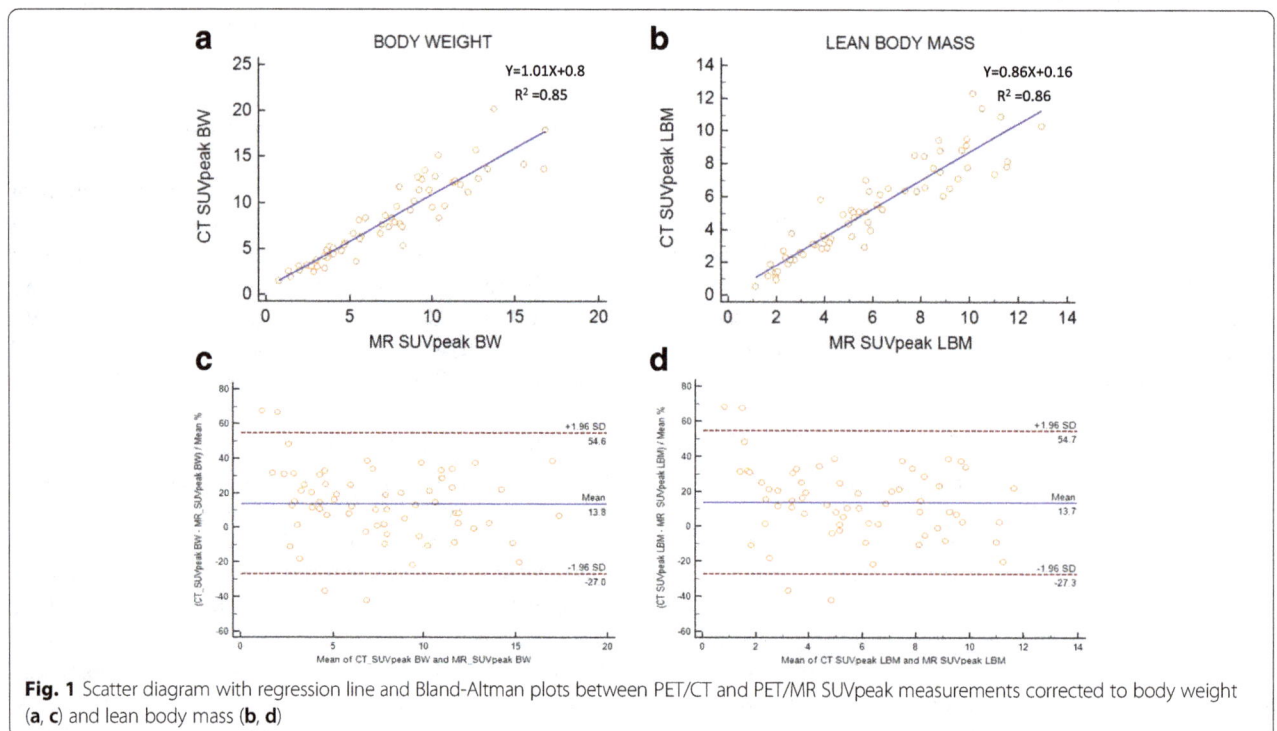

Fig. 1 Scatter diagram with regression line and Bland-Altman plots between PET/CT and PET/MR SUVpeak measurements corrected to body weight (**a**, **c**) and lean body mass (**b**, **d**)

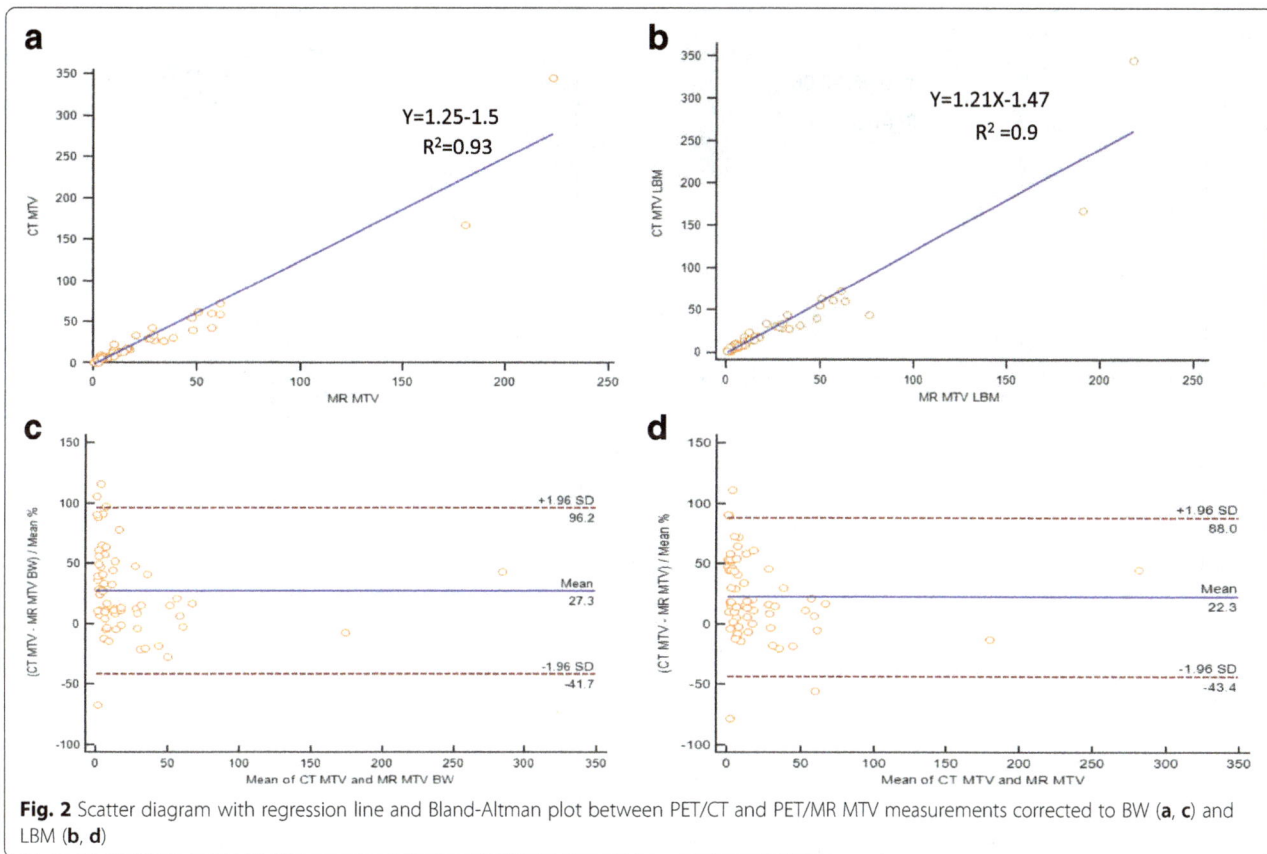

Fig. 2 Scatter diagram with regression line and Bland-Altman plot between PET/CT and PET/MR MTV measurements corrected to BW (**a**, **c**) and LBM (**b**, **d**)

Table 3 Two sequential PET/MR SUV and SUL measurements of tumor, liver and tumor to liver ratio

	Tumor	Liver	Ratio
SUV max			
PET/MR 1st	9.71 ± 5.35	2.28 ± 0.45	4.48 ± 2.74
PET/MR 2nd	10.33 ± 5.19	2.24 ± 0.44	4.78 ± 2.56
SUV mean			
PET/MR 1st	5.39 ± 2.86	1.82 ± 0.38	3.11 ± 1.82
PET/MR 2nd	5.92 ± 2.89	1.79 ± 0.37	3.42 ± 1.71
SUV peak			
PET/MR 1st	7.09 ± 3.93	2.03 ± 0.41	3.65 ± 2.21
PET/MR 2nd	7.42 ± 4.01	1.98 ± 0.39	3.86 ± 2.22
SUL max			
PET/MR 1st	7.17 ± 3.96	1.65 ± 0.31	4.55 ± 2.79
PET/MR 2nd	7.62 ± 3.81	1.62 ± 0.31	4.96 ± 2.93
SUL mean			
PET/MR 1st	3.98 ± 2.12	1.32 ± 0.27	3.16 ± 1.86
PET/MR 2nd	4.37 ± 2.13	1.28 ± 0.24	3.56 ± 1.89
SUL peak			
PET/MR 1st	5.23 ± 2.89	1.48 ± 0.28	3.69 ± 2.24
PET/MR 2nd	5.47 ± 2.9	1.43 ± 0.27	3.92 ± 2.23

volume less than 10ml the 95% limits of agreement ranged from -29.5 to 38.8 with a mean of 4.6 and -34 to 41.8 with a mean of 3.9 corrected to BW and LBM (Fig. 5).

Discussion

Our study demonstrates strong correlation of lesional PET metrics between same day PET/CT and PET/MR and between two sequential PET/MR with good lesional SUV/L peak agreement between two sequential PET/MR.

As a new modality PET/MR test-retest repeatability and agreement with regard to SUV/L's measurements has to be validated. Furthermore, reproducibility and agreement of PET-based variables between PET/MR and PET/CT must also be assessed as patients may swap between these modalities on follow-up studies. Principal factors that differ between PET/CT and PET/MR and might affect reliability include: different methods to create attenuation correction maps, scanning time, different PET detectors and MR hardware. Data regarding the reliability of FDG PET/MR metrics is sparse.

Reproducibility between PET/CT with PET/MR

With regard to *lesional reproducibility*, there are conflicting results in the literature. Al-Nabhani et al. [8] have shown that lesional SUVmean measurements were approximately 10% higher on PET/MR. Pace et al. [13]

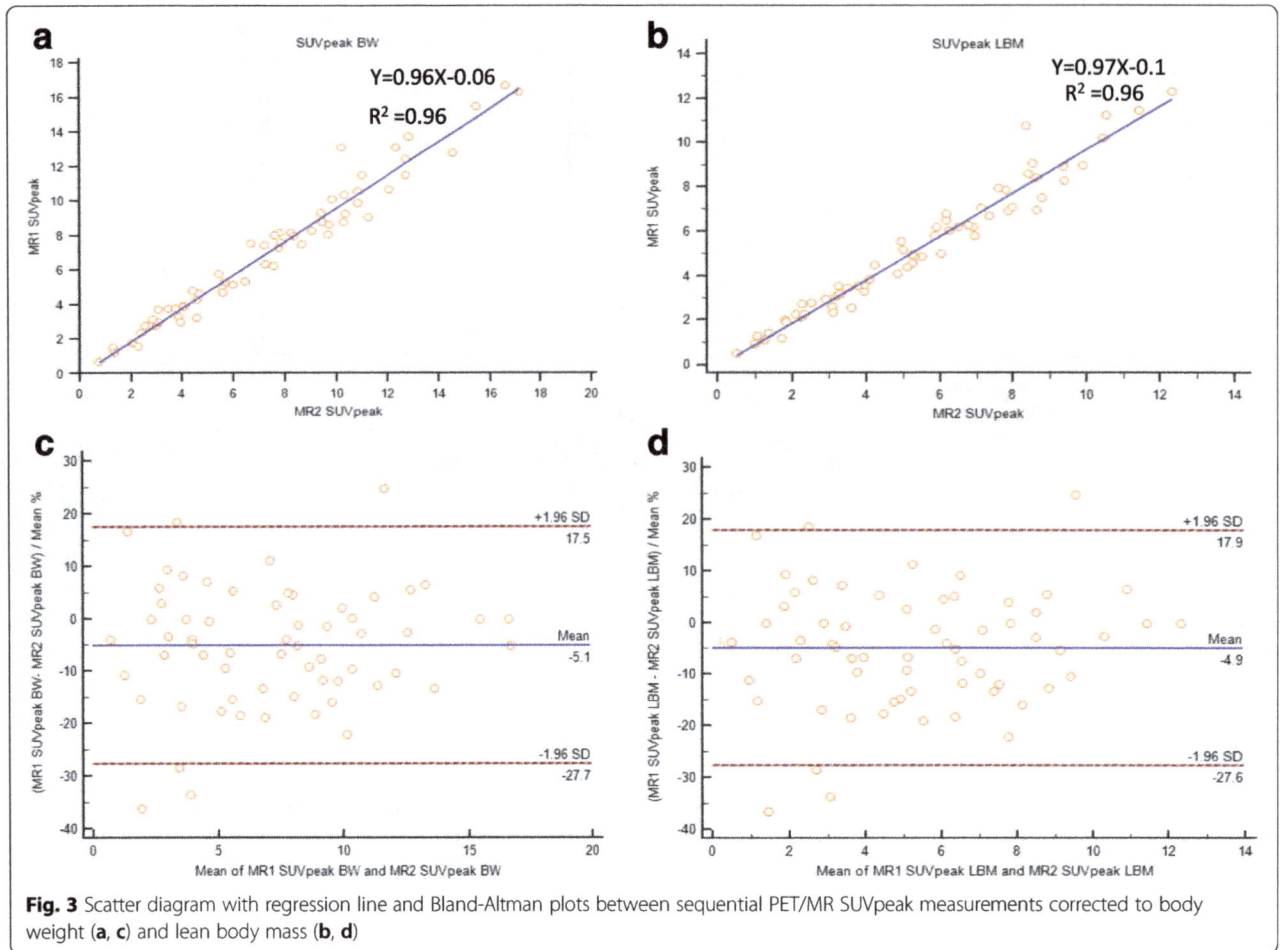

Fig. 3 Scatter diagram with regression line and Bland-Altman plots between sequential PET/MR SUVpeak measurements corrected to body weight (**a**, **c**) and lean body mass (**b**, **d**)

Table 4 Lower and upper 95% limits of agreement and mean difference expressed as percentages for lesional SUV max, peak and mean corrected to BW and LBM

		Mean difference (%)	Limits of agreement (%)	
			Lower	Upper
PET/CT vs PET/MR				
Corrected to BW	SUVmax	7	−43.7	57.7
	SUVpeap	13.9	−27.3	55
	SUVmean	8.3	−41.1	57.6
Corrected to LBM	SUVmax	36.1	−17.2	89.3
	SUVpeak	13.7	−27.3	54.7
	SUVmean	8.4	−40.6	57.4
PET/MR vs PET/MR				
Corrected to BW	SUVmax	−7.4	−36.8	22
	SUVpeak	−5.1	−27.7	17.5
	SUVmean	−10.5	−41.8	20.7
Corrected to LBM	SUVmax	−7.2	−36.7	22.4
	SUVpeak	−4.9	−27.6	17.9
	SUVmean	−10.6	−41.5	20.4

have also shown that PET/MR SUVmax and SUVmean were higher in primary lesions, lymph nodes and distant metastases in the range of 34 and 21%, respectively. On the contrary, Wiesmuller et al. [6] has shown a decrease of 22% and 10% in SUVmax and SUVmean, respectively. In all studies, patients underwent PET/CT followed by PET/MR on the same day. One major assumed factor that may have influenced these results is the time interval from the radiotracer injection to scanning that was longer for PET/MR in those studies. In order to reduce the effect of injection to scan time interval we randomized the order of studies. We found good correlation of PET metrics between PET/CT and PET/MR but a wide range of limits was demonstrated on Bland-Altman plots which is considered to be clinically unaccepted.

Repeatability between two sequential PET/MR

We found strong positive correlation for all PET metrics with clinically acceptable agreement only for lesional SUV/Lpeak. This is in accordance with Rasmussen et al. [16] who found 95% limits of agreement ranging from -12.5 to 20.4 for the different lesional SUV between two PET/MR that lies within a clinically acceptable range. A

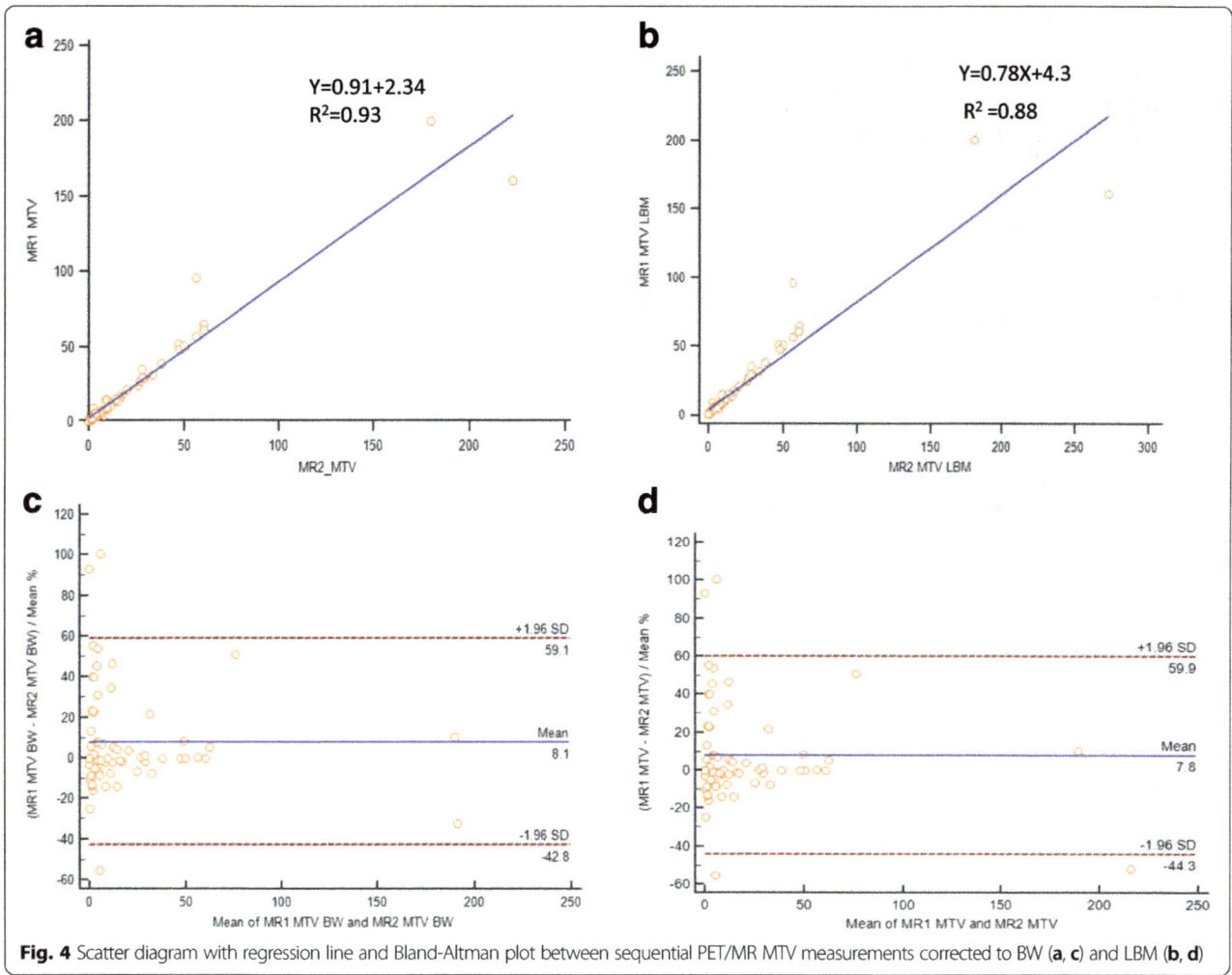

Fig. 4 Scatter diagram with regression line and Bland-Altman plot between sequential PET/MR MTV measurements corrected to BW (**a, c**) and LBM (**b, d**)

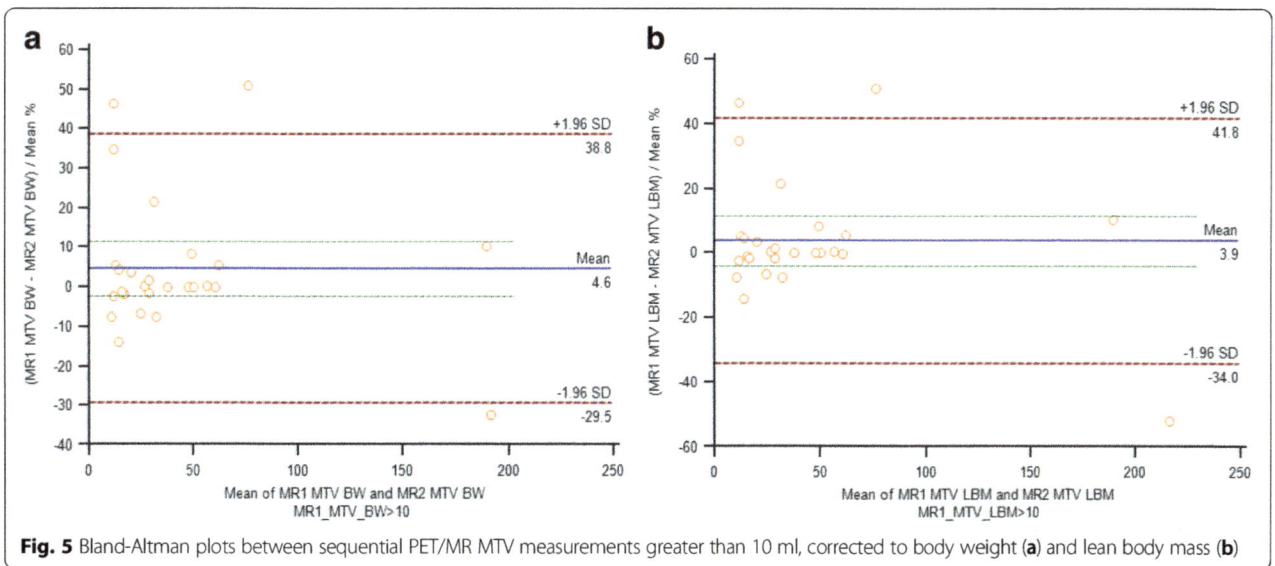

Fig. 5 Bland-Altman plots between sequential PET/MR MTV measurements greater than 10 ml, corrected to body weight (**a**) and lean body mass (**b**)

similar repeatability performance of PET/CT lesional FDG uptake was found in a meta-analysis performed by Langen et al. [17] for which 25% and 20% were found to be the limits for SUVmax and SUVmean, respectively.

Volumetric parameters have gained increasingly interest as prognostic factors for various cancers [18]. However, to date, only few studies have focused on MTV repeatability. We found a strong linear correlation of lesional MTV corrected to BW and LBM between PET/CT and PET/MR and between two sequential PET/MR. However, the range of 95% limits of agreement was far beyond the clinically acceptable range. Our findings are in accordance with several studies. For example, Fring et al. [19] demonstrated a repeatability range for metabolic tumor volume between two PET/CT up to 37% in non-small cell tumors greater than 4.2 ml and a range of 36% for gastrointestinal tumors [20]. Rasmussen et al. [16] found similar range between two PET/CT for head and neck squamous cell carcinoma. Interestingly, they found that the range between two PET/MR was lower than 30%. We have found similar results after exclusion of tumors with volume less than 10ml (Fig. 5).

We believe that there are two strength points in our study. First, randomization of the order of studies reduces the effect of the time interval from the radiotracer injection to scanning which has an effect on FDG uptake in lesions. Second, performing sequential PET/MR studies on the same day evaluates scanner performance with minimal effect of factors that are seen in longer interval that may influence reliability such as changes in body habitus, changes in tissues and lesional texture as a result of therapy.

Our study has several limitations. First, the number of patients is relatively small. Second, lesions determination relied on imaging findings and not on histopathology or follow up studies. Third, image analyses were performed by a single reader although with extensive experience and meticulous assessment of studies. Fourth, PET acquisition time was different between PET/CT and PET/MR which may affect SUV measurements. This, however, resembles reality where PET acquisition time in PET/MR is determined by the length of MR sequences and is longer than PET/CT.

Conclusions

PET/MR SUV/L peak has a clinically acceptable repeatability performance and can be used to evaluate the response to treatment. PET/MR MTV measurements have a larger limit range that is inversely related to the volume of the lesion. Further studies are warranted to evaluate the reproducibility and repeatability of other imaging systems and to consolidate our findings.

Abbreviations

BW: Body weight; CTAC: PET/CT attenuation correction; FDG: Fluorine 18 fluorodeoxyglucose; FS: Fat suppression; HASTE: Half-fourier acquisition single shot turbo spin echo; IR: Inversion recovery; LBM: Lean body mass; MRAC: PET/MR attenuation correction; MTV: Metabolic tumor volume; OSEM: Ordered subset expectation maximization; SUL: SUV for lean body mass; SUV: SUV for body weight; T/L: Tumor to liver ratio; VIBE: Volumetric interpolated breath-hold examination; VOI: Volume of interest

Acknowledgements

NA.

Funding

NA.

Authors' contributions

DG—Study conception and design, Analysis and interpretation of data, Drafting of manuscript, Critical revision. HB—Study conception and design, Acquisition of data, Analysis and interpretation of data. NG—Acquisition of data, Drafting of manuscript. MN and DS—Study conception and design, Analysis and interpretation of data. IAK—Study conception and design, Drafting of manuscript. LD—Study conception and design, Acquisition of data, Analysis and interpretation of data, Drafting of manuscript, Critical revision. All authors read and approved the final manuscript.

Competing interests

The authors declare that they have no competing interests.

Author details

[1]Department of Nuclear Medicine, Assuta Medical Center, 20 habarzel st., 6971028 Tel-Aviv, Israel. [2]Sackler Faculty of Medicine, Tel Aviv University, Tel-Aviv, Israel.

References

1. Quick HH, von Gall C, Zeilinger M, et al. Integrated whole-body PET/MR hybrid imaging: clinical experience. Invest Radiol. 2013;48:280–9.
2. Cheson BD. Staging and response assessment in lymphomas: the new Lugano classification. Chin Clin Oncol. 2015;4:5.
3. Li X, Heber D, Rausch I, et al. Quantitative assessment of atherosclerotic plaques on (18)F-FDG PET/MRI: comparison with a PET/CT hybrid system. Eur J Nucl Med Mol Imaging. 2016;43(8):1503–12.
4. Teuho J, Johansson J, Liden J, et al. Effect of attenuation correction on regional quantification between PET/MR and PET/CT: a multicentr study using a 3-dimensional brain phantom. J Nucl Med. 2016;57:818–24.
5. Schwenzer NF, Schraml C, Müller M, Brendle C, Sauter A, Spengler W, Pfannenberg AC, Claussen CD, Schmidt H. Pulmonary lesion assessment: comparison of whole-body hybrid MR/PET and PET/CT imaging–pilot study. Radiology. 2012;264:551–8.
6. Wiesmüller M, Quick HH, Navalpakkam B, Lell MM, Uder M, Ritt P, Schmidt D, Beck M, Kuwert T, von Gall CC. Comparison of lesion detection and quantitation of tracer uptake between PET from a simultaneously acquiring whole-body PET/MR hybrid scanner and PET from PET/CT. Eur J Nucl Med Mol Imaging. 2013;40:12–21.
7. Tian J, Fu L, Yin D, Zhang J, Chen Y, An N, Xu B. Does the novel integrated PET/MRI offer the same diagnostic performance as PET/CT for oncological indications? PLoS One. 2014;9:e90844.
8. Al-Nabhani KZ, Syed R, Michopoulou S, Alkalbani J, Afaq A, Panagiotidis E, O'Meara C, Groves A, Ell P, Bomanji J. Qualitative and quantitative comparison of PET/CT and PET/MR imaging in clinical practice. J Nucl Med. 2014;55:88–94.

9. Varoquaux A, Rager O, Poncet A, Delattre BMA, Ratib O, Becker CD, Dulguerov P, Dulguerov N, Zaidi H, Becker M. Detection and quantification of focal uptake in head and neck tumours: (18)F-FDG PET/MR versus PET/CT. Eur J Nucl Med Mol Imaging. 2014;41:462–75.

10. Ripa RS, Knudsen A, Hag AMF, Lebech A-M, Loft A, Keller SH, Hansen AE, von Benzon E, Højgaard L, Kjær A. Feasibility of simultaneous PET/MR of the carotid artery: first clinical experience and comparison to PET/CT. Am J Nucl Med Mol Imaging. 2013;3:361–71.

11. Eiber M, Takei T, Souvatzoglou M, et al. Performance of whole-body integrated 18F-FDG PET/MR in comparison to PET/CT for evaluation of malignant bone lesions. J Nucl Med. 2014;55:191–7.

12. Drzezga A, Souvatzoglou M, Eiber M, et al. First clinical experience with integrated whole-body PET/MR: comparison to PET/CT in patients with oncologic diagnoses. J Nucl Med. 2012;53:845–55.

13. Pace L, Nicolai E, Luongo A, Aiello M, Catalano OA, Soricelli A, Salvatore M. Comparison of whole-body PET/CT and PET/MRI in breast cancer patients: lesion detection and quantitation of 18F-deoxyglucose uptake in lesions and in normal organ tissues. Eur J Radiol. 2014;83:289–96.

14. Karlberg AM, Sæther O, Eikenes L, Goa PE. Quantitative comparison of PET performance-Siemens Biograph mCT and mMR. EJNMMI Phys. 2016;3:5.

15. Wahl RL, Jacene H, Kasamon Y, Lodge MA. From RECIST to PERCIST: Evolving Considerations for PET response criteria in solid tumors. J Nucl Med. 2009;50 Suppl 1:122S–50S.

16. Rasmussen JH, Fischer BM, Aznar MC, et al. Reproducibility of (18)F-FDG PET uptake measurements in head and neck squamous cell carcinoma on both PET/CT and PET/MR. Br J Radiol. 2015;88:20140655.

17. de Langen AJ, Vincent A, Velasquez LM, et al. Repeatability of 18F-FDG uptake measurements in tumors: a metaanalysis. J Nucl Med. 2012;53:701–8.

18. Domachevsky L, Groshar D, Galili R, Saute M, Bernstine H. Survival Prognostic Value of Morphological and Metabolic variables in Patients with Stage I and II Non-Small Cell Lung Cancer. Eur Radiol. 2015;25:3361–7.

19. Frings V, de Langen AJ, Smit EF, van Velden FHP, Hoekstra OS, van Tinteren H, Boellaard R. Repeatability of metabolically active volume measurements with 18F-FDG and 18F-FLT PET in non-small cell lung cancer. J Nucl Med. 2010;51:1870–7.

20. Frings V, van Velden FHP, Velasquez LM, Hayes W, van de Ven PM, Hoekstra OS, Boellaard R. Repeatability of metabolically active tumor volume measurements with FDG PET/CT in advanced gastrointestinal malignancies: a multicenter study. Radiology. 2014;273:539–48.

11

CT-perfusion measurements in pancreatic carcinoma with different kinetic models: Is there a chance for tumour grading based on functional parameters?

Sven Schneeweiß[†], Marius Horger[†], Anja Grözinger, Konstantin Nikolaou, Dominik Ketelsen, Roland Syha and Gerd Grözinger[*]

Abstract

Background: To evaluate the interchangeability of perfusion parameters obtained with help of models used for post-processing of perfusion-CT images in pancreatic adenocarcinoma and to determine the mean values and ranges of perfusion in different tumour gradings.

Methods: Perfusion-CT imaging was performed prospectively in 48 consecutive patients with pancreatic adenocarcinoma. In 42 patients biopsy-proven tumor grading was available (4 × G1/24 × G2/14 × G3/6× unknown). Images were post-processed using a model based on the maximum-slope (MS) approach (blood flow-BFMS) + Patlak analysis (P) (blood volume [BVP] and permeability [k-transP]), as well as a model with deconvolution-based (D) analysis (BFD, BVD and k-transD). 50 mL contrast agent were applied with a delay time of 7 s. Perfusion parameters were compared using intraclass correlation coefficient (ICC), the Wilcoxon matched-pairs test and Bland-Altman plots.

Results: Forty eight VOIs of tumours were outlined and analysed. Moderate to good ICC values were found for the perfusion parameters (ICC = 0.62–0.75). Wilcoxon matched-pairs revealed significantly lower values ($P < .001$ and 0.008), for the BF and BV values obtained using the maximum-slope approach + Patlak analysis compared to deconvolution based analysis. For k-trans measurement, deconvolution revealed significantly lower values ($P < 0.001$). Different histologic subgroups (G1-G3) did not show significantly different functional parameters.

Conclusion: There were significant differences in the perfusion parameters obtained using the different calculation methods, and therefore these parameters are not directly interchangeable. However, the magnitude of pairs of parametric values is in constant relation to each other enabling the use of any of these methods. VPCT parameters did not allow for histologic classification.

Keywords: Pancreatic carcinoma, Volume perfusion-CT, Kinetic calculation models, Grading

Background

Pancreatic cancer is one of the leading malignancies of the digestive tract [1]. It also has the poorest prognosis of all gastro-intestinal cancers. Over the last decades, there has been a continuous increase in diagnosed patients in Western industrialized nations. Only 2% of annually diagnosed patients outlive the following 5 years [2]. The most common pancreatic cancer is the adenocarcinoma of the pancreatic head [1]. Tumour characterization and accurate delineation is essential for staging and preoperative planning, as in addition to TNM staging, the degree of malignancy, called tumour grading is a decisive parameter of survival [3, 4]. So far, tumour grading is done histologically, which requires invasive biopsy sampling. Hence the development of a non-invasive method of tumour grading would be highly desirable.

Volume perfusion CT (VPCT) is a relatively new modality that has been increasingly used for oncologic

* Correspondence: gerd.groezinger@med.uni-tuebingen
[†]Equal contributors
Department of Diagnostic Radiology, Eberhard-Karls-University,
Hoppe-Seyler-Str.3, 72076 Tübingen, Germany

imaging over the last years [5]. Based on repetitive scanning of a tissue volume after contrast injection, VPCT enables the measurement of functional parameters of tumour vascularity like blood flow (BF), blood volume (BV) and the permeability of capillaries (permeability surface area product, or k-trans).

Recent studies show the capability of perfusion CT to evaluate tumour vascularization and monitor chemotherapy, radiation therapy or even effect of novel functional drugs affecting tumour environment and angiogenesis [6–10]. One preliminary study suggested that even a non-invasive tumour grading with VPCT might be possible in the case of pancreatic adenocarcinoma [6].

There are different calculation methods for the post-processing of perfusion-CT images: the compartment analysis assuming one (maximum slope) or two compartments (Patlak) and the deconvolution analysis. In other tumour tissues, several studies have already demonstrated significant differences in the calculated perfusion values between the different mathematical models [11–13].

For this purpose, reliability of CT-perfusion data is imperative. Besides an optimized CT-examinational protocol, standardization of perfusion quantification methods (post-processing) is essential, as well as knowledge about comparability of results using these different mathematical methods for perfusion calculation.

However, for reproducibility of studies and for determining cut-off values it is important to know if the different models deliver comparable results. For this reason this study explored for pancreas adenocarcinoma to which extent both models (maximum slope + Patlak and deconvolution) are comparable and if these functional parameters allow for a reliable tumour grading.

Methods
Clinical data
Inclusion criteria for the VPCT study were: Patients with suspicion of pancreatic cancer before treatment who agreed to take part in this study after informed consent. Exclusion criteria for VPCT were: Poor kidney function (GFR < 45 ml/min), pregnancy, allergy to contrast agent or iodine and incompliant patient unable to hold their breath.

Between September 2011 and November 2014, a total of 48 patients (28 male, 20 female; mean age: 69 ± 9 years, range: 39–84, respectively) were eligible for VPCT data analysis and prospectively enrolled in the study. In 42 of these patients, histologic data was available. In 4 cases patients refused a biopsy. In two cases, the biopsy did not contain sufficient diagnostic specimen for the pathologist. However, in time diagnosis of pancreatic cancer could be clearly made due to the presence of tumour markers and available imaging.

VPCT of the entire pancreas was performed. All biopsy specimens were examined by a pathologist and graded according to the AJCC Classification [14] and as described by Hruban et al.[15].

CT Perfusion scanning technique
All examinations were performed on a 128-row CT scanner (Somatom Definition AS+, Siemens Healthcare, Forchheim, *Germany*). The CT protocol consisted of a non-enhanced abdominal low-dose CT (NECT) (40 mAs, 100 kV, 5.0 mm slice thickness, collimation 128*0.6 mm, tube rotation time 0.5 s, pitch 0.6), which was obtained to localize the pancreas. Subsequently, a VPCT of the tumour using adaptive spiral scanning technique was performed. In the adaptive spiral mode the z-range is scanned continuously with a shuttle movement of the patient table. Perfusion parameters were: 80 kV, 100/120mAs (for patients </> 70 kg, respectively), collimation 64 × 0.6 mm with z-flying focal spot (Z coverage 6.9 cm) and 26 CT-whole coverages of the pancreas within a total scan time of 40s. Patients were asked to resume shallow breathing for the entire duration of the study. 50 ml Ultravist 370 (Bayer Vital Leverkusen, Germany) were injected at a flow rate of 5 mL/s in an antecubital vein followed by a saline flush of 50 ml NaCl at 5 mL/s, and a fixed start delay of 7 s. Contrast medium was administered by using a dual-head pump injector (Stellant, Medtron, Saarbruecken, Germany). One set of axial images with a slice thickness of 3 mm for perfusion analysis was reconstructed without overlap, using a smooth tissue convolution kernel (B10f). All images were transferred to an external workstation (Multi-Modality Workplace, Siemens) for analysis. The mean effective whole-body dose values for VPCT examinations of the pancreas are estimated 7.0 mSv for men and 7.1 for women [16].

CT Perfusion analysis
All data sets were transferred to a dedicated workstation (Syngo MMWP, VE 36A, Siemens Healthcare, Forchheim, Germany) and quantitative data evaluation was performed with a commercial software (Syngo Volume Perfusion CT Body). Automated motion correction and noise reduction of all datasets were applied by using an integrated motion correction algorithm with non-rigid deformable registration for anatomic alignment. A circular region of interest (ROI) was placed in the abdominal aorta, which provided the arterial input function for the computations. A second volume of interest (VOI) was placed in the pancreatic carcinoma for calculating the tumour perfusion. The VOI were chosen as large as possible and placed to avoid vessels and artefacts in a slice by slice approach (Fig. 1). For perfusion calculation we used two mathematical calculation methods (models): Compartmental analytic models (maximum slope (BFMS) + Patlak analysis

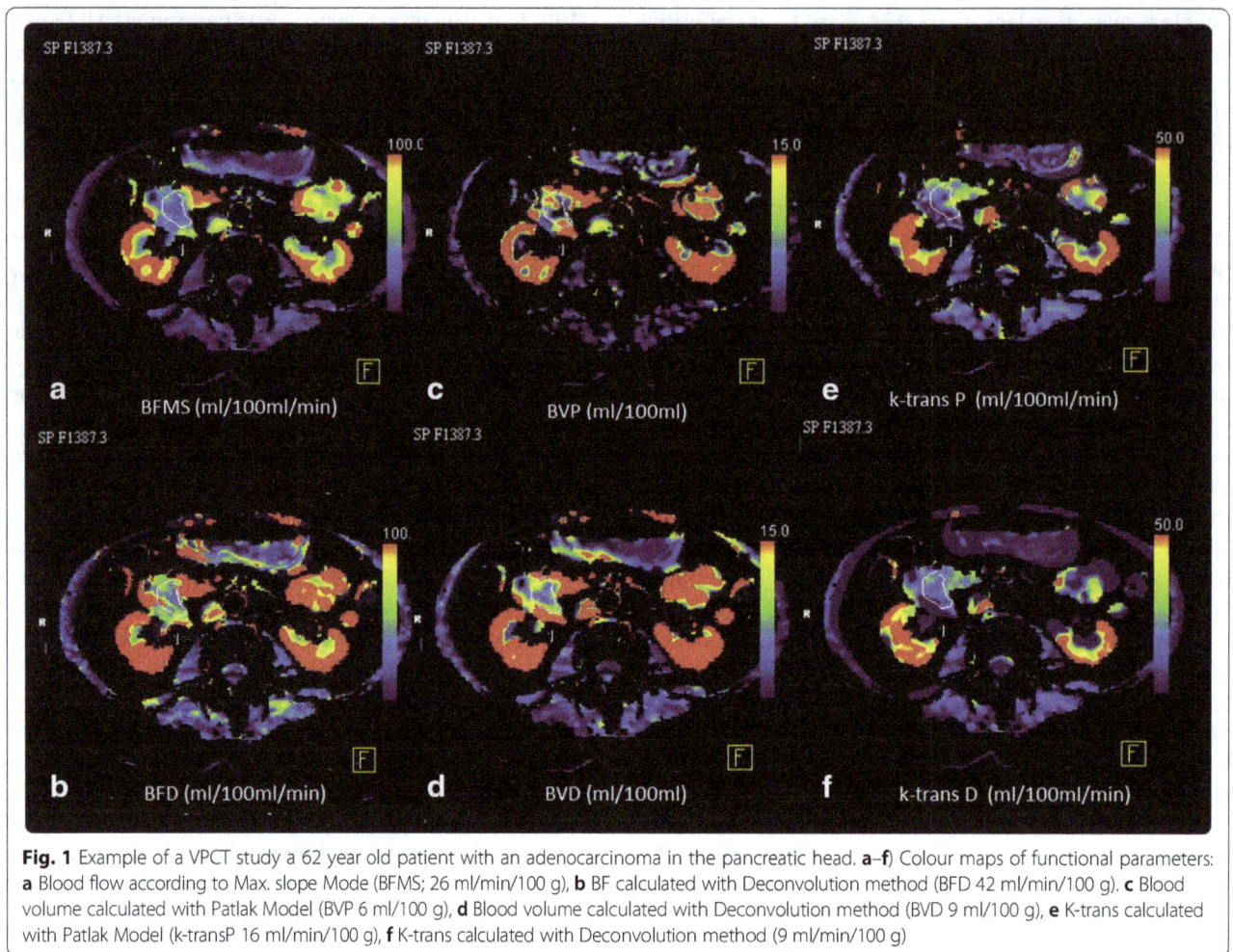

Fig. 1 Example of a VPCT study a 62 year old patient with an adenocarcinoma in the pancreatic head. **a–f)** Colour maps of functional parameters: **a** Blood flow according to Max. slope Mode (BFMS; 26 ml/min/100 g), **b** BF calculated with Deconvolution method (BFD 42 ml/min/100 g). **c** Blood volume calculated with Patlak Model (BVP 6 ml/100 g), **d** Blood volume calculated with Deconvolution method (BVD 9 ml/100 g), **e** K-trans calculated with Patlak Model (k-transP 16 ml/min/100 g), **f** K-trans calculated with Deconvolution method (9 ml/min/100 g)

(BVP, k-transP) vs. deconvolution model (BFD, BVD and k-transD). These two different kinetic calculation software programs used are both FDA approved and are part of the post-processing software recommended by the vendor. Perfusion parameters (BF, BV and k-trans) of both models were compared.

Statistical analysis

Statistical calculation was performed using JMP 11 (SAS Institute, Cary NC, USA) and SPSS 23 (Chicago, IL, USA). Mean values of BF, BV and k-trans as well as of their standard deviations (SD) are reported. Differences between the functional parameters were compared using the Wilcoxon matched-pairs test and Bland-Altman plots. Second, the mean difference, SD of the differences and the 95% limits of agreement (mean difference $-2 \times$ SD and mean difference $+2 \times$ SD) were calculated for each of the perfusion parameters. If Bland-Altman plots showed a linear relation a linear regression analysis was performed. Statistical significance was established at a P value <0.05.

Agreement between the different perfusion measures was assessed using the intra-class correlation coefficient

(ICC) as discussed by Shrout and Fleiss [17]. A value close to 1 indicates excellent agreement between the two readings. Additionally the Pearson's linear correlation coefficient was calculated for the corresponding functional parameter values obtained with the different methods. Parameters for different histological grading were compared using an ANOVA analysis.

Results and discussion

Forty eight Patients (28 men, 20 women, mean age: 69, range: 49–85 years) with untreated pancreatic adenocarcinoma were outlined and analysed. In total 28/48 tumours were localized in the head, 10/48 in the corpus and 10/48 in the pancreatic tail. In 42 patients biopsy-proven pathologic tumour grading was available (4 G1, 24 G2, 14 G3). The mean tumour size (measured the largest diameter) was 4.0 cm (range: 1.7–8.1 cm).

The calculated values of the *blood flow* (mL/100 g tissue/') in the compartment analysis (maximum slope, BFMS) were significantly lower than the calculated values in the deconvolution (BFD) method, with values of 20.4 ± 9.7 ml/min/100 g (range: 1.6–48.22 ml/min/100 g) in the maximum slope respectively 36.9 ± 16.0 ml/min/100 g (range: 5.54–68.61 ml/min/100 g) in the deconvolution method ($p < 0.004$) (Table 1).

The calculations of *blood volume* (BVMS vs. BVD) (mL/100 g tissue) showed similar results, with significantly higher values in the deconvolution method ($p = 0.004$). We calculated a mean blood volume value of 5.6 ± 5.5 ml/100 g (range: 0.81–25.71 ml/100 g) with the compartment analysis (Patlak analysis), whereas the deconvolution method yielded a mean value of 7.3 ± 4.7 ml/100 g (range: 1.56–21.58 ml/100 g). This difference was also significant ($p < 0.001$).

The calculated vessel wall *permeability* (*k-transP* vs. *k-transD*, mL/100 g tissue) showed a different trend. This parameter yielded higher values for the compartment analysis (Patlak analysis) than for the deconvolution method, with values of 18.9 ± 9.8 (range: 4.86–41.77), respectively 12.4 ± 8.2 (range: 0.5–30.34) ($p < 0.001$).

The Bland-Altman plots of the perfusion parameters showed no systematic errors for higher or lower mean values in BV and k-trans (Fig. 2). For BF, Bland-Altman Plots showed a linear relation with higher differences at high absolute values. Subsequent linear regression analysis showed a good linear fit with a resulting slope of 1.5. (Fig. 3a).

Despite significant differences in the calculated perfusion parameters between the different models, moderate to good correlation between the functional perfusion-based parameters with regard to ICC and Pearson's linear correlation coefficient (Table 2 and Fig. 3) were found.

Among the three histological differentiation subgroups (G1-G3), functional parameters did not vary significantly. No functional fingerprints could be established for less differentiated lesions. This was consistent between the mathematical models (Table 3).

CT perfusion imaging is evolving rapidly. Based on a recently published review recommending how to optimize CT-perfusion protocols in the light of current knowledge about strengths and limitations of the available mathematical calculation models and suggesting ways to standardize the state of the art examinational protocols, the aim of the study was to make a comparison of results obtained with the recommended perfusion protocol and available calculation methods and report about the magnitude of obtained perfusion values as well as of their ranges and correlations with the histologic differentiation grade [18].

Our results clearly show that quantification of pancreatic carcinoma perfusion is feasible with the proposed VPCT-examinational protocol and that the measured perfusion values are in line with those reported in previous works dealing with this issue and using comparable perfusion protocols [19]. Moreover, they confirm the knowledge that results of the two used mathematical calculation methods significantly differ from each other and are thus not directly interchangeable, but that the magnitude of their pairs of calculated parametric values stays in constant relation to each other for BV and k-trans values. BF values show a linear relationship with higher values for the deconvolution method and a linear relationship with a slope of 1.5. These differences are systematic differences explainable by the different underlying mathematical models. The Maximum slope model underestimates BF because venous outflow is not considered by the model. This error is proportional to the absolute BF. Accordingly the relation between BFMS and BFD is a constant ratio. The presented cohort comprising 48 cases is currently the largest VPCT series of pancreatic adenocarcinoma. There is a growing amount of data from the literature reporting perfusion values of the pancreas. However this data is very heterogeneous with regard to technical parameters and included subjects. Accordingly literature values are hard to compare. In line with previous reports, in our study, blood flow values were found to be significantly lower when calculated with the compartment model compared to values obtained with the deconvolution method. The same trend was observed also for the measured absolute values of blood volume which proved to be significantly lower when calculated with the compartment model vs. the deconvolution method. Expectedly, the calculated k-trans values were lower for the deconvolution method vs. the two-compartment model (Patlak model). Xu et al. reported blood flow and blood volume values in the tumour tissue of 29.5 ml/min/100 g and 59.72 ml/100 g, respectively, both measured with the deconvolution method [20]. The blood flow value was thus lower in their study, but still in the same range with our deconvolution measured values. However, the blood volume was noticeably higher than in our study (59.7 ml/100 g vs. 7.3 ml/100 g). Similar results were reported also by Klauß et al. who reported BF values for pancreatic

Table 1 Functional VPCT values for adenocarcinomas

Parameter	Max. slope	Patlak	Deconvolution	Mean Difference	95% limits of agreement	p-value[a]
BF (ml/min/100 g)	20.4 ± 9.7		36.9 ± 16.0	16.5 ± 8.9	−0.9;33,9	<0.001
BV (ml/100 g)		5.6 ± 5.5	7.3 ± 4.7	-1.7 ± 4.6	−10.7;7.3	0.004
k-trans (ml/min/100 g)		18.9 ± 9.8	12.4 ± 8.2	6.5 ± 5.8	−4.9;17.9	<0.001

Mean values of functional perfusion parameters for $n = 48$ adenocarcinomas obtained with Maximum slope-, Patlak- and deconvolution models
[a]for Wilcoxon matched-pairs test
Abbreviations: BF blood flow, *BV* blood volume, *G1-3* tumor grading

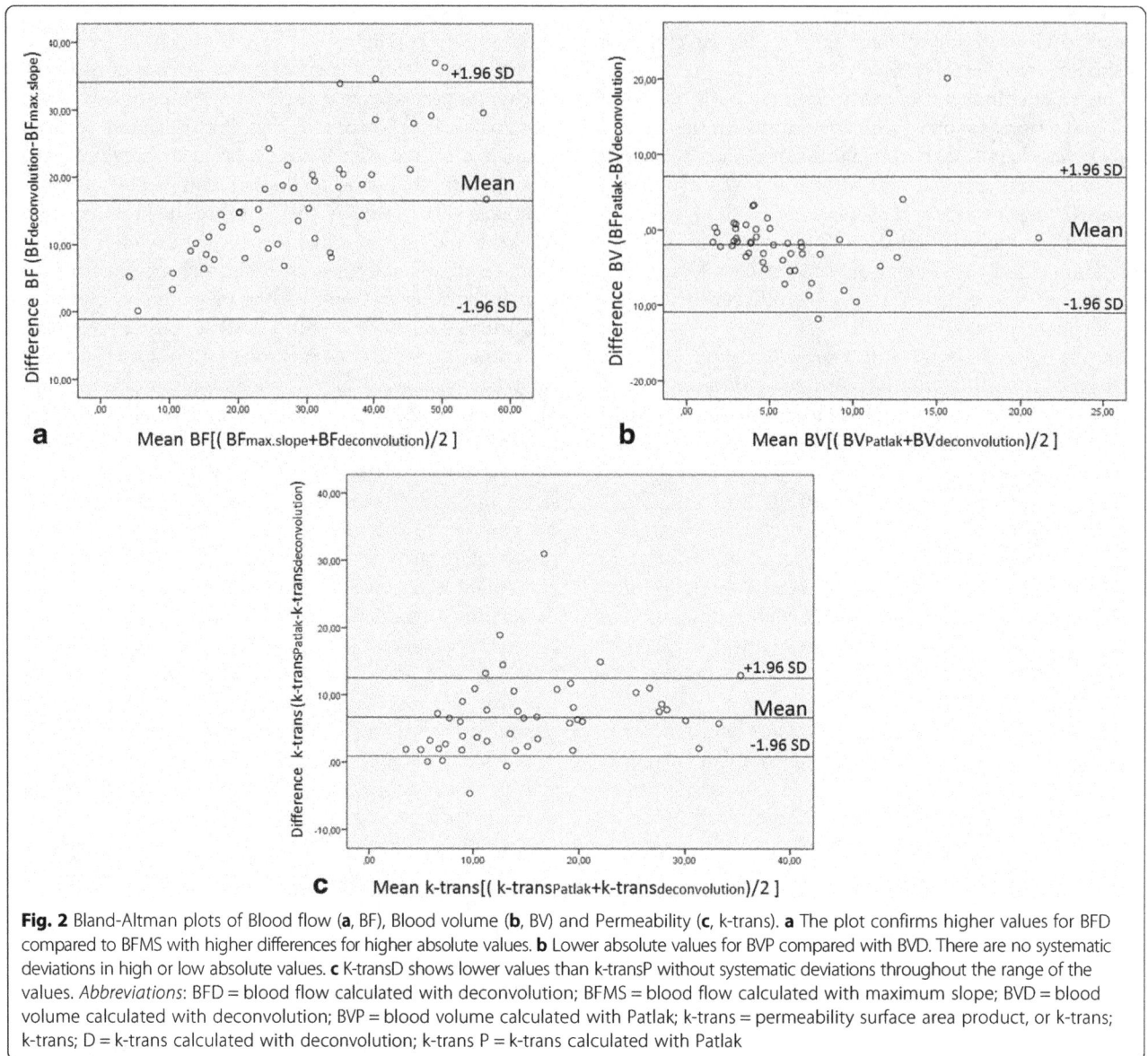

Fig. 2 Bland-Altman plots of Blood flow (**a**, BF), Blood volume (**b**, BV) and Permeability (**c**, k-trans). **a** The plot confirms higher values for BFD compared to BFMS with higher differences for higher absolute values. **b** Lower absolute values for BVP compared with BVD. There are no systematic deviations in high or low absolute values. **c** K-transD shows lower values than k-transP without systematic deviations throughout the range of the values. *Abbreviations*: BFD = blood flow calculated with deconvolution; BFMS = blood flow calculated with maximum slope; BVD = blood volume calculated with deconvolution; BVP = blood volume calculated with Patlak; k-trans = permeability surface area product, or k-trans; k-trans; D = k-trans calculated with deconvolution; k-trans P = k-trans calculated with Patlak

adenocarcinoma calculated with the Patlak analysis that were in the same range with ours; however, calculated BV values proved again significantly higher than in our population (38.9 ml/100 g vs. 5.6 ml/100 g) [21]. These discrepancies highlight the imperative of using robust examinational protocols as well as kinetic calculation

Table 2 Correlation between VPCT parameters obtained with different calculation models

Parameter	ICC	Pearsons r
Blood Flow (BF) (ml/min/100 g)	0.62	0.89
Blood Volume (BV) (ml/100 g)	0.62	0.60
Permeabilty (k-trans) (ml/min/100 g)	0.75	0.80

ICC and Pearson's linear correlation coefficient of the functional parameters obtained with Maximum slope-, Patlak- and deconvolution models
Abbreviations: *BF* blood flow, *BV* blood volume, *G1-3* tumor grading

models. According to our experience, a blood volume significantly higher than the corresponding blood flow is difficult to explain, in particular in a tumour with known desmoplastic stroma and lowered vascularisation. Notably, the data of Klauß et al. was obtained using a dual-energy perfusion protocol. On the contrary, Tan et al. obtained considerably higher BF values 60 ± 15.3 ml/min/100 g using lower temporal resolution during the first pass phase [22]. In particular, in the maximum slope model, temporal resolution between the start of contrast agent administration and the peak enhancement should be kept as high as technical feasible in order to avoid false high miscalculation [18]. Accordingly, the report by Li et al. using a reduced-dose examinational CT-perfusion protocol comparable to ours yielded similar results for BF, BV as well as for k-trans using the Patlak calculation

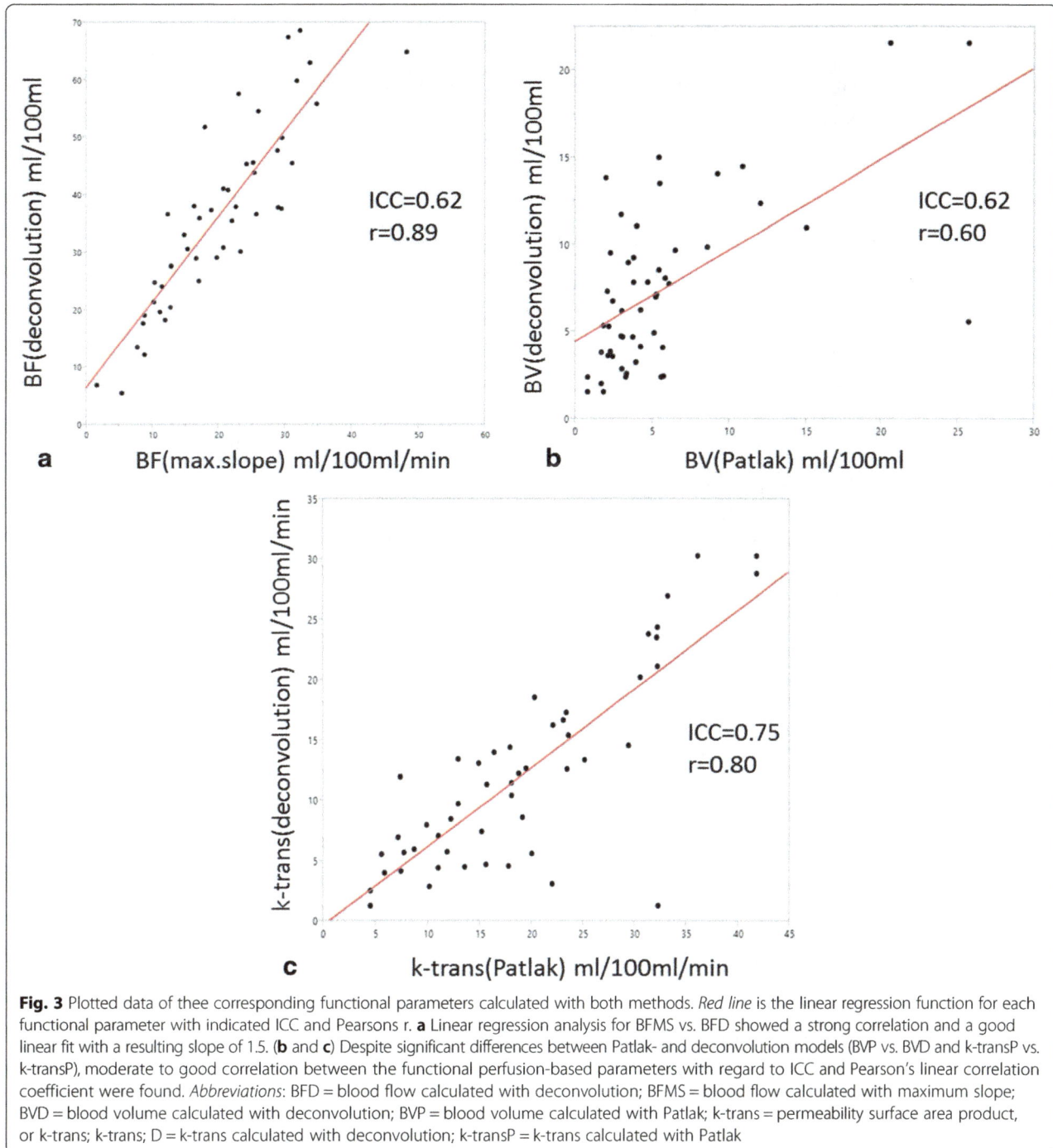

Fig. 3 Plotted data of thee corresponding functional parameters calculated with both methods. *Red line* is the linear regression function for each functional parameter with indicated ICC and Pearsons r. **a** Linear regression analysis for BFMS vs. BFD showed a strong correlation and a good linear fit with a resulting slope of 1.5. (**b** and **c**) Despite significant differences between Patlak- and deconvolution models (BVP vs. BVD and k-transP vs. k-transP), moderate to good correlation between the functional perfusion-based parameters with regard to ICC and Pearson's linear correlation coefficient were found. *Abbreviations*: BFD = blood flow calculated with deconvolution; BFMS = blood flow calculated with maximum slope; BVD = blood volume calculated with deconvolution; BVP = blood volume calculated with Patlak; k-trans = permeability surface area product, or k-trans; k-trans; D = k-trans calculated with deconvolution; k-transP = k-trans calculated with Patlak

model [23]. Another essential aspect with perfusion-CT is that concerning the total examination time. This is in particular essential for the calculation of k-trans. Spira et al. demonstrated significant decrease of BV values and concomitantly significant increase of k-trans-values with progressively shortened measurement time (down to 39 s) in lung carcinomas [24]. Accordingly it can be assumed that difference between k-transD and k-transP is caused partly by the limited scan time.

The use of perfusion-CT in other tumour tissues as reported by several previous studies has already demonstrated significant differences between the different mathematical models [11–13, 25]. A study from Djuric-Stojanovic et al., examining the perfusion parameters of oesophageal carcinoma, yielded a similar tendency with blood flow values showing significantly higher values for the compartmental analysis [13]. Similar to our study on pancreatic lesions, a good correlation for the blood

Table 3 Influence of histologic grading on perfusion parameters

Grading	BF		BV		k-trans	
	Max.slope (BFMS) (ml/min/100 g)	Deconvolution (BFD) (ml/min/100 g)	Patlak (BVP) (ml/100 g)	Deconvolution (BVD) (ml/100 g)	Patlak (k-transP) (ml/min/100 g)	Deconvolution (k-transD) (ml/min/100 g)
G1 (n = 4)	20.6 ± 8.6	33.5 ± 10.3	8.9 ± 11.3	6.4 ± 1.3	19.3 ± 4.5	11.5 ± 6.4
G2 (n = 24)	21.9 ± 10.4	37.7 ± 16.6	5.5 ± 4.5	7.9 ± 5.0	21.0 ± 10.2	13.7 ± 8.8
G3 (n = 14)	19.1 ± 8.4	35.6 ± 13.9	3.9 ± 2.4	6.1 ± 3.9	17.4 ± 8.7	11.9 ± 7.4
p-value (ANOVA)	0.71	0.94	0.42	0.68	0.55	0.71

Influence of histologic grading on perfusion parameters in n = 42 patients with histologic grading available
Abbreviations: BF blood flow, BV blood volume, G1-3 tumor grading

volume between the compartment- and the deconvolution model has also been shown for malignancy in the lung (0.86), spleen (0.9) and brain (0.79) [26].

It has been suggested that perfusion-based tumour characterisation could be a non-invasive tumour grading method in pancreatic adenocarcinoma [6, 27]. This is a highly interesting topic as tumour grading is a very important prognostic factor in patients suffering from pancreatic carcinoma [3]. However despite using a similar protocol, in the present study none of the applied models based on perfusion parameters proved able to reliably discriminate between degrees of tumour differentiation. However, even in this respect, the studies are not directly comparable as the applied parameters Peak Enhancement Intensity (PEI) which indicates the peak attenuation reached by the tissue after contrast media injection and BV vs. BF, BV and k-trans and the histologic subdivisions were different. We believe that in the above mentioned study, the temporal resolution (every 5 s) may have been too low in order to accurately determine the PEI and BF [6]. However, we agree that grading does not seem to be possible if based solely on the parameter BF. The reason for the inconclusiveness of the present data remains unclear. However there are also some concerns with regard to histologic analysis which might have led to these results. At first the histologic specimen is usually very small and limited to a small part of the tumor. It is known that the pancreatic adenocarcinoma consists of several parts of varying dedifferentiation [15]. Accordingly, the histologic specimen might not be representative for the whole tumour. Second, the perfusion values in pancreatic adenocarcinoma are generally very low, sometimes only slightly above noise level. By this, the measurement of relative differences within this group is intrinsically difficult as differences are expected to be very small.

Conclusions

In summary, both perfusion calculation methods seem to be applicable, but cannot be directly compared. Nevertheless, the magnitude of pairs of parametric values is in constant relation to each other enabling the use of any of these methods for clinical trials.

Abbreviations
BF: Blood flow; BFD: Blood flow calculated with deconvolution; BFMS: Blood flow calculated with maximum slope; BV: Blood volume; BVD: Blood volume calculated with deconvolution; BVP: Blood volume calculated with Patlak; ICC: Intraclass correlation coefficient; k-trans: Permeability surface area product, or k-trans; k-transD: k-trans calculated with deconvolution; k-transP: k-trans calculated with Patlak; MS: Maximum-slope; NECT: Non-enhanced abdominal low-dose CT; PA: Patlak analysis; PEI: Peak enhancement; ROI: Region of interest; SD: Standard deviations; VOI: Volume of interest; VPCT: Volume perfusion CT

Acknowledgements
Not applicable.

Funding
There is no funding in connection with this study.

Authors' contributions
SS: Contributed to conception Acquisition of data, Manuscript writing. MH: Development of protocols. Manuscript editing. AG: Acquisition of data. KN: Manuscript editing. RS: Statistical analysis. Manuscript editing. DK: Acquisition of data. Manuscript editing. GG: Statistical analysis, Manuscript editing. All authors read and approved the final manuscript.

Competing interests
The authors declare that they have no conflict of interest or competing interests in connection with the manuscript.

References
1. Schima W, Ba-Ssalamah A, Kolblinger C, Kulinna-Cosentini C, Puespoek A, Gotzinger P. Pancreatic adenocarcinoma. Eur Radiol. 2007;17:638–49.
2. Keane MG, Horsfall LJ, Rait G, Pereira SP. Sociodemographic trends in the incidence of pancreatic and biliary tract cancer in UK primary care. PLoS ONE. 2014;9, e108498.
3. Rochefort MM, Ankeny JS, Kadera BE, Donald GW, Isacoff W, Wainberg ZA, Hines OJ, Donahue TR, Reber HA, Tomlinson JS. Impact of tumor grade on pancreatic cancer prognosis: validation of a novel TNMG staging system. Ann Surg Oncol. 2013;20:4322–9.
4. Wasif N, Ko CY, Farrell J, Wainberg Z, Hines OJ, Reber H, Tomlinson JS. Impact of tumor grade on prognosis in pancreatic cancer: should we include grade in AJCC staging? Ann Surg Oncol. 2010;17:2312–20.
5. Mazzei MA, Squitieri NC, Sani E, Guerrini S, Imbriaco G, Di Lucia D, Guasti A, Mazzei FG, Volterrani L. Differences in perfusion CT parameter values with commercial software upgrades: a preliminary report about algorithm consistency and stability. Acta Radiol. 2013;54:805–11.
6. D'Onofrio M, Gallotti A, Mantovani W, Crosara S, Manfrin E, Falconi M, Ventriglia A, Zamboni GA, Manfredi R, Pozzi Mucelli R. Perfusion CT can predict tumoral grading of pancreatic adenocarcinoma. Eur J Radiol. 2013; 82:227–33.

7. Khan ML, Halfdanarson TR, Borad MJ. Immunotherapeutic and oncolytic viral therapeutic strategies in pancreatic cancer. Future Oncol. 2014;10:1255–75.

8. Silvestris N, Gnoni A, Brunetti AE, Vincenti L, Santini D, Tonini G, Merchionne F, Maiello E, Lorusso V, Nardulli P, et al. Target therapies in pancreatic carcinoma. Curr Med Chem. 2014;21:948–65.

9. Nishikawa Y, Tsuji Y, Isoda H, Kodama Y, Chiba T. Perfusion in the tissue surrounding pancreatic cancer and the patient's prognosis. Biomed Res Int. 2014;2014:648021.

10. Sahani DV, Kalva SP, Hamberg LM, Hahn PF, Willett CG, Saini S, Mueller PR, Lee TY. Assessing tumor perfusion and treatment response in rectal cancer with multisection CT: initial observations. Radiology. 2005;234:785–92.

11. Goh V, Halligan S, Bartram CI. Quantitative tumor perfusion assessment with multidetector CT: are measurements from two commercial software packages interchangeable? Radiology. 2007;242:777–82.

12. Bisdas S, Konstantinou G, Surlan-Popovic K, Khoshneviszadeh A, Baghi M, Vogl TJ, Koh TS, Mack MG. Dynamic contrast-enhanced CT of head and neck tumors: comparison of first-pass and permeability perfusion measurements using two different commercially available tracer kinetics models. Acad Radiol. 2008;15:1580–9.

13. Djuric-Stefanovic A, Saranovic D, Masulovic D, Ivanovic A, Pesko P. Comparison between the deconvolution and maximum slope 64-MDCT perfusion analysis of the esophageal cancer: is conversion possible? Eur J Radiol. 2013;82:1716–23.

14. AJCC. Cancer Staging Manual. 7tth ed. New York: Springer; 2010.

15. Hruban RH, Fukushima N. Pancreatic adenocarcinoma: update on the surgical pathology of carcinomas of ductal origin and PanINs. Mod Pathol. 2007;20 Suppl 1:S61–70.

16. Ketelsen D, Horger M, Buchgeister M, Fenchel M, Thomas C, Boehringer N, Schulze M, Tsiflikas I, Claussen CD, Heuschmid M. Estimation of radiation exposure of 128-slice 4D-perfusion CT for the assessment of tumor vascularity. Korean J Radiol. 2010;11:547–52.

17. Shrout PE, Fleiss JL. Intraclass correlations: uses in assessing rater reliability. Psychol Bull. 1979;86:420–8.

18. Klotz E, Haberland U, Glatting G, Schoenberg SO, Fink C, Attenberger U, Henzler T. Technical prerequisites and imaging protocols for CT perfusion imaging in oncology. Eur J Radiol. 2015;84:2359–67.

19. Kandel S, Kloeters C, Meyer H, Hein P, Hilbig A, Rogalla P. Whole-organ perfusion of the pancreas using dynamic volume CT in patients with primary pancreas carcinoma: acquisition technique, post-processing and initial results. Eur Radiol. 2009;19:2641–6.

20. Xu J, Liang Z, Hao S, Zhu L, Ashish M, Jin C, Fu D, Ni Q. Pancreatic adenocarcinoma: dynamic 64-slice helical CT with perfusion imaging. Abdom Imaging. 2009;34:759–66.

21. Klauss M, Stiller W, Pahn G, Fritz F, Kieser M, Werner J, Kauczor HU, Grenacher L. Dual-energy perfusion-CT of pancreatic adenocarcinoma. Eur J Radiol. 2013;82:208–14.

22. Tan Z, Miao Q, Li X, Ren K, Zhao Y, Zhao L, Li X, Liu Y, Chai R, Xu K. The primary study of low-dose pancreas perfusion by 640- slice helical CT: a whole-organ perfusion. Springerplus. 2015;4:192.

23. Li HO, Sun C, Xu ZD, Miao F, Zhang DJ, Chen JH, Li X, Wang XM, Liu C, Zhao B. Low-dose whole organ CT perfusion of the pancreas: preliminary study. Abdom Imaging. 2014;39:40–7.

24. Spira D, Gerlach JD, Spira SM, Schulze M, Sauter A, Horger M. Effect of scan time on perfusion and flow extraction product (K-trans) measurements in lung cancer using low-dose volume perfusion CT (VPCT). Acad Radiol. 2012;19:78–83.

25. Kaufmann S, Schulze M, Horger T, Oelker A, Nikolaou K, Horger M. Reproducibility of VPCT parameters in the normal pancreas: comparison of two different kinetic calculation models. Acad Radiol. 2015;22:1099–105.

26. Miles KA, Griffiths MR. Perfusion CT: a worthwhile enhancement? Br J Radiol. 2003;76:220–31.

27. Spira D, Neumeister H, Spira SM, Hetzel J, Spengler W, Von Weyhern CH, Horger M. Assessment of tumor vascularity in lung cancer using volume perfusion CT (VPCT) with histopathologic comparison: a further step toward an individualized tumor characterization. J Comput Assist Tomogr. 2013;37:15–21.

12

Review of targeted therapy in chronic lymphocytic leukemia: what a radiologist needs to know about CT interpretation

Babina Gosangi[1]* (iD), Matthew Davids[2,3], Bhanusupriya Somarouthu[4], Francesco Alessandrino[5], Angela Giardino[6], Nikhil Ramaiya[6] and Katherine Krajewski[6]

Abstract

The last 5 years have been marked by profound innovation in the targeted treatment of chronic lymphocytic leukemia (CLL) and indolent lymphomas. Using CLL as a case study, we present a timeline and overview of the current treatment landscape for the radiologist, including an overview of clinical and radiological features of CLL, discussion of the targeted agents themselves, and the role of imaging in response and toxicity assessment. The goal is to familiarize the radiologist with multiple Food and Drug Administration (FDA)-approved targeted agents used in this setting and associated adverse events which are commonly observed in this patient population.

Keywords: Indolent lymphoma, Chronic lymphocytic leukemia, Targeted therapy, Drug related toxicity

Background

Chronic lymphocytic leukemia (CLL)/ small lymphocytic lymphoma (SLL) is the most prevalent leukemia in older adults in the Western hemisphere, with an estimated 19,000 new cases diagnosed per year in the United States [1]. The treatment landscape of CLL has evolved dramatically in the last 5 years, with the approval of multiple new targeted agents leading to prolonged survival of affected patients. Many of the therapies are also approved by the United States FDA for treatment of other indolent lymphomas, including follicular lymphoma and lymphoplasmacytic lymphoma/ Waldenstrom's macroglobulinemia [2, 3]. Given the sizable population of patients being treated with these agents and the role of imaging in CLL/ lymphoma management, radiologists should gain familiarity with the drugs and especially, imaging manifestations of drug toxicity.

At present, the spectrum of CLL therapy options includes traditional chemotherapies, multiple antibodies (anti-CD20, anti-CD52) as well as small molecule inhibitors (Bruton tyrosine kinase, phosphatidylinositol 3-

kinase, and B cell leukemia/lymphoma-2 inhibitors). In CLL, individualized treatment selection and management decisions are based on the integration of several factors, including genomic assessment, patient co-morbidities and preference, and other factors contributing to prognostication and risk stratification [4]. When patients develop indications for treatment, such as cytopenias, massive or symptomatic splenomegaly or lymphadenopathy, therapeutic agents are generally selected based on patient age, co-morbidities and disease-related biological characteristics [5]. In younger CLL patients with few co-morbidities, chemoimmunotherapy regimens such as fludarabine, cyclophosphamide, and rituximab (FCR) have been standard first-line therapy [6]. In older patients, bendamustine and rituximab (BR), chlorambucil and obinutuzumab, and ibrutinib are all now considered to be reasonable standard first-line therapy options [7]. Other targeted agents have been approved in the relapsed/refractory setting, and several other therapies remain under active investigation.

The magnitude of the economic impact of the available targeted therapies is just starting to manifest [8]. As the targeted agents become more commonly used in both academic and community settings, it is necessary for radiologists to remain abreast of the radical changes in CLL and indolent lymphoma management. In this review, using CLL as a case study, we summarize the

* Correspondence: bgosangi@bwh.harvard.edu
[1]Thoracic Radiology, Brigham and Women's Hospital, 45 Francis Street, Boston, MA 02115, USA
Full list of author information is available at the end of the article

clinical and radiological features of this disease and discuss the various targeted therapies used to treat CLL and other indolent lymphomas, with emphasis on the role of imaging in toxicity assessment.

Chronic Lymphocytic Leukemia (CLL)/ Small Lymphocytic Lymphoma (SLL)

CLL and SLL are most common cancers of the elderly, with an average age of presentation of 71 years [5]. CLL and SLL represent a spectrum of the same disease, with CLL manifesting in the peripheral blood and marrow and defined by $> 5 \times 10^{9}$ monoclonal lymphocytes/L, while SLL manifests predominantly in the lymph nodes and spleen, with $< 5 \times 10^{9}$ monoclonal lymphocytes/L in the blood [4]. The lymph nodes and spleen are involved in both entities, however (Fig. 1), and the prognosis and management of both CLL and SLL is the same.

Patients are commonly referred for evaluation on the basis of peripheral lymphocytosis. Less commonly, patients may present with lymphadenopathy, splenomegaly, frequent infections and/or autoimmune disease. Diagnosis is based on the International Workshop on CLL (iwCLL) 2008 guidelines describing the precise immunophenotype of the blood or marrow lymphocytes, including expression of CD5, CD19, CD20 and usually CD23, among others [5]. Fluorescence in situ hybridization (FISH) is commonly performed, and has important prognostic and predictive power. For example, patients with chromosome 17p deletions and young patients with 11q deletions have been found to have a poorer prognosis as compared to patients with 13q deletion, trisomy 12, or normal FISH [9]. Additional markers with prognostic significance in this disease include presence or absence of somatic mutations of the immunoglobulin heavy chain variable region genes (*IGHV*), expression of the zeta-associated protein 70 (ZAP-70), and somatic mutations of genes such as *TP53*, *NOTCH1*, and *SF3B1* [10, 11]. Older serum markers such as B_2-microglobulin also have retained prognostic significance.

Staging is clinical and is assessed through physical examination and laboratory studies, using the Rai (US) or Binet (Europe) systems [12, 13]. According to NCCN guidelines, imaging is not necessary, but is commonly performed in advanced stage patients (stage III and IV, characterized by anemia and thrombocytopenia, respectively. A study by Muntanola et al. demonstrated that in Rai stage 0 patients, abdominal disease identified on CT was a predictor of progression, highlighting the possible utility of imaging even in early disease [14]. In this study, abnormal CT was defined by lymph nodes in the abdomen measuring > 10 mm in diameter, multiple clustered nodes in an anatomically defined region measuring < 10 mm in diameter, and/or splenomegaly. In practice, imaging in early stage CLL is generally reserved for patients with high risk disease biology, in particular, those with del (17p) or

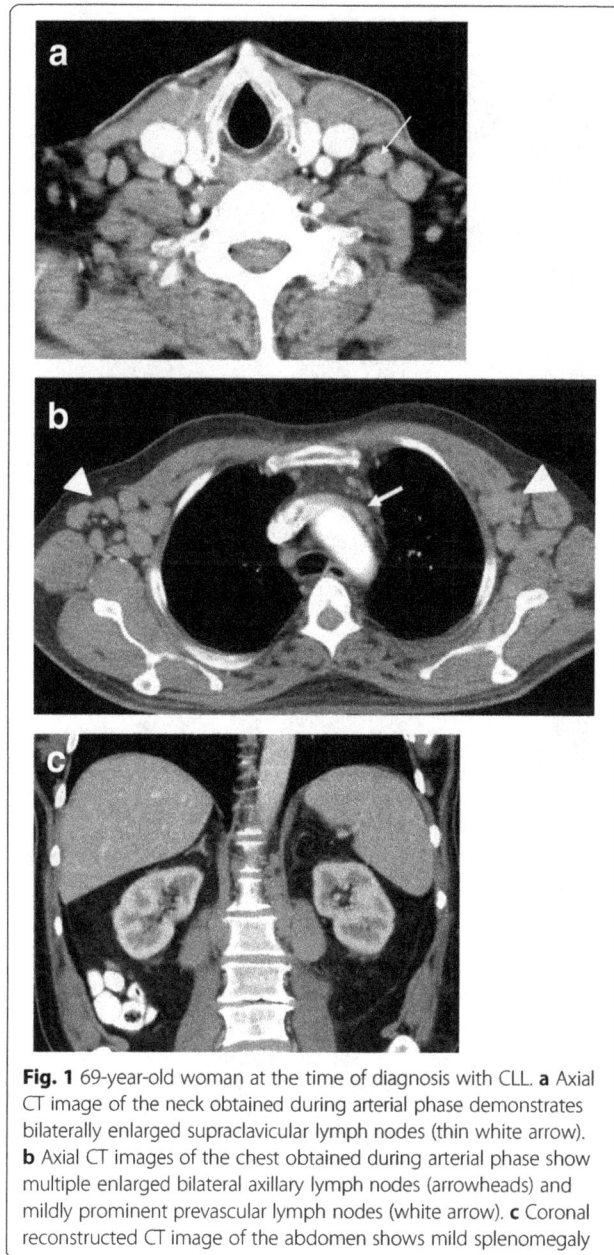

Fig. 1 69-year-old woman at the time of diagnosis with CLL. **a** Axial CT image of the neck obtained during arterial phase demonstrates bilaterally enlarged supraclavicular lymph nodes (thin white arrow). **b** Axial CT images of the chest obtained during arterial phase show multiple enlarged bilateral axillary lymph nodes (arrowheads) and mildly prominent prevascular lymph nodes (white arrow). **c** Coronal reconstructed CT image of the abdomen shows mild splenomegaly

del (11q), who not infrequently can have bulky abdominal lymphadenopathy out of proportion to their palpable lymphadenopathy on physical examination.

Contrast-enhanced CT (CECT) is the imaging modality of choice in CLL/SLL. Most commonly, CLL/SLL patients demonstrate multi-station mildly to moderately enlarged lymph nodes, with or without splenomegaly or hepatomegaly. Bulky nodes and confluent adenopathy is commonly seen during relapses or, as noted above, in patients at presentation with 17p or 11q deletion (Fig. 2) [15, 16]. Rare sites of CLL involvement have been reported, including the central nervous system [17, 18]. PET-CT is not commonly performed in CLL as it is not

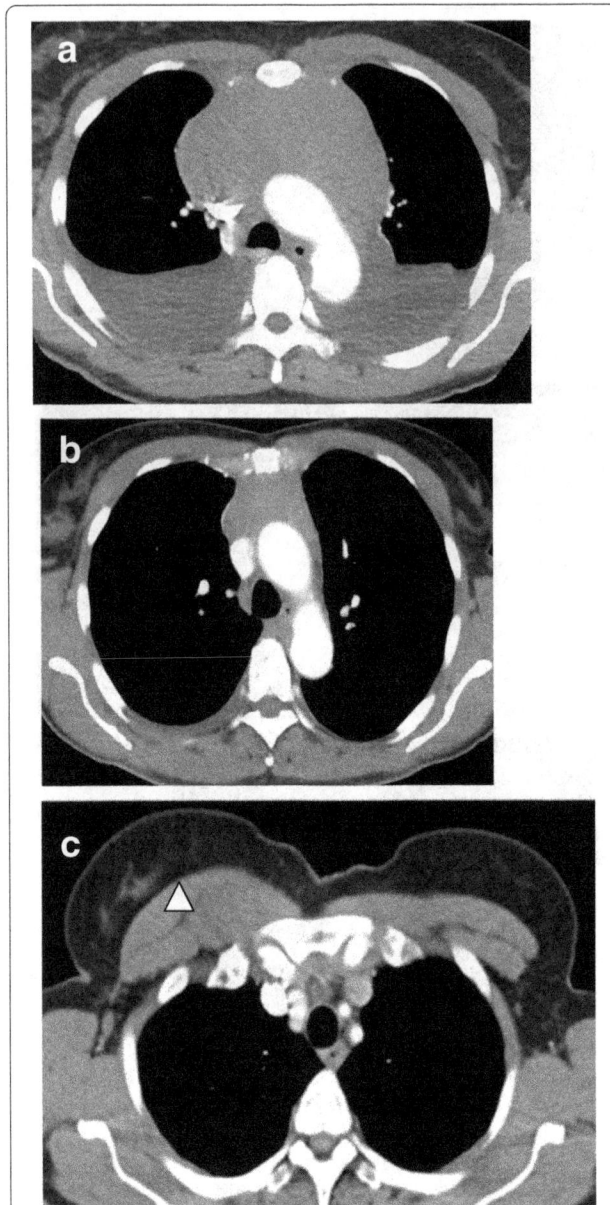

Fig. 2 76-year-old woman with chronic lymphocytic leukemia with 11q deletion and unmutated IGHV. **a** Axial CT images of the chest acquired during arterial phase at the time of initial presentation shows a large anterior mediastinal mass measuring up to 10 cm in its largest dimension with bilateral moderate pleural effusions. **b** Axial CT image of the chest obtained during arterial phase 4 months after initiating R-CHOP demonstrates significant decrease in size of the anterior mediastinal mass and improvement of bilateral pleural effusion. **c** Axial CT image of the chest obtained during arterial phase 4 years later demonstrates a new mass in the right sub pectoral region measuring up to 3.5 cm in its largest dimension suspicious for CLL (arrowheads). The lesion was biopsied and was consistent for recurrence of CLL

development of "B" symptoms (fevers, drenching night sweats, or unintentional weight loss) or markedly elevated serum lactate dehydrogenase (LDH) (Fig. 3). In these situations, PET-CT is helpful in identifying the most FDG-avid site of disease for tissue sampling and diagnosis [19]. Importantly, SUVmax likely reflects tumor aggressiveness, with or without Richter transformation. In one study of over 300CLL patients imaged with PET-CT, SUVmax ≥10 was a useful discriminator of outcomes, associated with median overall survival 6. 9 months compared to patients with SUVmax< 10 and median overall survival 56.7 months [20].

Indications for treatment are defined by the 2008 iwCLL guidelines, including progressive cytopenias, symptomatic or massive splenomegaly or lymphadenopathy, refractory autoimmune disease (usually autoimmune cytopenias), and constitutional symptoms driven by disease progression [5]. It is helpful to perform imaging at baseline prior to the onset of treatment and after the administration of

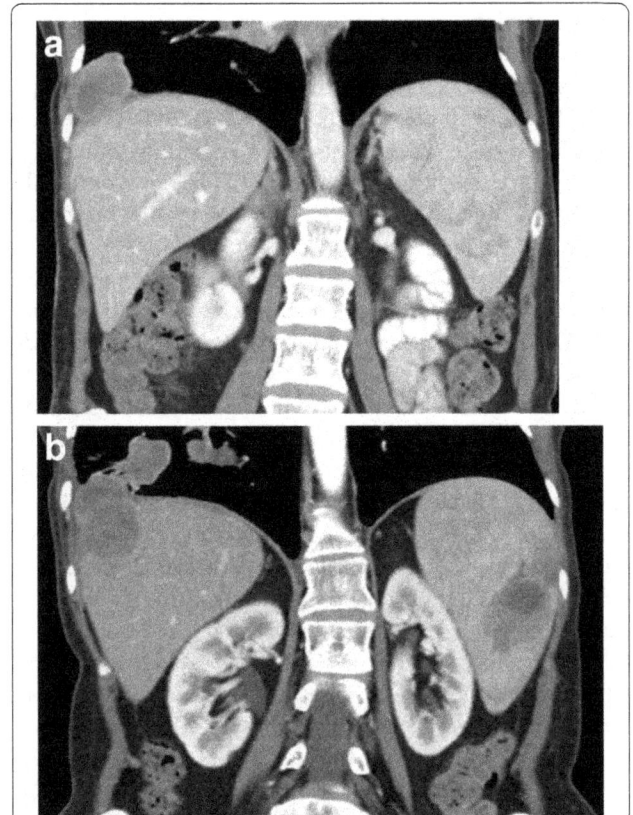

Fig. 3 55-year-old woman with CLL treated with rituximab with pain abdomen and fatigue. **a** Coronal reconstructed contrast enhanced CT image of the abdomen and pelvis acquired 4 months before developing new symptoms reveals perihepatic implant with no focal liver or splenic lesions. **b** Coronal reconstructed images of the abdomen and pelvis reveal new focal hypodense lesions in the liver and the spleen with increase in the perihepatic implant and new pulmonary masses. Liver lesion was biopsied and histologic evaluation showed transformation into diffuse large B cell lymphoma

often FDG-avid, unless transformation to a higher grade lymphoma (Richter transformation) is suspected, based on the presence of rapidly enlarging lymph nodes,

therapy to assess response. Response is also defined according to the 2008 iwCLL guidelines using clinical and imaging criteria. Imaging findings associated with complete response (CR) include no lymph node measuring > 1.5 cm in long axis diameter and no hepatosplenomegaly. Imaging features of partial remission (PR) include a decrease of 50% or more of the sum products of up to 6 nodes, with no increase (> 25%) or newly enlarged node, and/or decreased hepatosplenomegaly by ≥50%. In patients with minimal residual disease (sensitivity of 1 leukemic cell in 10,000 benign lymphocytes), residual splenomegaly after fludarabine, cyclophosphamide, rituximab (FCR) has been shown to have no prognostic significance [21]. A newly-described response category is PR with lymphocytosis (PR-L), which indicates patients who would otherwise meet PR criteria but have a residual lymphocytosis. This situation commonly occurs in patients on B cell receptor (BCR) pathway inhibitors such as ibrutinib or idelalisib who are responding well clinically to therapy and as such it was recognized that the persistent lymphocytosis represents a biological effect of these drugs rather than a sign of resistant disease. Progressive disease is indicated on imaging by the appearance of any new lesion, such as enlarged lymph nodes (> 1.5 cm), splenomegaly, hepatomegaly, or other organ infiltrate, or an increase by 50% or more in greatest determined diameter of any previous site.

Treatment strategies in CLL/SLL

In the last several years, there has been rapid evolution in the treatment strategies of CLL to a more personalized approach with newly available precision therapy [22]. In the 1990s, CLL was generally treated with alkylating agents like chlorambucil and cyclophosphamide and later the purine analog fludarabine. In the 2000's, combination regimens of first fludarabine plus cyclophosphamide (FC) and then FC plus the anti-CD20 monoclonal antibody rituximab (FCR) became used more widely. The anti-CD52 monoclonal antibody alemtuzumaband the second generation anti-CD20 monoclonal antibody ofatumumab also came into the clinic and had utility in higher risk and refractory patients. Bendamustine, another alkylating agent, used with or without rituximab, also became another important treatment option at this time. However, despite an excellent initial response to chemoimmunotherapy approaches in most patients, the progression free survival on repeated administration was significantly shorter.

In the last 5 years, targeted novel agents have expanded the available CLL treatment armamentarium dramatically, in particular small molecule inhibitors and newer monoclonal antibodies, providing excellent new treatment options for all CLL patients and particular those who are older and have multiple co-morbidities, poor prognostic features, or relapsed/refractory disease. For example, ibrutinib is now considered the standard of care as first-line therapy for del (17p) CLL [2]. In the following section, we reviewsome of the key monoclonal antibodies and also the recently approved targeted agents employed in the management of CLL, with attention to efficacy and toxicity features relevant to radiologists.

Rituximab (Anti-CD-20 antibody)

Rituximab is a monoclonal antibody which binds to CD20 expressed on the surface of B cells and causes depletion of malignant B cells primarily through antibody-dependent cellular cytotoxicity and complement-dependent cytotoxicity [23]. It was one of the first targeted drugs approved by the FDA for any cancer, with initial FDA approval for B-cell non Hodgkin lymphomas resistant to other regimens in 1997 [24]. Its label was subsequently broadened in 2006 to be included in combination with cyclophosphamide, vincristine and prednisone (R-CVP regimen), which became the standard of care first line treatment for follicular lymphoma [25]. Rituximab was subsequently approved in 2010 as a first line agent in CLL when given in combination with fludarabine and cyclophosphamide (FCR). Rituximab may be administered along with other agents in both fitter patients (for example, with bendamustine) and in older patients with co-morbid conditions (for example, with chlorambucil) [2]. As in other indolent NHLs, rituximab is sometimes utilized as monotherapy in CLL; however, unlike in those other diseases, response rates and durability of response in CLL are modest, and as such rituximab should not routinely be used as monotherapy in CLL.

On imaging, response to therapy occurs in the form of decreased size of lymph nodes, spleen, liver and other sites of lymphoma. In a clinical trial that led to FDA approval of rituximab (FCR) for CLL, at 3 years after randomization, 65% of patients in the FCR group were free of progression compared with 45% in the FC group [26].

Rituximab toxicities can manifest on imaging (Figs. 4 and 5). Notably, lung toxicities in the form of interstitial pneumonitis and acute respiratory distress syndrome (ARDS) have been well-described, and although they are rare, they can be life threatening [27–29]. Three time-to-onset patterns have been described: ARDS within hours of first infusion, acute/subacute hypoxemic organizing pneumonia within 2 weeks of last infusion, and macronodular organizing pneumonia with insidious/longer onset [27]. On high resolution computed tomography (HRCT), findings include focal or diffuse ground glass opacities and consolidation (Fig. 4) [28]. Rituximab is also known to increase the risk of hepatitis B reactivation in carriers, which can result in acute liver injury, andmanifestson CT with decreased liver attenuation, gallbladder wall edema > 3 mm and mild periportal

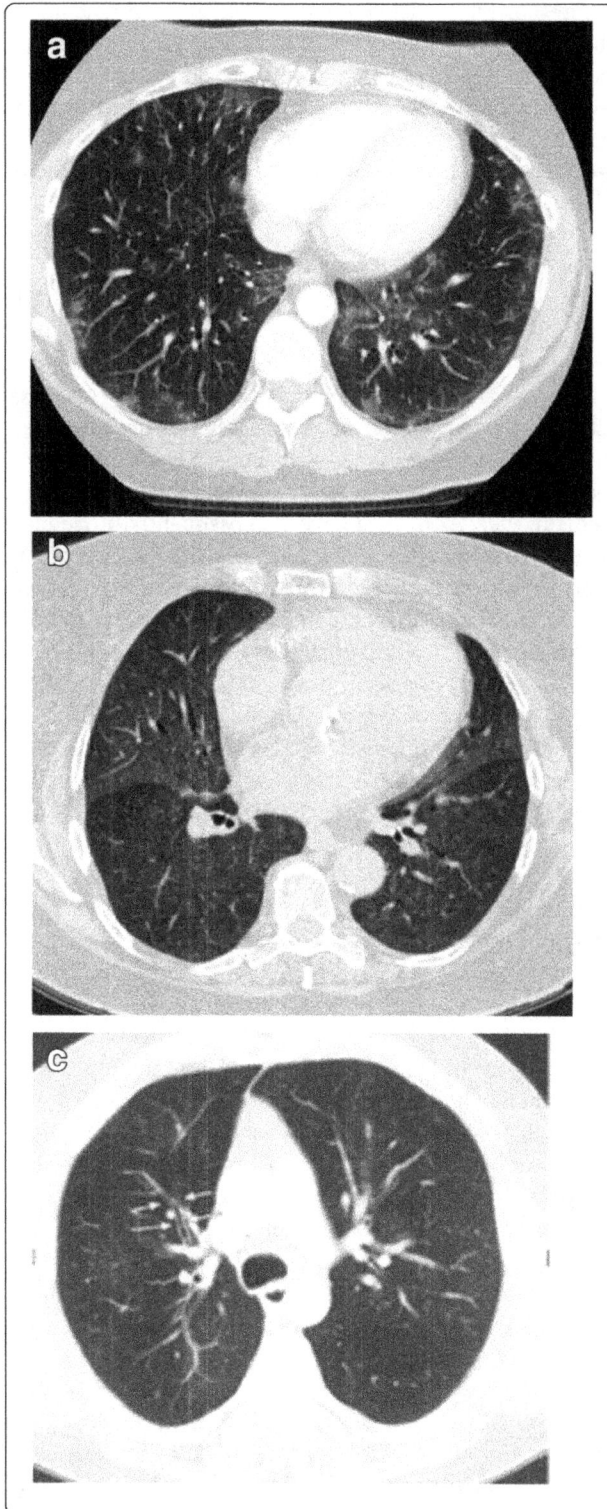

edema [30]. Progressive multifocal leukoencephalopathy (PML) has also been reported in rituximab-treated CLL patients, which is a rare demyelinating condition caused by JC virus reactivation [31]. On brain MRI, PMLmanifests as FLAIR hyperintense white matter lesions.

Alemtuzumab (Anti-CD-52 antibody)

Alemtuzumab is an anti-CD52 antibody, directed against the CD52 antigen expressed on the surface of B-cells, T-cells, natural killer cells, eosinophils and macrophages [32]. This antibody acts through complement-mediated and/or antibody-dependent cytotoxicity, and may cause direct apoptosis of B cells [33]. In 2001, alemtuzumab attained initial FDA-approvalunder accelerated approval regulations for B-cell CLL, and full approval was attained in 2007. According to the current NCCN guidelines, alemtuzumab may be employed as a single agent or in combination with rituximab, in the setting of CLL with 17p deletion or relapsed/refractory cases [2].

In the clinical trial that lead to alemtuzumab FDA approval, 297 patients were randomized to either alemtuzumab or chlorambucil. There was a higher overall response rate of 83% in patients treated with alemtuzumab compared to 55% in the chlorambucil arm [34, 35]. Adverse effects in alemtuzumab treated patients included infections, particularly with cytomegalovirus (CMV). The spectrum of severe infectious complications is thought to be related to profound lymphocyte depletion [36]. CMV pneumonitis can be appreciated on CT as bilateral patchy areas of ground glass opacities with centrilobular nodules, consolidation, as well as septal thickening and pleural effusion in some cases [37]. CMV colitis demonstrates a non-specific appearance on CT, associated with wall thickening, edema, mucosal hyperenhancement and perienteric stranding [38]. Additionally, infection with pneumocystis jiroveci pneumonia (PJP), fungal organisms and cerebral toxoplasmosis have been associated with alemtuzumab.

Ofatumumab (New anti-CD20 antibody)

Ofatumumab is a second generation, type I anti-CD20 antibody with better activation of complement-dependent

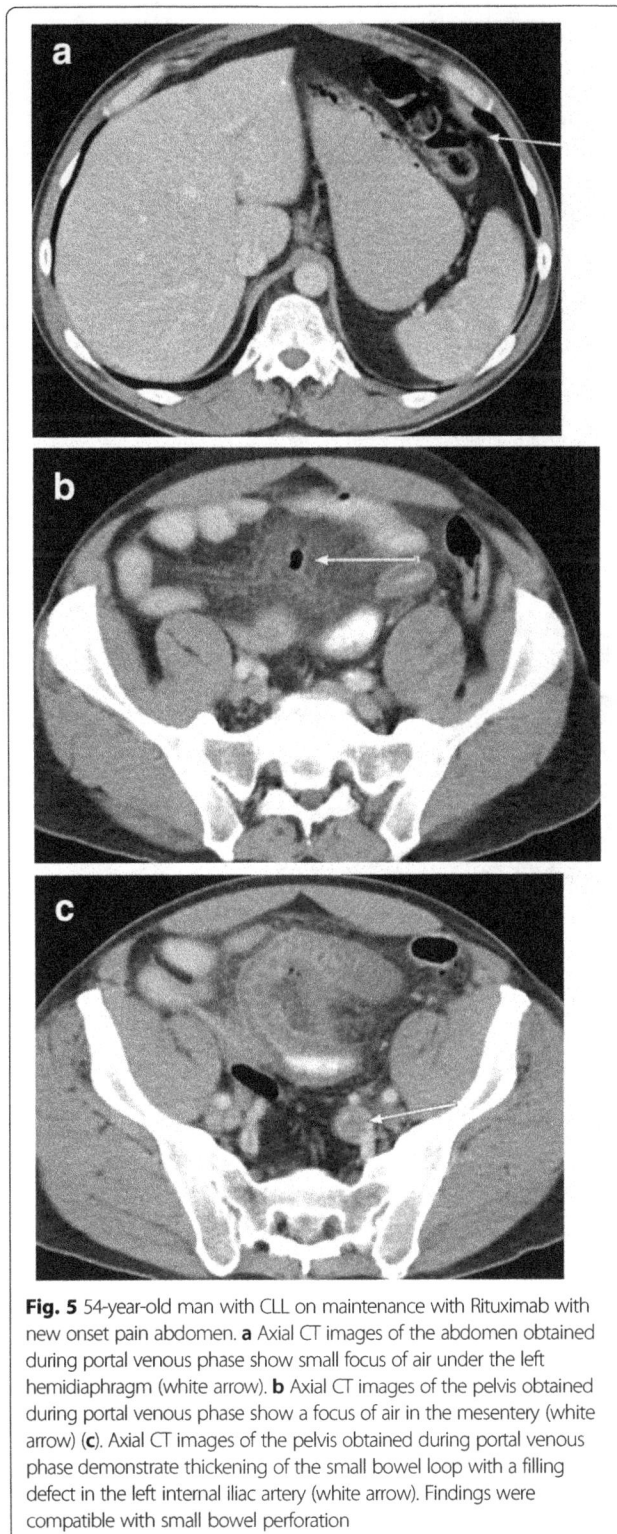

Fig. 5 54-year-old man with CLL on maintenance with Rituximab with new onset pain abdomen. **a** Axial CT images of the abdomen obtained during portal venous phase show small focus of air under the left hemidiaphragm (white arrow). **b** Axial CT images of the pelvis obtained during portal venous phase show a focus of air in the mesentery (white arrow) (**c**). Axial CT images of the pelvis obtained during portal venous phase demonstrate thickening of the small bowel loop with a filling defect in the left internal iliac artery (white arrow). Findings were compatible with small bowel perforation

cytotoxicity and thereby better activity in some cell lines resistant to rituximab and in cells with low CD20 expression [39]. In 2009, ofatumumab was FDA-approved for patients with previously treated CLL. In 2014, ofatumumab was approved in combination with chlorambucil in previously untreated patients, in whom fludarabine is not appropriate [40]. In 2016, ofatumumab was FDA-approved for extended treatment of patients with recurrent or progressive CLL who are in complete or partial response following at least two lines of therapy [41].

Ofatumumab has been evaluated in clinical trials of elderly CLL patients. In a large phase III study comparing ofatumumab plus chlorambucil with chlorambucil alone, the overall response rate has higher in patients treated with combination therapy (82% versus 69%) and 14% demonstrated complete responses in the ofatumumab plus chlorambucil group [42]. In the patients receiving combination therapy, cytopenias, infections and infusion reactions were the most common toxicities; these adverse effects are similar in other ofatumumab studies. As seen with rituximab, pneumonitis is a rare potential toxicity associated with treatment (Fig. 6) [43, 44].

Obinutuzumab (New anti-CD-20 antibody)

Obinutuzumab is a type II, glycoengineered antibody which has a slightly different orientation in binding to the CD20 receptor expressed on the B cell surface than rituximab, which produces greater apoptosis and more antibody mediated cytotoxicity [45]. It was FDA-approved in 2013 as a first line treatment (in combination with chlorambucil) in older CLL patients or in those with multiple co-morbidities.

In a phase III study of 781 CLL patients treated with chlorambucil alone, rituximab plus chlorambucil, or obinutuzumab plus chlorambucil, obinutuzumab with chlorambucil was superior to the rituximab containing regimen, with prolongation of progression free survival and higher rate of complete response (20.7% versus 7%) (Fig. 7). Common adverse events associated with obinutuzumab include cytopenias and infusion reactions. Infections, especially pneumonia, have occurred in association with treatment. Similar to the previously cited adverse events associated with rituximab, reactivation of hepatitis B and progressive multifocal leukoencephalopathy have also been reported with obinutuzumab [46].

Ibrutinib (Bruton Tyrosine Kinase Inhibitor)

Although antibody therapies have made an important contribution to the improvement in CLL therapy, small molecule targeted inhibitors such as ibrutinib have truly revolutionized the field in the last 5 years. One important difference between traditional chemoimmunotherapy and the newer targeted agents is that while the former are given as time-limited regimens (typically 6 months), the latter are typically given continuously until time of progression or unacceptable toxicity.

Ibrutinib is a small molecule which irreversibly inhibits the Bruton tyrosine kinase (BTK), by covalently binding to the cysteine-481 residueof BTK. It prevents downstream

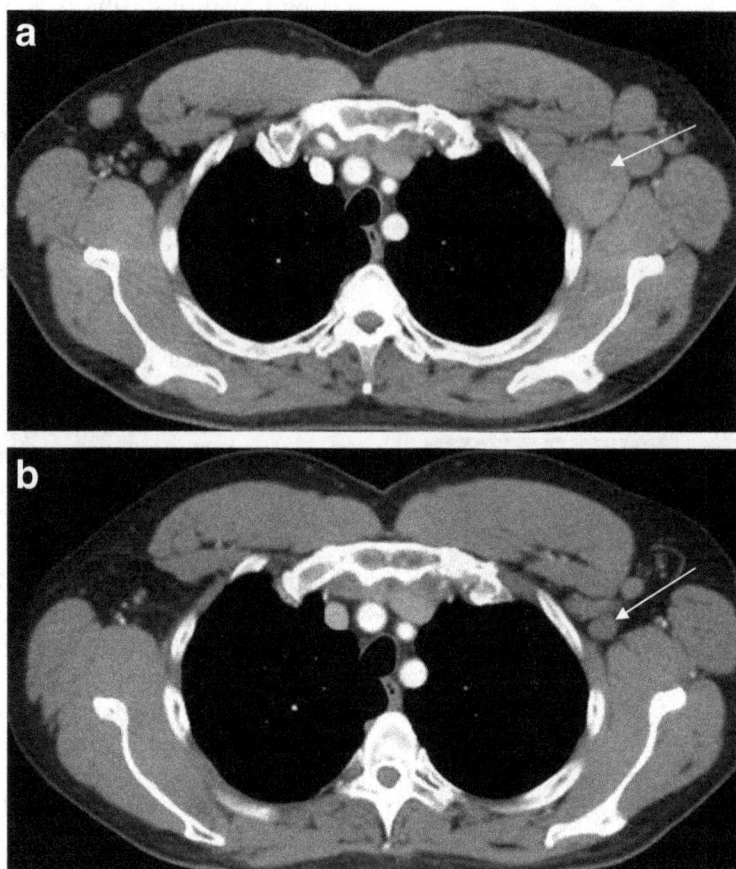

Fig. 6 59-year-old male with follicular lymphoma was observed initially for 6 months after diagnosis but he progressed with increasing left axillary lymphadenopathy. **a** Axial CT images of the chest acquired during arterial phase reveal left axillary lymphadenopathy with the largest lymph node measuring 5 cm in short axis (white arrow). **b** Axial CT images of the chest acquired during arterial phase after 1 year on Ofatumumab demonstrate decrease in the size of left axillary lymph node which now measures less than 1 cm in short axis

activation of transcription factors through blockade of the B cell receptor signaling pathway, which therefore inhibits CLL-cell survival and proliferation [47]. Ibrutinib is FDA-approved to treat any CLL patient in any line of therapy, including patients with del (17p) for whom it has become the standard of care for frontline therapy, and for those who have relapsed or progressed on prior treatments. A study by Burger et al. examined ibrutinib as a first line drug in CLL and compared to chlorambucil. In this report, 86% patients on ibrutinib monotherapy achieved an objective response compared to 35% on chlorambucil (Fig. 8) [48], and patients treated on the ibrutinib arm had a significant improvement in overall survival.

Ibrutinib is associated with a spectrum of adverse effects. For example, there is an associated 5–8% risk of atrial fibrillation, and increased risk of major and minor bleeding [49]. Ibrutinib should be held 3–7 days prior to and after any invasive procedure, due to the risk of periprocedural bleeding [50]. Other common adverse effects associated with ibrutinib include skin rash, diarrhea, hypertension and fatigue. Rarer complications include life-threatening central nervous system or gastrointestinal hemorrhage [51], as well as pneumonitis, which has been documented on chest CT, evidenced by diffuse bilateral ground glass opacities with or without consolidation (Fig. 8c) [52]. Ibrutinib is also associated with increased risk of infection with Pneumocystis jirovecii pneumonia and invasive aspergillosis [53]. Pneumocystis pneumonia commonly presents with interlobular septal thickening and diffuse ground glass opacities which are more predominant in the upper lobes [54]. Invasive pulmonary aspergillosis presents with nodules with central cavitation and aspergillosis of CNS presents as peripherally enhancing brain mass [55].

Idelalisib (Delta-isoform phosphatidylinositol 3-kinaseinhibitor)

Idelalisib is a small molecule that selectively inhibits the delta isoform (δ) of phosphatidylinositol 3-kinase (PI3K), a form restricted primarily to leukocytes [56]. Inhibition of PI3Kδ inhibits the B cell receptor pathway, thereby inhibits B cell activation, proliferation and survival [56].

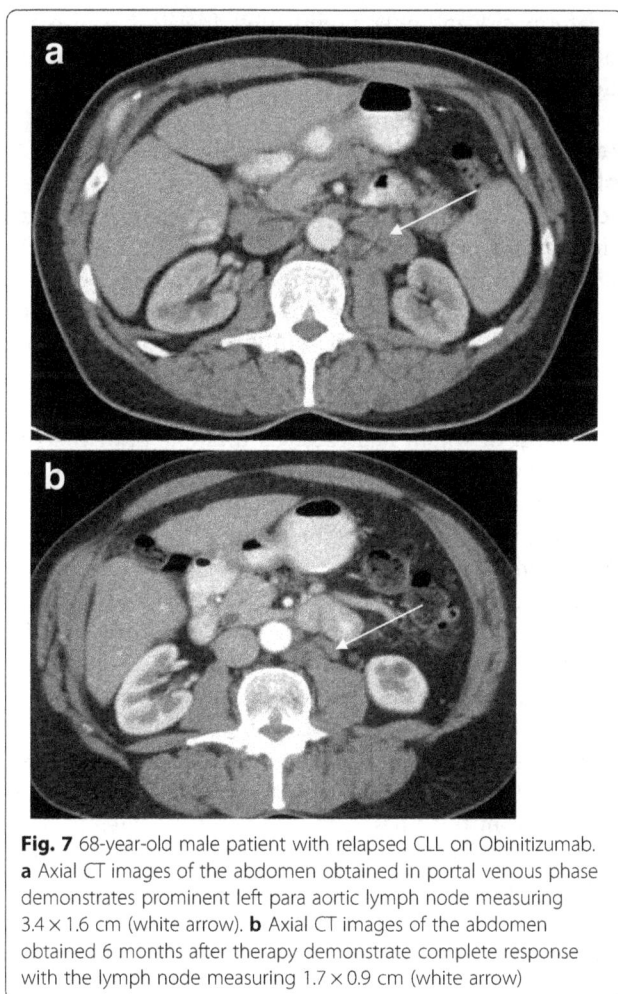

Fig. 7 68-year-old male patient with relapsed CLL on Obinitizumab. **a** Axial CT images of the abdomen obtained in portal venous phase demonstrates prominent left para aortic lymph node measuring 3.4 × 1.6 cm (white arrow). **b** Axial CT images of the abdomen obtained 6 months after therapy demonstrate complete response with the lymph node measuring 1.7 × 0.9 cm (white arrow)

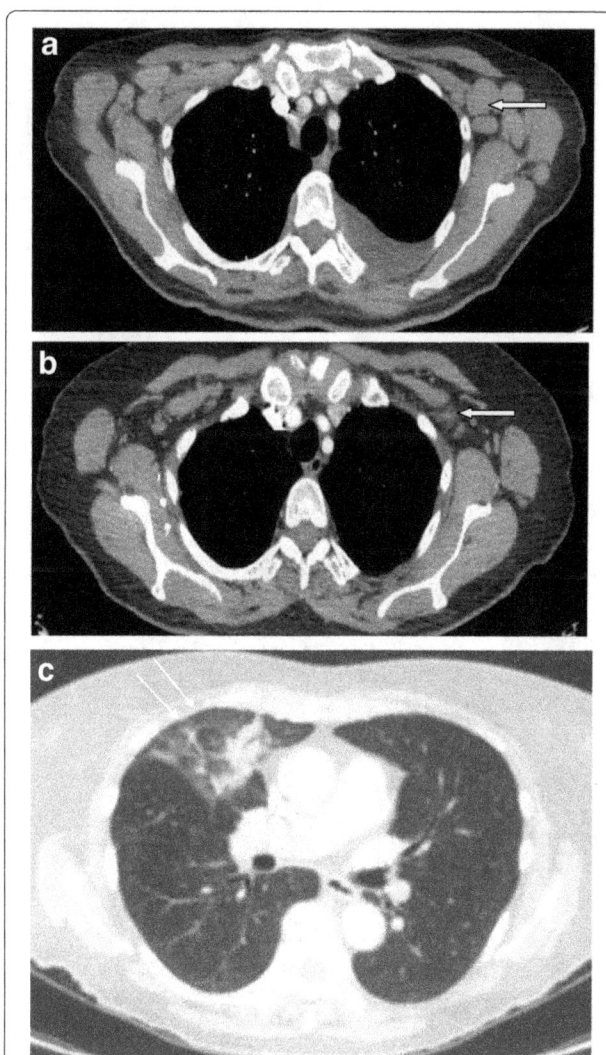

Fig. 8 A 68-year-old female with CLL with 13q deletion on watchful waiting with progression of CLL **a** Axial CT of the chest obtained in arterial phase demonstrates bilateral axillary lymphadenopathy with the largest left axillary lymph node measuring 2 cm in short axis (white arrow). **b** Axial CT of the chest obtained 3 months after initiating Ibrutinib therapy reveals significant decrease in the lymphadenopathy with the axillary node now measuring less than a centimeter in short axis (white arrow). **c** Axial CT of the chest obtained in arterial phase as a part of restaging examination in the same patient reveals focal ground glass opacity in the right upper lobe (double arrows) raising concern for Ibrutinib pneumonitis

In 2014, the FDA approved idelalisib in combination with rituximab for relapsed or refractory CLL [2]. In a phase 2 study of idelalisib in 125 previously treated patients (median of four prior treatments) with indolent lymphoma (follicular, SLL, marginal zone lymphoma or lymphoplasmacytic lymphoma), 90% of the patients demonstrated decreased lymph node size, with 57% achieving complete or partial response [56], and the greatest efficacy in this study was seen in SLL patients.

Idelalisib is associated with several immune-mediated toxicities which are worthy of discussion. Common adverse events in the phase 2 study above include, but are not limited, to diarrhea, nausea, fatigue, cough, abdominal pain, pneumonia, elevated liver function tests, infection and cytopenias [56]. Idelalisib- related pneumonitis has been described in literature, and manifests as cough, dyspnea and fever at any time in the course of treatment. CT findings including diffuse bilateral ground glass opacities, consolidations, diffuse micronodules and pleural effusions (Fig. 9a) [57]. Idelalisib-associated colitis has been noted to typically occur after patients have been on drug for 6 to 9 months or later [58], and we

have observed as case with CT findings of short segment colonic wall thickening, enlarged mesenteric lymph nodes and panniculitis (Fig. 9b and c). Another patient treated at our center with idelalisib was noted to have elevated liver function tests, and we observed imaging findings of decreased liver echogenicity and mild pericholecystic fluid on ultrasound. The multiple, potentially severe immune-mediated toxicities associated with this medication are delineated in a black box warning, for serious diarrhea, colitis, intestinal perforation,

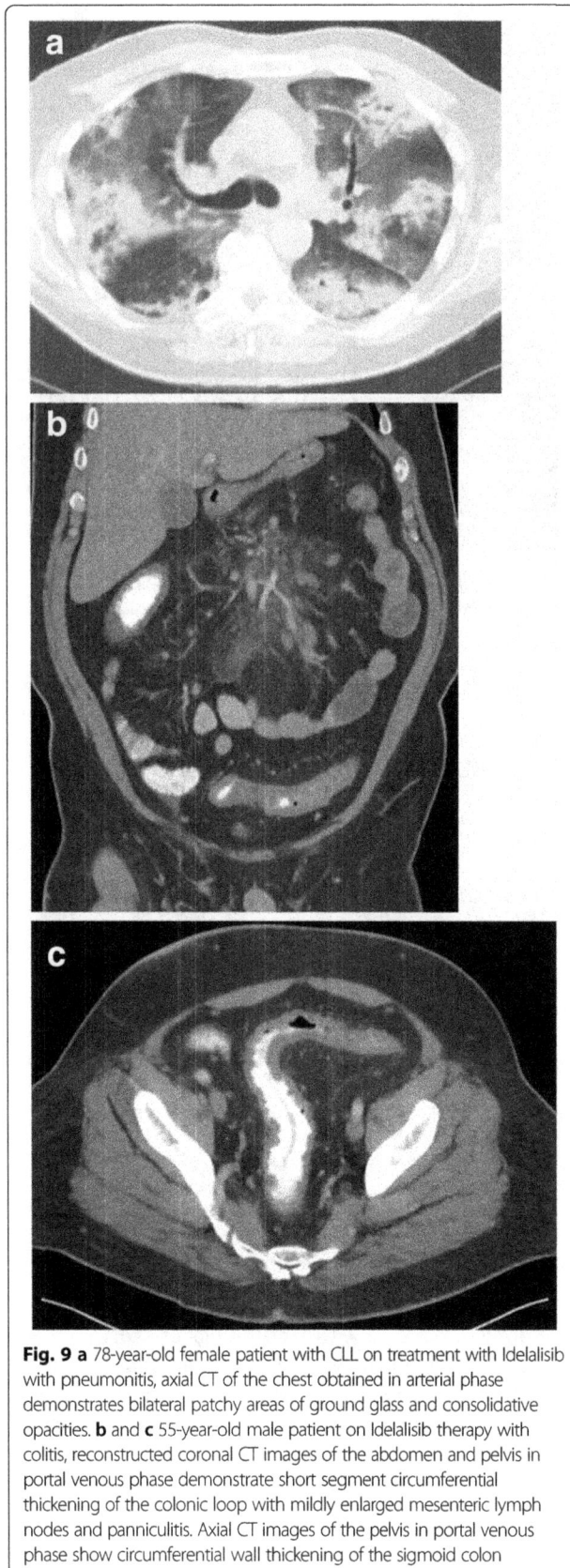

Fig. 9 a 78-year-old female patient with CLL on treatment with Idelalisib with pneumonitis, axial CT of the chest obtained in arterial phase demonstrates bilateral patchy areas of ground glass and consolidative opacities. **b** and **c** 55-year-old male patient on Idelalisib therapy with colitis, reconstructed coronal CT images of the abdomen and pelvis in portal venous phase demonstrate short segment circumferential thickening of the colonic loop with mildly enlarged mesenteric lymph nodes and panniculitis. Axial CT images of the pelvis in portal venous phase show circumferential wall thickening of the sigmoid colon

hepatotoxicity and pneumonitis [59]. Idelalisib is also associated with increased risk of opportunistic infections such as pneumocystis jirovecii [60].

Venetoclax (B-cell leukemia/lymphoma-2 inhibitor)

Venetoclax binds to anti-apoptotic B-cell leukemia/lymphoma-2 protein (Bcl-2) and displaces pro-apoptotic BH3-only proteins, which then induce rapid apoptosis in CLL cells [61]. Venetoclax was FDA-approved in 2016, to treat CLL with 17p deletion, refractory to treatment with at least one prior regimen [2]. In the phase 1 first in human studyin patients with relapsed or refractory CLL, most of whom had received multiple prior therapies and many of whom had del (17p), 116 patients received venetoclax. An overall response rate of 79% was reported, with complete response in 20% of the patients [61]. Tumor lysis syndrome (TLS) was noted in several patients and in some cases was severe, indicating the power of this drug but also requiring careful risk stratification, prophylaxis, and management of TLS. Other adverse associated events in the study patients included diarrhea, upper respiratory tract infection and nausea. Grade 3/4 neutropenia occurred in about 40% of patients, but the rate of febrile neutropenia was low. The findings from this phase I study were subsequently confirmed in a landmark study of 107 CLL patients with relapsed or refractory del (17p) disease, and the response rates in this high risk population were similar to those seen in the broader population in the phase I study [62].

Conclusion

The last 5 years have witnessed an exciting evolution of targeted therapy in CLL/SLL. Relatively few radiology-based papers have been written on this expansive subject; rather, case series have reported on the various drug-associated toxicities attributed to specific agents. Considering the logical development of the targeted agents and class-specific mechanisms of action, it becomes easier to appreciate the class-specific toxicities related to the drugs.

In general, indolent lymphoma patients on treatment are at risk of infectious complications. More specifically, the anti-CD20 antibodies rituximab, ofatumumab and obinutuzumab have been associated with reactivation of hepatitis B and rarely, progressive multifocal leukoencephalopathy. Pneumonitis has also been noted with these antibodies. The anti-CD52 antibody alemtuzumab has been associated with various infectious complications, especially CMV. Small molecule inhibitors have distinct adverse event profiles, including bleeding, atrial fibrillation and diarrhea with ibrutinib, potentially severe colitis, hepatotoxicity and pneumonitis with idelalisib, and tumor lysis syndrome, neutropenia, and diarrhea with venetoclax. Despite these potential toxicities, each of these agents is well-tolerated for the majority of patients and each has demonstrated dramatically improved response rates and progression free survival compared to chemoimmunotherapy in heavily-pretreated patients, leading to substantial improvements in overall survival, particularly for those patients with high risk del (17p) CLL. Ongoing studies combining these novel agents hold promise to further revolutionize the treatment of CLL and hold the potential to even further reduce or possibly even eliminate the need for chemoimmunotherapy in many patients. It is worth noting that although these new drugs also have activity in other low grade B cell non-Hodgkin lymphomas, their efficacy is generally lower than in CLL, and as such it is likely that these conditions will also benefit from combination therapeutic strategies, which is already being explored in the clinic.

Given the indolent nature of CLL and other low grade lymphomas, the spectrum of available treatments today and the associated prolonged survival of affected patients, it is likely that radiologists will encounter more imaging studies of patients treated with these novel drugs. It is necessary to be familiar with the expected response patterns and common toxicities associated with targeted agents to optimize care of this growing population.

Abbreviations
ARDS: Acute respiratory distress syndrome; Bcl2: B-cell leukemia/lymphoma 2; BCR: B-cell receptor; BR: Bendamustine, rituximab; BTK: Bruton tyrosine kinase; CECT: Contrast-enhanced CT; CLL: Chronic lymphocytic leukemia; CMV: Cytomegalovirus; CNS: Central nervous system; CR: Complete response; FCR: Foscarnet, cyclophosphamide, rituximab; FDA: Food and Drug Administration; FISH: Florescence in-situ hybridization; HRCT: High resolution CT; IGHV: Immunoglobulin heavy chain variable; iwCLL: International Workshop on Chronic Lymphocytic Leukemia; LDH: Lactate dehydrogenase; MRD: Minimal residual disease; PI3K: Phosphotidylionositol 3 kinase; PR: Partial response; PR-L: Partial response with lymphocytosis; RCVP: Rituximab, cyclophosphamide, vincristine, prednisone; SLL: Small lymphocytic leukemia; TLS: Tumor lysis syndrome; ZAP-70: Zeta-associated protein 70

Authors' contributions
BG- Conceived the idea, drafted the manuscript, worked on figures, edited the manuscript. MD- Drafted the manuscript, edited the manuscript. BS- Helped with figures, helped in editing the manuscript. FA- Helped with figures, edited the manuscript. AG- Edited the manuscript. NR- Conceived the idea, edited the manuscript. KK- Conceived the idea, drafted the manuscript, edited the manuscript. All authors have contributed to drafting the manuscript. All authors have read and approved the submission.

Competing interests
The authors declare that they have no competing interests.

Author details
[1]Thoracic Radiology, Brigham and Women's Hospital, 45 Francis Street, Boston, MA 02115, USA. [2]Harvard Medical School, 25 Shattuck Street, Boston, MA 02115, USA. [3]Chronic Lymphocytic Leukemia, Dana Farber Cancer Institute, 450 Brookline Avenue, Boston 02284, USA. [4]Radiology, Massachusetts General Hospital, 55 Fruit Street, Boston, MA 02114, USA. [5]Emergency Radiology, Brigham and Women's Hospital, 45 Francis Street, Boston, MA 02115, USA. [6]Department of Radiology, Dana Farber Cancer Institute, Boston, MA 02284, USA.

References
1. Surveillance Epidemiology and End Results (SEER). (2017). Cancer stat facts – chronic lymphocytic leukemia. Accessed 11 July 17 athttps://seer.cancer.gov/statfacts/html/clyl.html.
2. Wierda WG, Zelenetz AD, Gordon LI, et al. NCCN guidelines insights: chronic lymphocytic leukemia/small lymphocytic leukemia, version 1.2017. J Natl Compr Cancer Netw. 2017;15(3):293–311.
3. http://www.cancernetwork.com/review-article/indolent-b-cell-non-hodgkins-lymphomas. Accessed 13 Apr 2018.
4. Rai KR, Jain P. Chronic lymphocytic leukemia (CLL)-then and now. Am J Hematol. 2016;91(3):330–40.
5. Hallek M, Cheson BD, Catovsky D, et al. Guidelines for the diagnosis and treatment of chronic lymphocytic leukemia: a report from the International Workshop on Chronic Lymphocytic Leukemia updating the National Cancer Institute-Working Group 1996 guidelines. Blood. 2008;111(12):5446–56.
6. Keating MJ, O'Brien S, Albitar M, et al. Early results of a chemoimmunotherapy regimen of fludarabine, cyclophosphamide, and rituximab as initial therapy for chronic lymphocytic leukemia. J Clin Oncol. 2005;23(18):4079–88.
7. Goede V, Fischer K, Busch R, et al. Obinutuzumab plus chlorambucil in patients with CLL and coexisting conditions. N Engl J Med. 2014;370(12):1101–10.
8. Chen Q, Jain N, Ayer T, et al. Economic burden of chronic lymphocytic leukemia in the era of oral targeted therapies in the United States. J Clin Oncol. 2017;35(2):166–74.
9. Döhner H, Stilgenbauer S, Benner A, et al. Genomic aberrations and survival in chronic lymphocytic leukemia. N Engl J Med. 2000;343(26):1910–6.
10. Damle RN, Wasil T, Fais F, et al. Ig V gene mutation status and CD38 expression as novel prognostic indicators in chronic lymphocytic leukemia. Blood. 1999;94(6):1840–7.
11. Hamblin TJ, Davis Z, Gardiner A, Oscier DG, Stevenson FK. Unmutated Ig V(H) genes are associated with a more aggressive form of chronic lymphocytic leukemia. Blood. 1999;94(6):1848–54.
12. Rai KR, Sawitsky A, Cronkite EP, et al. Clinical staging of chronic lymphocytic leukemia. Blood. 1975;46(2):219–34.
13. Binet JL, Auquier A, Dighiero G, et al. A new prognostic classification of chronic lymphocytic leukemia derived from a multivariate survival analysis. Cancer. 1981;48(1):198–206.
14. Muntañola A, Bosch F, Arguis P, et al. Abdominal computed tomography predicts progression in patients with Rai stage 0 chronic lymphocytic leukemia. J Clin Oncol. 2007;25(12):1576–80.
15. Šimković M, Motyčková M, Belada D, et al. Five years of experience with rituximab plus high-dose dexamethasone for relapsed/refractory chronic lymphocytic leukemia. Arch Med Sci. 2016;12(2):421–7.
16. Döhner H, Stilgenbauer S, James MR, et al. 11q deletions identify a new subset of B-cell chronic lymphocytic leukemia characterized by extensive nodal involvement and inferior prognosis. Blood. 1997;89(7):2516–22.
17. Kakimoto T, Nakazato T, Hayashi R, et al. Bilateral occipital lobe invasion in chronic lymphocytic leukemia. J Clin Oncol. 2010;28(3):e30–2.
18. Strati P, Uhm JH, Kaufmann TJ. Prevalence and characteristics of central nervous system involvement by chronic lymphocytic leukemia. Haematologica. 2016;101(4):458–65.
19. Shaikh F, Janjua A, Van Gestel F, Ahmad A. Richter transformation of chronic lymphocytic leukemia: a review of fluorodeoxyglucose positron emission tomography-computed tomography and molecular diagnostics. Cureus. 2017;9(1):e968.
20. Falchi L, Keating MJ, Marom EM, et al. Correlation between FDG/PET, histology, characteristics, and survival in 332 patients with chronic lymphoid leukemia. Blood. 2014;123(18):2783–90.
21. Kovacs G, Robrecht S, Fink AM, et al. Minimal residual disease assessment improves prediction of outcome in patients with Chronic Lymphocytic

Leukemia (CLL) who achieve partial response: comprehensive analysis of two phase III studies of the German CLL study group. J Clin Oncol. 2016; 34(31):3758–65.

22. Byrd JC, Jones JJ, Woyach JA, et al. Entering the era of targeted therapy for chronic lymphocytic leukemia: impact on the practicing clinician. J Clin Oncol. 2014;32(27):3039–47.

23. Weiner GJ. Rituximab: mechanism of action. Semin Hematol. 2010;47(2):115–23.

24. Scott SD. Rituximab: a new therapeutic monoclonal antibody for non-Hodgkin's lymphoma. Cancer Pract. 1998;6(3):195–7.

25. https://www.cancer.gov/about-cancer/treatment/drugs/fda-rituximab#b. Accessed 23 Mar 17.

26. Hallek M, Fischer K, Fingerle-Rowson G, et al. Addition of rituximab to fludarabine and cyclophosphamide in patients with chronic lymphocytic leukaemia: a randomised, open-label, phase 3 trial. Lancet. 2010;376(9747): 1164–74.

27. Lioté H, Lioté F, Séroussi B, Mayaud C, Cadranel J. Rituximab-induced lung disease: a systematic literature review. Eur Respir J. 2010;35(3):681–7.

28. Wagner SA, Mehta AC, Laber DA. Rituximab-induced interstitial lung disease. Am J Hematol. 2007;82(10):916–9.

29. Burton C, Kaczmarski R, Jan-Mohamed R. Interstitial pneumonitis related to rituximab therapy. N Engl J Med. 2003;348:2690–1.

30. Niscola P, Del Principe MI, Maurillo L, et al. Fulminant B hepatitis in a surface antigen-negative patient with B-cell chronic lymphocytic leukaemia after rituximab therapy. Leukemia. 2005;19(10):1840–1.

31. Garrote H, de la Fuente A, Oña R, et al. Long-term survival in a patient with progressive multifocal leukoencephalopathy after therapy with rituximab, fludarabine and cyclophosphamide for chronic lymphocytic leukemia. Exp Hematol Oncol. 2015;4:8.

32. Fraser G, Smith CA, Imrie K, et al. Alemtuzumab in chronic lymphocytic leukemia. Curr Oncol. 2007;14(3):96–109.

33. Schweighofer CD, Wendtner CM. First-line treatment of chronic lymphocytic leukemia: role of alemtuzumab. Onco Targets Ther. 2010;3:53–67.

34. Demko S, Summers J, Keegan P. Pazdur R.FDA drug approval summary: alemtuzumab as single-agent treatment for B-cell chronic lymphocytic leukemia. Oncologist. 2008;13(2):167–74.

35. Hillmen P, Skotnicki AB, Robak T, et al. Alemtuzumab compared with chlorambucil as first-line therapy for chronic lymphocytic leukemia. J Clin Oncol. 2007;25:5616–23.

36. Nosari A, Montillo M, Morra E. Infectious toxicity using alemtuzumab. Haematologica. 2004;89(12):1415–9.

37. Moon JH, Kim EA, Lee KS, Kim TS, Jung KJ, Song JH. Cytomegalovirus pneumonia: high-resolution CT findings in ten non-AIDS immunocompromised patients. Korean J Radiol. 2000;1(2):73–8.

38. Knollmann FD, Grünewald T, Adler A, et al. Intestinal disease in acquired immunodeficiency: evaluation by CT. Eur Radiol. 1997;7(9):1419–29.

39. Barth MJ, Czuczman MS. Ofatumumab: a novel, fully human anti-CD20 monoclonal antibody for the treatment of chronic lymphocytic leukemia. Future Oncol. 2013;9(12):1829–39.

40. https://www.cancer.gov/about-cancer/treatment/drugs/fda-ofatumumab. Accessed 23 Mar 17.

41. van Oers MH, Kuliczkowski K, Smolej L, et al. Ofatumumab maintenance versus observation in relapsed chronic lymphocytic leukaemia (PROLONG): an open-label, multicentre, randomised phase 3 study. Lancet Oncol. 2015; 16(13):1370–9.

42. Hillmen P, Robak T, Janssens A, et al. Chlorambucil plus ofatumumab versus chlorambucil alone in previously untreated patients with chronic lymphocytic leukaemia (COMPLEMENT 1): a randomised, multicentre, open-label phase 3 trial. Lancet. 2015;385(9980):1873–83.

43. Coiffier B, Lepretre S, Pedersen LM, et al. Safety and efficacy of ofatumumab, a fully human monoclonal anti-CD20 antibody, in patients with relapsed or refractory B-cell chronic lymphocytic leukemia: a phase 1-2 study. Blood. 2008;111(3):1094–100.

44. Barber NA, Ganti AK. Pulmonary toxicities from targeted therapies: a review. Target Oncol. 2011;6(4):235–43. https://doi.org/10.1007/s11523-011-0199-0. Epub 2011 Nov 11

45. Cartron G, Hourcade-Potelleret F, Morschhauser F, et al. Rationale for optimal obinutuzumab/GA101 dosing regimen in B-cell non-Hodgkin lymphoma. Haematologica. 2016;101(2):226–34.

46. Raisch DW, Rafi JA, Chen C, Bennett CL. Detection of cases of progressive multifocal leukoencephalopathy associated with new biologicals and targeted cancer therapies from the FDA's adverse event reporting system. Expert Opin Drug Saf. 2016;15(8):1003–11.

47. Wiestner A. Targeting B-cell receptor signaling for anticancer therapy: the Bruton's tyrosine kinase inhibitor ibrutinib induces impressive responses in B-cell malignancies. J Clin Oncol. 2013;31(1):128–30.

48. Burger JA, Tedeschi A, Barr PM, et al. Ibrutinib as initial therapy for patients with chronic lymphocytic leukemia. N Engl J Med. 2015;373(25):2425–37.

49. Thompson PA, Lévy V, Tam CS, et al. Atrial fibrillation in CLL patients treated with ibrutinib. An international retrospective study. Br J Haematol. 2016; 175(3):462–6.

50. Brown JR. How I treat CLL patients with ibrutinib. Blood. 2018;131:379–86.

51. Seiter K, Stiefel MF, Barrientos J, et al. Successful treatment of ibrutinib-associated central nervous system hemorrhage with platelet transfusion support. Stem Cell Investig. 2016;3:27.

52. Mato AR, Islam P, Daniel C, et al. Ibrutinib-induced pneumonitis in patients with chronic lymphocytic leukemia. Blood. 2016;127(8):1064–7.

53. Ghez D, Calleja A, Protin C, et al. Early-onset invasive aspergillosis and other fungal infections in patients treated with ibrutinib. Blood. 2018; https://doi.org/10.1182/blood-2017-11-818286. [Epub ahead of print]

54. Bollée G, Sarfati C, Thiéry G, Bergeron A, de Miranda S, Menotti J, de Castro N, Tazi A, Schlemmer B, Azoulay E. Clinical picture of pneumocystis jiroveci pneumonia in cancer patients. Chest. 2007;132(4):1305–10.

55. Peri AM, Bisi L, Cappelletti A, Colella E, Verga L, Borella C, Foresti S, Migliorino GM, Gori A, Bandera A. Invasive aspergillosis with pulmonary and central nervous system involvement during ibrutinib therapy for relapsed chronic lymphocytic leukaemia: case report. Clin Microbiol Infect. 2018; https://doi.org/10.1016/j.cmi.2018.01.028. [Epub ahead of print]

56. Gopal AK, Kahl BS, de Vos S, et al. PI3Kδ inhibition by idelalisib in patients with relapsed indolent lymphoma. N Engl J Med. 2014;370(11):1008–18.

57. Haustraete E, Obert J, Diab S, et al. Idelalisib-related pneumonitis. Eur Respir J. 2016;47(4):1280–3.

58. Weidner AS, Panarelli NC, Geyer JT, et al. Idelalisib-associated colitis: histologic findings in 14 patients. Am J Surg Pathol. 2015;39(12):1661–7.

59. Coutré SE, Barrientos JC, Brown JR, et al. Management of adverse events associated with idelalisib treatment: expert panel opinion. Leuk Lymphoma. 2015;56(10):2779–86.

60. Reinwald M, Silva JT, Mueller NJ, Fortún J, Garzoni C, de Fijter JW, Fernández-Ruiz M, Grossi P, Aguado JM. ESCMID Study group for infections in Compromised Hosts (ESGICH) consensus document on the safety of targeted and biological therapies: an infectious diseases perspective (Intracellular signaling pathways: tyrosine kinase and mTOR inhibitors). Clin Microbiol Infect. 2018; https://doi.org/10.1016/j.cmi.2018.02.009. [Epub ahead of print]

61. Roberts AW, Davids MS, Pagel JM, et al. Targeting BCL2 with venetoclax in relapsed chronic lymphocytic leukemia. N Engl J Med. 2016;374(4):311–22.

62. Stilgenbauer S, Eichhorst B, Schetelig J, et al. Venetoclax in relapsed or refractory chronic lymphocytic leukaemia with 17p deletion: a multicentre, open-label, phase 2 study. Lancet Oncol. 2016;17(6):768–78.

13

Intravoxel incoherent motion DWI of the pancreatic adenocarcinomas: monoexponential and biexponential apparent diffusion parameters and histopathological correlations

Chao Ma[1], Yanjun Li[1], Li Wang[1], Yang Wang[2], Yong Zhang[3], He Wang[3], Shiyue Chen[1] and Jianping Lu[1*]

Abstract

Background: To investigate the associations between the diffusion parameters obtained from multiple-b-values diffusion weighted imaging (DWI) of pancreatic ductal adenocarcinoma (PDAC) and the aggressiveness and local stage prediction, and assess the values of the quantitative parameters for the discrimination of tumors from healthy pancreas.

Methods: Fifty-one patients with surgical pathology-proven PDAC (size, 35 ± 12 mm) and fifty-seven healthy volunteers were enrolled. Diffusion parameters including monoexponential apparent diffusion coefficient (ADC_b and ADC_{total}) and biexponential intravoxel incoherent motion (IVIM) parameters (ADC_{slow}, ADC_{fast} and f) based on 9 b-values (0 to 1000s/mm^2) DWI were calculated for the lesions and the healthy pancreas. These parameters were compared by grades of differentiation, lymph node status, tumor stage and location. The diagnostic performances were calculated and compared by using the receiver operating characteristic curves (ROC) analyses.

Results: There was no statistically significant difference in ADC_b, ADC_{total}, ADC_{slow}, ADC_{fast} or f between PDAC stage T1/T2 and stage T3/T4 or moderately differentiated versus poorly differentiated PDAC ($p = 0.060\text{-}0.941$). In addition, no significant differences were observed for the quantitative parameters between tumors located in the pancreatic head versus other pancreatic regions ($p = 0.203\text{-}0.954$) or between tumors with and without metastatic peripancreatic lymph nodes ($p = 0.313\text{-}0.917$). $ADC_{25\text{-}600}$, ADC_{1000}, ADC_{total} and ADC_{fast} were significantly lower for PDAC compared the healthy pancreas (all $p < 0.05$). ROC analyses showed the area under curve for ADC_{20} was the largest (0.911) to distinguish PDAC from normal pancreas (cut-off value, 5.58×10^{-3}mm^2/s) and had the highest combined sensitivity (89.5%) and specificity (82.4%).

Conclusions: Multiple-b-values DWI derived monoexponential and biexponential parameters of PDAC do not exhibit significance dependence on tumor grade or tumor characteristics. ADC_{20} provided the best accuracy for differentiating PDAC from healthy pancreas in the study.

Keywords: IVIM, Apparent diffusion coefficient, Pancreatic cancer, DWI, Biexponential apparent diffusion

* Correspondence: cjr.lujianping@vip.163.com
[1]Department of Radiology, Changhai Hospital of Shanghai, The Second
Military Medical University, No.168 Changhai Road, Shanghai 200433, China
Full list of author information is available at the end of the article

Background

Pancreatic cancer accounts for about 3% of all cancer cases [1]. It is one of the few cancers which have shown little improvement in survival rate over the past 40 years [2]. Diagnosis of the early stages of pancreatic cancer is difficult even with powerful imaging techniques such as computed tomography (CT), magnetic resonance imaging (MRI), transabdominal and endoscopic ultrasonography (EUS) and endoscopic retrograde cholangiopancreatography (ERCP) [3, 4]. About 74% patients with pancreatic cancer die within the first year of diagnosis [1].

Diffusion-weighted magnetic resonance imaging (DWI) is the only noninvasive technique exploring the microscopic mobility of water molecules in the tissues without contrast administration. The diffusion of water molecules in the human body can be quantified by apparent diffusion coefficient (ADC) based on DWI [5]. Recent technique advancements allow DWI and ADC measurements to be increasingly used in the diagnosis of abdominal diseases [6–8]. Several studies have demonstrated significantly lower ADC in pancreatic cancer than in benign pancreas tissue [9–23]. There is still diagnostic challenge as described by Fukukura et al [13], also the published range of ADC values for both normal and neoplastic tissues varied dramatically as reported in different studies [9–23]. Recently, the role of ADC values in predicting adverse pathological features of pancreatic cancer were reported [12, 24, 25]. However, conflicting results have been described: significant association [24] and lack of association [12, 25] between the ADC and pathological grade of pancreatic cancer were reported. These reports, however, used only two b values (0, 500 or 800 s/mm^2) to measure ADC, which is influenced not only by the structures of the tissue, but also by the microcirculation of blood in the capillary network. Ideally, multiple-b-values DWI with intravoxel incoherent motion (IVIM) model should be set up for the separate estimation of tissue perfusion and diffusivity [26].

The objective of this study was to investigate potential associations between the DWI-derived IVIM parameters such as ADC$_{fast}$ (pseudo-diffusion coefficient), ADC$_{slow}$ (the tissue coefficient), f (perfusion fraction) and the commonly used DWI-derived monoexponential ADC in pancreatic cancer and the tumor grade as well as tumor characteristics including lymph node status, tumor stage and location [12]. In addition, we also investigated the values of multiple-b-values DWI derived parameters for the discrimination of tumors from healthy pancreas.

Methods

Subjects

This prospective study was approved by our Institutional Review Board. Signed written informed consent was obtained from all participants before MRI examinations.

We enrolled 133 patients with a suspect pancreatic mass seen in a CT or US between May 2011 and June 2013 from the inpatients (Fig. 1). Among them, 113 patients received surgery within 7 days after the time of inclusion in our study. 51 patients were pancreatic ductal adenocarcinomas (PDAC) (27 men, 24 women; mean age 59.6 years; range 36-76 years) with histopathologic diagnoses. We also enrolled 57 healthy volunteers (36 men and 21 women; mean age 45.0 years; range 21-68 years) as the control group. Exclusion criteria for the healthy volunteers included diseases which might affect normal pancreatic function, such as pancreatic disease, severe fatty liver and hepatic cirrhosis history.

Image Acquisition

All examinations were performed on a 3.0-Tesla MR (Signa HDxt V16.0, GE Healthcare, Milwaukee, USA) with an eight-element phased array coil. All the participants underwent MRI protocols including transverse respiratory triggered single-shot echo-planar DWI (weighted along three orthogonal gradient directions) with b values of 0, 20, 50, 100, 200, 400, 600, 800 and 1000 s/mm^2. Selective presaturation with inversion recovery (SPIR) was used for fat saturation; two saturation slabs were fixed on the A/P direction to reduce potential motion artifacts. The main scan parameters of MRI sequences were listed in the Table 1. Only the 51 patients underwent contrast-enhanced liver acceleration volume acquisition (LAVA) which was performed with Gadopentetate Dimeglumine injection (physiological saline, 10-15ml; media, 0.1-0.15 mmol/kg; injection rate, 2-3 ml/s) at the end of the study.

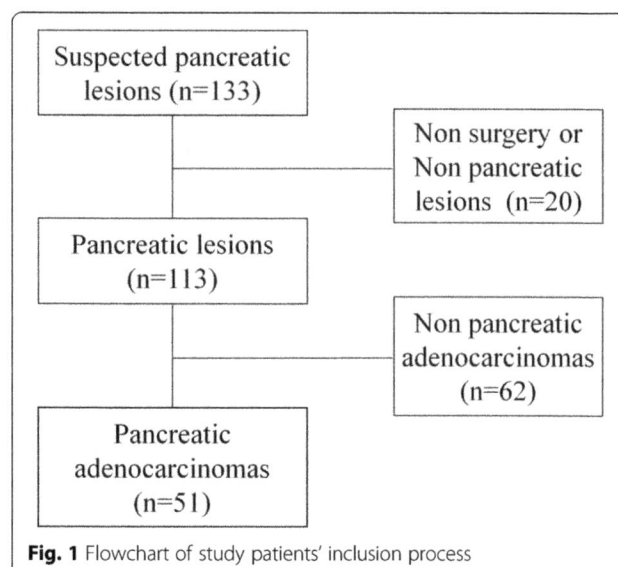

Fig. 1 Flowchart of study patients' inclusion process

Table 1 The main parameters of MR sequences

Sequences	TR/TE (ms)	FOV (mm)	Matrix	Thickness/gap (mm)	Flip angle (°)	slices	NEX	Band width (KHz)	Acceleration factor
2D Single-Shot Fast Spin Echo, SSFSE (MRCP)	7000/1221	300 × 300	288 × 288	64/0	–	6	0.92	31.3	–
Axial Fast Spin Echo, FSE (T2WI)	6316/72	360 ~ 400	320 × 192	5/1	90	20	2	83.3	2
Axial Single-Shot Echo Planar Imaging, ss DWEPI (DWI)	3333/66.8	360 ~ 400	192 × 160	5/1	90	20	4	250	2
3D fat-suppressed Gradient Echo, 3D GRE (LAVA)	2.5/1.1	440 × 418	256 × 180	5/0	11	76	0.71	125	2

Data analysis

DWI-data were processed using a standard software package (Function 6.3.1e, GE AW VolumeShare 2, GE Healthcare, Milwaukee, USA). The multiple-b-values DWI derived parameters were calculated for all slices voxel-by-voxel with the following three approaches, which have been presented in our previously study in details [27]:

1. Direct calculation of the ADC_b using only two b-values (zero and non-zero):

$$ADC_b = \frac{1}{b} \ln\left(\frac{S_0}{S}\right)$$

2. The ADC_{total} calculation by monoexponential fitting to the equation using all b-values:

$$\frac{S}{S_0} = \exp(-b \times ADC_{total})$$

3. Biexponential fitting on IVIM model gave ADC_{fast}, ADC_{slow}, f according to the following equation:

$$\frac{S}{S_0} = f \exp(-b \times ADC_{fast}) + (1-f) \exp(-b \times ADC_{slow})$$

Image Analysis

Quantitative analysis of DWI was performed by two readers (6-year and 4-year experience) in consensus. All available data, including the ADC_b-, ADC_{total}-, ADC_{slow}-, ADC_{fast}-, f maps and DWI images, were loaded in the software in conjunction. Region of interests (ROIs) were drawn on multiple slices of the images of b_{1000} and were directly co-localized on the diffusion parameters maps, respectively. For the tumor diffusion parameters measurements, mean values of $ADC_{20-1000}$, ADC_{total}, ADC_{fast}, ADC_{slow} and f were calculated from an oval ROI (mean 118 mm^2; range 55 - 308 mm^2), which was placed on the solid portion of the tumor (Fig. 2), avoiding pancreatic ducts and cystic lesions by referring to other MRI images such as T2WI or LAVA. In the healthy cases, conventional

MR sequences including T2WI, LAVA images did not show any diffuse parenchymal abnormalities. No substantial distortion artifacts were visible in the pancreas. The mean values of $ADC_{20-1000}$, ADC_{total}, ADC_{fast}, ADC_{slow} and f for normal pancreatic tissue were derived from an oval ROI (mean 64.5 mm^2; range 35-108 mm^2), which was drawn in the head of the pancreas and kept away from the border of the pancreas to prevent partial volume effect. An effort was made to avoid pancreatic duct, vessels, and the common bile duct.

Histological Analysis

Histopathological analyses were performed by a pathologist with 12 years of experience specifically for pancreatic diseases. Surgically resected specimens were used for the pathological evaluation of all tumors, which were subcategorized as well, moderately, and poorly differentiated adenocarcinomas according to the classification system of the World Health Organization (WHO) [28] and practical grading scheme for pathology [29] in the current study. Meantime, pathologically determined tumor size, T stage, and nodal status (whether metastatic peri-pancreatic lymph nodes were identified) were recorded for each case.

Statistical analysis

Statistical analyses were performed using the SPSS software for windows (Version 16.0, SPSS Inc., Chicago, IL, USA). The extracted parameters values were tested for significant differences between patients with PDAC of poorly and moderately differentiated; stage T3/T4 and stage T1/T2 tumors (given the infrequency of stage T1 and T4 tumors); tumors with and without metastatic peri-pancreatic lymph nodes; and tumors located in the pancreatic head versus body or tail using a Mann-Whitney U test, which also was used to compare the multi-b-values DWI derived parameters between pancreatic tumors and healthy pancreas. Spearman-rank correlations were used to assess the relationship between these quantitative parameters and tumor size. The

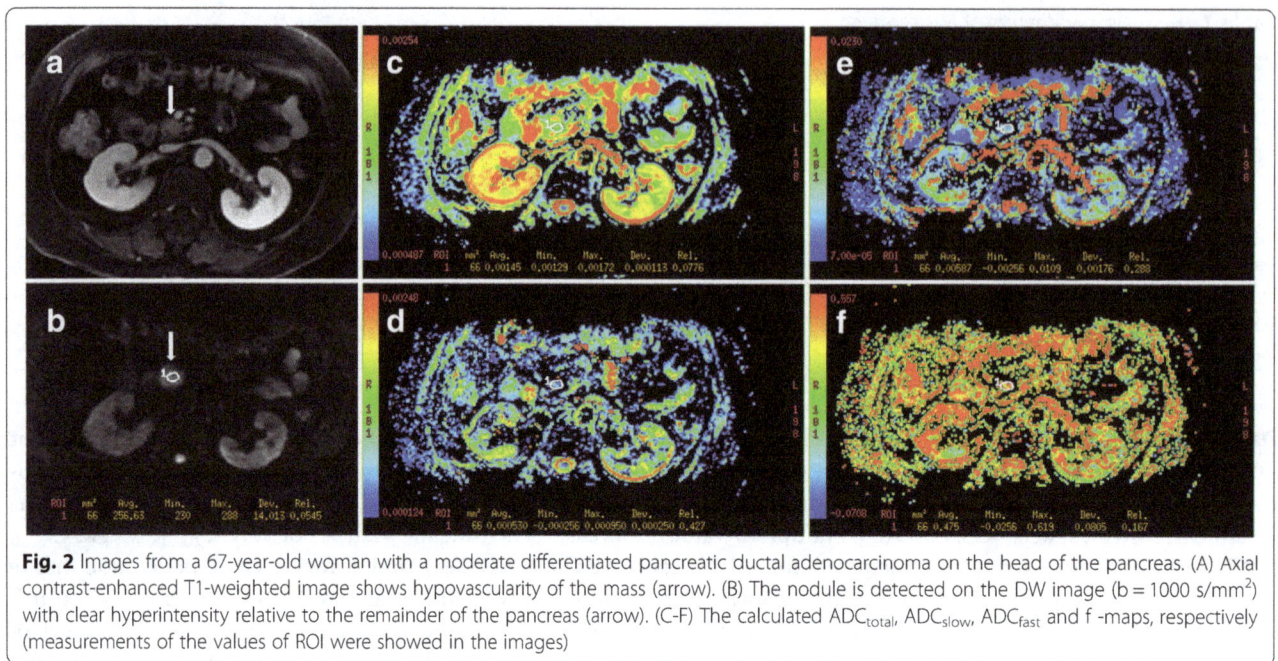

Fig. 2 Images from a 67-year-old woman with a moderate differentiated pancreatic ductal adenocarcinoma on the head of the pancreas. (A) Axial contrast-enhanced T1-weighted image shows hypovascularity of the mass (arrow). (B) The nodule is detected on the DW image (b = 1000 s/mm^2) with clear hyperintensity relative to the remainder of the pancreas (arrow). (C-F) The calculated ADC$_{total}$, ADC$_{slow}$, ADC$_{fast}$ and f -maps, respectively (measurements of the values of ROI were showed in the images)

comparison of mean ADC$_b$ values of the PDAC or the healthy pancreas among different b values was analyzed using Friedman tests. For the multiple comparisons of ADC values, post-hoc analyses were performed with Wilcoxon signed-rank tests and a Bonferroni correction applied. The statistical significance threshold of the Friedman test was set at a p-value below 0.05, while at a p-value below 0.0018 (0.05/28) for post hoc tests. In addition, receiver operating characteristics (ROC) analyses were used to identify the diagnostic performances of the multiple-b-values DWI derived parameters to distinguish pancreatic cancer from healthy pancreas tissue. A P-value of less than 0.05 was considered to indicate a statistically significant difference.

Results

Tumors

Based on the WHO classification criteria, 14 patients with poorly differentiated adenocarcinoma and 37 patients with moderately differentiated tumors were identified. The 51 tumors had a mean maximum lesion diameter at histopathological analyses of 35 ± 12 mm (range 15-90 mm). Among the 51 tumors, 30 (58.8%) were located in the pancreatic head; 38 (74.5%) were stage T3/T4 and 29 (56.9%) had metastatic peri-pancreatic lymph nodes.

Comparisons of IVIM DWI parameters between PDAC and healthy pancreas

The Friedman tests results demonstrated significant declines of the mean ADCs of the monoexponential DWI from b$_{20}$ to b$_{1000}$ for the PDAC or the healthy

pancreatic tissue (both P < 0.001, Table 2). The mean ADC$_{20-600}$, ADC$_{1000}$, ADCt$_{otal}$, ADC$_{fast}$ values were significantly lowers for PDAC than for healthy pancreas. The diagnostic performances of ADC$_{20-600}$, ADC$_{1000}$, ADCt$_{otal}$, ADC$_{fast}$ for differentiating PDAC form healthy pancreas was shown in Fig. 3 and the ROC analyses results were summarized in Table 3. The largest area under curve (AUC) was 0.911 for ADC$_{20}$ with a cut-off value of 5.58×10^{-3} mm^2/s, and ADC$_{20}$ also had the highest combined sensitivity (89.5%) and specificity (82.4%).

Table 2 Comparisons of multi-b-value DWI derived parameters (mean ± standard deviation) of healthy pancreas and pancreatic adenocarcinoma

Parameters	Pancreatic cancer	Healthy pancreas	P
ADC$_{20}$ ($\times10^{-3}$mm^2/s)	4.08 ± 2.19	9.01 ± 3.76	0.000
ADC$_{50}$ ($\times10^{-3}$mm^2/s)	2.62 ± 1.57	5.19 ± 2.07	0.000
ADC$_{100}$ ($\times10^{-3}$mm^2/s)	1.96 ± 0.92	3.72 ± 1.60	0.000
ADC$_{200}$ ($\times10^{-3}$mm^2/s)	1.86 ± 0.65	2.61 ± 0.82	0.000
ADC$_{400}$ ($\times10^{-3}$mm^2/s)	1.72 ± 0.43	2.03 ± 0.52	0.003
ADC$_{600}$ ($\times10^{-3}$mm^2/s)	1.61 ± 0.43	1.76 ± 0.38	0.037
ADC$_{800}$ ($\times10^{-3}$mm^2/s)	1.49 ± 0.33	1.61 ± 0.34	0.177
ADC$_{1000}$ ($\times10^{-3}$mm^2/s)	1.20 ± 0.28	1.31 ± 0.25	0.016
ADC$_{total}$ ($\times10^{-3}$mm^2/s)	1.38 ± 0.26	1.56 ± 0.30	0.003
ADC$_{fast}$ ($\times10^{-3}$mm^2/s)	6.39 ± 5.55	14.05 ± 8.31	0.000
ADC$_{slow}$ ($\times10^{-3}$mm^2/s)	0.84 ± 0.32	0.92 ± 0.26	0.235
f (%)	0.42 ± 0.15	0.39 ± 0.12	0.212

ADC indicates apparent diffusion coefficient; IVIM, intravoxel incoherent motion; SD, standard deviation; P < 0.05 was considered to indicate a statistically significant difference

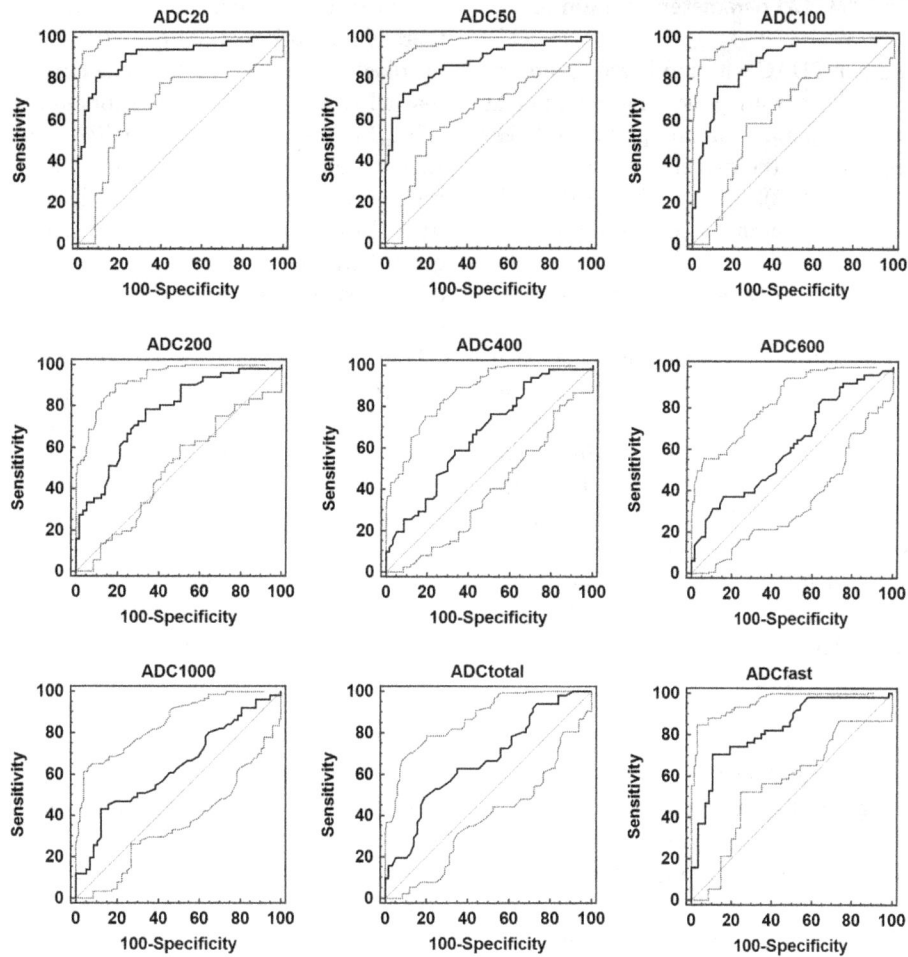

Fig. 3 ROC-curves for differentiating pancreatic cancer from healthy pancreas of ADC$_{20-600}$, ADC$_{1000}$, ADC$_{total}$, and ADC$_{fast}$. ADC$_{20}$ revealed significantly higher AUC than other multiple-b-values DWI derived parameters

Table 3 Results from the ROC analyses for the 9 parameters to distinguish between pancreatic adenocarcinoma and healthy pancreas

Parameters	Optimal cutoff values (×10^{-3}mm^2/s)	AUC	Sensitivities (%)	Spectificities (%)	PPV (%)	NPV (%)	ACC (%)
ADC$_{20}$	5.58	0.911	0.895	0.824	0.820	0.898	0.858
ADC$_{50}$	3.06	0.874	0.912	0.725	0.748	0.902	0.813
ADC$_{100}$	2.37	0.876	0.877	0.765	0.770	0.874	0.818
ADC$_{200}$	2.19	0.771	0.667	0.784	0.734	0.725	0.729
ADC$_{400}$	1.91	0.667	0.491	0.765	0.651	0.627	0.636
ADC$_{600}$	1.41	0.616	0.842	0.373	0.546	0.725	0.594
ADC$_{1000}$	1.09	0.634	0.877	0.431	0.580	0.797	0.642
ADC$_{total}$	1.36	0.664	0.807	0.490	0.586	0.739	0.640
ADC$_{fast}$	5.86	0.828	0.895	0.706	0.731	0.883	0.795

ROC, operating characteristic curve; AUC, area under curve; ADC, apparent diffusion coefficient; PPV, positive predictive value; NPV, negative predictive value; ACC, accuracy

Association between IVIM DWI parameters and tumor grade

The mean ADC values in PDAC with moderate differentiation were similar to those with poor differentiation at $b_{20\text{-}1000}$ ($p = 0.460\text{-}0.941$). In addition, no significant differences were observed between the two groups for ADC_{total} ($P = 0.720$), ADC_{slow} ($P = 0.658$), ADC_{fast} ($P = 0.326$) and f ($P = 0.941$). The results were summarized in Table 4.

Association between IVIM DWI parameters and tumor characteristics

There were no significant correlations between multiple-b-values DWI derived parameters values and tumor size ($P = 0.195\text{-}0.986$). There was no statistically significant difference in all of the multi-b-values DWI derived parameters between PDAC stage T1/T2 and stage T3/T4. ($p = 0.060\text{-}0.880$). In addition, all of the quantitative parameters were not significantly different between tumors located in the pancreatic head versus other pancreatic regions ($p = 0.203\text{-}0.954$) or between tumors with and without metastatic peri-pancreatic lymph nodes ($p = 0.313\text{-}0.917$).

Discussion

Our study showed that multiple-b-values DWI derived parameters including $ADC_{20\text{-}600}$, ADC_{1000}, $ADCt_{otal}$, ADC_{fast} might be useful markers to distinguish PDAC from healthy pancreas, and the ADC_{20} provided the highest accuracy. No associations between the mean ADC_b, ADC_{total}, ADC_{slow}, ADC_{fast} and f values of PDAC and the tumor grade were found. However, tumors with low values for all of the multiple-b-values DWI derived parameters had a tendency to be at advanced stage.

To the authors' knowledge, three studies investigated the potential associations between ADC values of PDAC and tumor grade [12, 24, 25]. Similar b values (0, 500 or 800 s/mm^2) and the same field strength of 1.5-T for DWI experiments to measure ADC values with a monoexponential model. Wang et al. reported significantly lower ADC in cases of PDAC that are poorly differentiated in comparison with well/moderately differentiated lesions [24]. However, no associations between ADC values of PDAC and tumor grade in other two studies were observed [12, 25]. As in the present study, we failed to observe a statistically lower ADC in PDAC of poorly differentiated in comparison with those of moderately differentiated lesions, which is consistent with the results of Rosenkrantz A.B. et al [12] and Hayano K. et al [25].It is possible that histological differences between cases included in the studies account for the discrepant conclusions under the given single maximal b-value (500 s/mm^2) [12].

Recently, IVIM DWI have been studied for pancreatic lesions [9, 18, 30]. Although IVIM parameters have been

shown to aid distinguishing tumors from normal tissue, there is no work that compared IVIM parameters for the histological grade of tumors. The current results indicated that all of the mean monoexponential ADC (ADC_b and ADC_{total}) and biexponential IVIM parameters (ADC_{slow}, ADC_{fast} and f) values for PDAC did not exhibit significance dependence on tumor grade or tumor characteristics. Thus, based on the present data, it seems that the quantitative parameters are currently unlikely to be of clinical values for the non-invasive prediction of adverse pathological features of newly detected cases of PDAC.

Four research groups reported the IVIM-based parameters measurements in PDAC [9, 18, 20, 30–33]. Klauss M et al. reported the ADC_b of PDAC obtained from monoexponential model ranging from 4.04 to 1.18×10^{-3} mm^2/s [30], which is in good agreement with our study. In addition, in the current study, the mean ADC_{total} values of PDAC is 1.37×10^{-3} mm^2/s, which is also in good agreement with two previous studies (1.28 and 1.31×10^{-3} mm^2/s, respectively) [13, 30]. Inconsistent with previous studies [11, 18], the perfusion fraction f was unable to distinguish PDAC from healthy pancreas. The main reason is that the IVIM DWI derived parameters are usually affected by the number and distribution of b values and postprocessing methods used.

In addition to pathological factors that may impact ADC values, MRI technique itself including field strength, method for respiratory compensation, parameter variance and ADC measurement technique also influenced ADC measurements. In the present study, we found a significant decline of the mean ADC values of the monoexponential DWI from b_{20} to b_{1000} for the PDAC or the healthy pancreatic tissue. The mean ADC_b values were significantly lower for PDAC than for healthy pancreatic tissue except ADC_{800}. Some previous studies showed significant difference in ADC_{800} values between PDAC and normal pancreatic tissue at 1.5-T [18, 25], the underlying reason for no significant difference in ADC_{800} at 3T as observed in this study maybe the variations in the data acquisition [33]. We also found that the ADC_{20} provided the highest accuracy to distinguish PDAC from healthy pancreas. It is necessary to optimize the low b values to differentiate pancreatic diseases in future studies, despite the perfusion effect on ADC values were obvious.

The present study had some limitations. Firstly, the number of subjects was limited, as many cases were PDAC with moderate differentiation or stage T3/T4. Further studies with larger samples size are needed to confirm our results. Secondly, our previous study had clarified that the effect of age and gender on ADCs in the normal adult pancreas can be excluded [34]. In the current study, we did not take into account the effect of age and gender on the ADC values of the control group,

Table 4 Comparisons of multi-b-value DWI derived parameters (mean ± standard deviation) of pancreatic adenocarcinoma with tumor characteristics

Parameters	Grades of differentiation			Tumor locations			Tumor grades			lymph node status		
	well/moderately differentiated	poorly differentiated	P	Head	Elsewhere in pancreas	P	T1/T2	T3/T4	P	Present	Absent	P
ADC_{20} ($\times10^{-3}mm^2/s$)	4.15 ± 2.24	3.92 ± 2.13	0.849	4.05 ± 2.12	4.13 ± 2.35	0.901	4.24 ± 2.78	4.06 ± 2.04	0.846	3.97 ± 2.37	4.17 ± 2.09	0.419
ADC_{50} ($\times10^{-3}mm^2/s$)	2.62 ± 1.69	2.62 ± 1.23	0.665	2.44 ± 1.36	2.87 ± 1.83	0.358	3.04 ± 1.33	2.50 ± 1.65	0.098	2.64 ± 1.79	2.60 ± 1.40	0.897
ADC_{100} ($\times10^{-3}mm^2/s$)	2.03 ± 1.01	1.77 ± 0.65	0.499	1.89 ± 0.71	2.06 ± 1.18	0.954	2.19 ± 0.81	1.88 ± 0.96	0.107	1.95 ± 0.96	1.97 ± 0.92	0.775
ADC_{200} ($\times10^{-3}mm^2/s$)	1.89 ± 0.74	1.77 ± 0.29	0.460	1.86 ± 0.51	1.85 ± 0.82	0.599	2.10 ± 0.44	1.79 ± 0.70	0.060	1.93 ± 0.79	1.81 ± 0.53	0.827
ADC_{400} ($\times10^{-3}mm^2/s$)	1.73 ± 0.49	1.68 ± 0.19	0.768	1.69 ± 0.35	1.76 ± 0.52	0.811	1.80 ± 0.27	1.70 ± 0.46	0.496	1.74 ± 0.43	1.70 ± 0.43	0.732
ADC_{600} ($\times10^{-3}mm^2/s$)	1.63 ± 0.49	1.57 ± 0.23	0.941	1.53 ± 0.28	1.73 ± 0.57	0.320	1.73 ± 0.29	1.59 ± 0.46	0.226	1.65 ± 0.51	1.58 ± 0.36	0.662
ADC_{800} ($\times10^{-3}mm^2/s$)	1.51 ± 0.36	1.44 ± 0.19	0.486	1.43 ± 0.26	1.57 ± 0.40	0.235	1.60 ± 0.27	1.46 ± 0.34	0.256	1.51 ± 0.29	1.47 ± 0.35	0.917
ADC_{1000} ($\times10^{-3}mm^2/s$)	1.22 ± 0.31	1.14 ± 0.17	0.506	1.16 ± 0.23	1.25 ± 0.32	0.203	1.21 ± 0.17	1.20 ± 0.30	0.880	1.18 ± 0.29	1.21 ± 0.27	0.337
ADC_{total} ($\times10^{-3}mm^2/s$)	1.38 ± 0.29	1.35 ± 0.16	0.720	1.34 ± 0.22	1.43 ± 0.31	0.450	1.47 ± 0.20	1.36 ± 0.27	0.399	1.37 ± 0.19	1.38 ± 0.30	0.387
ADC_{fast} ($\times10^{-3}mm^2/s$)	6.98 ± 6.28	4.81 ± 2.38	0.326	6.87 ± 6.49	5.70 ± 3.88	0.612	8.89 ± 9.15	5.58 ± 3.74	0.154	5.63 ± 3.6	6.96 ± 6.67	0.634
ADC_{slow} ($\times10^{-3}mm^2/s$)	0.86 ± 0.32	0.81 ± 0.33	0.658	0.80 ± 0.31	0.91 ± 0.33	0.343	0.86 ± 0.37	0.84 ± 0.31	0.689	0.80 ± 0.36	0.88 ± 0.29	0.313
f (%)	0.42 ± 0.15	0.42 ± 0.14	0.941	0.41 ± 0.16	0.43 ± 0.13	0.653	0.43 ± 0.17	0.42 ± 0.14	0.854	0.43 ± 0.16	0.41 ± 0.14	0.562

ADC indicates apparent diffusion coefficient; IVIM, intravoxel incoherent motion; SD, standard deviation

which may affect the results. Thirdly, in the current study, 58.8% of cancers were located in the pancreatic head. In these cases, it is difficult to find any normal tissue to compare with for there is obstruction of the pancreatic duct, which leads to significant atrophy of the rest of the pancreatic gland. So we did not analyze the DWI derived parameters of the PDAC tissue versus adjacent pancreatic parenchyma. Fourthly, for IVIM DWI, a navigator-triggered technique was employed to achieve higher SNR and decrease motion artifacts. Despite that the participants recruited were required to perform regular breathing training prior to scanning to decrease the misalignment between images, image registration at different b-values was not performed, which may affect the results. Finally, our findings were similar to the results of Rosenkrantz A.B. et al [12], but inconformity with the results of Wang et al[24]. It is possible that histological differences between cases included in the two studies account for the discrepant conclusions.

Conclusions
Our results demonstrate that there were no associations between multiple-b-values DWI derived monoexponential and biexponential diffusion parameters of PDAC and tumor grade or tumor characteristics, and ADC_{20} provided the best accuracy for differentiating PDAC from healthy pancreas. This finding suggests that the clinical use of multiple-b-values DWI derived parameters to predict the prognosis of newly diagnosed PDAC is not advisable.

Abbreviations
ADC: Apparent diffusion coefficient; AUC: Area under curve; CT: Computed tomography; DWI: Diffusion-weighted magnetic resonance imaging; ERCP: Endoscopic retrograde cholangiopancreatography; EUS: Endoscopic ultrasonography; IVIM: Intravoxel incoherent motion; LAVA: Liver acceleration volume acquisition; MRI: Magnetic resonance imaging; PDAC: Pancreatic ductal adenocarcinomas; ROC: Receiver operating characteristic; ROI: Region of interest; SPIR: Selective presaturation with inversion recovery; WHO: World Health Organization

Acknowledgements
Not applicable.

Funding
Supported by Grants from the 1255 Academic Discipline Project of Shanghai Changhai Hospital, No. CH125520800; the Youth Scientific Research Funds of Shanghai Changhai Hosptial, No. 201302.

Authors' contributions
MC, LYJ, WL, WY and CSY performed the majority of experiments, made substantial contributions to the data analysis and interpretation, and wrote the manuscript draft; ZY and WH participated in the design of the study and made substantial contribution to data analysis; Lu JP made substantial contributions to the study conception and design, critically revised the manuscript draft for important intellectual content, and gave final approval of the version to be published; all the authors read and approved the final manuscript.

Competing interests
The authors declare that they have no competing interests.

Author details
[1]Department of Radiology, Changhai Hospital of Shanghai, The Second Military Medical University, No.168 Changhai Road, Shanghai 200433, China. [2]Department of Pathology, Changhai Hospital of Shanghai, The Second Military Medical University, No.168 Changhai Road, Shanghai, China. [3]MR Group, GE Healthcare, No. 1 Huatuo Road, Shanghai, China.

References
1. International Agency for Research on Cancer, WHO. http://eco.iarc.fr/eucan/Cancer.aspx?Cancer. Accessed September 9, 2013
2. Siegel R, Naishadham D, Jemal A. Cancer Statistics, 2013. CA CANCER J CLIN. 2013;63:11–30.
3. Muniraj T, Jamidar PA, Aslanian HR. Pancreatic cancer: A comprehensive review and update. Diease-a-month. 2013;59:368–402.
4. Garcea G, Dennison AR, Pattenden CJ, Neal CP, Sutton CD, Berry DP. Survival following curative resection for pancreatic ductal adenocarcinoma. A systematic review of the literature. JOP. 2008;9:99–132.
5. Bammer R. Basic principles of diffusion-weighted imaging. Eur J Radiol. 2003;45:169–84.
6. Dale BM, Braithwaite AC, Boll DT, Merkle EM. Field strength and diffusion encoding technique affect the apparent diffusion coefficient measurements in diffusion-weighted imaging of the abdomen. Invest Radiol. 2010;45:104–8.
7. Mürtz P, Flacke S, Träber F, Van den Brink JS, Gieseke J, Schild HH. Abdomen: diffusion-weighted MR imaging with pulse-triggered single-shot sequences. Radiology. 2002;224:258–64.
8. Thoeny HC, De Keyzer F. Extracranial applications of diffusion-weighted magnetic resonance imaging. Eur Radiol. 2007;17:1385–93.
9. Kang KM, Lee JM, Yoon JH, Kiefer B, Han JK, Choi BI. Intravoxel Incoherent Motion Diffusion-weighted MR Imaging for Characterization of Focal Pancreatic Lesions. Radiology. 2014;270:444–53.
10. Koc Z, Erbay G. Optimal b value in diffusion-weighted imaging for differentiation of abdominal lesions. J Magn Reson Imaging. 2014;40:559–66.
11. Concia M, Sprinkart AM, Penner AH, Brossart P, Gieseke J, Schild HH, et al. Diffusion-weighted magnetic resonance imaging of the pancreas: diagnostic benefit from an intravoxel incoherent motion model-based 3 b-value analysis. Invest Radiol. 2014;49:93–100.
12. Rosenkrantz AB, Matza BW, Sabach A, Hajdu CH, Hindman N. Pancreatic cancer: Lack of association between apparent diffusion coefficient values and adverse pathological features. Clin Radiol. 2013;68:e191–7.
13. Fukukura Y, Takumi K, Kamimura K, Shindo T, Kumagae Y, Tateyama A, et al. Pancreatic adenocarcinoma: variability of diffusion-weighted MR imaging findings. Radiology. 2012;263:732–40.
14. Wiggermann P, Grützmann R, Weissenböck A, Kamusella P, Dittert DD, Stroszczynski C. Apparent diffusion coefficient measurements of the pancreas, pancreas carcinoma, and mass-forming focal pancreatitis. Acta Radiol. 2012;53:135–9.
15. Wang Y, Miller FH, Chen ZE, Merrick L, Mortele KJ, Hoff FL, et al. Diffusion-weighted MR imaging of solid and cystic lesions of the pancreas. Radio Graphics. 2011;31:E47–64.
16. Kamisawa T, Takuma K, Anjiki H, Egawa N, Hata T, Kurata M, et al. Differentiation of autoimmune pancreatitis from pancreatic cancer by diffusion-weighted MRI. Am J Gastroenterol. 2010;105:1870–5.
17. Fattahi R, Balci NC, Perman WH, Hsueh EC, Alkaade S, Havlioglu N, et al. Pancreatic diffusion-weighted imaging (DWI): comparison between mass-forming focal pancreatitis (FP), pancreatic cancer (PC), and normal pancreas. J Magn Reson Imaging. 2009;29:350–6.
18. Lemke A, Laun FB, Klauss M, Re TJ, Simon D, Delorme S, et al. Differentiation of pancreas carcinoma from healthy pancreatic tissue using multiple b-values: comparison of apparent diffusion coefficient and intravoxel incoherent motion derived parameters. Invest Radiol. 2009;44:769–75.
19. Kartalis N, Lindholm TL, Aspelin P, Permert J, Albiin N. Diffusion-weighted magnetic resonance imaging of pancreas tumours. Eur Radiol. 2009;19:1981–90.

20. Lee SS, Byun JH, Park BJ, Park SH, Kim N, Park B, et al. Quantitative analysis of diffusion-weighted magnetic resonance imaging of the pancreas: usefulness in characterizing solid pancreatic masses. J Magn Reson Imaging. 2008;28:928–36.

21. Muraoka N, Uematsu H, Kimura H, Imamura Y, Fujiwara Y, Murakami M, et al. Apparent diffusion coefficient in pancreatic cancer: characterization and histopathological correlations. J Magn Reson Imaging. 2008;27:1302–8.

22. Matsuki M, Inada Y, Nakai G, Tatsugami F, Tanikake M, Narabayashi I, et al. Diffusion-weighed MR imaging of pancreatic carcinoma. Abdom Imaging. 2007;32:481–3.

23. Ichikawa T, Erturk SM, Motosugi U, Sou H, Iino H, Araki T, et al. High-b value diffusion weighted MRI for detecting pancreatic adenocarcinoma: preliminary results. Am J Roentgenol. 2007;188:409–14.

24. Wang Y, Chen ZE, Nikolaidis P, McCarthy RJ, Merrick L, Sternick LA, et al. Diffusion-weighted magnetic resonance imaging of pancreatic adenocarcinomas: association with histopathology and tumour grade. J Magn Reson Imaging. 2011;33:136–42.

25. Hayano K, Miura F, Amano H, Toyota N, Wada K, Kato K, et al. Correlation of apparent diffusion coefficient measured by diffusion-weighted MRI and clinicopathologic features in pancreatic cancer patients. J Hepatobiliary Pancreat Sci. 2013;20:243–8.

26. Le Bihan D, Breton E, Lallemand D, Grenier P, Cabanis E, Laval-Jeantet M. MR imaging of intravoxel incoherent motions: application to diffusion and perfusion in neurologic disorders. Radiology. 1986;161:401–7.

27. Ma C, Liu L, Li YJ, Chen LG, Pan CS, Zhang Y, et al. Intravoxel incoherent motion MRI of the healthy pancreas: Monoexponential and biexponential apparent diffusion parameters of the normal head, body and tail. J Magn Reson Imaging. 2015;41:1236–41.

28. Bosman FT, Carneiro F, Hruban RH, Theise ND. International Agency for Research on Cancer, Lyon. 4th ed. 2010.

29. American Joint Committee on Cancer (AJCC) TNM staging system, September 6, 2013. American Cancer Society. Available at http://www.cancer.org/cancer/pancreaticcancer/detailedguide/pancreatic-cancer-staging. Accessed September 9, 2013

30. Klauss M, Lemke A, Grünberg K, Simon D, Re TJ, Wente MN, et al. Intravoxel incoherent motion MRI for the differentiation between mass forming chronic pancreatitis and pancreatic carcinoma. Invest Radiol. 2011;46:57–63.

31. Re TJ, Lemke A, Klauss M, Laun FB, Simon D, Grünberg K, et al. Enhancing pancreatic adenocarcinoma delineation in diffusion derived intravoxel incoherent motion f-maps through automatic vessel and duct segmentation. Magn Reson Med. 2011;66:1327–32.

32. Klauss M, Gaida MM, Lemke A, Grünberg K, Simon D, Wente MN, et al. Fibrosis and pancreatic lesions: counterintuitivebehavior of the diffusion imaging-derived structural diffusion coefficient D. Invest Radiol. 2013;48:129–33.

33. Partridge SC, McDonald ES. Diffusion weighted magnetic resonance imaging of the breast: protocol optimization, interpretation, and clinical applications. Magn Reson Imaging Clin N Am. 2013;21:601–24.

34. Ma C, Pan CS, Zhang HG, Wang H, Wang J, Chen SY, et al. Diffusion-weighted MRI of the normal adult pancreas: the effect of age on apparent diffusion coefficient values. Clin Radiol. 2013;68:e532–7.

14

Whole-body MRI in pediatric patients with cancer

Marcos Duarte Guimarães[1,2], Julia Noschang[3*], Sara Reis Teixeira[4], Marcel Koenigkam Santos[4], Henrique Manoel Lederman[5], Vivian Tostes[6], Vikas Kundra[7], Alex Dias Oliveira[3], Bruno Hochhegger[8] and Edson Marchiori[9]

Abstract

Cancer is the leading cause of natural death in the pediatric populations of developed countries, yet cure rates are greater than 70% when a cancer is diagnosed in its early stages. Recent advances in magnetic resonance imaging methods have markedly improved diagnostic and therapeutic approaches, while avoiding the risks of ionizing radiation that are associated with most conventional radiological methods, such as computed tomography and positron emission tomography/computed tomography. The advent of whole-body magnetic resonance imaging in association with the development of metabolic- and function-based techniques has led to the use of whole-body magnetic resonance imaging for the screening, diagnosis, staging, response assessment, and post-therapeutic follow-up of children with solid sporadic tumours or those with related genetic syndromes. Here, the advantages, techniques, indications, and limitations of whole-body magnetic resonance imaging in the management of pediatric oncology patients are presented.

Keywords: Neoplasm, Pediatrics, Magnetic resonance imaging, Whole body MRI, Whole body imaging

Background

Cancer is currently the leading cause of natural death in the pediatric populations of developed countries [1]. However, the cure rates for cancers are greater than 70% in some cases when a cancer is diagnosed in its early stages. To increase the cure rates for cancer patients, diagnostic and therapeutic advances are needed. To select the most appropriate treatment for a child with cancer, the type, location, and staging of the tumour should be completely assessed [2–4]. Ideally, imaging protocols should be rapid, provide high quality images, have a low radiation, and provide clinically significant information [5–7]. In addition, every effort should be made to avoid redundant examinations that do not provide additional information relevant to therapeutic decision making [8]. There are many imaging modalities that are currently used to characterise the extent of local and distant disease. For example, ultrasonography, computed tomography (CT), magnetic resonance imaging (MRI),

metaiodobenzylguanidine (MIBG) scans, and bone scintigraphy (BS) are most frequently performed [8, 9]. However, modalities that deposit radiation, such as BS and CT, should be used with caution in pediatric patients due to the risk of complications, including the risk of developing secondary malignancies.

Positron emission tomography/computed tomography (PET/CT) has recently been used in children with cancer because it provides whole-body (WB) coverage and information regarding the metabolic stage of tumours. Regarding the latter, an intravenous injection of the radiopharmaceutical, ^{18}F-fluorodeoxyglucose (^{18}F-FDG), allows regions of abnormal glucose metabolism to be detected with hybrid systems such as PET/CT and correlated with possible morphological changes on anatomic images [10, 11]. PET/CT also plays an important role in tumour staging, in assessing response to treatment, and can potentially predict treatment success in certain oncology settings [12]. Operational limitations of PET/CT include its restricted availability to specialised centers in many countries; the short half life of ^{18}F which requires prompt delivery and use [13]; and the radiation burden to a patient.

* Correspondence: julia_noschang@hotmail.com
[3]Department of Imaging, AC Camargo Cancer Center, Rua Prof. Antônio Prudente, 211, Liberdade, Sao Paulo/SP 01509-010, Brazil
Full list of author information is available at the end of the article

In contrast, MRI can provide exquisite anatomic detail and functional information without radiation to patients. In addition, technological advances, particularly in the development of fast imaging sequences, allow MRI to provide WB coverage in a reasonable time frame [14, 15]. Thus, with the fusion of morphological sequences and functional techniques, such as diffusion-weighted imaging (DWI) and WB morphological/functional mapping, relevant information regarding disease activity can be obtained [16, 17]. The aim of this review is to discuss the advantages, techniques, indications, and limitations of WB MRI in evaluations of pediatric patients with cancer.

Main Text
Advantages of WB MRI

WB MRI provides a single examination of the entire body without the use of ionizing radiation. In addition to the excellent contrast and spatial resolution of WB MRI, functional information is obtained which improves the capacity of this method to differentiate normal tissues from pathological tissues. MRI equipment is often available at both large and small centers, thereby facilitating the implementation of more advanced studies, such as MRI diffusion, perfusion, and WB studies [18, 19]. Furthermore, a complete disease assessment in the oncology setting, including detection of metastasis sites, in a single examination helps to reduce the number of patient visits to an imaging service, thereby reducing related costs [20].

Exposure to ionizing radiation is a major concern in pediatric patients with cancer [7]. However, imaging methods that use ionizing radiation sources, such as X-ray, CT, BS, and PET/CT, are often routinely employed [21, 22]. The risk of tumour development due to ionizing radiation exposure is related to the amount, intensity, and accumulation of the applied radiation over an individual's life [23]. Newer CT scanners use iterative image reconstruction which reduces radiation exposure, although, exposure still occurs and repeated studies can incur a significant radiation dose for a patient. This risk increases when radiation exposure occurs at younger ages, especially exposure during childhood. In a recent study that examined the risks associated with the use of imaging methods that employ ionizing radiation for

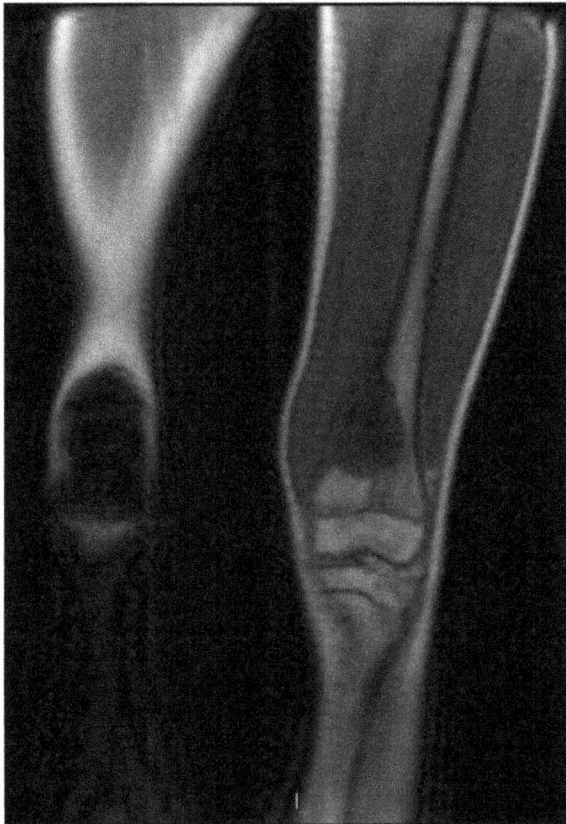

Fig. 1 A 15-year-old male patient follow up whole-body MRI examination by bilateral retinoblastoma and osteosarcoma in right femur, in the last exam, the T1-weighted image demonstrated a lesion with low signal intensity in distal left femur. Histological diagnosis of second osteosarcoma

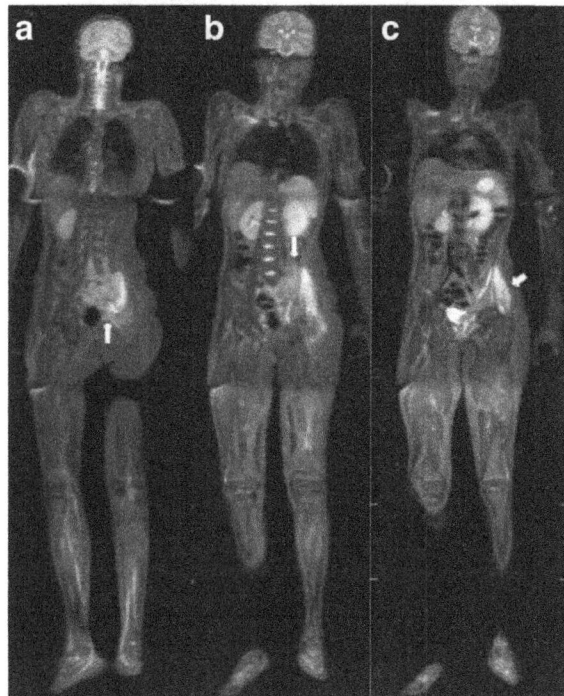

Fig. 2 An 18-year-old female patient with a voluminous lesion in the *left* hemi-pelvis (a, *arrow*) and histologically confirmed chondrosarcoma underwent whole-body MRI with a coronal STIR sequence for staging. The examination revealed involvement in the sacrum (a, *arrow*) and *left* ilium (b, *arrow*) and the presence of soft-tissue components adjacent to marked hyperintensity (c, *arrow*). Note the antalgic position, with slight body deviation to the *right*. No other lesion suspicious of malignancy was noted

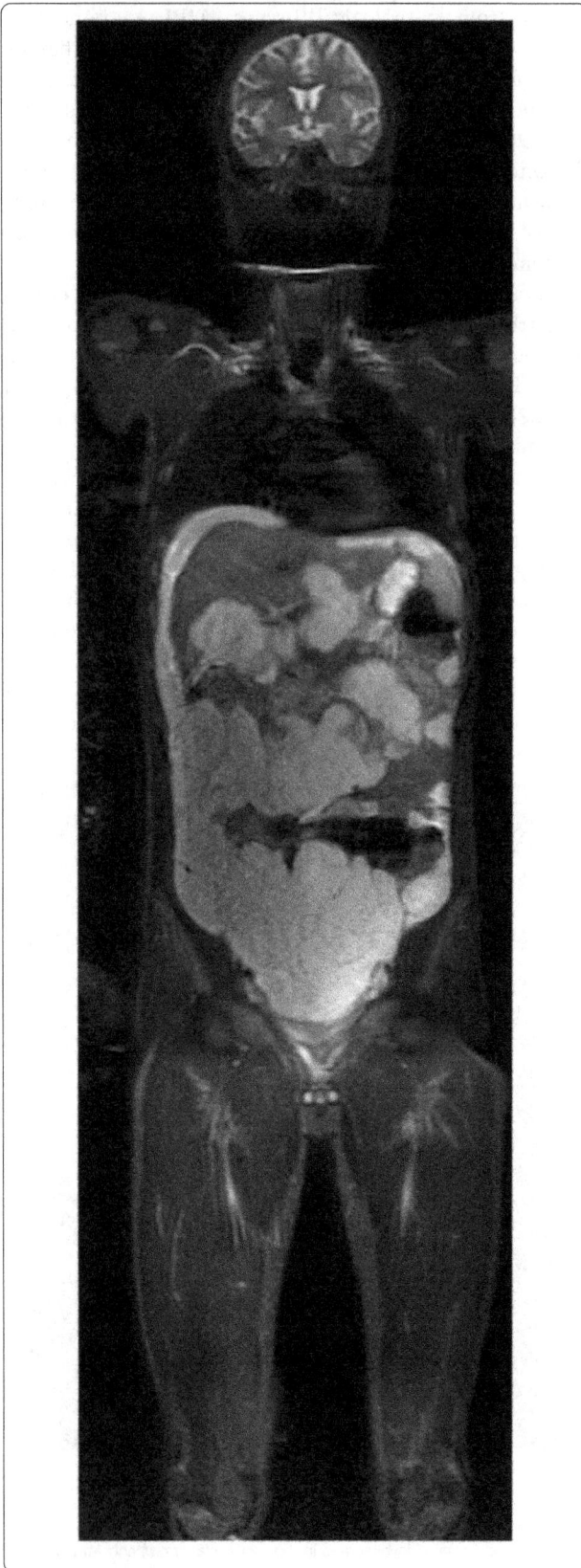

Fig. 3 Whole-body MRI with a coronal STIR sequence in a 17-year-old male patient with multiple lesions disseminated in the peritoneal cavity and a histological diagnosis of mucinous adenocarcinoma of high-grade colonic with abdominal implants

diagnostic purposes, an estimated 29,000 new cancer cases were found to be related to the number of CT scans performed in the United States in 2007, with 15% of the estimated cancers associated with scans that were performed on patients younger than 18 years [24, 25]. An advantage of WB MRI is that it can be applied to at-risk populations, including those that may be affected by familial syndromes, to conduct cancer screenings. Advances in genetics have enabled the identification of patients with hereditary syndromes related to the development of neoplasms. The goal of performing WB MRI for cancer screenings is to detect malignancies in their early stages when the effectiveness of treatments and cure rates are optimal [26, 27]. Ideally, screenings should be applied to apparently healthy populations that are at high risk for tumour development. Examples of inherited syndromes that are associated with increased risks of cancer include: multiple endocrine neoplasias I and II (e.g., endocrine tumours), Von Hippel-Lindau syndrome (e.g., renal carcinomas), familial adenomatous polyposis (e.g., colorectal tumours), and Li-Fraumeni syndrome (e.g., various types of tumours including sarcomas) (Fig. 1) [28–31]. Correspondingly, a new screening protocol that involves WB MRI has recently been proposed for patients with Li-Fraumeni syndrome [32].

Magnetic resonance technique / protocol
To date, there is no overall consensus regarding a WB MRI protocol for children. Typically, T1 and T2 imaging are performed with free-breathing, suspended respiration, or physiological motion control. It is also widely accepted that short tau inversion recovery (STIR) sequences and diffusion add diagnostic value to WB MRI examinations. Depending on a pediatric patient's age and size, a complete set of images are obtained in a single acquisition (e.g., for infants), or in two or more segmental acquisitions (e.g., for older children and adolescents). The images are subsequently aligned using specific software to enable visualization of the entire body [20, 33]. WB MRI should be performed with high-field ($\geq$1.5 Tesla) equipment with surface and/or body coils. Dedicated pediatric receiver coils are currently being introduced and will progressively have increased availability. Patients should be examined from head to toe in a supine position with their arms parallel to the body and their legs together. Coronal acquisition, which is more rapid than other approaches, is preferred, although at least one sequence (e.g., diffusion) should be acquired in the axial plane to compensate for the

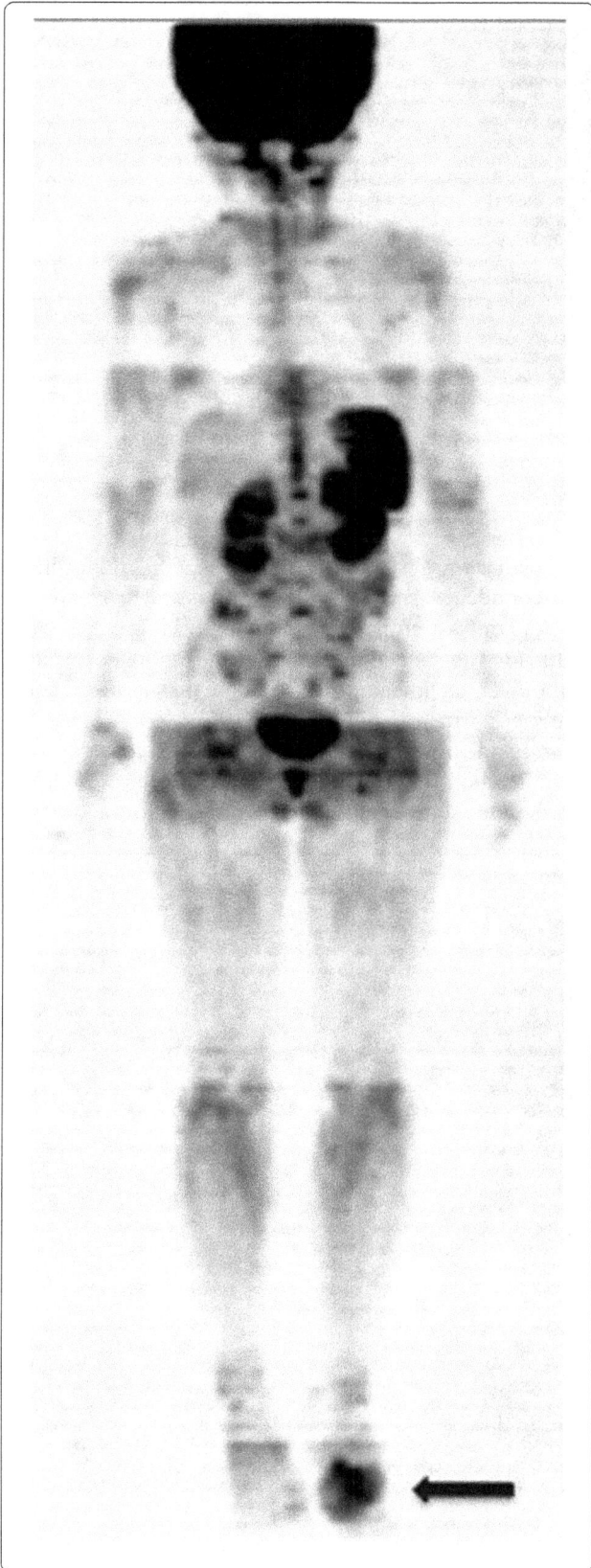

Fig. 4 A 9-year-old male patient with a histological diagnosis of osteosarcoma in the left foot (*arrow*) underwent whole-body MRI with diffusion sequences with three-dimensional reconstruction for staging, which showed no other lesion site

limitations associated with coronal acquisition (e.g., for the ribs, sternum, cranium, and spine) [34]. Sagittal acquisition is helpful for evaluating the spine. However, depending on the manufacturer, it is possible to perform axial T1-weighted acquisitions without wasting time. Moreover, synchronization of respiratory and cardiac movements can be achieved with external gates to avoid physiological motion artifacts [5, 33].

Conventional sequences, including T1- and T2-weighted spin-echo sequences, are usually performed without the administration of a paramagnetic contrast medium. Malignant lesions are usually hypointense (low signal intensity) on T1-weighted images (Fig. 1) and have a high signal intensity on T2-weighted images [35].

The STIR sequence is highly sensitive for the detection of pathologic lesions. Bone marrow lesions, including marrow infiltration from lymphoma, metastases, and tumour-related edema, exhibit high signal intensity on STIR sequences (Figs. 2 and 3). Focal parenchymal lesions can be distinguished by their slightly different signal intensity in STIR sequences, while pathologic lymph nodes cannot be differentiated from normal nodes on the basis of signal intensity. The STIR technique also cannot be used to differentiate benign conditions from malignant neoplastic lesions. The latter limitation restricts the application of STIR in WB MRI in oncologic patients after treatment, since therapy-induced marrow changes, such as edema, necrosis, fibrosis, or red marrow hyperplasia, cannot be differentiated from viable tumours. However, STIR may be very useful in staging pediatric tumours; although, additional clinical experience and data are needed to determine its efficacy [36, 37].

Diffusion-weighted MRI sequences are increasingly being employed for WB evaluations of patients with cancer (Fig. 4). These sequences detect the random motion of water molecules, also known as Brownian motion, through biological tissues by detecting the protons in the water molecules. The movement of the water molecules causes a phasic dispersion of proton spin, thereby resulting in signal loss due to diffusion sensitivity. The signal intensity of an object of study is analyzed quantitatively by calculating the absolute apparent diffusion coefficient (ADC, in mm²/s) of the object relative to the diffusion of water molecules in the proximal region [16, 38]. This qualitative and quantitative analysis is primarily influenced by the presence of barriers that restrict the diffusion of water molecules in their microenvironment, and this produces imaging contrast between tissues. Thus, the signal

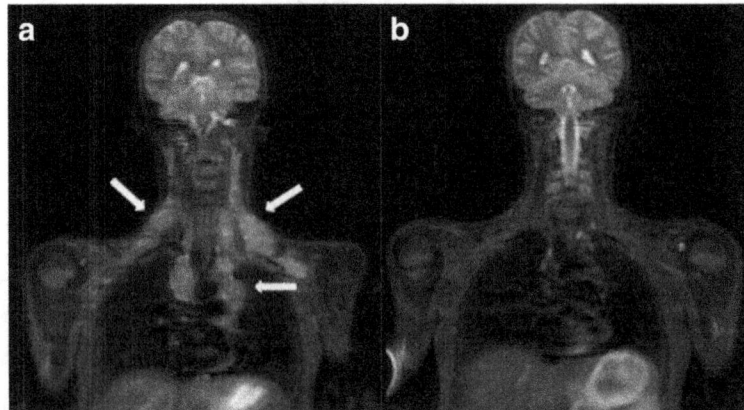

Fig. 5 Whole-body MRI with a coronal STIR sequence highlighting the cervical and thoracic regions of a17-year-old female patient with histologically confirmed non-Hodgkin lymphoma. **a** Multiple cervical lymphadenopathies in the supraclavicular and anterior mediastinal regions (*arrows*) were detected at diagnosis. **b** A follow-up examination performed 15 days after chemotherapy showed that the lesions had disappeared

intensities and ADCs of different tissues are distinct as a result of their structural characteristics. The restricted diffusion of water molecules that characterises malignant tumours is potentially due to the increased cell density of these tumours, thereby resulting in increased signal intensity in DWI and reduced ADCs, both of which facilitate detection of malignant lesions [16]. However, it should be noted that particularly in children, a high signal in DWI with body background suppression (DWIBS) can be a normal finding in the bony pelvis and lumbar spine. The different types of tissues with high cellularity that are present within these bones contribute to this high signal [39].

Currently, paramagnetic contrast agents can be used in WB MRI examinations, although they are not always indicated. It has been considered that the addition of post-contrast sequences significantly increases examination time and that the behavioral characteristics of lesion enhancement cannot be examined in the arterial, venous, and equilibrium phases simultaneously in WB scans, especially when multiple organs are involved [40]. However, strategies have been developed to address these limitations. For example, the Dixon technique achieves a uniform separation of water and fat that is resistant to large-field inhomogeneities compared to fat suppression by chemical shift selective saturation (CHESS) [41]. Furthermore, when properly implemented, the Dixon technique can be used to acquire either T1-weighted [42] or T2-weighted [43] images within a single breath hold. These rapid Dixon sequences have been successfully incorporated into a WB MRI protocol that is capable of providing multisequence and multiplanar scans, including triphasic (arterial, portal-venous, and equilibrium or delayed) contrast-enhanced imaging of the liver, in approximately 1 h [44]. This Dixon-based WB MRI with multisequence and

multiplanar images are also complementary and facilitate high-confidence reading, while multisequence and triphasic contrast-enhanced abdominal imaging is very useful for the detection and characterization of lesions in the liver, an imaging examination that is more commonly performed in adult examinations [44, 45]. On the other hand, however, it is important to consider that administration of paramagnetic contrast agents are associated with some risks, such as those for accidental

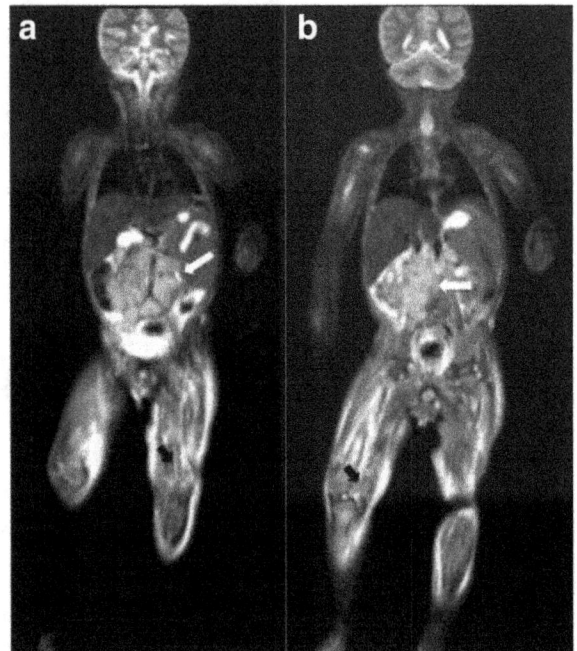

Fig. 6 Whole-body MRI with a coronal STIR sequence was performed in a 3-year-old male patient with histologically confirmed neuroblastoma. **a** and **b** The primary lesion appears as an extensive retroperitoneal mass (*white arrows*), and multiple bone metastases (*black arrows*) are present in the femoral

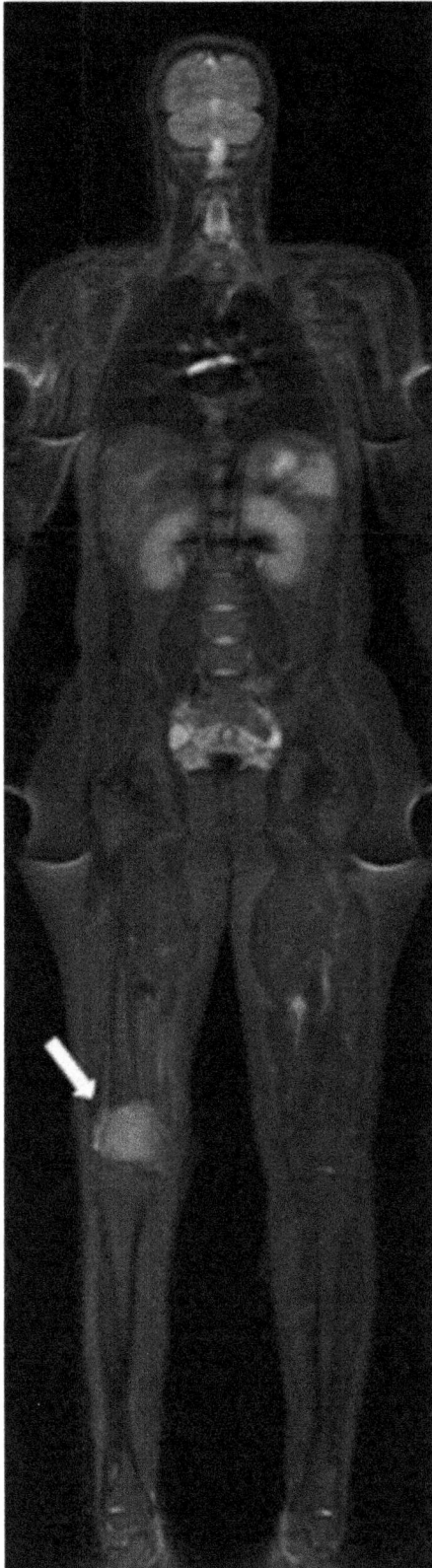

Fig. 7 Whole-body MRI with a coronal STIR sequence in a15-year-old male patient with a lesion in the right distal femur and a histological diagnosis of Ewing's sarcoma showed surrounding soft-tissue components (*arrow*), but no other area of abnormal signal intensity suggestive of malignancy

puncture, allergic reaction, renal failure, and nephrogenic systemic fibrosis [46]. Consequently, the prudent use of gadolinium-based contrast agents to avoid or minimise the risk of nephrogenic systemic fibrosis cannot be overemphasised, as pediatric oncologic patients are more likely to have impaired renal function secondary to anti-cancer therapy [47]. Pediatric patients should also be examined for hepatic lesions following the administration of paramagnetic contrast reagents, despite hepatic lesions being less frequent in children than in adults.

For patients who are unable to receive gadolinium-based contrast agents, ferumoxytol may be a useful MRI contrast agent. Ferumoxytol is an ultrasmall superparamagnetic iron oxide (USPIO) that is comprised of iron oxide particles surrounded by a carbohydrate coat. Initially, this agent was used to treat anemia in patients with chronic renal failure [48]. However, more recently, ferumoxytol has been investigated as an intravenous contrast agent in MRI. The advantages of ferumoxytol include its ability to be administered as a bolus injection, allergic and idiosyncratic reactions with its administration have been limited, and it is not associated with a risk for nephrogenic systemic fibrosis [48, 49]. Femuroxytol also has a long intravascular half-life of 14–15 h [50], and thus, can be used to obtain different types of images. However, there is currently a paucity of data available regarding its use as a paramagnetic contrast agent.

Clinical indications

WB MRI can be applied for lesion detection/staging, evaluation of treatment response, and follow-up and screening of children with cancer predisposition syndromes.

Lesion detection / staging

Clinical indications for WB MRI in pediatric patients with cancer depend on the disease type and stage of management. For several types of neoplasms, WB MRI has been shown to be a valid alternative to CT, PET/CT, and scintigraphic studies [20, 35, 47]. Many studies have also shown that WB MRI can be applied at different times during cancer management, including during the screening, staging, response evaluation, and post-therapeutic follow-up stages [5, 20].

The capacity for WB MRI to detect lesions depends on several factors, including the anatomic site, size, histological type, and differentiation grade of the lesions being examined. WB MRI has exhibited good diagnostic accuracy in the staging of a variety of tumours, including both lymphomas and solid tumours [51]. In fact, staging of these neoplasms contributed to the development of this examination technique [5, 51]. Currently, WB MRI can detect lesions present in various anatomical sites, such as the brain, cervical region, thoracic organs, abdomen, bone marrow, and musculoskeletal system. The performance of WB MRI has also been shown to be similar to that of PET/CT in the staging of different cancers, and superior to CT, BS, and scintigraphy with gallium in evaluations of certain osseous and extra-osseous metastases [35, 52, 53].

WB MRI enables a proper assessment of WB bone marrow and the detection of compromised neoplastic sites, including primary tumours and metastases arising from diffusion [37]. However, since normal red marrow impedes diffusion, this may confound disease detection in younger children. Patients with melanoma and Langerhans cell histiocytosis may be evaluated with WB MRI. In fact, the sensitivity, specificity, and accuracy of this method in these cases has been found to similar or superior to those of other methods, including those employing MIBG [20, 54]. WB MRI has also been shown to perform well in the detection of bone metastases, with a higher positive predictive value (94 vs. 76%, respectively) and greater sensitivity (99 vs. 26%, respectively) observed compared with bone scintigraphy [35]. The use of WB MRI is limited in the detection of rib and skull lesions, although the use of respiratory synchronization (triggering) has been shown to reduce the occurrence of motion artifacts, thereby improving

the ability of WB MRI to evaluate these anatomic sites [20, 55].

MRI provides different image contrasts that represent specific tissue characteristics. This is important for evaluations of primary tumours and metastases in the brain. Furthermore, if a lesion is detected in the brain or in another part of the body during a WB MRI exam, then a region-specific exam also needs to be conducted. Thus, for patients with Li-Fraumeni syndrome who have an elevated risk of brain tumours, a brain-specific protocol should be added to a WB MRI protocol.

Oncologic patients may undergo multiple MRI, thereby receiving repeated administrations of a gadolinium-based contrast agent. A high signal in the dentate nucleus and globus pallidus on unenhanced T1-weighted images should be cautiously evaluated in these patients, since the signal observed may be a consequence of the number of times that a gadolinium-based contrast material was administered, and not due to the presence of pathologic lesions [56, 57].

Currently, the most important clinical applications of WB MRI in children include the staging of malignant disease and screening for metastatic spread. These applications are particularly relevant in cases involving lymphoma and solid tumours.

Lymphoma

Diagnostic imaging provides important information regarding the staging and response assessment of lymphomas. Recently, a combination of CT and PET was applied to lymphoma staging and evaluations of treatment response [58]. However, both PET and CT involve substantial radiation exposure, and children often undergo

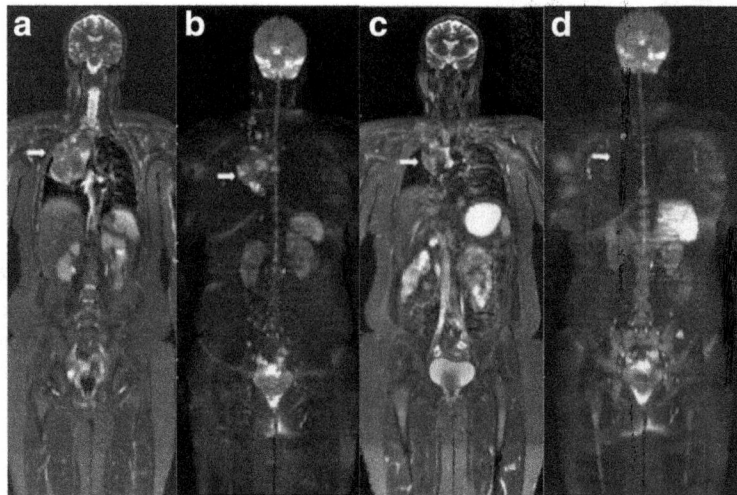

Fig. 8 A 16-year-old female patient with primary mediastinal Hodgkin lymphoma (stage III-B) underwent whole-body MRI with STIR (**a**, **c**) and diffusion (**b**, **d**) sequences. **a** and **b** Examinations performed for pre-therapeutic staging showed a voluminous anterior mediastinal lesion (*arrows*). **c** and **d** Post-therapeutic imaging showed the presence of a residual mediastinal lesion with no sign of activity (*arrows*)

several PET/CT examinations during a treatment course. Thus, WB MRI represents a radiation-free alternative for lymphoma staging and follow-up (Fig. 5). Furthermore, when WB MRI and CT were compared in their capacity to provide staging of lymphoma, WB MRI was able to provide disease staging, detect lymph nodes greater than 1.2 cm (with sensitivity and specificity values of 92.0 and 99.9%, respectively), and evaluate the presence or absence of disease spread to bone marrow [58]. In a study of eight children with lymphoma, WB MRI with a coronal STIR sequence was also more sensitive than conventional imaging (e.g., radiography, nuclear medicine studies - bone scintigraphy and gallium scintigraphy - and CT) in detecting bone marrow involvement in the initial stages of disease [15]. Following treatment, however, residual and therapy-induced bone marrow signal abnormalities could not be differentiated from lymphomatous involvement [15].

Solid tumours

In various pediatric studies, the sensitivity of WB MRI for the detection of distant metastases has been compared with the sensitivities of radiography, CT, conventional MRI, nuclear medicine studies, and PET/CT [53, 54, 59]. Additional studies have suggested that WB MRI is a promising method for the detection of metastases in patients with small cell tumours, and that WB MRI provides at least equivalent information to conventional

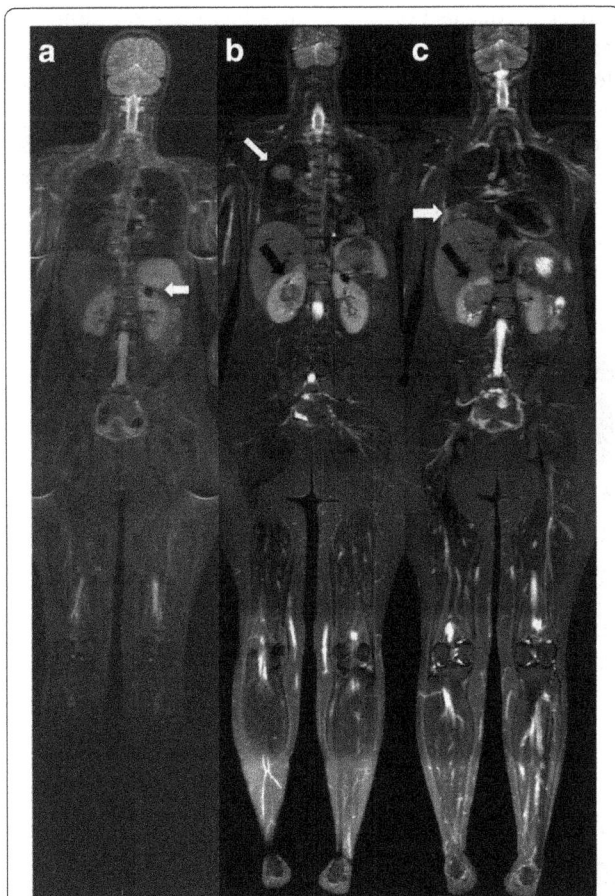

Fig. 9 A 20-year-old female patient with Li-Fraumeni syndrome in whom multiple neoplasms had developed since childhood, including lymphoma, soft-tissue sarcomas in the back and thigh, malignant fibrous histiocytoma in the buttock, and adrenal carcinoma. Follow up whole-body MRI examination since 2013, in the last the coronal STIR sequence demonstrated the presence that new lung lesions and kidney nodule. Histological diagnosis suggestive that metastasis of pleomorphic undifferentiated sarcoma in lung and renal cell carcinoma in kidney. Current Whole-body MRI with a coronal STIR sequence demonstrate the presence of multiple lesions in lung (b, c *white arrows*) and the kidney nodule (b, c *black arrows*), compared to previous exam which demonstrated only the presence of simple renal cyst (*arrow*), with no other change suggestive of malignancy (a)

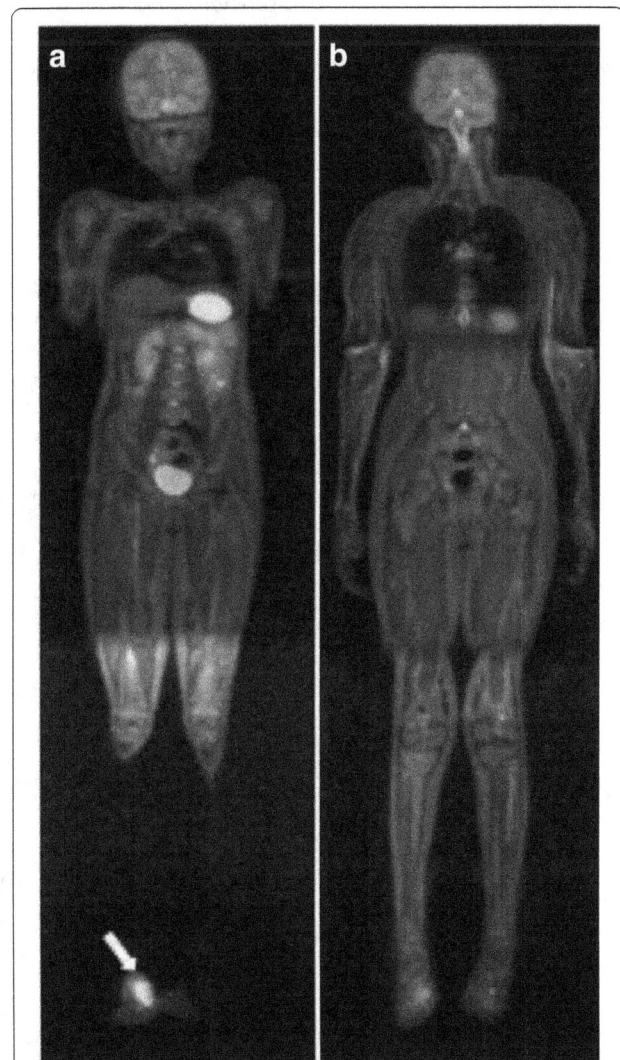

Fig. 10 A 16-year-old male patient with histologically confirmed osteosarcoma on the dorsum of the right foot underwent whole-body MRI with a coronal STIR sequence for staging. a Note the lesion in the right foot (*arrow*). b No skip metastasis or distant lesion was detected

imaging studies [53, 59]. Neuroblastoma (Fig. 6), primitive neuroectodermal tumour, rhabdomyosarcoma, and Ewing's sarcoma (Fig. 7) are small round-cell malignancies that have been found to occur in the pediatric population. For the detection of metastases to bone, most investigators have reported a sensitivity of more than 97% for WB MRI, and WB MRI has consistently exhibited a sensitivity comparable to, or greater than, that of skeletal scintigraphy with technetium 99 m (^{99m}Tc) medronate disodium [35, 53, 59].

Evaluation of treatment response and follow-up

WB MRI can be used to evaluate therapeutic response in pediatric oncology patients [51, 60, 61], and the information obtained can be used in combination with Response Evaluation Criteria in Solid Tumors (RECIST) [61]. For example, WB MRI can provide a morphological assessment of target lesions by measuring their major axes according to RECIST, while also providing a functional evaluation of lesions with diffusion sequences. Several studies have described the use of WB MRI to identify partial or complete responses, including increased absolute ADC, after the application of chemo-

or radiotherapy to brain tumours, liver tumours, and sarcomas [62, 63]. Similar to CT and PET/CT, WB MRI can also be useful in evaluating significant morphological and functional improvements in lymphomas (Fig. 8), and these are often characterised by an inverse correlation between the tendency toward increased ADC and reduced tumour volume [35, 52]. Furthermore, WB MRI can help distinguish between abnormal scarring and recurrence after therapy [64], thereby enabling the detection of any complications that are related or unrelated to disease or treatment.

Screening of children with cancer predisposition syndromes

Cancer predisposition syndromes include a multitude of cancers in which a mode of familial inheritance has been clearly established, although a specific genetic defect may not have been identified [65]. WB MRI has been useful in the screenings of children with cancer predisposition syndromes, and it also has the potential to provide a preclinical diagnosis of any associated tumours. For example, at some institutions, WB MRI is performed annually to screen for tumours in children with Li-

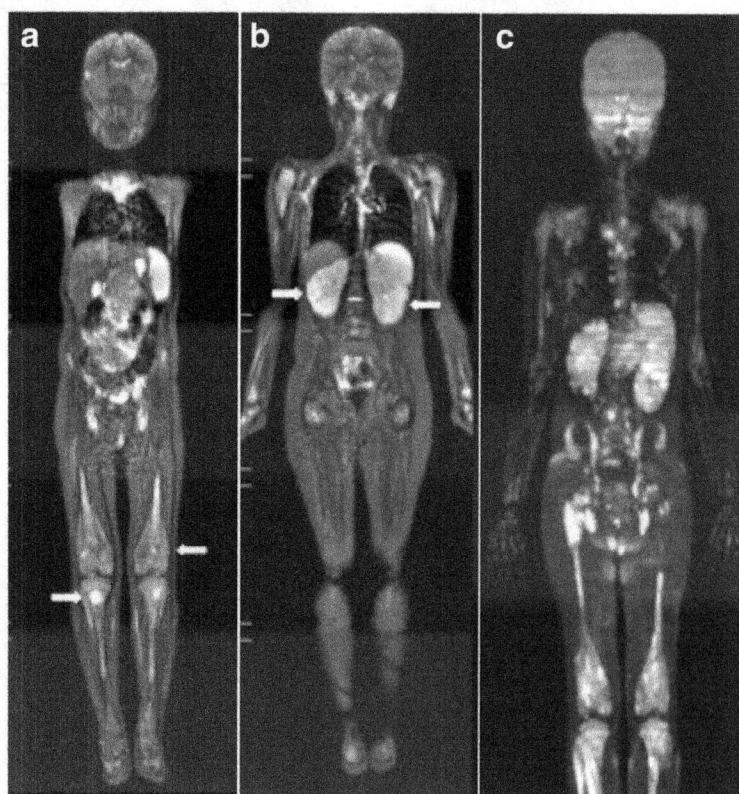

Fig. 11 Whole-body MRI was performed in a 6-year-old male patient with acute lymphoblastic leukemia for staging. **a** Diaphyseal and metaphyseal lesions in the distal femoral and proximal tibial regions are represented by hyperintense signals in a coronal STIR sequence (*arrows*). **b** Signs of bilateral renal infiltration by the underlying pathology (*arrows*) were observed. **c** A diffusion sequence demonstrated multiple hyperintense foci, consistent with leukemic infiltration

Fraumeni syndrome (Fig. 9). Li-Fraumeni syndrome is an autosomal dominant hereditary syndrome that is caused by a loss-of-function mutation in the *TP53* gene and affected individuals have a lifelong increased risk of osteosarcoma (Fig. 10), soft-tissue sarcoma, leukemia (Fig. 11), breast cancer, brain tumour, melanoma, and adrenal cortical tumours [65]. Similarly, individuals with hereditary retinoblastoma (RB) have a very high risk of developing subsequent malignant neoplasms, with osteosarcoma being the most common. When WB MRI screening tests were performed for survivors of hereditary RB, the sensitivity and specificity of detecting subsequent malignant neoplasms was 66.7 and 92.1%, respectively [66].

Limitations

The use of WB MRI in pediatric oncological clinical practice is limited in some cases. For example, standard contraindications to conventional MRI, such as the presence of metallic body implants or history of claustrophobia, can also preclude the use of WB MRI. Due to the examination time of WB MRI (which can range from 30 min to 1 h), the use of sedation or general anesthesia is typically needed in a significant proportion of pediatric patients, especially those who are young or uncooperative. Thus, the risks associated with these agents must be considered. Immobilization during the examination is also essential for preventing motion artifacts which can impair image acquisition and interpretation of the findings. In addition, physiological artifacts related to respiratory movements, heartbeat, and intestinal peristalsis can impair image acquisition [67]. To minimise the occurrence of these artifacts, multi-channel equipment, body coils, and parallel imaging can be employed. Furthermore, single-shot acquisition, the use of presaturation bands in the anterior body, and mechanisms of synchronization with respiratory and cardiac movements can reduce the time needed for an examination and facilitate the acquisition of highquality images [67, 68]. Finally, the occurrence of false-positive results is another limiting factor in the use of WB MRI. For example, inflammatory abnormalities, infections, and even benign lesions such as simple cysts or vascular lesions have been found to simulate malignant lesions [67].

Conclusion

Currently, WB MRI is able to provide total body coverage, high tissue contrast, and good spatial resolution without the use of radiation. Moreover, the ability to obtain relevant morphological and functional information in a single examination represents a key advantage of this method in the management of pediatric oncology patients.

Abbreviation

18F-FDG: 18F-fluorodeoxyglucose; 99mTc: Technetium 99m; ADC: Absolute apparent diffusion coefficient; ADC: Absolute apparent diffusion coefficient; BS: Bone scintigraphy; CHESS: Chemical shift selective saturation; CT: Computed tomography; DWI: Diffusion- weighted imaging; DWIBS: Diffusion-weighted imaging with body background suppression; MIBG: Metaiodobenzylguanidine; MRI: Magnetic resonance imaging; PET/CT: Positron emission tomography/ computed tomography; RB: Retinoblastoma; RECIST: Response Evaluation Criteria in Solid Tumors; STIR: Short tau inversion recovery; USPIO: Ultrasmall superparamagnetic iron oxide; WB: Whole body

Acknowledgements
None.

Funding
Not applicable.

Authors' contributions
MDG conceived of the topic for the review and the methodology used in this work. MDG, JN, SRT, MKS, HML VST, ADO, EM, BH undertook the literature search and manuscript drafting. MDG, VK controlled and checked the manuscript. All authors have read, edited and approved the final manuscript.

Competing interests
The authors declare that they have no competing interests.

Author details
1Department of Imaging, AC Camargo Cancer Center, Rua Prof. Antônio Prudente, 211, Liberdade, São Paulo/SP 01509-010, Brazil. 2Universidade Federal do Vale do São Francisco (UNIVASF), Av. José de Sá Maniçoba, Petrolina, PE 56304-917, Brazil. 3Department of Imaging, AC Camargo Cancer Center, Rua Prof. Antônio Prudente, 211, Liberdade, Sao Paulo/SP 01509-010, Brazil. 4Division of Radiology, Department of Internal Medicine, Ribeirao Preto Medical School, University of Sao Paulo, Av. Bandeirantes, 3900, Ribeirao Preto/ SP 14049-090, Brazil. 5Universidade Federal de São Paulo, Departamento de Diagnóstico Por Imagem, Disciplina de Diagnóstico por Imagem em Pediatria, Rua Napoleão de Barros, 800, Vila Clementino, Sao Paulo/SP 04024002, Brazil. 6Universidade Federal de São Paulo, Centro de Diagnóstico por Imagem do Instituto de Oncologia Pediátrica e Médica Radiologista do Centro de Diagnóstico por Imagem do Instituto de Oncologia Pediátrica, Rua Napoleão de Barros, 800, Vila Clementino, Sao Paulo/SP 04024002, Brazil. 7Department of Diagnostic Radiology, The University of Texas MD Anderson Cancer Center, 1515 Holcombe Blvd, Houston, TX 77030, USA. 8Department of Radiology, Universidade Federal de Ciências da Saúde de Porto Alegre, Rua Professor Anes Dias, 285, Centro Histórico, Porto Alegre/RS 90020-090, Brazil. 9Department of Radiology, Universidade Federal do Rio de Janeiro, Rua Thomaz Cameron, 438, Valparaíso, Petrópolis/RJ 25685-129, Brazil.

References
1. Chatenoud L, Bertuccio P, Bosetti C, Levi F, Negri E, La Vecchia C. Childhood cancer mortality in America, Asia and Oceania, 1970 through 2007. Cancer. 2010;116(21):5063–74.
2. Kleis M, Daldrup-Link H, Matthay K, Goldsby R, Lu Y, Schuster T, et al. Diagnostic value of PET/CT for the staging and restaging of pediatric tumors. Eur J Nucl Med Mol Imaging. 2009;36(1):23–36.

3. Federico SM, Spunt SL, Krasin MJ, Billup CA, Wu J, Shulkin B, et al. Comparison of PET-CT and conventional imaging in staging pediatric rhabdomyosarcoma. Pediatr Blood Cancer. 2013;60(7):1128–34.

4. Hernandez-Pampaloni M, Takalkar A, Yu JQ, Zhuang H, Alavi A. F-18 FDG-PET imaging and correlation with CT in staging and follow-up of pediatric lymphomas. Pediatr Radiol. 2006;36(6):524–31.

5. Ley S, Ley-Zaporozhan J, Schenk JP. Whole-body MRI in the pediatric patient. Eur J Radiol. 2009;70(3):442–51.

6. Schmidt GP, Haug A, Reiser MF, Rist C. Whole-body MRI and FDG-PET/CT imaging diagnostics in oncology. Radiologe. 2010;50(4):329–38.

7. Alzen G, Benz-Bohm G. Radiation protection in pediatric radiology. Dtsch Arztebl Int. 2011;108(24):407–14.

8. Oltmann SC, Garcia NM, Barber R, Hicks B, Fischer AC. Pediatric ovarian malignancies: how efficacious are current staging practices? J Pediatr Surg. 2010;45(6):1096–102.

9. Shapiro NL, Bhattacharyya N. Staging and survival for sinus cancer in the pediatric population. Int J Pediatr Otorhinolaryngol. 2009;73(11):1568–71.

10. Miller E, Metser U, Avrahami G, Dvir R, Valdman S, Sira LB, et al. Role of 18F-FDG PET/CT in staging and follow-up of lymphoma in pediatric and young adult patients. J Comput Assist Tomogr. 2006;30(4):689–94.

11. Völker T, Denecke T, Steffen I, Misch D, Schönberger S, Plotkin M, et al. Positron emission tomography for staging of pediatric sarcoma patients: results of a prospective multicenter trial. J Clin Oncol. 2007;25(34):5435–41.

12. von Falck C, Maecker B, Schirg E, Boerner AR, Knapp WH, Klein C, et al. Post transplant lymphoproliferative disease in pediatric solid organ transplant patients: a possible role for [18F]-FDG-PET(/CT) in initial staging and therapy monitoring. Eur J Radiol. 2007;63(3):427–35.

13. Truong MT, Erasmus JJ, Macapinlac HA, Marom EM, Mawlawi O, Gladish GW, et al. Integrated positron emission tomography/computed tomography in patients with non-small cell lung cancer: normal variants and pitfalls. J Comput Assist Tomogr. 2005;29(2):205–9.

14. Kavanagh E, Smith C, Eustace S. Whole-body turbo STIR MR imaging: controversies and avenues for development. Eur Radiol. 2003;13(9):2196–205.

15. Kellenberger CJ, Miller SF, Khan M, Gilday DL, Weitzman S, Bayn PS. Initial experience with FSE STIR whole-body MR imaging for staging lymphoma in children. Eur Radiol. 2004;14(10):1829–41.

16. Eiber M, Dütsch S, Gaa J, Fauser C, Rummeny EJ, Holzapfel K. Diffusion-weighted magnetic resonance imaging (DWI-MRI): a new method to differentiate between malignant and benign cervical lymph nodes. Laryngorhinootologie. 2008;87(12):850–1.

17. Koh DM, Padhani AR. Diffusion-weighted MRI: a new functional clinical technique for tumour imaging. Br J Radiol. 2006;79(944):633–5.

18. Blomqvist L, Torkzad MR. Whole-body imaging with MRI or PET/CT: the future for single-modality imaging in oncology ? JAMA. 2003;290(24):3248–9.

19. Chen W, Jian W, Li HT, Li C, Zhang YK, Xie B, et al. Whole-body diffusion-weighted imaging vs. FDG-PET for the detection of non small-cell lung cancer. How do they measure up? Magn Reson Imaging. 2010;28(5):613–20.

20. Goo HW. Regional and whole-body imaging in pediatric oncology. Pediatr Radiol. 2011;41(1):S186–94.

21. Hall EJ, Brenner DJ. Cancer risks from diagnostic radiology. Br J Radiol. 2008;81(965):362–78.

22. Davies HE, Wathen CG, Gleeson FV. The risks of radiation exposure related to diagnostic imaging and how to minimise them. BMJ. 2011;342:d947.

23. Brenner DJ, Shuryak I, Einstein AJ. Impact of reduced patient life expectancy on potential cancer risks from radiologic imaging. Radiology. 2011;261(1):193–8.

24. Berrington de Gonzalez A, Mahesh M, Kin KP, Bhargavan M, Lewis R, Mettler F, et al. Projected cancer risks from computed tomographic scans performed in the United States in 2007. Arch Intern Med. 2009;169(22):2071–7.

25. Chawla SC, Federman N, Zhang D, Nagata K, Nuthakki S, McNitt-Gray M, et al. Estimated cumulative radiation dose from PET/CT in children with malignancies: a 5-year retrospective review. Pediatr Radiol. 2010;40(5):681–6.

26. Egger M, Zwahlen M. Tumor screening. Ther Umsch. 2013;70:193–4.

27. Ducreux M, Mateus C, Planchard D, Fizazi K. Screening and early diagnosis of other cancers (non-small cell lung carcinoma, urologic cancers, liver cancer and melanoma). Rev Prat. 2010;60(2):219–23.

28. Sweed MF, Vig HS. Hereditary colorectal cancer syndromes. Start risk assessment in primary care. Adv Nurse Pract. 2007;15(7):49–52.

29. Digweed M. Human genetic instability syndromes: single gene defects with increased risk of cancer. Toxicol Lett. 1993;67(1–3):259–81.

30. Malkin D. Li-fraumeni syndrome. Genes Cancer. 2011;2(4):475–84.

31. Testa JR, Malkin D, Schiffman JD. Connecting molecular pathways to hereditary cancer risk syndromes. Am Soc Clin Oncol Educ Book. 2013;33:81–90.

32. Villani A, Tabori U, Schiffman J, Schilien A, Beyene J, Druker H, et al. Biochemical and imaging surveillance in germline TP53 mutation carriers with Li-Fraumeni syndrome: a prospective observational study. Lancet Oncol. 2011;12(6):559–67.

33. Schaefer JF, Kramer U. Whole-body MRI in children and juveniles. Rofo. 2011;183(1):24–36.

34. Koh DM, Collins DJ. Diffusion-weighted MRI in the body: applications and challenges in oncology. AJR Am J Roentgenol. 2007;188(6):1622–35.

35. Goo HW, Choi SH, Ghim T, Moon HN, Seo JJ. Whole-body MRI of paediatric malignant tumours: comparison with conventional oncological imaging methods. Pediatr Radiol. 2005;35(8):766–73.

36. Kellenberger CJ, Epelman M, Miller SF, Babyn PS. Fast STIR whole-body MR imaging in children. Radiographics. 2004;24(5):1317–30.

37. Karmazyn B, Cohen MD, Jennings SG, Robertson KA. Marrow signal changes observed in follow-up whole-body MRI studies in children and young adults with neurofibromatosis type 1 treated with imatinib mesylate (Gleevec) for plexiform neurofibromas. Pediatr Radiol. 2012;42(10):1218–22.

38. Takahara T, Imai Y, Yamashita T, Yasuda S, Nasu S, Van Cauteren M. Diffusion weighted whole body imaging with background body signal suppression (DWIBS): technical improvement using free breathing, STIR and high resolution 3D display. Radiat Med. 2004;22(4):275–82.

39. Ording Müller LS, Avenarius D, Olsen ØE. High signal in bone marrow at diffusion-weighted imaging with body background suppression (DWIBS) in healthy children. Pediatr Radiol. 2011;41(2):221–6.

40. Hasebroock KM, Serkova NJ. Toxicity of MRI and CT contrast agents. Expert Opin Drug Metab Toxicol. 2009;5(4):403–16.

41. Glover GH, Schneider E. Three-point Dixon technique for true water/fat decomposition with B0 inhomogeneity correction. Magn Reson Med. 1991;18(2):371–83.

42. Ma J, Vu AT, Son JB, Choi H, Hazle JD. Fat-suppressed three-dimensional dual echo Dixon technique for contrast agent enhanced MRI. J Magn Reson Imaging. 2006;23(1):36–41.

43. Ma J, Son JB, Zhou Y, Le-Petross H, Choi H. Fast spin-echo triple-echo dixon (fTED) technique for efficient T2-weighted water and fat imaging. Magn Reson Med. 2007;58(1):103–9.

44. Ma J, Costelloe CM, Madewell JE, Hortobagyi GN, Green MC, Cao G, et al. Fast dixon-based multisequence and multiplanar MRI for whole-body detection of cancer metastases. J Magn Reson Imaging. 2009;29(5):1154–62.

45. Costelloe CM, Kundra V, Ma J, Chasen BA, Rohren EM, Bassett RL, et al. Fast Dixon whole-body MRI for detecting distant cancer metastasis: a preliminary clinical study. J Magn Reson Imaging. 2012;35(2):399–408.

46. Juluru K, Vogel-Claussen J, Macura KJ, Kamel IR, Steever A, Bluemke DA. MR imaging in patients at risk for developing nephrogenic systemic fibrosis: protocols, practices, and imaging techniques to maximize patient safety. Radiographics. 2009;29(1):9–22.

47. Siegel MJ, Acharyya S, Hoffer FA, Wyly JB, Friedmann AM, Snyder BS, et al. Whole-body MR imaging for staging of malignant tumors in pediatric patients: results of the American College of Radiology Imaging Network 6660 Trial. Radiology. 2013;266(2):599–609.

48. Bashir MR, Bhatti L, Marin D, Nelson RC. Emerging Applications for Ferumoxytol as a Contrast Agent in MRI. J Magn Reson Imaging. 2015;41(4):884–98.

49. Weinstein JS, Varallyay CG, Dosa E, Gahramanov S, Hamilton B, Rooney WD, et al. Superparamagnetic iron oxide nanoparticles: diagnostic magnetic resonance imaging and potential therapeutic applications in neurooncology and central nervous system inflammatory pathologies, a review. J Cereb Blood Flow Metab. 2010;30(1):15–35.

50. McCullough BJ, Kolokythas O, Maki JH, Green DE. Ferumoxytol in Clinical Practice: Implications for MRI. J Magn Reson Imaging. 2013;37(6):1476–9.

51. Darge K, Jaramillo D, Siegel MJ. Whole-body MRI in children: current status and future applications. Eur J Radiol. 2008;68(2):289–98.

52. Punwani S, Taylor SA, Bainbridge A, Prakah V, Bandula S, De Vita E, et al. Pediatric and adolescent lymphoma: comparison of whole-body STIR half-Fourier RARE MR imaging with an enhanced PET/CT reference for initial staging. Radiology. 2010;255(1):182–90.

53. Kumar J, Seith A, Kumar A, Sharma R, Bakhshi S, Kumar R, et al. Whole-body MR imaging with the use of parallel imaging for detection of skeletal metastases in pediatric patients with small-cell neoplasms:

comparison with skeletal scintigraphy and FDG PET/CT. Pediatr Radiol. 2008;38(9):953–62.

54. Krohmer S, Sorge I, Krausse A, Kluge R, Bierbach U, Marwede D, et al. Whole-body MRI for primary evaluation of malignant disease in children. Eur J Radiol. 2010;74(1):256–61.

55. Goo HW. State-of-the-art pediatric chest imaging. Pediatr Radiol. 2013;43(3):261.

56. Roberts DR, Holden KR. Progressive increase of T1 signal intensity in the dentate nucleus and globus pallidus on unenhanced T1-weighted MR images in the pediatric brain exposed to multiple doses of gadolinium contrast. Brain Dev. 2016;38(3):331–6.

57. Kanda T, Ishii K, Kawagichi H, Kitajima K, Takenaka D. High signal intensity in the dentate nucleus and globus pallidus on unenhanced T1-weighted MR images: relationship with increasing cumulative dose of a gadolinium-based contrast material. Radiology. 2014;270(3):834–41.

58. Brennan DD, Gleeson T, Coate LE, Cronin C, Carney D, Eustace SJ. A comparison of whole-body MRI and CT for the staging of lymphoma. AJR Am J Roentgenol. 2005;85(3):711–6.

59. Mazundar A, Siegel MJ, Narra V, Luchtman-Jones L. Whole-body fast inversion recovery MR imaging of small cell neoplasms in pediatric patients: a pilot study. AJR Am J Roentgenol. 2002;179(5):1261–6.

60. Li SP, Padhani AR. Tumor response assessments with diffusion and perfusion MRI. J Magn Reson Imaging. 2012;35(4):745–63.

61. Padhani AR, Koh DM. Diffusion MR imaging for monitoring of treatment response. Magn Reson Imaging Clin N Am. 2011;19(1):181–209.

62. Padhani AR, Khan AA. Diffusion-weighted (DW) and dynamic contrast-enhanced (DCE) magnetic resonance imaging (MRI) for monitoring anticancer therapy. Target Oncol. 2010;5(1):39–52.

63. Padhani AR, Liu G, Koh DM, Chenevert TL, Thoeny HC, Takanara T, et al. Diffusion-weighted magnetic resonance imaging as a cancer biomarker: consensus and recommendations. Neoplasia. 2009;11(2):102–25.

64. Herman M, Paucek B, Raida L, Myslivecek M, Zapletalová J. Comparison of magnetic resonance imaging and (67)gallium scintigraphy in the evaluation of posttherapeutic residual mediastinal mass in the patients with Hodgkin's lymphoma. Eur J Radiol. 2007;64(3):432–8.

65. Monsalve J, Kapur J, Malkin D, Babyn PS. Imaging of cancer predisposition syndromes in children. Radio Graphics. 2011;31(1):263–80.

66. Friedman DN, Lis E, Sklar CH, Oeffinger KC, Reppucci M, Fleischut MH, et al. Whole-body magnetic resonance imaging (WB-MRI) as surveillance for subsequent malignancies in survivors of hereditary retinoblastoma: a pilot study. Pediatr Blood Cancer. 2014;61(8):1440–4.

67. Koh DM, Blackledge M, Padhani AR, Takahara T, Kwee TC, Leach MO, et al. Whole-body diffusion-weighted MRI: tips, tricks, and pitfalls. AJR Am J Roentgenol. 2012;199(2):252–62.

68. Koh DM, Takahara T, Imai Y, Collins DJ. Practical aspects of assessing tumors using clinical diffusion-weighted imaging in the body. Magn Reson Med Sci. 2007;6(4):211–24.

15

^{68}Ga PSMA-11 PET with CT urography protocol in the initial staging and biochemical relapse of prostate cancer

Amir Iravani[1]*[iD], Michael S. Hofman[1,2], Tony Mulcahy[1], Scott Williams[3], Declan Murphy[4], Bimal K. Parameswaran[1] and Rodney J. Hicks[1,2]

Abstract

Background: ^{68}Ga-labelled prostate specific membrane antigen (PSMA) ligand PET/CT is a promising modality in primary staging (PS) and biochemical relapse (BCR) of prostate cancer (PC). However, pelvic nodes or local recurrences can be difficult to differentiate from radioactive urine. CT urography (CT-U) is an established method, which allows assessment of urological malignancies. The study presents a novel protocol of ^{68}Ga-PSMA-11 PET/CT-U in PS and BCR of PC.

Methods: A retrospective review of PSMA PET/CT-U preformed on 57 consecutive patients with prostate cancer. Fifty mL of IV contrast was administered 10 min (range 8–15) before the CT component of a combined PET/CT study, acquired approximately 60 min (range 40–85) after administration of 166 MBq (range 91–246) of ^{68}Ga-PSMA-11. PET and PET/CT-U were reviewed by two nuclear medicine physicians and CT-U by a radiologist. First, PET images were reviewed independently followed by PET/CT-U images. Foci of activity which could not unequivocally be assessed as disease or urinary activity were recorded. PET/CT-U was considered of potential benefit in final interpretation when the equivocal focal activity in PET images corresponded to opacified ureter, bladder, prostate bed, seminal vesicles, or urethra. Student's T test and Pearson's correlation coefficient was used for assessment of variables including lymph node size and standardized uptake value.

Results: Overall 50 PSMA PET/CT-U studies were performed for BCR and 7 for PS. Median PSA with BCR and PS were 2.0 ± 11.4 ng/ml (0.06–57.3 ng/ml) and 18 ± 35.3 ng/ml (6.8–100 ng/ml), respectively. The median Gleason-score for both groups was 7 (range 6–10). In BCR group, PSMA PET was reported positive in 36 (72%) patients, CT-U in 11(22%) patients and PET/CT-U in 33 (66%) patients. In PS group, PSMA PET detected the primary site in all seven patients, of which one patient with metastatic nodal disease had negative CT finding. Of 40 equivocal foci (27/57 patients) on PET, 11 foci (10/57 patients, 17.5%) were localized to enhanced urine on PET/CT-U, hence considered of potential benefit in interpretation. Of those, 3 foci (3 patients) were solitary sites of activity on PSMA imaging including two local and one nodal site and 4 foci (3 patients) were in different nodal fields.

Conclusions: PET/CT-U protocol is a practical approach and may assist in interpretation of ^{68}Ga-PSMA-11 imaging by delineation of the contrast opacified genitourinary system and matching focal PSMA activity with urinary contrast.

Keywords: PSMA PET/CT, PSMA-HBED PET, ^{68}Ga-PSMA-11 PET, CT urogram, Prostate cancer, Biochemical recurrence

* Correspondence: amir.iravani@petermac.org
[1]Centre for Molecular Imaging, Department of Cancer Imaging, Peter MacCallum Cancer Centre, 305 Grattan Street, Melbourne, Australia
Full list of author information is available at the end of the article

Background

Worldwide, prostate cancer (PC) is the most common malignancy in men [1]. Accurate staging of PC is of high importance for patient management as treatment selection is mainly influenced by the presence or absence of metastases [2]. Of all patients with PC undergoing therapeutic regimens with curative intent, about a quarter will ultimately have BCR with rise in PSA level. Of those, 50% will have local recurrence and 50% systemic disease with or without local recurrence [3, 4]. For an optimized and timely management, accurate primary staging (PS) of the disease and location of recurrence is essential. But at low PSA levels, small lymph nodes below the size threshold are commonly missed by conventional imaging [5]. The European Association of Urology (EAU) advocates bone scan and abdominopelvic CT only for patients with BCR after radical prostatectomy(RP) who have PSA level of higher than 10 ng/ml or PSA doubling time less than six months or bone pain [6]. Therefore, salvage radiotherapy (SRT) after RP is commonly decided on the basis of BCR, without imaging [6].To date, early and accurate localization of BCR remains a major challenge for all conventional imaging methods [7–9].

Prostate-specific membrane antigen (PSMA) is a type II membrane glycoprotein that is highly expressed by many PCs and correlates with tumor aggressiveness, metastatic and recurrent disease [10]. Positron Emission Tomography (PET)/CT imaging using Glu-NH-CO-NH-Lys-(Ahx)-[68Ga(HBED-CC)] (68Ga-PSMA-11) as a 68Ga-labelled PSMA ligand can detect PC metastases and relapses and with high contrast and specificity by binding to the extracellular domain of PSMA [11, 12]. The sensitivity and specificity of 68Ga-PSMA-11 PET/CT for detection of nodal metastases in PS is 75% and 96%, respectively and, both 86% in BCR [13, 14]. However, 68Ga-PSMA-11 PET/CT is limited by intense radiotracer activity in the kidneys, ureters and urinary bladder due to urinary excretion [12]. Ureters also not infrequently have abrupt turns and kinks throughout the course with associated urinary pooling, particularly as they cross major vascular structures. Bladder diverticulae, postsurgical resection cavities, post-instrumentation urethral dilatation and refluxed urine into the ejaculatory duct or retained seminal vesicles following prostatectomy can also retain urine. Excreted radioactivity in the urine can be difficult to differentiate from small pelvic nodes or local recurrence lying close to these structures. Acquisition of contrast-enhanced CT in the urogram phase as part of PET/CT protocol may potentially overcome this problem by distinguishing urinary activity from radiotracer activity. In this manuscript we present our experience and diagnostic utility of incorporating CT urography (CT-U) protocol in 68Ga-PSMA-11 PET imaging in primary staging (PS) and BCR of PC.

Methods

Patients

This study is a retrospective analysis of 68Ga-PSMA-11 PET/CT on consecutive patients referred to our center from July 2015 to October 2015 with histopathological diagnosis of PC after introduction of this CT methodology as a standard of care in patients with adequate renal function and without prior contrast allergy. Overall, 57 patients were included in the study. Of those, 50 patients with mean age of 64 years (range 47–78) were referred with BCR following prostatectomy, external beam radiation, brachytherapy or combination of these administered with curative intent. Seven patients with newly diagnosed PC were referred for initial staging prior to curative intent treatment with mean age of 64 years (range 58–78). This research has been approved by the institutional ethics committee and patient consent was waived (approval number: 15/46R). All investigations were performed as part of routine clinical care.

Image acquisition and protocol

For PET, 2 MBq/kg of 68Ga-PSMA-11 were injected intravenously (mean 166 MBq, range 91–246 MBq). This was followed by an uptake period of mean 62 min (range 40–85 min). Using the same intravenous line, 50 ml of Omnipaque 300 mg/ml contrast medium (GE Healthcare, Princeton, NJ) was administered a mean of 10 min (range 8–15) minutes prior to CT acquisition in order to obtain a pyelogram phase CT. The conventional unenhanced or nephrographic phases of CT-U [15] were not acquired. Renal function was assessed by estimated glomerular filtration rate (eGFR) on peripheral blood test prior to contrast injection. Prior history of allergic reaction to intravenous iodine contrast was sought. Oral hydration was encouraged during uptake time. Patients were asked to void before imaging. Sequential CT and PET acquisition was then performed on an integrated PET/CT device (GE Discovery PET/CT 690, GE Healthcare, Milwaukee, WI or Siemens Biograph 16 PET/CT, Siemens Healthcare, Erlangen, Germany). The CT portion of the study was acquired in cranio-caudal direction encompassing vertex to mid-thigh with patient supine with slice thickness of 5 mm, increment of 1.5 mm, 140 keV, 220 mAs and 0.6 pitch. PET acquisition was subsequently acquired in caudo-cranial direction to minimize mis-registration in the pelvis as the primary region of interest. 3-D acquisition was performed with emission data corrected for randoms, scatter and decay. Reconstruction was conducted with an ordered subset expectation maximization (OSEM) algorithm with 2 iterations/8 subsets and Gauss-filtered to a transaxial resolution of 5 mm at full-width at half-maximum (FWHM). Attenuation correction was performed using above mentioned CT-U data. PET and CT-U were performed using the same protocol for every patient on both cameras.

Image analysis

Image analysis was performed using an appropriate workstation and software (Syngo MMWP VE31A, TrueD, Siemens, Berlin, Germany) for the stand-alone CT assessment and (MIM 5.4.4; MIM Software, Cleveland, OH) for the combined PET/CT study. Two nuclear physicians, with prior experience of more than 1000 PSMA PET/CT, reviewed PET and PET/CT-U data and reached consensus on cases. First, PET images (three planes and MIP image) were reviewed and the number of focal (not linear or curvilinear) abnormalities, which could not unequivocally be determined to represent urinary activity was recorded. These were regarded as suspicious for prostate cancer. Then PET/CT-U images were reviewed and number of equivocal foci which corresponded to the contrast-enhanced urine were recorded.

Maximum standardized uptake values (SUVmax) were calculated from manually drawn regions of interest over the sites of focal increased uptake including in the prostate, lymph nodes, ureters at the same level as any identified lymph nodes or distant metastatic sites. Short-axis, long-axis and volume of each positive PSMA lymph node was measured on co-registered PET/CT-U images semi-automatically by using PET edge tool of MIM software (MIM 5.4.4; MIM Software, Cleveland, OH), which was based on tumor gradient for segmentation. Distance between the opacified ureter and the ipsilateral lymph node was measured to assess the proximity of these foci (fig.1).

One radiologist reviewed the standalone CT-U images independently. Number and size of lymph nodes and site of local recurrence was recorded. Criteria for metastatic lymph nodes on CT-U was short axis larger than 8 mm. An osseous or soft tissue lesion which did not have all characteristics of a PC metastasis, was considered equivocal. These were considered negative for the final statistical analysis. Based on length of contrast opacified ureters, four groups were defined as follows; proximal ureters from renal pelvis to common iliac bifurcation, distal ureters from common iliac bifurcation to the vesicoureteral junction, entire length of both ureters, and patchy/unilateral ureter.

Statistical analysis

All results were expressed as mean ± SD. Student's T test was used to assess the difference between the mean values. Pearson correlation coefficients (r) were measured. For statistical analysis Excel software was used (Microsoft Office 2013, Redmond, WA). A p value lower than 0.05 was considered statistically significant.

Results

Overall, 50 ^{68}Ga-PSMA-11 PET/CT-U studies were performed for BCR and 7 for PS of PC. The median PSA value for patients with BCR and PS was 2.0 ± 11.4 ng/ml (0.06–57.3 ng/ml) and 18 ± 35.3 ng/ml (6.8–100 ng/ml), respectively. The most common GS for both groups was 7 (range 6–10).

^{68}Ga-PSMA-11 PET, PET/CT and CT-U

Overall in BCR group, PSMA PET alone was reported positive in 36 patients (72%), CT-U in 11 patients (22%), PSMA PET/CT-U in 33 patients (66%) and in 36 patients (72%) at least one of the above modalities. Figure 2 shows the proportion of positive results of each modality stratified by PSA level. Patients' characteristics and modality based results are presented in Additional file 1: Table S3 and S4.

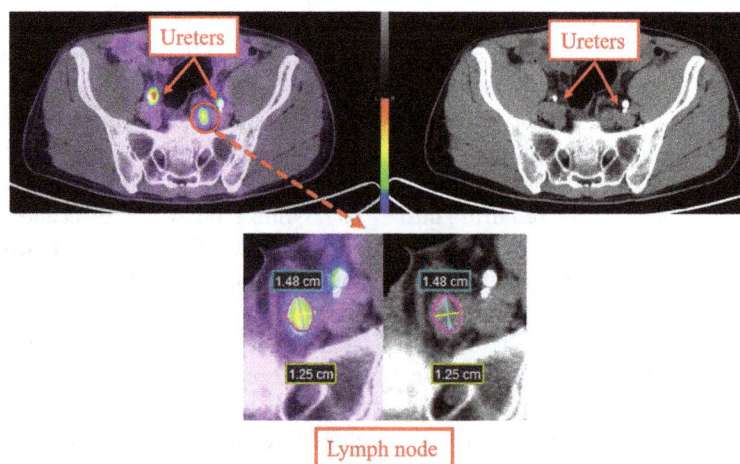

Fig. 1 Top row. PET/CT-U and CT-U images show PSMA activity corresponding to opacified ureters and a left pelvic lymph node. The high-density focus posterior to the left ureter is a phlebolith in the iliac vessel. Bottom row. Magnified PET/CT-U and CT-U with semi-automatic PET edge detection with lymph node measurements

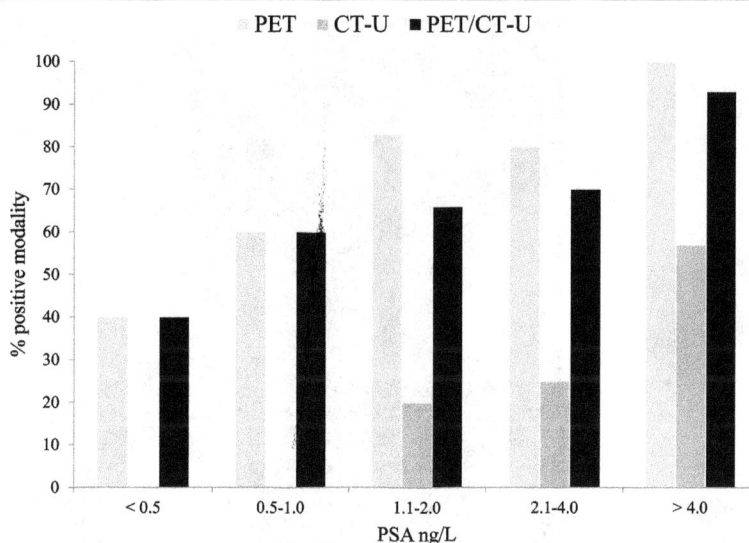

Fig. 2 Percentage of positive result of each modality stratified by PSA level demonstrates an increasing likelihood of a positive imaging result with increasing PSA level. Most discordant cases between CT and PSMA PET positivity were in patients with a PSA <4ng/L

PSMA PET detected PC in all seven patients for PS, which was confirmed either by histopathology or MRI. PSMA PET and PSMA PET/CT-U detected nodal metastasis in one patient while CT-U was negative in all seven patients. The mean SUVmax of prostate lesions was 14 ± 7.5 (range 7–26.1).

Overall 40 equivocal foci of activity were recorded in review of standalone PET images in 27/57 (47%) patients. On review of PET/CT-U, 11 foci in 10 patients (17.5%) corresponded to enhanced urine in the ureters, bladder, prostate bed, seminal vesicle or urethra. Of these, 3 foci (3 patients) were solitary sites of activity on PSMA imaging including two local and one nodal site. 4 foci (3 patients) were in different nodal fields, either contralateral pelvis or ipsilateral pelvis but above or below common iliac vessels bifurcation (figs. 3, 4, 5). In addition, in one patient in PS group, PSMA activity in one side of prostate was attributed to refluxed urinary activity in the prostate capsule which was subsequently confirmed by histopathology (fig. 6).

Table 1 shows the breakdown of the sites of recurrence in these patients. 75% (25/33) of patients with recurrence had at least one nodal metastasis. Overall 48 PSMA-expressing pelvic or para-aortic lymph nodes were detected in 25 patients. In 13 patients, there was only one positive lymph node. The parameters for ureters, lymph nodes and the distance between lymph nodes and ipsilateral ureters are detailed in the Table 2. No statistically significant difference is noted between the SUVmax of ureteric tracer activity and lymph nodes ($p = 0.5$). Low to moderate correlation was found between the SUVmax and short-axis diameter, long- axis diameter and the volume of the lymph nodes ($r = 0.43$,

0.5 and 0.4, respectively). The mean PSA value of the patients with positive scan was statistically higher than the patients with negative scan ($p = 0.038$) (fig. 7).

CT-U

In subgroup of patients with BCR, standalone CT detected 12 lymph nodes in 8 patients. The mean short axis of these lymph nodes was 12.8 ± 3.5 mm (9–18.9). Overall CT reported metastatic disease in 11 (22%) patients, all of whom also had confirmatory PSMA PET finding. In addition, PSMA PET did not show increased uptake in CT-reported equivocal findings in 5 patients. These included 4 patients with osseous abnormalities which did not have all characterics of PC metastases and one with enlarged retroperitoneal lymph nodes, which were subsequently proven to be lymphoma. 54.5% (31/57) of studies showed opacification of entire bilateral ureters, 31.5% (18/57) patchy or unilateral, 12% (7/57) proximal ureters and 2%(1/57) distal ureters. The mean distance between PSMA avid lymph nodes and opacified ureters, bladder, prostate bed, urethra or seminal vesicles was 12.6 ± 9.5 mm (range 2–41).

Discussion

An important characteristic of prostate cancer is the expression of PSMA, which makes the tumors ideal targets for functional imaging [16–18]. ^{68}Ga-PSMA-11 specifically binds to PSMA and an increasing number of studies suggest that PSMA PET/CT imaging is useful in detection of PC lesions [11, 12]. In a recent meta-analysis involving 1309 patients, detection rate for the PSA categories 0–0.2, 0.2–1, 1–2, and >2 ng/ml were 42%, 58%, 76%, and 95% scans, respectively [14]. Therefore,

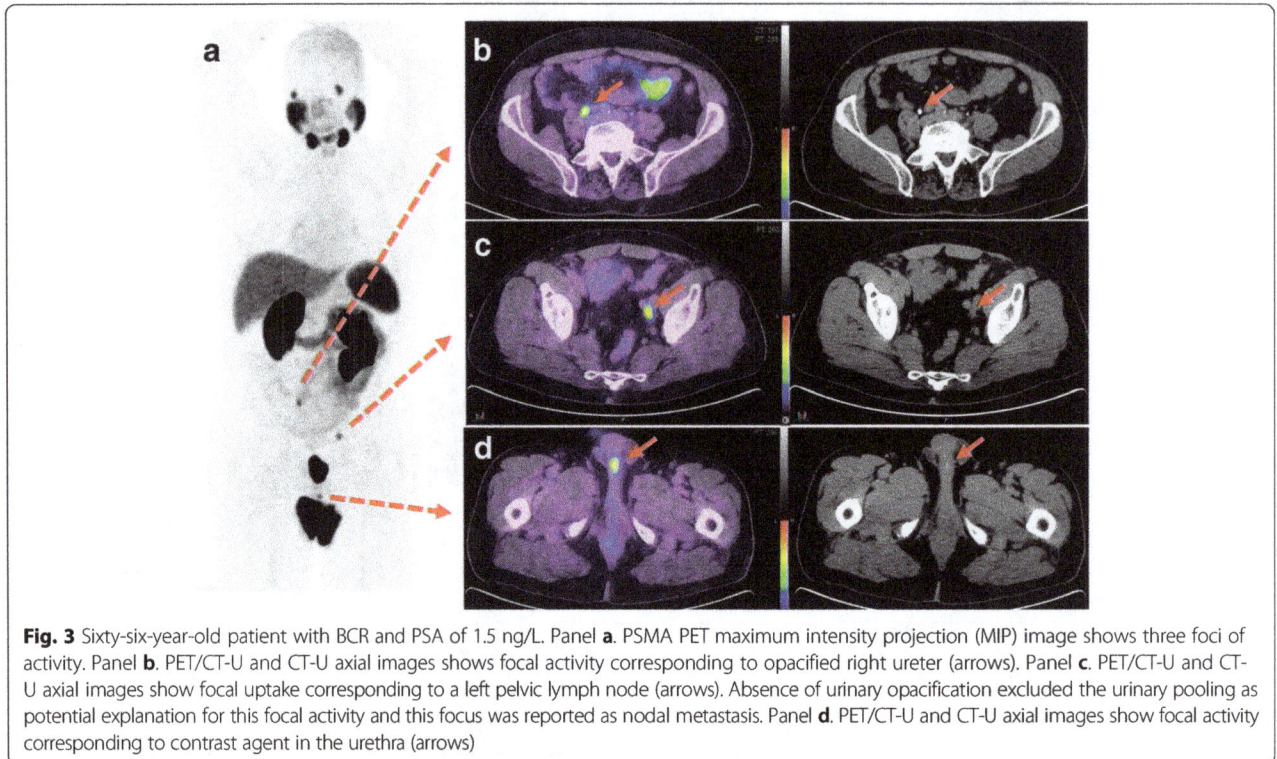

Fig. 3 Sixty-six-year-old patient with BCR and PSA of 1.5 ng/L. Panel **a**. PSMA PET maximum intensity projection (MIP) image shows three foci of activity. Panel **b**. PET/CT-U and CT-U axial images shows focal activity corresponding to opacified right ureter (arrows). Panel **c**. PET/CT-U and CT-U axial images show focal uptake corresponding to a left pelvic lymph node (arrows). Absence of urinary opacification excluded the urinary pooling as potential explanation for this focal activity and this focus was reported as nodal metastasis. Panel **d**. PET/CT-U and CT-U axial images show focal activity corresponding to contrast agent in the urethra (arrows)

due to the very high positive predictive value and high detection rate even at low PSA values, PSMA PET could be considered as the standard of reference in BCR.

There is, however, significant ^{68}Ga-PSMA-11 accumulation in the ureters and urinary bladder due to radiotracer excretion through kidneys [19]. This poses significant challenge in the assessment of the small lymph nodes in the proximity of the ureters or small local recurrence in peri-vesical region, prostate bed and urethra, particularly when potentially distorted by intervention. In our facility, we have adopted a new protocol using a modified CT-U with PET/CT imaging. In this approach, the CT was acquired at the time of ureteric and bladder opacification followed by PET acquisition and replaces the non-contrast or portal venous phase CT that is typically used for anatomical correlation and attenuation correction of PET data. In our experience, this technique is practical and could potentially assist in the final interpretation of about

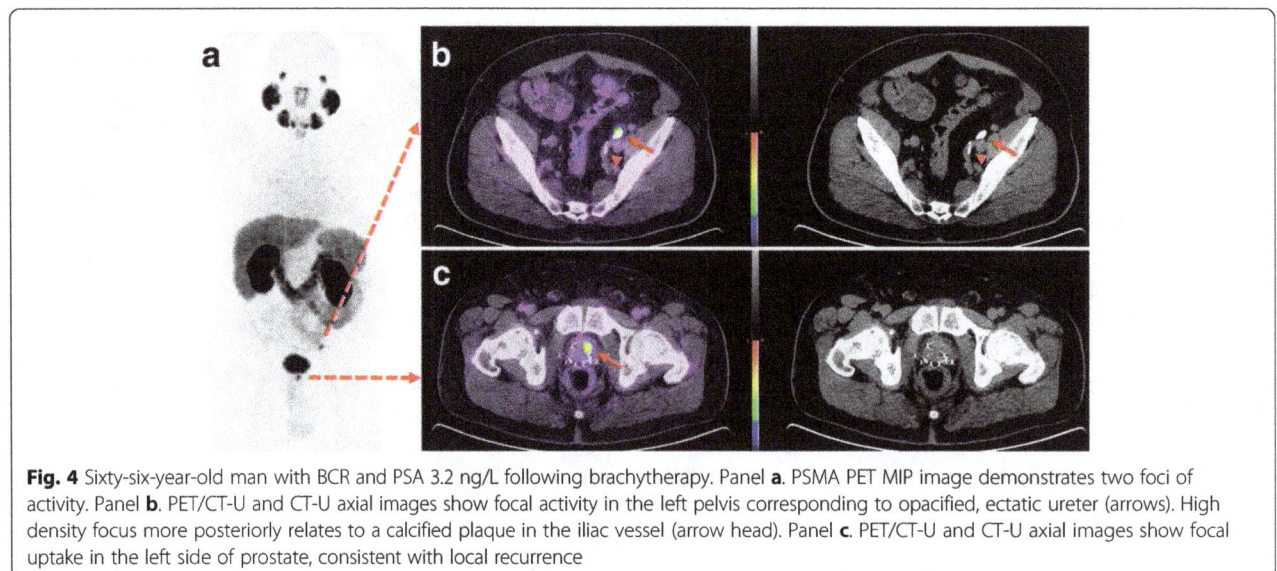

Fig. 4 Sixty-six-year-old man with BCR and PSA 3.2 ng/L following brachytherapy. Panel **a**. PSMA PET MIP image demonstrates two foci of activity. Panel **b**. PET/CT-U and CT-U axial images show focal activity in the left pelvis corresponding to opacified, ectatic ureter (arrows). High density focus more posteriorly relates to a calcified plaque in the iliac vessel (arrow head). Panel **c**. PET/CT-U and CT-U axial images show focal uptake in the left side of prostate, consistent with local recurrence

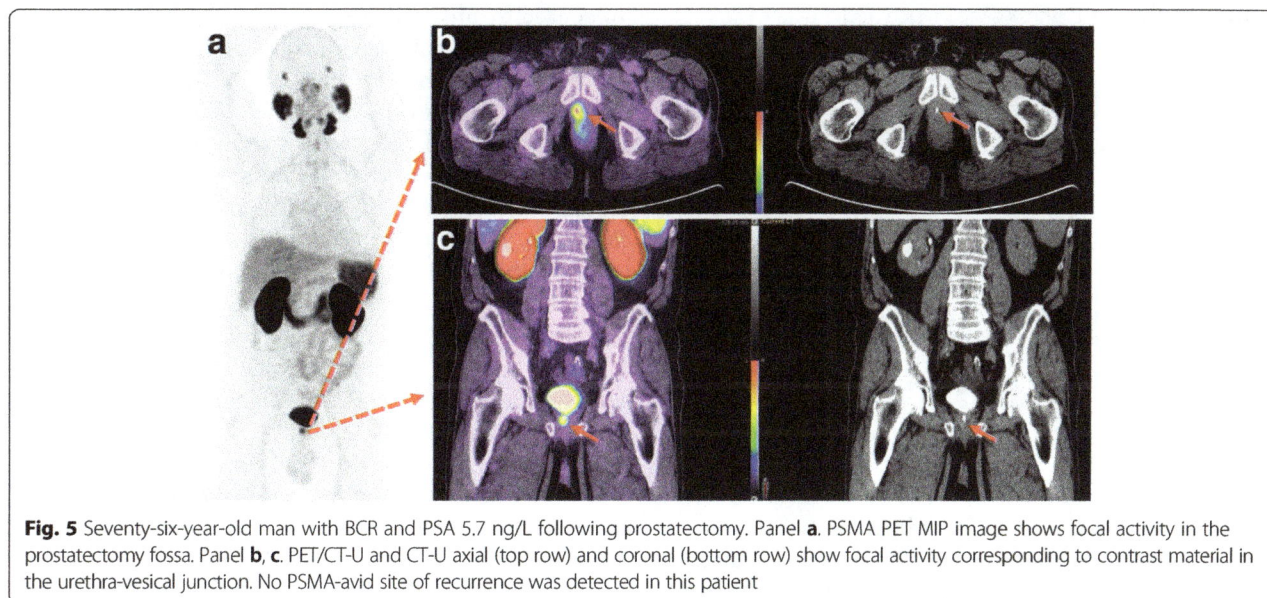

Fig. 5 Seventy-six-year-old man with BCR and PSA 5.7 ng/L following prostatectomy. Panel **a**. PSMA PET MIP image shows focal activity in the prostatectomy fossa. Panel **b**, **c**. PET/CT-U and CT-U axial (top row) and coronal (bottom row) show focal activity corresponding to contrast material in the urethra-vesical junction. No PSMA-avid site of recurrence was detected in this patient

17.5% of studies by localizing the focal tracer activity to the contrast enhanced urine. Especially, in three studies interpretation was changed from positive on PET to negative on PET/CT-U for site of recurrence. Multiple imaging protocols have been used to overcome this issue, which is not unique to ^{68}Ga-PSMA imaging. Kamel et al. adopted a protocol including hydration and forced diuresis before FDG PET imaging for staging and restaging of urogenital malignancies such as bladder cancer. In this study, there was good visualization of the primary bladder cancer [20]. Rauscher et al. proposed injection of diuretic at the time of tracer injection to reduce artefacts associated with high tracer activity in the urinary collecting system and bladder [21]. This approach could also be added to our protocol,

however would be more technically demanding with especial attention to the patient's hydration status. Kabasakal et al. assessed the value of early pelvic imaging in the PSMA PET imaging in a retrospective study. PET/CT images of the pelvis were performed at 5 min followed by whole body images at 60 min post tracer injection. Comparison between early and late pelvic images revealed no difference in the number of lesions. Due to lack of bladder activity in early images, assessment of primary tumor and local lesions were easier but was potentially compromised by significantly lower lesional uptake in early images [22]. Furthermore, fitting multiple time-point imaging into the schedule of a busy PET department is difficult while our protocol provide one time point imaging. However, it

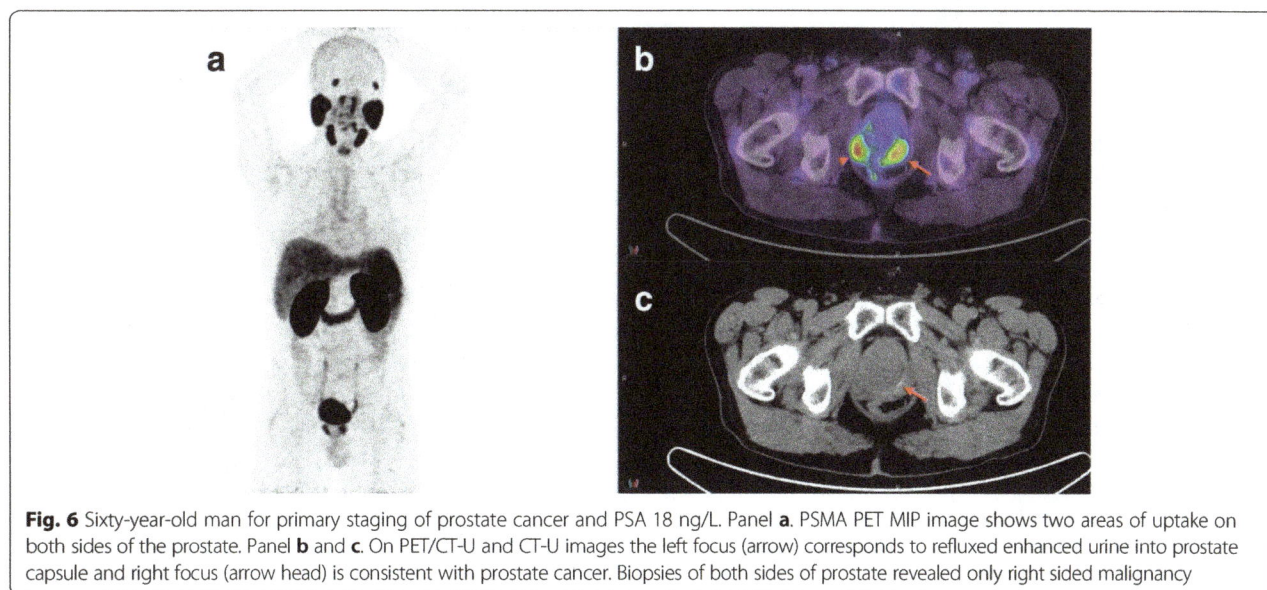

Fig. 6 Sixty-year-old man for primary staging of prostate cancer and PSA 18 ng/L. Panel **a**. PSMA PET MIP image shows two areas of uptake on both sides of the prostate. Panel **b** and **c**. On PET/CT-U and CT-U images the left focus (arrow) corresponds to refluxed enhanced urine into prostate capsule and right focus (arrow head) is consistent with prostate cancer. Biopsies of both sides of prostate revealed only right sided malignancy

Table 1 Breakdown of sites of recurrence in the patients with positive PSMA scan

Number of patients	Local	Lymph node	Bone	Other (liver)
16		+		
4	+			
3	+	+		
3		+	+	
2	+	+	+	
1	+	+	+	+

Some patients had multiple sites of recurrence as indicated by "+" sign

should be noted, as we have not performed head to head comparison between PET/CT-U and PET/CT protocol, incremental value of the PET/CT-U or diagnostic advantage of this approach could not inferred from our data.

When imaging the ureter with CT-U, it can be difficult to achieve complete opacification and adequate distention with a single excretory phase [23]. We also experienced the same issue as only 54% of the CT-U images showed complete opacification of the entire length of bilateral ureters. Several techniques have been proposed to address this concern, such as oral or intravenous hydration; intravenous furosemide; use of abdominal compression devices; prone patient positioning; and additional delayed phase imaging but none have been universally effective in practice [23]. In addition, incorporating these techniques in PET/CT protocol can be impractical or potentially harmful but oral hydration remains the simplest approach. However, in our experience, even if the ureters do not completely opacify, CT-U helps in better delineation of the ureteric course. In addition, in the absence of corresponding focal contrast hold-up, an equivocal focal PSMA activity would be more likely interpreted as a lymph node (fig. 4, panel C).

Local recurrence is most frequently located near the vesico-urethral anastomosis or less commonly in the retained seminal vesicles, posterior bladder wall, rectovesical region and at the resection site of the vas deferens [24]. Multi parametric(mp) MRI of the prostate can distinguish prostate cancer recurrence from residual healthy glandular tissue, post-treatment changes including scar/fibrosis or granulation tissue [25]. In a study by Freitag et al., mpMRI was compared to PSMA PET/MRI and PET/CT in detection of local recurrence. In this study, 50% of the patients with local recurrence on mpMRI were missed by PET and detection of local recurrence using the PET-component was significantly

influenced by proximity to the bladder [26]. We have also observed pooling of the urinary activity in the proximal part of urethra, penile urethra and refluxed urine into the retained seminal vesicles particularly following prostatectomy (fig. 5). Even prior to prostatectomy, we have observed refluxed urinary contrast in the seminal vesicles or prostate capsule (fig. 6). These potentially pose significant challenges in differentiating local PSMA-avid disease from urinary activity. In our experience, contrast opacification of the bladder, bladder neck and urethra is, perhaps, the major advantage of this protocol in discriminating urinary activity from local recurrence. Evolving fluorinated PSMA agents with little or no early urinary excretion, however, could overcome this challenge [27].

In this study, standard dose CT was acquired for PSMA PET/CT-U protocol. The mean calculated effective radiation dose to patients form this imaging protocol was 18 mSv (16-20 mSv). CT acquisition during PET/CT imaging is often performed for a variety of purposes including diagnosis, anatomic localization of the PET images and attenuation correction of the PET images. CT for diagnosis purposes (110-200mAs) imparts more radiation dose (effective dose of 11-20 mSv) than CT for anatomic localization (30-60mAs) with effective radiation dose of 3-6 mSv [28, 29]. Therefore, if CT is performed only for anatomic localization of the PET images radiation often could be reduced by 50–80% [28–30]. In our study, stand-alone diagnostic CT detected metastatic disease in only 30% (11/33) of patients. It is unclear whether standard dose CT would have additional diagnostic value and this protocol could potentially be used with low dose CT.

A typical CT-U protocol has three phases including an initial unenhanced acquisition, nephrographic phase 90–100 seconds following administration of contrast agent and pyelographic phase images 5–15 minutes after contrast administration [15]. This is an excellent technique for the assessment of urothelial malignancies. In this study, however, for the purpose of the ureteric and bladder opacification, only pyelogram phase of this imaging protocol has been acquired and referred to CT-U. In addition, we administered only 50 ml of contrast agent in this protocol whereas in the standard technique 100-150 ml of the nonionic contrast is commonly used [15]. A modification to this protocol is also possible by dual-bolus intravenous contrast administration with simultaneous nephrographic phase (portal-venous enhancement) and pyelographic phase in a single CT acquisition. Notwithstanding small risk of allergic reaction has to be considered. However, only two patients were not able to

Table 2 Parameters in patients with BCR

Ureteric SUVmax	Lymph node SUVmax	Short axis (mm)	Long axis (mm)	Volume (ml)	Distance to ureter (mm)
8.8 ± 6.5 (3.8–31.4)	9.5 ± 6.6 (2.8–31.2)	8.3 ± 4.2 (1.5–18.9)	12 ± 5.5 (4.2–23)	0.94 ± 1.3 (0.05–6)	12.6 ± 9.5 (2–41)

All values are in mean ± SD (range)

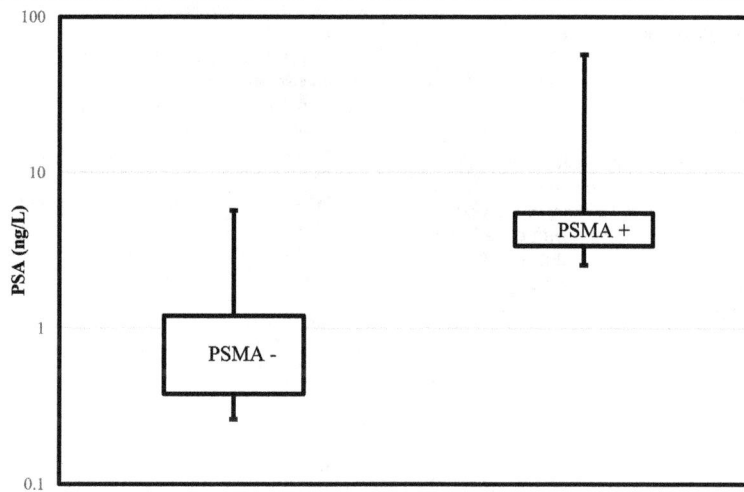

Fig. 7 Logarithmic PSA values of patients with positive and negative PSMA PET

undergo this protocol due to prior contrast allergy or impaired renal function.

It has been reported that up to 80% of metastatic lymph nodes in PC have a short-axis diameter less than 7 mm [8, 9]. In a retrospective study of 21 patients Giesel et al. reported the mean short axis of 5.8 mm for the PSMA positive lymph nodes [31]. However, in our study, the mean short axis of PSMA positive lymph nodes was slightly higher at 8.3 mm. Nonetheless, this demonstrates the incremental value of the PMSA PET/CT over CT alone for assessment of BCR.

In our study, the overall detection rate for the any site of recurrence or metastasis was 66%. Afshar-Oromieh et al. reported the detection rate of 86.6% for PSMA PET in a retrospective study of 37 patients with BCR. The lower detection rate in our study could potentially be explained by the lower mean PSA levels of 2.0 ng/ml compared to 11.1 ng/ml [32]. This also may reflect referral of patients with BCR for investigation by PSMA PET with lower PSA levels and slower PSA kinetics than in prior series, based on the encouraging results recently presented in the literature.

This study has certain limitations. Firstly, there was no comparison group to demonstrate additional value of PET/CT-U to non-enhanced PET/CT. We instituted the CT-U protocol because of the uncertainty we experienced using non-contrast CT with PSMA PET. Our experience in the transition from a non-contrast to a CT-U protocol, however, is consistent with the findings in this study. The data provided, however, cannot quantify the incremental value of CT-U compared to unenhanced or standard portal venous phase CT. Lack of pathologic confirmation of lesions detected by ^{68}Ga-PSMA PET/CT imaging or follow-up imaging is another limitation. It was not possible to obtain histologic verification because of ethical and practical reasons. However, given high positive predicative value of PSMA PET, this is becoming widely accepted as the standard of imaging.

Conclusions

PSMA PET/CT-U is a practical protocol that can help in the interpretation these studies by distinguishing focal urinary activity in the ureters, bladder, prostate bed, seminal vesicles and urethra from low volume PC.

Abbreviations
BCR: Biochemical relapse; CT: Computed tomography; CT-U: CT urography; eGFR: Estimated glomerular filtration rate; FWHM: Full-width at half-maximum; GS: Gleason score; mp: Multi parametric; MRI: Magnetic resonance; OSEM: Ordered subset expectation maximization; PC: Prostate cancer; PET: Positron emission tomography; PS: Primary staging; PSA: Prostate-specific antigen; PSMA: Prostate-specific membrane antigen; SUVmax: Maximum standardized uptake value

Acknowledgements
Not applicable.

Funding
Not applicable.

Authors' contributions
AI: design of the study, collection of data, analysis and interpretation, writing of the manuscript. MSH: analysis and interpretation of data, critical reviewing of the manuscript. TM: design of the CT-U protocol as part of PET/CT, critical reviewing of the manuscript. SW and DM, acquisition of data and critical reviewing of the manuscript. BKP, analysis and interpretation of CT data and reviewing of the manuscript. RJH, design of the study, development of protocol, critical reviewing of the manuscript. All authors read the manuscript and approved of the contents.

Competing interests

The authors declare that they have no competing interests.

Author details

[1]Centre for Molecular Imaging, Department of Cancer Imaging, Peter MacCallum Cancer Centre, 305 Grattan Street, Melbourne, Australia. [2]Sir Peter MacCallum Department of Oncology, University of Melbourne, 305 Grattan Street, Melbourne, Australia. [3]Sir Peter MacCallum Department of Radiation Oncology, University of Melbourne, 305 Grattan Street, Melbourne, Australia. [4]Sir Peter MacCallum Department of Surgical Oncology, University of Melbourne, 305 Grattan Street, Melbourne, Australia.

References

1. Siegel R, Ma J, Zou Z, Jemal A. Cancer statistics, 2014. CA Cancer J Clin. 2014;64:9–29.
2. Heidenreich A, Bastian PJ, Bellmunt J, Bolla M, Joniau S, van der Kwast T, Mason M, Matveev V, Wiegel T, Zattoni F, et al. EAU guidelines on prostate cancer. Part II: treatment of advanced, relapsing, and castration-resistant prostate cancer. Eur Urol. 2014;65:467–79.
3. Hodolic M. Role of (18)F-choline PET/CT in evaluation of patients with prostate carcinoma. Radiol Oncol. 2011;45:17–21.
4. Horvat A, Kovač V, Strojan P. Radiotherapy in palliative treatment of painful bone metastases. Radiol Oncol. 2009;43:213–24.
5. Heidenreich A, Bellmunt J, Bolla M, Joniau S, Mason M, Matveev V, Mottet N, Schmid HP, van der Kwast T, Wiegel T, et al. EAU guidelines on prostate cancer. Part 1: screening, diagnosis, and treatment of clinically localised disease. Eur Urol. 2011;59:61–71.
6. Cornford P, Bellmunt J, Bolla M, Briers E, De Santis M, Gross T, Henry AM, Joniau S, Lam TB, Mason MD, et al. EAU-ESTRO-SIOG guidelines on prostate cancer. Part II: treatment of relapsing, metastatic, and castration-resistant prostate cancer. Eur Urol. 2017;71:630–42.
7. Kosuri S, Akhtar NH, Smith M, Osborne JR, Tagawa ST. Review of salvage therapy for biochemically recurrent prostate cancer: the role of imaging and rationale for systemic salvage targeted anti-prostate-specific membrane antigen radioimmunotherapy. Adv Urol. 2012;2012:921674.
8. Hovels AM, Heesakkers RA, Adang EM, Jager GJ, Strum S, Hoogeveen YL, Severens JL, Barentsz JO. The diagnostic accuracy of CT and MRI in the staging of pelvic lymph nodes in patients with prostate cancer: a meta-analysis. Clin Radiol. 2008;63:387–95.
9. Flanigan RC, McKay TC, Olson M, Shankey TV, Pyle J, Waters WB. Limited efficacy of preoperative computed tomographic scanning for the evaluation of lymph node metastasis in patients before radical prostatectomy. Urology. 1996;48:428–32.
10. Eder M, Eisenhut M, Babich J, Haberkorn U. PSMA as a target for radiolabelled small molecules. Eur J Nucl Med Mol Imaging. 2013;40:819–23.
11. Afshar-Oromieh A, Haberkorn U, Eder M, Eisenhut M, Zechmann CM. [68Ga]gallium-labelled PSMA ligand as superior PET tracer for the diagnosis of prostate cancer: comparison with 18F-FECH. Eur J Nucl Med Mol Imaging. 2012;39:1085–6.
12. Afshar-Oromieh A, Malcher A, Eder M, Eisenhut M, Linhart HG, Hadaschik BA, Holland-Letz T, Giesel FL, Kratochwil C, Haufe S, et al. PET imaging with a [68Ga]gallium-labelled PSMA ligand for the diagnosis of prostate cancer: biodistribution in humans and first evaluation of tumour lesions. Eur J Nucl Med Mol Imaging. 2013;40:486–95.
13. Eiber M, Maurer T, Beer AJ, Souvatzoglou M, Weirich G, Kubler H: Prospective evaluation of PSMA-PET imaging for preoperative lymph node staging in prostate cancer J Nucl Med 2014 55 (Supplement 1).
14. Perera M, Papa N, Christidis D, Wetherell D, Hofman MS, Murphy DG, Bolton D, Lawrentschuk N. Sensitivity, specificity, and predictors of positive 68Ga-prostate-specific membrane antigen positron emission tomography in advanced prostate cancer: a systematic review and meta-analysis. Eur Urol. 2016;70:926–37.
15. O'Connor OJ, Fitzgerald E, Maher MM. Imaging of hematuria. AJR Am J Roentgenol. 2010;195:W263–7.
16. Reinhardt JM, Maleike D, Pluim JPW, Fabel M, Tetzlaff R, von Tengg-Kobligk H, Heimann T, Meinzer H-P, Wolf I. Lymph node segmentation on CT images by a shape model guided deformable surface methodh. Proc SPIE. 2008;6914:69141S.
17. Sterzing F, Fiedler H, Stefanova M, Afshar-Oromieh A, Kratochwil C, Debus J, Haberkorn U, Giesel F. Impact of 68Ga-PSMA PET/CT in Staging of Prostate Cancer Patient Prior to Radiation Therapy. International Journal of Radiation Oncology*Biology*Physics. 2014;90:S449.
18. Wright GL Jr, Grob BM, Haley C, Grossman K, Newhall K, Petrylak D, Troyer J, Konchuba A, Schellhammer PF, Moriarty R. Upregulation of prostate-specific membrane antigen after androgen-deprivation therapy. Urology. 1996;48:326–34.
19. Silver DA, Pellicer I, Fair WR, Heston WD, Cordon-Cardo C. Prostate-specific membrane antigen expression in normal and malignant human tissues. Clin Cancer Res. 1997;3:81–5.
20. Kamel EM, Jichlinski P, Prior JO, Meuwly JY, Delaloye JF, Vaucher L, Malterre J, Castaldo S, Leisinger HJ, Delaloye AB. Forced diuresis improves the diagnostic accuracy of 18F-FDG PET in abdominopelvic malignancies. J Nucl Med. 2006;47:1803–7.
21. Rauscher I, Maurer T, Fendler WP, Sommer WH, Schwaiger M, Eiber M. (68)Ga-PSMA ligand PET/CT in patients with prostate cancer: how we review and report. Cancer Imaging. 2016;16:14.
22. Kabasakal L, Demirci E, Ocak M, Akyel R, Nematyazar J, Aygun A, Halac M, Talat Z, Araman A. Evaluation of PSMA PET/CT imaging using a 68Ga-HBED-CC ligand in patients with prostate cancer and the value of early pelvic imaging. Nucl Med Commun. 2015;36:582–7.
23. Potenta SE, D'Agostino R, Sternberg KM, Tatsumi K, Perusse K, Urography CT. For evaluation of the ureter. Radiographics. 2015;35:709–26.
24. Cirillo S, Petracchini M, Scotti L, Gallo T, Macera A, Bona MC, Ortega C, Gabriele P, Regge D. Endorectal magnetic resonance imaging at 1.5 tesla to assess local recurrence following radical prostatectomy using T2-weighted and contrast-enhanced imaging. Eur Radiol. 2009;19:761–9.
25. Panebianco V, Barchetti F, Grompone MD, Colarieti A, Salvo V, Cardone G, Catalano C. Magnetic resonance imaging for localization of prostate cancer in the setting of biochemical recurrence. Urol Oncol. 2016;34:303–310.
26. Freitag MT, Radtke JP, Afshar-Oromieh A, Roethke MC, Hadaschik BA, Gleave M, Bonekamp D, Kopka K, Eder M, Heusser T, et al. Local recurrence of prostate cancer after radical prostatectomy is at risk to be missed in 68Ga-PSMA-11-PET of PET/CT and PET/MRI: comparison with mpMRI integrated in simultaneous PET/MRI. Eur J Nucl Med Mol Imaging. 2017;44:776–87.
27. Giesel FL, Hadaschik B, Cardinale J, Radtke J, Vinsensia M, Lehnert W, Kesch C, Tolstov Y, Singer S, Grabe N, et al. F-18 labelled PSMA-1007: biodistribution, radiation dosimetry and histopathological validation of tumor lesions in prostate cancer patients. Eur J Nucl Med Mol Imaging. 2017;44:678–88.
28. Brix G, Lechel U, Glatting G, Ziegler SI, Munzing W, Muller SP, Beyer T. Radiation exposure of patients undergoing whole-body dual-modality 18F-FDG PET/CT examinations. J Nucl Med. 2005;46:608–13.
29. Alessio AM, Kinahan PE, Manchanda V, Ghioni V, Aldape L, Parisi MT. Weight-based, low-dose pediatric whole-body PET/CT protocols. J Nucl Med. 2009;50:1570–7.
30. Gelfand MJ, Lemen LC. PET/CT and SPECT/CT dosimetry in children: the challenge to the pediatric imager. Semin Nucl Med. 2007;37:391–8.
31. Giesel FL, Fiedler H, Stefanova M, Sterzing F, Rius M, Kopka K, Moltz JH, Afshar-Oromieh A, Choyke PL, Haberkorn U, Kratochwil C. PSMA PET/CT with Glu-urea-Lys-(Ahx)-[(6)(8)Ga(HBED-CC)] versus 3D CTvolumetric lymph node assessment in recurrent prostate cancer. Eur J Nucl Med Mol Imaging. 2015;42:1794-1800.
32. Afshar-Oromieh A, Zechmann CM, Malcher A, Eder M, Eisenhut M, Linhart HG, Holland-Letz T, Hadaschik BA, Giesel FL, Debus J, Haberkorn U. Comparison of PET imaging with a (68)Ga-labelled PSMA ligand and (18)F-choline-based PET/CT for the diagnosis of recurrent prostate cancer. Eur J Nucl Med Mol Imaging. 2014;41:11–20.

16

DEB TACE for Intermediate and advanced HCC – Initial Experience in a Brazilian Cancer Center

Jose Hugo Mendes Luz[1*], Paula M. Luz[2], Henrique S. Martin[1], Hugo R. Gouveia[1], Raphal Braz Levigard[3], Felipe Diniz Nogueira[3], Bernardo Caetano Rodrigues[4], Tiago Nepomuceno de Miranda[1] and Marcelo Henrique Mamede[5]

Abstract

Background: According to Barcelona Clinic Liver Cancer classification transarterial chemoembolization is indicated in patients with Hepatocellular Carcinoma in the intermediate stage. Drug-eluting microspheres can absorb and release the chemotherapeutic agent slowly for 14 days after its intra-arterial administration. This type of transarterial chemoembolization approach appears to provide at least equivalent effectiveness with less toxicity.

Methods: This is a prospective, single-center study, which evaluated 21 patients with intermediate and advanced hepatocellular carcinoma who underwent transarterial chemoembolization with drug-eluting microspheres. The follow up period was 2 years. Inclusion criteria was Child-Pugh A or B liver disease patients, intermediate or advanced hepatocellular carcinoma and performance status equal or below 2. Transarterial chemoembolization with drug-eluting microspheres was performed at 2-month intervals during the first two sessions. The third and subsequent sessions were performed according to the image findings on follow-up, on a "demand schedule". Tumor response and time to progression were evaluated along the two-year follow up period.

Results: Of the 21 patients 90% presented with liver cirrhosis, 62% had Barcelona Clinic Liver Cancer stage B and 38% had Barcelona Clinic Liver Cancer stage C hepatocellular carcinoma. Average tumor size was 6.9 cm. The average number of Transarterial chemoembolization with drug-eluting microspheres procedures was 3 with a total of 64 sessions. The predominant toxicity was mild. Liver function was not significantly affected in most patients. Two deaths occurred within 90 days after Transarterial chemoembolization with drug-eluting microspheres (ischemic hepatitis and hydropic decompensation). Technical success was achieved in 63 of 64 procedures. The mean hospital stay was 1.5 days. The progression free and overall survival at 1 and 2 years were 73.0% and 37.1%, 73.7% and 41.6%, respectively.

Conclusion: Transarterial chemoembolization with drug-eluting microspheres is able to deliver significant tumor response and progression free survival rate with acceptable toxicity. Larger studies are needed to identify exactly which subset of advanced hepatocellular patients may benefit from this treatment.

* Correspondence: jhugoluz@gmail.com
[1]Department of Interventional Radiology, Radiology Division, National Cancer Institute, INCA, Praça Cruz Vermelha 23, Centro, Rio de Janeiro CEP 20230-130, Brazil
Full list of author information is available at the end of the article

Background

Hepatocellular carcinoma (HCC) has become one of the most common tumors worldwide with approximately 500,000 new cases per year [1]. The main risk factors are infection with hepatitis B and C viruses. Approximately 1.4 to 2.5% of cirrhotic patients with hepatitis C and 1.5 to 6.6% of patients with hepatitis B viruses develop HCC [1]. Other risk factors are toxins (alcohol and aflatoxin B1), metabolic disorders (hemochromatosis, alpha 1-antitrypsin deficiency, cutaneous porphyria, etc.), anabolic steroids consumption and other causes of cirrhosis [1]. One of the most frequently used staging criteria for HCC is the BCLC algorithm (Barcelona Clinic Liver Cancer Staging Classification). Patients are classified accordingly to tumor size, number of hepatic tumors, PS (Karnofsky performance status scale), vascular invasion and extrahepatic spread. Those with a PS of zero, a single tumor larger than 5 cm or three tumors larger than 3 cm without vascular invasion or extra-hepatic disease are classified as intermediate HCC (BCLC stage B) and TACE is the treatment of choice. Patients with PS equal or greater than 1 and/or with portal invasion and/or extrahepatic disease are classified as advanced HCC (BCLC stage C) and Sorafenib was recently approved for the treatment of this subset of patients [2]. Those with advanced liver cirrhosis or PS greater than 2 are classified as terminals (BCLC stage D) and receive supportive therapy [3–5]. Treatments for patients allocated in BCLC stage B and C are considered palliative, differing from surgery, ablation and transplant, the therapeutics options for BCLC stage A HCC, which are recognized curative treatments.

Developed in the last decade, "drug eluting beads" (DEB) for TACE, made with superabsorbent polymers, have the property of absorbing the chemotherapy and slowly release it over several days (up to 14 days) in a steadily sustained manner. In conventional TACE there is a peak on the bloodstream of the chemotherapeutic agent right after the procedure [6, 7]. With DEB TACE there is a slow release of the chemotherapeutic agent into the hepatic tumor, limiting the systemic exposure of the drug and thus potentially reducing the occurrence of side effects. Another important change with this new approach is that TACE protocols are now standardized (diluting instructions are designed by the manufacturers [6]). One of the DEB TACE devices available is DC-Beads® which are precisely calibrated microspheres that are capable of absorbing chemotherapy (eg. doxorubicin). After its administration in liver tumor by intra-arterial injection, these microspheres begin to slowly release chemotherapy in a controlled and sustained manner for 14 days [7]. Experimental studies have shown that TACE with DEB has a secure pharmacokinetic profile and determines effective tumor destruction in animal models [8, 9].

With DEB TACE, chemotherapy plasma concentration is maintained low and constant throughout 14 days. In addition, the chemotherapy agent is maintained longer in contact with the tumor in the case of DEB TACE, but in the conventional technique chemotherapy is quickly eliminated from the liver [9–13].

Methods

This is a prospective non-randomized study where 21 patients with intermediate and advanced HCC, from a tertiary referral cancer center, were selected and submitted to DEB TACE loaded with doxorubicin from September 2009 thru April 2010. Our primary endpoint of interest was tumor response and progression-free survival and the secondary endpoint was to evaluate the occurrence of adverse events. The DEB TACE procedures were done at 2-month intervals during the first two sessions. From this point on new DEB TACE sessions were performed on demand accordingly to response in magnetic resonance (MR) and clinical outcome. Tumor response was evaluated with liver dedicated dynamic-enhanced MR of the abdomen and interpreted by body-imaging radiologists. Patients unable to perform MR were schedule to undergo computed tomography (CT). Clinical and laboratory tests were performed before and after each session and during hospitalizations, targeting the evaluation of the toxicity and quantification of adverse effects. For the inclusion criteria patients had to be 18 years old or above, present a Child-Pugh A or B (Child-Pugh Classification) status, a PS equal or less than 2, a liver tumor compatible with a BCLC stage B or C HCC which had not been previously submitted to TACE or any intra-arterial treatment.

TACE with DEB – the procedure

Procedures, DEB TACE, were done by a staff member of our interventional radiology team with experience with oncology interventions. Two vials of the DEB TACE product DC Beads (2 mL, BioCompatibles Ltd., UK) with a diameter of 100 to 300 μm or 300 to 500 μm were loaded, per vial, with 75 mg of doxorubicin hydrochloride (37,5 mg/mL). Thru the common femoral artery and using a diagnostic catheter (eg. Cobra 5 F) a microcatheter was placed as selective as possible to the vessel irrigating the hepatic tumor. After the tip of the microcatheter achieved a secure point we performed the injection of the DC Beads loaded with doxorubicin mixed with contrast media in a smooth fashion. Our endpoint was to administer the whole two DC Beads vials or when flow of the tumor-nourishing artery reduced markedly. Total stasis of the tumor vascularity was avoided so it wouldn't disturb the subsequent DEB TACE sessions (Figs. 1, 2 and 3).

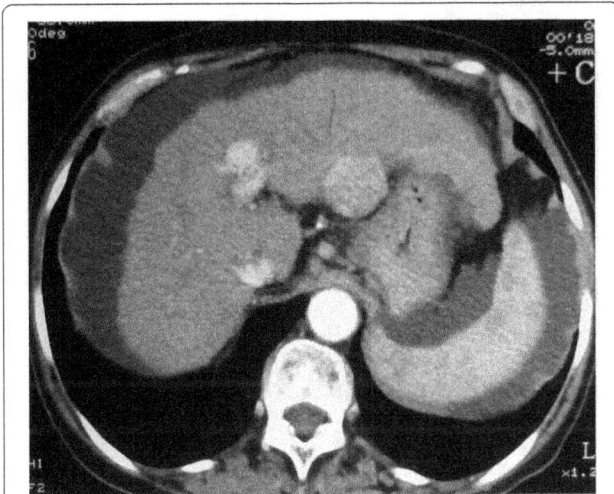

Fig. 1 Computed tomography before DEB TACE. Computed tomography showing a hypervascular liver tumor in the left lobe compatible with Hepatocellular Carcinoma in a 71 year-old female patient with liver cirrhosis and hepatitis C

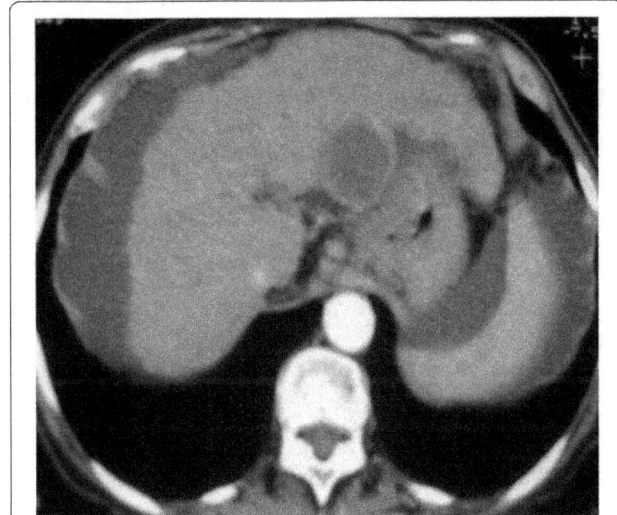

Fig. 3 Computed tomography after DEB TACE. Computed tomography 30 days after DEB TACE showing lack of enhancement in the liver tumor consistent with complete response accordingly to the EASL criteria

Criteria for therapeutic response

Traditionally the RECIST criteria is used for evaluation of tumor response in solid tumors. According to this criteria it is possible to measure response to treatment by quantifying tumor size reduction and its been validated as a valuable tool in assessing the efficacy of anti-tumor cytotoxic drugs [12]. But strictly anatomical criteria that only take into account the reduction of the size of the tumor to assess response can be misleading when applied to targeted molecular therapies or locoregional treatment (eg. TACE). Frequently HCC liquefies and becomes avascular after a favorable response to TACE, even thought initially it may not show a significant size

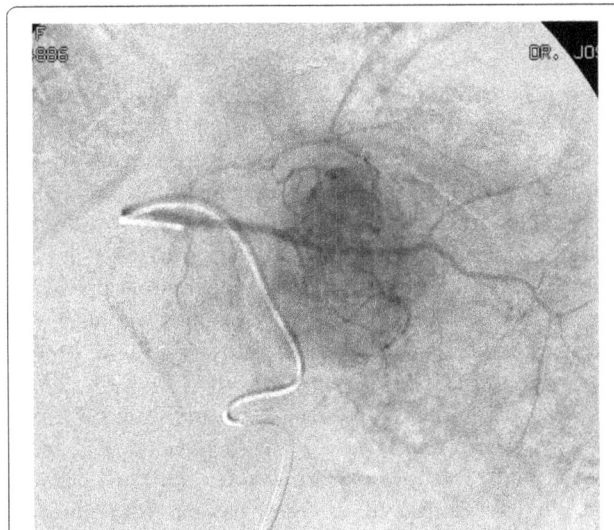

Fig. 2 Angiography during DEB TACE. During the DEB TACE procedure the angiography shows the hypervascular lesion

reduction or no size reduction at all. On this account, in the year 2000, a panel of experts through the European Association for the study of the Liver - EASL [3] - and later in 2008 through the American Association for the Study of Liver Diseases - AASLD [5] - established a series of guidelines for tumor response which included the degree of tumor necrosis for HCC [14]. Therefore, in this current study, the EASL criteria (tumor viability and tumor necrosis) was used. According to this guideline a Partial Response (PR) and Disease Progression (PD) were defined as more than 50% reduction or more than 25% increase, respectively, in the size of the contrast enhancement tumor area of the target lesions. The appearance of new lesions at least 1 cm in size consistent with HCC indicated PD. The enhancement analysis was always performed in the CT or MR contrast arterial [5] phase. An experienced body diagnostic radiologist performed all evaluations (Figs. 4, 5 and 6).

Progression-free survival and overall survival were recorded according to imaging studies and clinical outcomes. Statistical analysis was performed by the Kaplan Meyer method and log-rank using S-plus software. The Kaplan-Meier method was used to describe two outcomes of interest: the probability of survival and the probability of not progressing. The log-rank and Peto test were used to assess whether the survival curves were statistically different between strata of variable categories.

Assessment of toxicity

Toxicity was assessed after each DEB-TACE session by recording the patient's clinical status and complete laboratory evaluation. The pain in the immediate postoperative period was registered on a scale of 0 to 10 (0

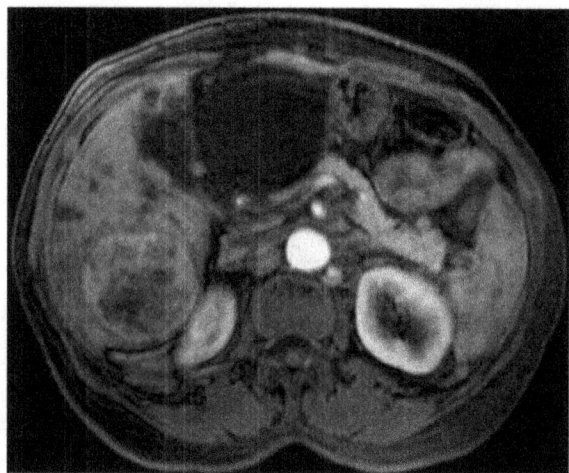

Fig. 4 Magnetic Resonance before DEB TACE. A 62 year-old male with alcoholic liver cirrhosis and a large HCC in the right hepatic lobe. At magenetic resonance the lesion is hypervascular with its central portion showing some areas of no contrast enhancement suggestive of necrosis

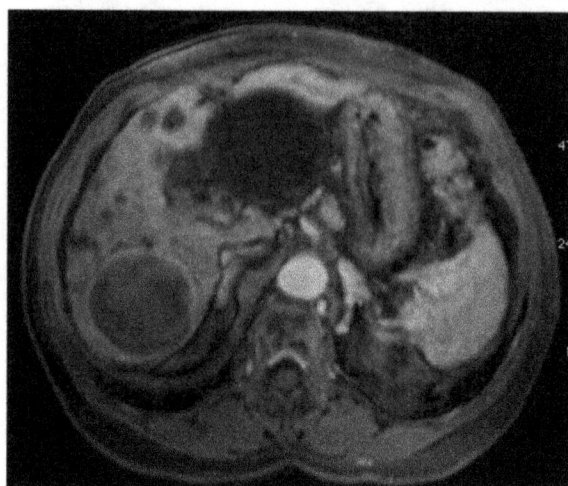

Fig. 6 Magnetic resonance after DEB TACE. Magnetic Resonance done four months after DEB TACE showed that the tumor is now avascular. By the EASL criteria there is a complete response but with the Recist criteria the analysis would be just of stable disease

being no pain and 10 being pain of highest intensity). Adverse events were assessed according to the definitions of the NCI-CTC version 3.0. The occurrence of post-embolization syndrome was also recorded after all treatments [15].

Results

DEB-TACE was done 52 times in 21 patients. Thirteen patients had BCLC B (62%) HCC and eight patients had BCLC C (38%) HCC with a mean population age of 61 years. Liver cirrhosis was present in 20 patients

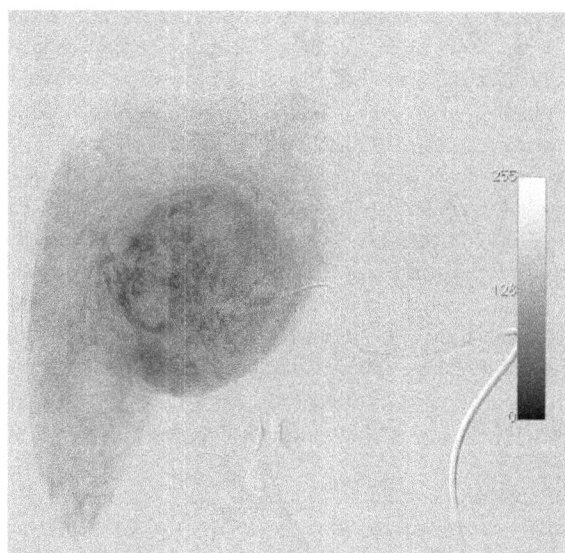

Fig. 5 Angiography during DEB TACE. The angiography during TACE shows the large tumor occupying a central position in the liver

(95%). The average tumor size was 6.7 cm (range from 3.5 cm to 12 cm). The average number of DEB-TACE procedures per patient was 3 (ranging from 1 to 6 sessions). The mean follow-up was 16.6 months (range 6–30 months). Technical success was achieved in 52 of the 53 DEB-TACE procedures (98%, 52/53). In this single procedure without technical success it was already the fourth DEB-TACE session. During the procedure we identified a complete occlusion of the proper hepatic artery thus preventing the catheter to be placed in suitable position for administration of microspheres loaded with doxorubicin. An average dose of 110 mg (range 75 to 150 mg) of doxorubicin was administered in 52 procedures. The microcatheter was used in all DEB-TACE procedures. The average hospital stay was 1.5 days (range 1–14 days). Only one patient had moderate and persistent pain after DEB-TACE and needed continuous use of analgesics. This patient had partial portal vein thrombosis. We attributed the persistent symptom to the extensive tumor necrosis and wedge shaped areas of suggestive liver parenchyma infarction seen on his MR studies. Overall pain was reported to be minimal to mild (pain intensity score reported averaged at 2.5). Two patients showed hydropic decompensation that were reversed with diuretic therapy. Two patients had increased bilirubin above 3.5 (maximum 4.9), which were also reverted to pre-treatment values in both.

At two years follow-up 12 patients had died. Of those deaths 3 were unrelated to the hepatic cancer (one patient died of acute myocardial infarction, one from a severe pneumonia and a third patient who showed tumor response on imaging studies nevertheless experienced worsening of liver function related to the return of alcohol ingestion). Of the 8 patients who are alive at the 2 years follow-up 7 showed a complete response and 1 patient with partial response. These patients are in clinical and radiological follow-up and no DEB TACE session are scheduled for them in the next 30 days. The patient who had a partial response is currently being evaluated for liver surgery or liver transplant.

Time to progression and survival

The median survival time estimated by the Kaplan-Meier method was 19.6 months. The median time to progression estimated by the Kaplan-Meier procedure was 17.4 months. The progression free and overall survival at 1 and 2 years were 73.0% and 37.1%, 73.7% and 41.6%, respectively (Graphic 1). There was a trend towards a increased survival in patients with BCLC stage B compared to those patients with BCLC stage C (Graphic 2) and patients with lower bilirubin levels (value of bilirubin lower than 2.5), however, without reaching statistical significance ($p = 0.10$ and $p = 0.11$ respectively). Other risks were assessed and showed no association such as gender, race, age, tumor size, portal invasion, alpha-feto protein (AFP) levels, Child-Pugh classification, PS and number of DEB TACE sessions performed (Figs. 7 and 8).

Security

On average, the toxicity was low to moderate, with a small frequency of grade 2 events (CTCAE v3.0). No Grade 3 or 4 events were reported. Post-embolization syndrome [15] occurred in approximately 50% of patients and was mainly characterized by low-grade fever (up to 38 °C) and malaise lasting an average of 15 days after DEB TACE. In all cases treatments were directed to the symptoms reported and successfully controlled. The laboratory parameters of liver function were not

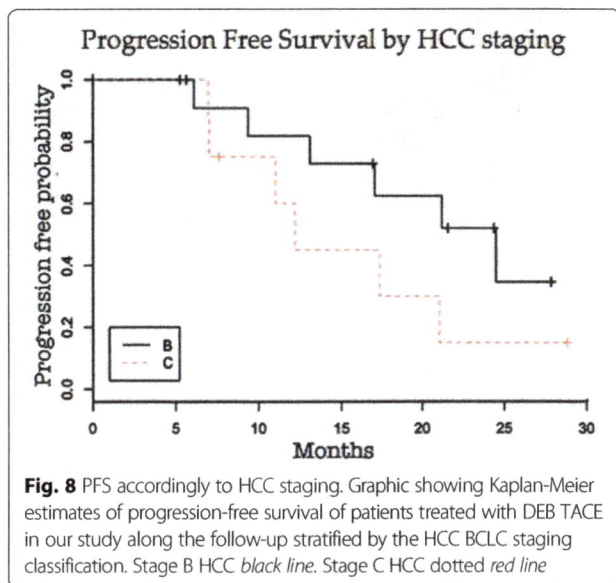

Fig. 8 PFS accordingly to HCC staging. Graphic showing Kaplan-Meier estimates of progression-free survival of patients treated with DEB TACE in our study along the follow-up stratified by the HCC BCLC staging classification. Stage B HCC *black line*. Stage C HCC dotted *red line*

significantly altered after most of the procedures (eg. Liver enzymes usually up to 3 times baseline). No patient died within the first thirty days after DEB TACE. Two patients died within 60 days after the procedure. One of them was discharged 3 days after the procedure with well-compensated liver disease. He was re-admitted 39 days later with liver failure due to worsening of hepatic cirrhosis also associated to the return ethyl derivatives consumption. He remained hospitalized for 21 days and died of progressive worsening of liver function and multiple organ failure. The other patient was discharged 24 h after the procedure. Re-hospitalized 50 days after DEB TACE due to a severe lung infection and died within 7 days.

Alpha-fetoprotein values

Only 7 patients had augmentation of AFP leves above 200 ng/ml (median 667, range 335–1500). We were able to identify a reduction of approximately 80% in AFP levels after DEB TACE sessions, falling to an average of 133 ng/ml overall. There was a tendency of positive correlation in the reduction of AFP levels and tumor response identified by MR.

Discussion

TACE is one of the principal medical managements for HCC, being responsible for the treatment of nearly half of all patients with this liver cancer at some point during their disease course [13]. TACE has a limited ability to maintain the chemotherapeutic agent in the liver tumor vascularization. Besides that conventional TACE was the first treatment to show survival benefit in BCLC stage B HCC [4]. Nonetheless it is known that in this conventional approach a chemotherapy blood peak occurs

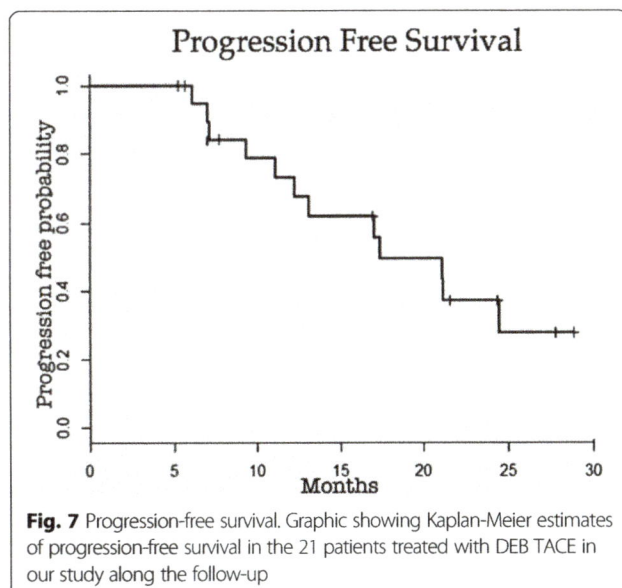

Fig. 7 Progression-free survival. Graphic showing Kaplan-Meier estimates of progression-free survival in the 21 patients treated with DEB TACE in our study along the follow-up

immediately after TACE mainly due to the inability of its well-established vector, lipiodol, to slowly release the drug [14]. The use of embolization material is (eg. Gelfoam particles, PVA) associated with chemotherapy and lipiodol to obtain an acceptable degree of response, often causing a not inconsiderable damage to adjacent non-tumor liver parenchyma speeding deterioration of liver function and increasing the toxicity of this therapeutic modality.

DEB TACE represents an approach to perform chemoembolization employing the administration of microspheres loaded with chemotherapy [17]. Once administered through the catheter, these microspheres in addition to obstruction blood flow also release chemotherapy into tumor vascularity in a controlled and sustained manner for 14 days [18]. This sustained release allows greater exposure of the chemotherapy to cancer cells and thus increasing the degree of tumor necrosis. Furthermore since it is possible to obtain a lower peak of the drug immediately in the systemic circulation after the procedure DEB TACE also appears to cause lower toxicity than the traditional method [14]. With this decrease in morbidity TACE can be repeated more often and thus might have the potential to treat more severe patients who would normally be excluded from conventional TACE (eg. patients with advanced HCC).

One of the feared complications during TACE is inadvertent embolization of non-target organs such as the stomach, gallbladder or the pancreas. One patient reported grade 2 abdominal pain in the right upper quadrant immediately after the completion of DEB TACE and this was attributed to the possible reflux of microspheres into the cystic artery causing acute cholecystitis. This patient was treated symptomatically with no surgical intervention and evolved with resolution of pain in 24 h. During our study the immediate postoperative pain reported was minimal to mild discomfort (pain intensity score reported average was 2.5). Post-embolization syndrome was reported in 50% of our patients. This syndrome is defined as pain, fever, nausea, vomiting and leukocytosis and may occur in up to 90% of patients treated with traditional TACE. Commonly patients do not present all symptoms and they occur in varying intensities [16, 19, 20]. While most patients who present this syndrome are successfully treated with medications directed to the symptoms, this is a complication that in some cases may prolong hospitalization and increase procedure related morbidity. In our study, DEB TACE was extremely well tolerated and all post-embolization syndromes identified were successfully managed in an outpatient approach. In conventional TACE it is not unusual to require powerful painkillers, sometimes narcotics in the postoperative period. In this study the pain reported by patients in the postoperative period was minimal, with the highest intensity observed in the first patient (pain graduated 4/10), which was controlled

within 24 h. These findings are consistent with the PRECISION V study [14], a randomized multicenter trial, which compared patients undergoing conventional TACE and DEB TACE. This study showed a significantly lower rate of post-embolization syndrome in patients treated with this new technique [14].

DEB TACE also appears to promote greater tumor response rate. The RECIST criteria, currently used to evaluate tumor response, is based solely in tumor size changes [21]. Criteria such as those from the EASL take into account not only changes in the size of the lesion but also modification in tumor enhancement [22]. The concept is that tumor necrosis is not always accompanied by tumor shrinkage nevertheless it is nearly always followed by reduction on tumor enhancement at contrasted imaging studies such as MR and CT. If we had used the RECIST criteria in our study we would've achieved lower response rates which probably would not correspond to the actual therapeutic outcome evaluation. Indeed, not rarely, absence of tumor contrast enhancement after TACE is seen with little or no reduction in the tumor size. This finding was present in 4 of 7 patients who achieved complete response in our study. Moreover, in our study tumor shrinkage was only attested after the second MR imaging follow-up corroborating that tumor response to TACE may not be accompanied by reduction in the size of the liver tumor.

Not infrequently patients responding well to TACE can become resectable or be included in transplantation list due to the occurrence of *downstaging*. In our study, three patients who showed complete response also had reduction of the tumor to less than five cm and thus were evaluated to be included in the liver transplantation list (according to the Brazilian legislation patients with HCC less or equal to 5 cm up to 69 years old may be listed for liver transplantation queue). However in our study, these three patients were over 69 years old and were not listed. One of these patients was also judged to be surgical candidate after evaluation by the Hepato-Biliary surgery team, but due to advanced age (76 years), presence of cirrhosis and some comorbidities surgery was contraindicated. This patient had complete response after 3 sessions of DEB TACE, has been monitored for 30 months with no signs of recurrence or new lesions.

Most of the patients (86%) that presented with an AFP above 200 ng/ml before DEB TACE ($n = 7$, mean AFP of 667, ranging from 335 to 1500) and had radiologic response, also showed a significant decrease on AFP values. The only patient who showed no decrease on AFP value, but had responded according to imaging criteria, also presented bone metastasis after DEB TACE treatment, thus suggesting that the persistently elevated AFP was due to the development of extrahepatic disease.

Time to progression at 1 year and 2 years was 73% and 37.1% respectively and the survival rate at 1 and 2 years was 73.7% and 41.6% respectively. This is similar to the rates published for TACE [23–25]. However, studies evaluating TACE with the new microspheres loaded with chemotherapy, DEB TACE, showed significantly higher survival rates [14, 18]. The lower survival rate in our study could be related to patient selection. Of the 21 treated patients, 8 presented with stage C HCC according to the BCLC criteria. Most studies evaluating DEB TACE and conventional TACE included a significant number of patients with stage A [12, 14, 27]. In addition, in our study, there was a trend of an improved time to progression and survival rate in stage B patients treated with DEB TACE in comparison to stage C patients. Other risks were assessed and showed no association: gender, race, age, tumor size, portal invasion, AFP levels, Child classification, PS and number of DEB TACE sessions performed. According to the BCLC criteria patients with stage C HCC are generally not treated with TACE being referred for treatment with systemic chemotherapy, specifically Sorafenib [8]. This can be a criticism to our study since we didn't offer the treatment option of Sorafenib for patients with advanced HCC. Patient enrollment happened when Sorafenib was not available for stage C HCC in our institution. Although patients with advanced HCC are usually excluded from TACE because of questionable benefit and unacceptable toxicity, in our group of patients with advanced HCC we didn't identify any serious adverse event within 30 days after DEB TACE. Of the two patients who died within 60 days after DEB TACE one of them was due to acute myocardial infarction and the other to progression of cirrhosis (patient returned to alcohol consumption and developed rapid deterioration of liver function). These two deaths were not directly related to the procedure performed. Therefore the lower adverse events incidence seen in our stage C HCC patients treated with DEB TACE may indicate that this particular approach might have an acceptable toxicity profile in this population, as been demonstrated in other studies [14, 26, 27].

Although only some few studies evaluated the efficacy of TACE in the treatment of patients with stage C HCC they were able to show benefit in tumor response as well as in survival for patients who underwent TACE when comparing it to supportive treatment [26–28]. In the randomized, multicenter PRECISION V [13] study, which compared conventional TACE with DEB TACE, the subgroup analysis showed that more advanced disease such as Child B and PS 1 patients with tumors in both hepatic lobes or relapsing disease, the incidence of objective response and stable disease was higher, with statistical significance, in patients treated with DEB TACE. The most significant difference was found in the

subgroups of patients with PS 1 (Stage C HCC) and Child-Pugh B classification where 63% of patients treated with DEB TACE showed radiological response compared to only 32% of patients treated with conventional TACE [14]. In our study it was also possible to obtain significant tumor response in patients with advanced HCC treated with DEB TACE. Of the 8 patients with advanced HCC, 1 patient had complete response, 4 patients had partial response, 2 patients showed stable disease and 1 patient presented disease progression on imaging studies at 6 months follow-up. 4 patients died at 1 year, 2 patients died at 2 years and 2 patients are still alive on follow-up. In our study, thru the DEB approach it was possible to deliver TACE with low toxicity even to BCLC HCC advanced patients. Nevertheless, because of the inherent higher cost of this treatment we understand that there is not enough evidence to replace conventional TACE for less grave patients or when a not to large liver area is expected to be treated.

Conclusions

Transarterial chemoembolization with drug-eluting microspheres is able to deliver significant tumor response and progression free survival rate with acceptable toxicity. Larger studies are needed to identify exactly which subset of advanced hepatocellular patients may benefit from this treatment.

Abbreviations

AASLD: American association for the study of liver diseases; AFP: alpha-feto protein; BCLC: Barcelona clinic liver cancer; CT: Computed tomography; DEB TACE: Drug-eluting beads transarterial chemoembolization; DEB: Drug-eluting beads; EASL: European associantion for the study of the Liver; HCC: Hepatocellular carcinoma; MR: Magnetic ressonance; PD: Disease progression; PR: Partial response; PS: Karnofsky performance status scale; TACE: Transarterial chemoembolization

Acknowledgements

We have the moral obligation to acknowledge the hole nurse group at our department that with their enthusiasm and good will accepted this extra work. We also acknowledge the patients for participating and collaborating with this project.

Funding

There was no funding for this work.

Authors' contributions

JHML: MD. MSc. Interventional Radiologist. Contributed to the conception and design of this work. Performed part of the interventional procedures. He is a contributor responsible for the overall content as guarantor. Reviewed the manuscript. Approved the final version to be published. Agreed to be accountable to all aspects of this work. PML: MD. PhD. Contributed in the analyses and interpretation of data. Reviewed the manuscript. She is a contributor responsible for the overall content as guarantor. Approved the final version to be published. Agreed to be accountable to all aspects of this work. HSM: MD. Interventional Radiologist. Contributed to the conception and design of this work. Established the ideal technique for the DEB-TACE procedure. Performed part of the interventional procedures. Reviewed the manuscript. Approved the final version to be published. Agreed to be accountable to all aspects of this work. HRG: MD. Interventional Radiologist. Contributed to the conception and design of this work. Established the ideal technique for the DEB-TACE procedure. Performed part of the interventional procedures. Reviewed the manuscript. Approved the final version to be published. Agreed to be accountable to all aspects of this work. RBL: MD. Interventional Radiology fellow at the time of the study conduction. Contributed to the conception and design of this work. Performed part of the DEB-TACE procedures. Reviewed the manuscript. Approved the final version to be published. Agreed to be accountable to all aspects of this work. FD: MD. Interventional Radiology fellow at the time of the study conduction. Contributed in the analyses and interpretation of data. Reviewed the manuscript. Approved the final version to be published. Agreed to be accountable to all aspects of this work. BCR: MD. Interventional Radiology fellow at the time of the study conduction. Contributed in the analyses and interpretation of data. Reviewed the manuscript. Approved the final version to be published. Agreed to be accountable to all aspects of this work. MM: MD. PhD. Full Professor at the Anatomic and Radiology Department. Contributed in the analyses and interpretation of data. Reviewed the manuscript. Approved the final version to be published. Agreed to be accountable to all aspects of this work. All authors read and approved the final manuscript.

Authors' information
JHML: MD. MSc. Interventional Radiologist. Master Degree in Medical Oncology at INCA – Brazilian's National Cancer Institute – is the actual Coordinator of the Interventional Radiology Department at INCA. His main focus is research on liver diseases and oncology, having recently published our experience with partial splenic embolization to permit continuation of systemic chemotherapy at *Cancer Medicine* (doi: 10.1002/cam4.856).

Competing interests
The authors declare that they have no competing interests.

Author details
[1]Department of Interventional Radiology, Radiology Division, National Cancer Institute, INCA, Praça Cruz Vermelha 23, Centro, Rio de Janeiro CEP 20230-130, Brazil. [2]National Institute of Infectious Disease Evandro Chagas, Oswaldo Cruz Foundation, Avenida Brasil 4365, Manguinhos, Rio de Janeiro 21040-360, Brazil. [3]Department of Interventional Radiology, Radiology Division, Hospital Federal de Bonsucesso, Avenida Londres, 616, Bonsucesso, Rio de Janeiro 21041-030, Brazil. [4]Department of Interventional Radiology, Radiology Division, Hospital Federal de Ipanema, Rua Antônio Parreiras, 67, Ipanema, Rio de Janeiro 22411-020, Brazil. [5]Department of Anatomy and Radiology, Full Professor, Medicine School – UFMG, Avenida Presidente Antônio Carlos, 6627 Pampulha, Belo Horizonte, Minas Gerais 31270-901, Brazil.

References
1. Bosch FX, Ribes J, Borras J. Epidemiology of primary liver cancer. Semin Liver Dis. 1999;19:271–85.
2. Llovet JM, Ricci S, Mazzaferro V, et al. Sorafenib in advanced hepatocellular carcinoma. N Engl J Med. 2008;359:378–90.
3. Forner A, Reig ME, de Lope CR, Bruix J. Current strategy for staging and treatment: the BCLC update and future prospects. Semin Liver Dis. 2010;30:61–74.
4. Bruix J, Sherman M; American Association for the Study of Liver Diseases. Management of hepatocellular carcinoma: an up-date. Hepatology. 2011; 53(3):1020–2.
5. Bruix J, Sherman M, Llovet JM, et al. Clinical management of hepatocellular carcinoma: conclusions of the Barcelona-2000 EASL conference. European Association for the Study of the Liver. J Hepatol. 2001;35(3):421–30.
6. Lewis AL, Gonzalez MV, Lloyd AW, et al. DC bead: in vitro characterization of a drug-delivery device for transarterial chemoembolization. J Vasc Interv Radiol. 2006;17:335–42.
7. Hong K, Khwaja A, Liapi E, et al. New intra-arterial drug delivery system for the treatment of liver cancer: preclinical assessment in a rabbit model of liver cancer. Clin Cancer Res. 2006;12:2563–7.
8. Lee KH, Liapi EA, Cornell C, et al. Doxorubicin-loaded QuadraSphere microspheres: plasma pharmacokinetics and in- tratumoral drug concentration in an animal model of liver cancer. Cardiovasc Intervent Radiol 2010 33:576–82.
9. Jordan O, Denys A, De Baere T, Boulens N, Doelker E. Comparative study of chemoembolization loadable beads: in vitro drug release and physical properties of DC bead and hepasphere loaded with doxorubicin and irinotecan. J Vasc Interv Radiol. 2010;21:1084–90.
10. Varela M, Real MI, Burrel M, et al. Chemoembolization of hepatocellular carcinoma with drug eluting beads: efficacy and doxorubicin pharmacokinetics. J Hepatol. 2007;46:474–81.
11. Burrel M, Reig M, Forner A et al. Survival of patients with hepatocellular carcinoma treated by transarterial chemoembolisation (TACE) using Drug Eluting Beads. Implications for clinical practice and trial design. J Hepat. 2012;56(6):1330–35.
12. Martin R, Geller D, Espat J et al. Safety and efficacy of transarterial chemoembolization with drug-eluting beads in hepatocellular cancer: a systematic review. Hepatogastroenterology. 2012;59(113):255–60.
13. Geschwind JF, Kudo M, Marrero JA, Venook AP, Chen XP, Bronowicki JP, et al. TACE treatment in patients with sorafenib treated unresectable hepatocellular carcinoma in clinical practice: final analysis of GIDEON. Radiology. 2016;8:150667 [Epub ahead of print].
14. Lammer J, Malagari K, Vogl T, et al. Prospective randomised study of doxorubicin-eluting-bead embolization in the treatment of hepatocellular carcinoma: results of the PRECISION V study. Cardiovasc Intervent Radiol. 2010;33:41–52.
15. Lencioni R, Llovet JM. Modified RECIST (mRECIST) Assessment for Hepatocellular Carcinoma. Semin Liver Dis. 2010;30:52–60.
16. Patel NH, Hahn D, Rapp S, et al. Hepatic artery embolization: factors predisposing to postembolization pain and nausea. J Vasc Interv Radiol. 2000;11:453–60.
17. Brown DB, Geschwind JF, Soulen MC, et al. Society of Interventional Radiology position statement on chemoembolization of hepatic malignancies. J Vasc Interv Radiol. 2006;17(2 Pt 1):217–23.
18. Lewis AL, Gonzalez MV, Leppard SW, et al. Doxorubicin eluting beads–1: effects of drug loading on bead characteristics and drug distribution. J Mater Sci Mater Med. 2007;18:1691–9.
19. Chung JW, Park JH, Han JK, et al. Hepatic tumors: predisposing factors for complications of transcatheter oily chemoembolization. Radiology. 1996;198:33–40.
20. Leung DA, Goin JE, Sickles C, et al. Determinants of postembolization syndrome after hepatic chemoembolization. J Vasc Interv Radiol. 2001;12:321–6.
21. Joon OP, Lee SI, Song SY, et al. Measuring response in solid tumors: comparison of RECIST and WHO response criteria. Jpn J Clin Oncol. 2003; 33:533–7.
22. Shim H, Lee H, Won H, et al. Maximum number of target lesions required to measure responses to transarterial chemoembolization using the enhancement criteria in patients with intrahepatic hepatocellular carcinoma. J Hepatol. 2012;56(2):406–11.
23. Geschwind JF, Artemov D, Abraham S, et al. Chemoembolization of liver tumor in a rabbit model: assessment of tumor cell death with diffusion- weighted MR imaging and histologic analysis. J Vasc Interv Radiol. 2000;11:1245–55.
24. Ikeda M, Okada S, Yamamoto S, et al. Prognostic factors in patients with hepatocellular carcinoma treated by transcatheter arterial embolization. Jpn J Clin Oncol. 2002;32:455–60.
25. Llado L, Virgili J, Figueras J, et al. A prognostic index of the survival of patients with unresectable hepatocellular carcinoma after transcatheter arterial chemoembolization. Cancer. 2000;88:50–7.
26. Niu ZJ, Ma YL, Kang P, et al. Transarterial chemoembolization compared with conservative treatment for advanced hepatocellular carcinoma with portal vein tumor thrombus: using a new classification. Med Oncol. 2012; 29(4):2992–7.
27. Scartozzi M, Baroni GS, Faloppi L, et al. Trans-arterial chemo-embolization (TACE), with either lipiodol (traditional TACE) or drug-eluting microspheres (precision TACE, pTACE) in the treatment of hepatocellular carcinoma: efficacy and safety results from a large mono-institutional analysis. J Exp Clin Cancer Res. 2010;29:164.

17

Solid component proportion is an important predictor of tumor invasiveness in clinical stage $T_1N_0M_0$ ($cT_1N_0M_0$) lung adenocarcinoma

Meng Li[1], Ning Wu[1,2*], Li Zhang[1], Wei Sun[3], Ying Liu[2], Lv Lv[1], Jiansong Ren[4] and Dongmei Lin[3]

Abstract

Background: Preoperative tumor invasiveness in clinical stage $T_1N_0M_0$ lung adenocarcinoma is critical for optimal surgical procedure. The aim of the present study was to evaluate the relationship between the ground-glass opacity component (GGOc) / solid component (Sc) proportion measured using three-dimensional (3D) computer-quantified computer tomography (CT) number analysis to explore radiographic features for invasiveness prediction in $cT_1N_0M_0$ lung adenocarcinomas.

Methods: A total of 375 surgically resected $cT_1N_0M_0$ lung adenocarcinoma patients were included. The relativity between the GGOc/Sc proportion and lepidic growth pattern percentage was assessed using Spearman's rank analysis. Multiple logistic regression analysis was used to determine independent factors from radiographic features for tumor invasiveness. Prediction probability for tumor invasiveness was analysed using a receiver operating characteristic curve (ROC).

Results: We found that the GGOc proportion was positively correlated with lepidic growth pattern percentage ($r = 0.67$, $P < 0.01$), while the Sc proportion was negatively correlated with it ($r = -0.74$, $P < 0.01$). Multivariate analysis showed that tumor size and Sc proportion were identified as independent predictors for tumor invasiveness. The area under the ROC curve (AUC) of Sc proportion was 0.875, which was higher than that of tumor size (0.750) ($P < 0.001$), and had no significant difference with that of combination of these two factors (0.884) ($P = 0.28$).

Conclusions: The GGOc/Sc proportion measured using 3D computer-quantified CT number analysis reflects the lepidic growth pattern percentage in tumors, and the Sc proportion may be an important factor for the prediction of tumor invasiveness in $cT_1N_0M_0$ lung adenocarcinoma.

Keywords: Lung adenocarcinoma, Neoplasm invasiveness, Computer tomography, Positron-emission tomography, CT number analysis

Background

Lung adenocarcinoma (ADC) is the most common histologic subtype of lung cancer in most countries, and an upward trend in ADC incidence has been investigated [1, 2]. Many advances have occurred in oncology, molecular biology, pathologic examination, radiology, and surgery of lung ADC. With this background, the International Association for the Study of Lung Cancer, the American Thoracic Society and the European Respiratory Society (IASLC/ATS/ERS) proposed a new classification of lung ADC in 2011 [3, 4], which is closely related to clinical prognosis and has been identified as an independent prognostic factor in the disease-free survival and overall survival of patients [5]. Previous studies have documented that the 5-year disease-free survival of patients with adenocarcinoma in situ (AIS) was 100%, with minimally invasive adenocarcinoma (MIA) near 100% and invasive adenocarcinoma ranging from 40% to 85% [5–7].

* Correspondence: cjr.wuning@vip.163.com
[1]Department of Diagnostic Radiology, National Cancer Center/Cancer Hospital, Chinese Academy of Medical Sciences and Peking Union Medical College, Beijing, China
[2]PET-CT Center, National Cancer Center/Cancer Hospital, Chinese Academy of Medical Sciences and Peking Union Medical College, Beijing, China
Full list of author information is available at the end of the article

The difference in clinical prognosis is an important basis for individual treatment plan. Although the role of limited resection awaits the results of two randomized trials (JCOG 0802 in Japan and CALGB 140503 in North America) [8, 9], previous studies have suggested that sublobar (limited) resection alone without adjuvant therapy is the optimal choice for AIS/MIA because of the satisfactory prognosis, and some of the cases involved multiple primary adenocarcinoma [10, 11]. Invasive adenocarcinoma may need lobectomy and adjuvant therapy according to its pathological subtypes and other clinicopathological factors [3]. Therefore, pre- or intraoperative diagnosis is critical to select an optimal surgical procedure. However, it is difficult for pathologists to decide tumor invasion on preoperative and intraoperative frozen sections [3, 12]. Thus, preoperative radiography is necessary and important to help predict tumor invasiveness and determine the most appropriate surgical procedures.

Three-dimensional (3D) computer-quantified CT number analysis is used to determine the proportion of tissue component by calculating the proportion of one CT number or a range of CT numbers in the lesion [13–15]. We hypothesized that the tissue component proportion in CT images measured using a 3D computer-quantified CT number analysis is associated with the pathological constituents percentage, and this components proportion and other radiographic features can help predict tumor invasiveness. Therefore, the aim of the present study is to evaluate the relationship between the ground-glass opacity component (GGOc)/solid component (Sc) proportion measured using 3D computer-quantified CT number analysis to explore radiographic features for invasiveness prediction in $cT_1N_0M_0$ lung adenocarcinomas.

Methods

Patients

A total of 375 consecutive patients with surgically resected $cT_1N_0M_0$ lung adenocarcinoma at our hospital between January 2005 and December 2012 were included. The following inclusion criteria were considered for the present study: (a) single adenocarcinomas (3 cm or less in diameter at CT image) with no evidence of malignant satellite nodules (previously confirmed with imaging study or lung biopsy) and no hilar or mediastinal lymphadenopathy on imaging study or at mediastinoscopy, (b) first treatment with surgery alone, (c) either chest high-resolution computer tomography (HRCT) studies or integrated 18 fluorodeoxyglucose positron emission tomography (^{18}F-FDG PET)/CT acquired within 1 month for preoperative staging before resection, and (d) both pathological sections and clinical data are available for review.

Image acquisition

The CT images were obtained using an eight-(LightSpeed Ultra, GE Medical Systems), 16-(ProSpeed or Discovery ST, GE Medical Systems) or 64-(LightSpeed VCT, GE Medical Systems or Toshiba Aqulion, TOSHIBA Medical Systems) slice spiral CT scanner. CT images were obtained with 120 kVp, 250 ~ 350 mA, and a reconstruction kernel with standard algorithm. Reconstruction thicknesses were 1.0 or 1.25 mm, and the intervals were 0.8 or 1.0 mm. With enhanced CT examination, 80 ml intravenous contrast was administered at 2.5 mL/s, and images were obtained 25 to 30 s after contrast infusion.

PET/CT images were acquired using an integrated PET/CT device (Discovery ST 16, GE Medical Systems). After confirmation of normal blood glucose levels in the peripheral blood was ensured (≤8 mmol/L), the patients were administered an intravenous injection of ^{18}F-FDG at 3.70 ~ 4.44 MBq/kg and subsequently rested for approximately 60 ~ 70 min before undergoing the body scan. The whole body scan was performed from the head to root of the thigh, and the thoracic scan was performed from the super-clavicle to the adrenal gland. The patients who did not undergo chest CT examination within 10 days underwent a breath-hold thoracic spiral CT scan with 120 kV, 205 mA after the PET/CT scan.

Image interpretation

CT images were retrospectively assessed for visual morphological features. Two radiologists (M.L. and L.Z.), who had 11 and 8 years of experience, respectively, were informed that the involved patients had surgically treated adenocarcinomas but were blinded to histologic subtypes and conducted the analysis of the morphological features using a Carestream GCRIS 2.1 PACS workstation (Carestream Health) in consensus. The morphological features included CT appearance (solid nodules [SN], part solid nodules [PSN] or mGGO [mixed ground-glass opacity], pure ground-glass opacity [pGGO]), tumor size (the longest tumor diameter on the transverse lung window image, where the largest nodule dimension appeared), location (centre or periphery, periphery was defined as within 3 cm of the pleura), contour (smooth, lobular or spiculated), necrosis (necrosis of tumor was defined as low attenuation in tumor), and vacuole sign or cyst/cavity (vacuole sign was defined as a gas-filled space less than 0.5 cm in tumor while cyst/cavity was no less than 0.5 cm) [16, 17].

Two chest radiologists with PET/CT diagnostic experience (N.W. and Y.L.) retrospectively evaluated the integrated PET/CT images. For a semi-quantitative analysis of FDG uptake, regions of interest (ROI) were placed over the tumor site on the hottest trans-axial slice. In some patients, nodular FDG uptake could not be identified on the PET component images. For these patients, a

ROI was drawn in a presumed nodular location, considering the CT component images of PET/CT. The maximum standard uptake value (SUV_{max}) within the ROI was used as the reference measurement.

CT number analysis by three-dimensional computerized quantification

Three-dimensional computer-quantified CT number analysis was performed on an ADW 4.6 workstation (GE Medical Systems) to measure the proportion of GGOc and Sc. This measurement was performed in three steps as follows. **(a)** Nodule segmentation. The entire tumor mass was separated from surrounding anatomic structures using a computer-aided volume measurement software (Auto Contour in Volume Rendering). Subsequently, a radiologist visually inspected the computer-generated tumor boundaries for correctness and consistency. If any segmentation results were considered suboptimal, the radiologist edited the tumor contours superimposed on the original images. The mean CT value of tumor was automatically tallied up (Fig. 1). **(b)** Aaccording to the CT visual appearance (pGGO, PSN, SN), the threshold values of GGOc and Sc were obtained using receiver operating characteristic (ROC) curves. **(c)** As the second step, the entire tumor mass was separated using the same method in the first step, and the CT number histogram of the tumor was automatically generated by the computer software (3 Dimension Histogram). The proportion of GGOc/Sc was calculated based on the threshold values obtained in the second step (Fig. 2).

To examine the intra- and inter-observer agreement, two radiologists (M.L. and L.Z.) performed the same measurement on 50 randomly selected tumors and the second radiologist (L.Z.) performed the measurement again after one month. The workflow for all the 375 patients was completed by the second radiologist (L.Z.).

Pathologic evaluation

An experienced lung pathologist with 8 years of experience (W.S.) in lung pathology retrospectively reviewed all resected specimens according to the 2011 IASLC/ATS/ERS classification [3]. For each lesion, histologic subtypes were semiquantitatively recorded in 5% increments. For difficult cases (20 cases), histologic subtypes were assessed through consultation with a lung cancer pathology expert (D.L.). Based on the reported prognosis of lung adenocarcinoma [5–7, 18], AIS and MIA were referred to as non-invasive adenocarcinomas, and other subtypes of tumors were referred to as invasive adenocarcinomas in the present study.

Statistical analysis

Inter- and intraobserver agreements were assessed using 95% Bland-Altman limits of agreement and the intraclass correlation coefficient. An intraclass correlation coefficient greater than 0.75 represented good agreement. The difference in the CT value for pGGO, PSN, and SN between enhanced and non-enhanced CT imaging was accessed using an independent Student's t test. The relativity between the GGOc/Sc proportion in CT images and the

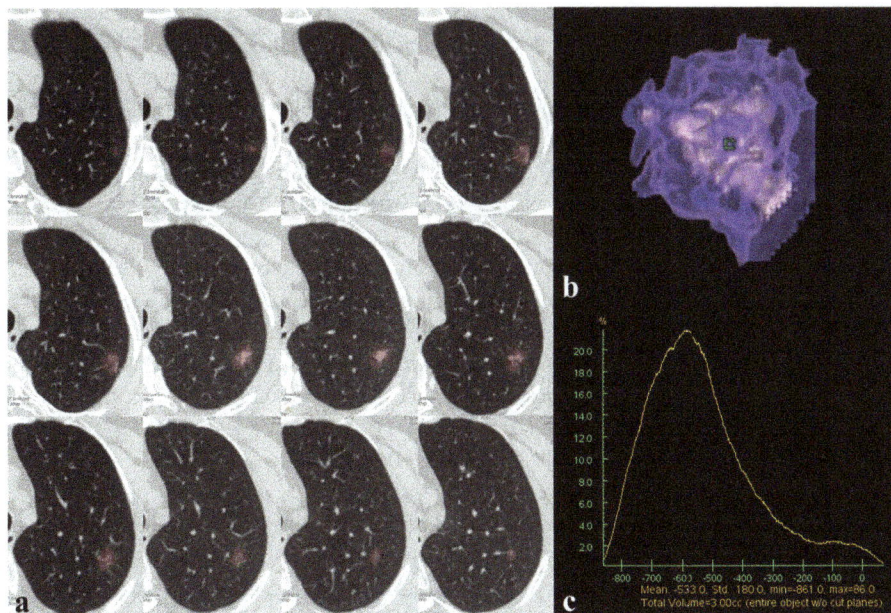

Fig. 1 Mean CT value calculated using three-dimensional (3D) computer-quantified CT number analysis. **a** CT images show computer-generated tumor boundaries that were inspected and edited slice-by-slice by radiologist for correctness and consistency. **b** 3D image of the tumor generated automatically by the computer. **c** CT number distribution curve of the tumor. The mean CT value of this tumor is − 533 HU ranging from − 861 HU to 86 HU

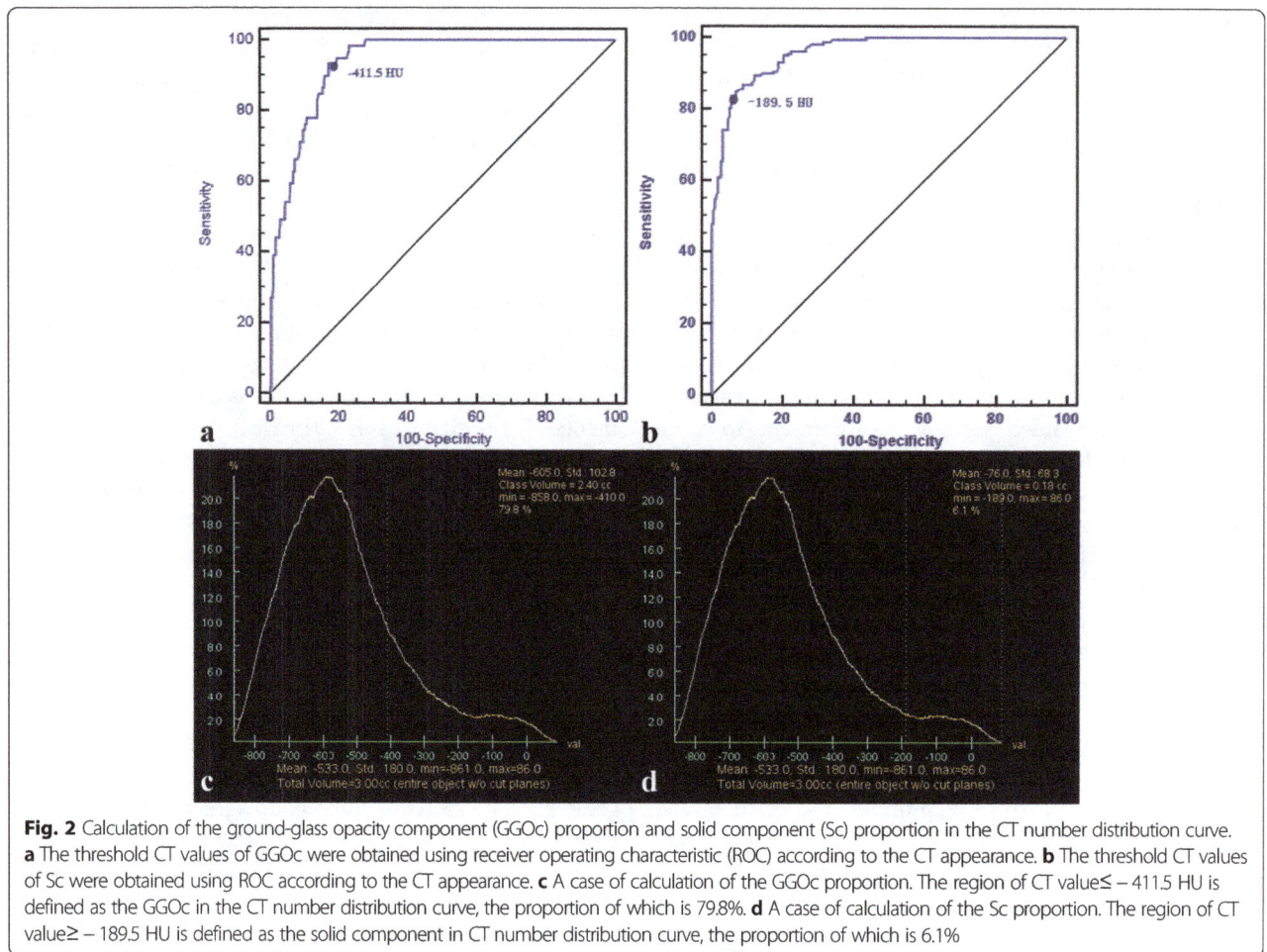

Fig. 2 Calculation of the ground-glass opacity component (GGOc) proportion and solid component (Sc) proportion in the CT number distribution curve. **a** The threshold CT values of GGOc were obtained using receiver operating characteristic (ROC) according to the CT appearance. **b** The threshold CT values of Sc were obtained using ROC according to the CT appearance. **c** A case of calculation of the GGOc proportion. The region of CT value≤ − 411.5 HU is defined as the GGOc in the CT number distribution curve, the proportion of which is 79.8%. **d** A case of calculation of the Sc proportion. The region of CT value≥ − 189.5 HU is defined as the solid component in CT number distribution curve, the proportion of which is 6.1%

lepidic growth pattern percentage in pathologic specimens was accessed using Spearman's rank correlation. The prevalence of nominal variables (e.g., tumor appearance, location, contour, intratumoral necrosis and vacuole sign or cavity/cyst in tumor) was compared using Fisher's exact test. Differences in the mean values between continuous variables (e.g., tumor size, GGOc proportion, Sc proportion and SUV_{max}) were compared using an independent Student's t test. Multivariate logistic regression analysis was used to identify the independent factors to predict adenocarcinoma invasiveness. Finally, ROC analysis was performed to evaluate the differentiating performance of logistic regression models in diagnosing invasive adenocarcinoma. All statistical analyses were performed using a commercial software package (SPSS, Inc., an IBM Company, Chicago, IL, USA). A P value of less than 0.05 indicated a significant difference.

Results

Patient demographics and pathologic evaluation

The clinicopathological characteristics of the 375 patients with lung adenocarcinomas included in the present study

are summarized in Table 1. Among all 375 patients, 92 patients (24.5%) had non-invasive adenocarcinomas and 273 patients (75.5%) had invasive adenocarcinomas.

Difference in the mean CT value between enhanced and non-enhanced CT imaging

All patients included in the present study underwent non-enhanced or enhanced chest CT. Among the 375 nodules analysed, 58 nodules showed pGGO, 159 samples were PSN, and 158 samples were SN. No significant difference was detected between non-enhanced and enhanced chest CT groups for pGGO ($t = − 1.76$, $P = 0.08$), PSN ($t = − 1.72$, $P = 0.09$) and SN ($t = − 0.84$, $P = 0.40$) (Table 2.).

Consistency between the GGOc and Sc proportions

The 95% limits of inter- and intra-observer agreements obtained using Bland-Altman analysis to measure the GGOc proportion were − 0.26 to 0.22 and − 0.03 to 0.03, with intraclass correlation coefficients of 0.954 (95% confidence interval [CI]: 0.918, 0.974) and 0.999 (95% CI: 0.999, 1.000), respectively ($P <$ 0.001). The

Table 1 Patient characteristics

Characteristic	No. of patients (%)
Median age (y)[a]	58.6 ± 9.8 (31 ~ 84)
Sex	
Male	157 (41.9)
Female	218 (58.1)
Smoking status	
Current or former smoker	119 (31.7)
Non-smoker	256 (68.3)
Invasive lobe	
RUL	152 (40.5)
RML	19 (5.1)
RLL	69 (18.4)
LUL	84 (22.4)
LLL	51 (13.6)
Surgical procedure	
Wedge resection	33 (8.8)
Segmentectomy	1 (0.3)
Lobectomy	341 (90.9)
Imaging technique[b]	
Enhanced CT	193 (51.5)
Non-enhanced CT	182 (48.5)
PET/CT	147 (39.2)
Subtype predominance	
AIS	41 (10.9)
MIA	51 (13.6)
Lepidic	49 (13.1)
Acinar	176 (46.9)
Papillary	32 (8.5)
Micropapillary	5 (1.3)
Solid	11 (2.9)
Variants	10 (2.7)
Pathologic Stage [c]	
IA	173 (47.5)
IB	148 (40.7)
IIA	22 (6.0)
IIIA	21 (5.8)

Note. Unless otherwise indicated, data are numbers, with percentages in parentheses. [a] The data are presented as the means ± standard deviation, with ranges in parentheses. [b] All patients underwent CT examination. [c] Eleven patients did not undergo lymph node dissection; the pathologic stage was made in 364 patients. AIS, adenocarcinoma in situ; MIA, minimally invasive adenocarcinoma; LLL, left lower lobe; LUL, left upper lobe; RLL, right lower lobe; RML, right middle lobe; RUL, right upper lobe

95% limits of inter- and intra-observer agreements in the measurement of the Sc proportion were – 0.016 to 0.016 and – 0.03 to 0.04, with intraclass correlation coefficients of 0.999 (95% *CI*: 0.998, 1.000) and 0.998 (95% *CI*: 0.997, 0.999), respectively (*P* < 0.001).

Table 2 Mean CT value of pGGO, PSN and SN between enhancement and non-enhancement CT scan

Tumor appearance	Number (%)	Mean CT value (HU)	*t*	*P*
pGGO	58	– 553.38 ± 101.1		
Enhancement	33 (56.9)	–533.36 ± 103.79	–1.764	0.083
Non-enhancement	25 (43.1)	– 579.80 ± 92.92		
PSN/mGGO	159	–364.87 ± 129.61		
Enhancement	94 (59.1)	– 379.49 ± 128.80	1.721	0.087
Non-enhancement	65 (40.9)	– 343.74 ± 128.82		
SN	158	–104.24 ± 93.05		
Enhancement	55 (34.8)	–95.67 ± 94.30	–0.845	0.399
Non-enhancement	103 (65.2)	– 108.82 ± 92.51		

CT, computer tomogram; pGGO, pure ground-glass opacity; PSN, part solid nodule; mGGO, mixed ground-glass opacity; SN, solid nodule; HU, hounsfield unit

Threshold values for GGOc and Sc

The optimal threshold value for GGOc was – 411.5 HU (area under the ROC curve [AUC], 0.93; 95% *CI*, 0.91–0.96) with a sensitivity of 93.2% and specificity of 82.9%, and the optimal threshold value for Sc was – 189.5 HU (AUC, 0.96; 95% *CI*, 0.94–0.97) with a sensitivity of 83.6% and specificity of 94%.

Relationship between the GGOc/Sc proportion and lepidic growth pattern percentage

The proportion of GGOc in the CT images was positively correlated with the lepidic growth pattern percentage in pathologic specimens ($r = 0.67$, $P < 0.01$), while the proportion of Sc was negatively correlated with the lepidic growth pattern percentage ($r = – 0.74$, $P < 0.01$).

Radiographic features analysis

Radiographic features of invasive adenocarcinoma and non-invasive adenocarcinoma are presented in Table 3. Tumor size, contour, necrosis, vacuole sign or cyst/cavity, GGOc proportion, Sc proportion (Fig. 3) and SUV_{max} showed significant differences between invasive adenocarcinoma and non-invasive adenocarcinoma ($P < 0.001$, $P < 0.001$, $P = 0.002$, $P < 0.001$, $P < 0.001$, $P < 0.001$, and $P = 0.018$, respectively). Among all 375 patients, only 147 patients underwent PET/CT, thus SUV_{max} was removed from the multivariate analysis. The results of the logistic regression analysis (Table 4) demonstrated that tumor size and Sc proportion were independent predictors of invasive adenocarcinomas (odds ratio [OR] = 2.79, $P = 0.002$, and $OR = 40.24$, $P < 0.001$, respectively).

Predictive probability of radiographic features for adenocarcinoma invasiveness

Based on multivariate analysis, two significant factors were combined (combination of tumor size and Sc proportion) for the prediction of invasive adenocarcinoma,

Table 3 Correlation between radiographic features and pathology

Radiographic features	Invasive adenocarcinoma	Non-invasive adenocarcinoma	χ^2/t	P
HRCT	283 (n)	92 (n)		
Size[a]	2.04±0.55	1.55 ± 0.51	−7.601	< 0.001
Location			0.295	0.587
Centre	50	14		
Periphery	233	78		
Contour			48.04	< 0.001
Smooth	36	40		
Lobular	143	42		
Spiculated	104	10		
Necrosis			9.415	0.002
Yes	33	1		
No	250	91		
Vacuole sign or cyst/cavity			16.346	< 0.001
No	172	77		
Vacuole sign	89	12		
Cyst/cavity	22	3		
Computer-quantified CT number analysis	283 (n)	92 (n)		
GGOc proportion[a]	(14 ± 17) %	(44 ± 29) %	9.461	< 0.001
Sc proportion[a]	(56 ± 30) %	(14 ± 21) %	−14.822	< 0.001
PET/CT	137 (n)	10 (n)		
SUV_{max}[a]	3.75 ± 2.85	1.54 ± 2.41	−2.21	0.018

Note. Unless otherwise indicated, the data are the number of patients. a The data are presented as the means ± standard deviation. *HRCT*, high-resolution computer tomography; *GGOc*, glass-ground-opacity component; *Sc*, solid component; *PET*, positron emission tomography; *SUV*, standard uptake value

whose AUC value of ROC was 0.884 (95% *CI*: 0.847 ~ 0. 922, *P* < 0.001), which was higher than that of tumor size (AUC: 0.750, 95% *CI*: 0.692 ~ 0.808, *P* < 0.001) with a significant difference (*Z* = 4.75, *P* < 0.001). However, no significant difference (*Z* = 1.07, *P* = 0.28) was detected between these combined factors and Sc proportion (AUC: 0.875, 95% *CI*: 0.832 ~ 0.917, *P* < 0.001) (Fig. 4). The optimal threshold for the detection of invasive adenocarcinoma in the Sc proportion was 25.8%, with 78.1% sensitivity and 82.6% specificity.

Discussions

In the new adenocarcinoma classification, adenocarcinomas with lepidic growth patterns included AIS, MIA, lepidic predominant invasive adenocarcinoma and other adenocarcinomas containing a lepidic growth component. In the lepidic growth pattern, neoplastic cells grow along pre-existing alveolar structures in a flat manner, without forming papillary or micropapillary structures and lacking of stromal, vascular or pleural invasion [3]. Multiple studies have shown that adenocarcinomas with lepidic growth patterns have favourable prognosis and low risk of recurrence [4, 19, 20]. A comparison of high-resolution computer tomography (HRCT) images with pathological sections revealed that areas of GGO in the

HRCT image reflect a growth pattern where tumor cells have replaced alveolar lining cells, as in lepidic growth without collapse. In contrast, areas of consolidation primarily represent the foci of fibrosis or tumors of a solid growth pattern, consistent with previous reports [21, 22]. In the present study, the GGOc/Sc proportion measured using 3D computer-quantified CT number analysis was related to the lepidic growth pattern percentage. Tumors with high lepidic growth pattern percentages have low Sc proportion and high GGOc proportion, suggesting that the GGOc/Sc proportion measured using the 3D computer-quantified CT number analysis is accurate and objective and reflects the lepidic growth pattern percentage in pathologic specimens.

To predict invasive adenocarcinoma, we accessed the potential risk factors of radiographic features. We observed that tumor size, contour, necrosis, vacuole sign or cyst/cavity, GGOc proportion, Sc proportion and SUV_{max} were significantly different between invasive adenocarcinoma and non-invasive adenocarcinoma. In the present study, the tumor size of invasive adenocarcinoma is significantly larger than the non-invasive adenocarcinoma, consistent with the current criteria for tumor stage (T stage). We also observed that compared

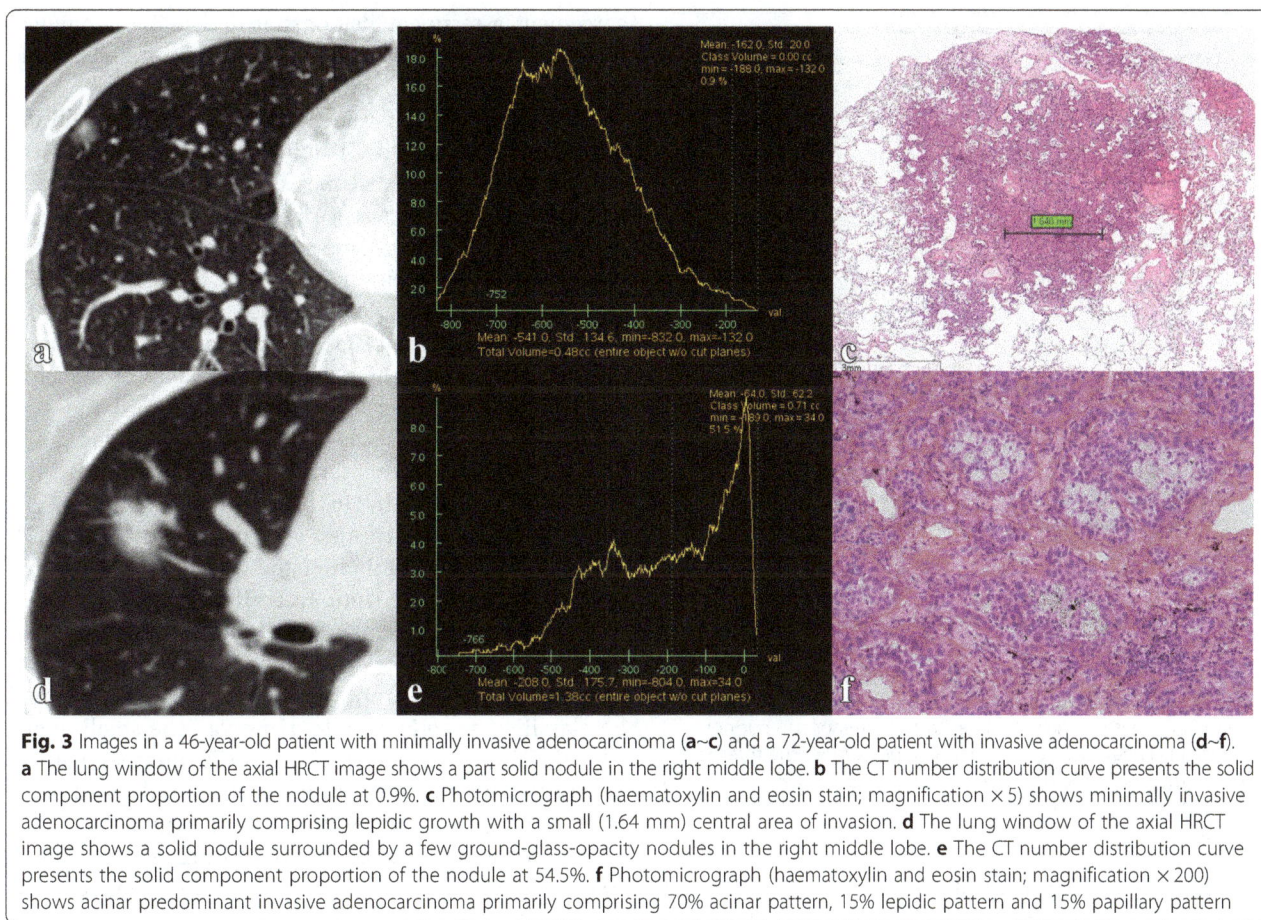

Fig. 3 Images in a 46-year-old patient with minimally invasive adenocarcinoma (**a~c**) and a 72-year-old patient with invasive adenocarcinoma (**d~f**). **a** The lung window of the axial HRCT image shows a part solid nodule in the right middle lobe. **b** The CT number distribution curve presents the solid component proportion of the nodule at 0.9%. **c** Photomicrograph (haematoxylin and eosin stain; magnification × 5) shows minimally invasive adenocarcinoma primarily comprising lepidic growth with a small (1.64 mm) central area of invasion. **d** The lung window of the axial HRCT image shows a solid nodule surrounded by a few ground-glass-opacity nodules in the right middle lobe. **e** The CT number distribution curve presents the solid component proportion of the nodule at 54.5%. **f** Photomicrograph (haematoxylin and eosin stain; magnification × 200) shows acinar predominant invasive adenocarcinoma primarily comprising 70% acinar pattern, 15% lepidic pattern and 15% papillary pattern

to non-invasive adenocarcinoma, invasive adenocarcinoma is more likely to present as lobular or speculate, necrotic lesion with vacuole sign or cyst/cavity, which demonstrated as malignant signs in lung nodule diagnosis. The GGOc proportion and Sc proportion are quantitative indicators of tumor appearance. In the present study, the GGOc proportion of invasive adenocarcinoma is lower than that of non-invasive adenocarcinoma, while the Sc proportion is higher, consistent with other

Table 4 Multivariate analysis for invasiveness of lung adenocarcinoma

Variable	Odds Ratio	95% CI	P
Size (X_1)	2.79	1.48 ~ 5.27	0.002
Contour (X_2)	1.11	0.68 ~ 1.82	0.67
Necrosis (X_3)	0.81	0.09 ~ 7.19	0.85
Vacuole sign or cyst/cavity (X_4)	1.72	0.96 ~ 3.09	0.07
GGOc proportion (X_5)	0.17	0.028 ~ 1.002	0.05
Sc proportion (X_6)	40.24	5.35 ~ 302.73	< 0.001

Note. CI, confidence interval; $GGOc$, glass-ground-opacity component; Sc, solid component

reports [18, 22, 23]. SUV_{max} is a semi-quantified index of FDG uptake, which is associated with tissue glucose metabolism. Previous studies [24, 25] have reported that SUV_{max} could be affected by cell differentiation and proliferative rate potential. The tumor with high SUV_{max} is more likely an invasive lesion and with an unfavourable prognosis. In the present study, the SUV_{max} of the invasive adenocarcinoma is significantly higher than that of non-invasive adenocarcinoma, which is consistent with previous studies [26, 27].

We analysed these factors, except SUV_{max}, using logistic multivariate analysis to assess the joint effects and interactions of the variables on adenocarcinoma invasiveness. These results showed that only tumor size and Sc proportion retained statistical significance, whereas contour, necrosis, vacuole sign or cyst/cavity and GGOc proportion had no significant difference. We proposed that their effects were substituted by the enrolled index. According to the ROC analysis, AUC of Sc proportion was 0.875, which was higher than that of tumor size (0.750, $P < 0.001$) and had no significant difference with that of combination of the two factors (0.884, $P = 0.28$). This result suggested that Sc proportion has higher predicted value than tumor size

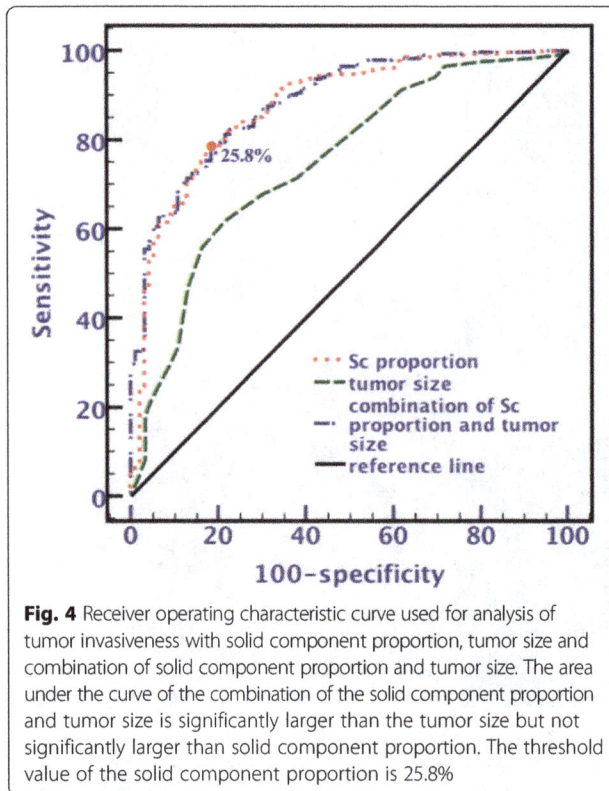

Fig. 4 Receiver operating characteristic curve used for analysis of tumor invasiveness with solid component proportion, tumor size and combination of solid component proportion and tumor size. The area under the curve of the combination of the solid component proportion and tumor size is significantly larger than the tumor size but not significantly larger than solid component proportion. The threshold value of the solid component proportion is 25.8%

and has equal efficacy as combined factors. Therefore, we recommend a threshold with an Sc proportion of no less than 25.8% to predict tumor invasiveness, not only because it has favourable efficacy but also because it has good clinical practicability and easy operation.

The major strength of the present study was the measurement of the GGOc/Sc proportion. In the present study, the GGOc and Sc proportions were measured using 3D computer-quantified CT number analysis. Until recently, several measuring methods of the GGOc proportion have been reported. Some researchers [28, 29] calculated the GGOc proportion by measuring the maximum cross-sectional tumor diameter on CT images, which is easy to operate but may only represent a single tumor cross-section instead of the entire tumor mass. In addition, although many studies have calculated the GGOc proportion using computer software for volumetric nodule segmentation, the classic technique has limitations on tumor boundary generation and segmentation on the inner components of tumor [30]. In the present study, the radiologist visually inspected computer-generated tumor boundaries to avoid the vessels and bronchial tubes around the tumor and ensure correctness and consistency; the GGOc and Sc in the tumor were identified using a CT number distribution curve with threshold values obtained from ROC curves, which improved segmentation on the inner composition of the tumor. Intra- and inter-observer

agreement assessment demonstrated that 3D computer-quantified CT number analysis is reproducible and reliable in measuring the GGOc/Sc proportion.

In this study, the CT values of SN obtained through the 3D computer-quantified CT number analysis software were much lower than manual measurement in routing work, and there were no difference between non-enhanced and enhanced group. There are several reasons to explain the results. First and foremost, the mean CT value obtained through the 3D computer-quantified CT number analysis was differing from manual measurement. The software measured the entire entire nodule, including the vacuole, cyst/cavity, bronchogram in the tumor, and the surrounding lung tissue, which cannot be excluded absolutely through segmentation automatically by the computer or manually in lung window. The air CT value (– 1000) interrupted and drove down the CT value of SN, and eliminated the influence of contrast injection at the same time. In addition, the partial volume effect in the pixel of the nodule edge will also exert an influence. Second, lung nodules with small quantity of GGO cannot be observed visually and will be classified as solid nodule. However, the small quantity of GGO with extremely low CT number will be accounted by the computer. Last, the delayed scan time is relatively short (25 to 30 s), which had little effect on the attenuation of small lung lesion. This is also why we did not analyse the non-enhanced and enhanced CT imaging separately.

The present study has several limitations. First, the CT examinations in the present study were conducted using different scanners from three companies that may influence the accuracy of the CT value. Second, the present study was conducted as a single-centre study, and additional studies in multiple centres are needed to confirm these results, particularly the threshold values of the GGOc and Sc. Last, we did not conduct survival analyses because the follow-up time for some cases was too short; thus, advanced study is warranted to analyse patient survival.

Conclusions

The results of this study support the idea that 3D computer-quantified CT number analysis is a reliable method to measure the GGOc/Sc proportion, potentially reflecting the lepidic growth pattern percentage in $cT_1N_0M_0$ lung adenocarcinoma, and a threshold with an Sc proportion of no less than 25.8% has satisfactory efficacy in tumor invasiveness prediction.

Abbreviations

ADC: Adenocarcinoma; AIS: Adenocarcinoma in situ; GGOc: Ground-glass opacity component; mGGO: Mixed ground-glass opacity; MIA: Minimally invasive adenocarcinoma; pGGO: Pure ground-glass opacity; PSN: Part solid nodules; Sc: Solid component; SN: Solid nodules; SUV_{max}: Maximum standard uptake value

Funding

M.L. was supported by National Natural Science Foundation of China (81601494) and PUMC Youth Fund/the Fundamental Research Funds for the Central Universities (3332016030). L.Z. was supported by PUMC Youth Fund/the Fundamental Research Funds for the Central Universities (2017320017). N.W. was supported by National key R&D Program of China (2017YFC1308700). The funding source had no involvement in study design, interpretation of data and in the writing of the article.

Authors' contributions

NW., ML. and LZ. conceived and designed the study. WS. and DL. contributed to pathologic evaluation of resected specimens. YL. contributed to PET/CT image analysis. JR. contributed to statistical analysis. LZ., ML. and LL. contributed collection, analysis of data and manuscript preparation. ML, LZ. and NW. wrote and revised the manuscript. All authors read and approved the final manuscript.

Consent for publication

Written informed consent for publication was obtained from all patients.

Author details

[1]Department of Diagnostic Radiology, National Cancer Center/Cancer Hospital, Chinese Academy of Medical Sciences and Peking Union Medical College, Beijing, China. [2]PET-CT Center, National Cancer Center/Cancer Hospital, Chinese Academy of Medical Sciences and Peking Union Medical College, Beijing, China. [3]Department of Pathology, Beijing Cancer Hospital, Beijing, China. [4]National Office for Cancer Prevention and Control, National Cancer Center/Cancer Hospital, Chinese Academy of Medical Sciences and Peking Union Medical College, Beijing, China.

References

1. Nakamura H, Saji H. Worldwide trend of increasing primary adenocarcinoma of the lung. Surg Today. 2014;44:1004–12.
2. Zhang L, Li M, Wu N, Chen Y. Time trends in epidemiologic characteristics and imaging features of lung adenocarcinoma: a population study of 21,113 cases in China. PLoS One. 2015;10:e0136727.
3. Travis WD, Brambilla E, Noguchi M, Nicholson AG, Geisinger KR, Yatabe Y, et al. International association for the study of lung cancer/american thoracic society/european respiratory society international multidisciplinary classification of lung adenocarcinoma. J Thorac Oncol. 2011;6:244–85.
4. Murakami S, Ito H, Tsubokawa N, Mimae T, Sasada S, Yoshiya T, et al. Prognostic value of the new IASLC/ATS/ERS classification of clinical stage IA lung adenocarcinoma. Lung Cancer. 2015;0:199–204.
5. Gu J, Lu C, Guo J, Chen L, Chu Y, Ji Y, et al. Prognostic significance of the IASLC/ATS/ERS classification in Chinese patients-a single institution retrospective study of 292 lung adenocarcinoma. J Surg Oncol. 2013; 107:474–80.
6. Yoshizawa A, Sumiyoshi S, Sonobe M, Kobayashi M, Fujimoto M, Kawakami F, et al. Validation of the IASLC/ATS/ERS lung adenocarcinoma classification for prognosis and association with EGFR and KRAS gene mutations: analysis of 440 Japanese patients. J Thorac Oncol. 2013;8:52–61.
7. Woo T, Okudela K, Mitsui H, Tajiri M, Yamamoto T, Rino Y, et al. Prognostic value of the IASLC/ATS/ERS classification of lung adenocarcinoma in stage I disease of Japanese cases. Pathol Int. 2012;62:785–91.
8. Nakamura K, Saji H, Nakajima R, Okada M, Asamura H, Shibata T, et al. A phase III randomized trial of lobectomy versus limited resection for small-sized peripheral non-small cell lung cancer (JCOG0802/WJOG4607L). Jpn J Clin Oncol. 2010;40:271–4.
9. Blasberg JD, Pass HI, Donington JS. Sublobar resection: a movement from the lung Cancer study group. J Thorac Oncol. 2010;5:1583–93.
10. Yang CF, D'Amico TA. Thoracoscopic segmentectomy for lung cancer. Ann Thorac Surg. 2012;94:668–81.
11. Yang CF, D'Amico TA. Open, thoracoscopic and robotic segmentectomy for lung cancer. Ann Cardiothorac Surg. 2014;3:142–52.
12. Yoshizawa A, Motoi N, Riely GJ, Sima CS, Gerald WL, Kris MG, et al. Impact of proposed IASLC/ATS/ERS classification of lung adenocarcinoma: prognostic subgroups and implications for further revision of staging based on analysis of 514 stage I cases. Mod Pathol. 2011;24:653–64.
13. Son JY, Lee HY, Lee KS, Kim JH, Han J, Jeong JY, et al. Quantitative CT analysis of pulmonary ground-glass opacity nodules for the distinction of invasive adenocarcinoma from pre-invasive or minimally invasive adenocarcinoma. PLoS One. 2014;9:e104066.
14. Ikeda K, Awai K, Mori T, Kawanaka K, Yamashita Y, Nomori H. Differential diagnosis of ground-glass opacity nodules: CT number analysis by three-dimensional computerized quantification. Chest. 2007;132:984–90.
15. Nomori H, Ohtsuka T, Naruke T, Suemasu K. Differentiating between atypical adenomatous hyperplasia and bronchioloalveolar carcinoma using the computed tomography number histogram. Ann Thorac Surg. 2003;76:867–71.
16. Hansell DM, Bankier AA, MacMahon H, McLoud TC, Muller NL, Remy J. Fleischner society: glossary of terms for thoracic imaging. Radiology. 2008; 246:697–722.
17. Onn A, Choe DH, Herbst RS, Correa AM, Munden RF, Truong MT, et al. Tumor cavitation in stage I non-small cell lung cancer: epidermal growth factor receptor expression and prediction of poor outcome. Radiology. 2005;237:342–7.
18. Takahashi M, Shigematsu Y, Ohta M, Tokumasu H, Matsukura T, Hirai T. Tumor invasiveness as defined by the newly proposed IASLC/ATS/ERS classification has prognostic significance for pathologic stage IA lung adenocarcinoma and can be predicted by radiologic parameters. J Thorac Cardiovasc Surg. 2014;147:54–9.
19. Sasada S, Miyata Y, Mimae T, Mimura T, Okada M. Impact of Lepidic Component Occupancy on Effects of Adjuvant Chemotherapy for Lung Adenocarcinoma. Ann Thorac Surg. 2015;100:2079–86.
20. Kadota K, Villena-Vargas J, Yoshizawa A, Motoi N, Sima CS, Riely GJ, et al. Prognostic significance of adenocarcinoma in situ, minimally invasive adenocarcinoma, and nonmucinous lepidic predominant invasive adenocarcinoma of the lung in patients with stage I disease. Am J Surg Pathol. 2014;38:448–60.
21. Hashizume T, Yamada K, Okamoto N, Saito H, Oshita F, Kato Y, et al. Prognostic significance of thin-section CT scan findings in small-sized lung adenocarcinoma. Chest. 2008;133:441–7.
22. Honda T, Kondo T, Murakami S, Saito H, Oshita F, Ito H, et al. Radiographic and pathological analysis of small lung adenocarcinoma using the new IASLC classification. Clin Radiol. 2013;68:e21–6.
23. Tsutani Y, Miyata Y, Nakayama H, Okumura S, Adachi S, Yoshimura M, et al. Prognostic significance of using solid versus whole tumor size on high-resolution computed tomography for predicting pathologic malignant grade of tumors in clinical stage IA lung adenocarcinoma: a multicenter study. J Thorac Cardiovasc Surg. 2012;143:607–12.
24. Uehara H, Tsutani Y, Okumura S, Nakayama H, Adachi S, Yoshimura M, et al. Prognostic role of positron emission tomography and high-resolution computed tomography in clinical stage IA lung adenocarcinoma. Ann Thorac Surg. 2013;96:1958–65.
25. Watanabe K, Nomori H, Ohtsuka T, Naruke T, Ebihara A, Orikasa H, et al. [F-18]Fluorodeoxyglucose positron emission tomography can predict pathological tumor stage and proliferative activity determined by Ki-67 in clinical stage IA lung adenocarcinomas. Jpn J Clin Oncol. 2006;36:403–9.
26. Iwano S, Kishimoto M, Ito S, Kato K, Ito R, Naganawa S. Prediction of pathologic prognostic factors in patients with lung adenocarcinomas: comparison of thin-section computed tomography and positron emission tomography/computed tomography. Cancer Imaging. 2014;14:3.
27. Nakamura H, Saji H, Shinmyo T, Tagaya R, Kurimoto N, Koizumi H, et al. Close association of IASLC/ATS/ERS lung adenocarcinoma subtypes with glucose-uptake in positron emission tomography. Lung Cancer. 2015;87:28–33.
28. Kim EA, Johkoh T, Lee KS, Han J, Fujimoto K, Sadohara J, et al. Quantification of ground-glass opacity on high-resolution CT of small peripheral adenocarcinoma of the lung: pathologic and prognostic implications. AJR Am J Roentgenol. 2001;177:1417–22.
29. Ohde Y, Nagai K, Yoshida J, Nishimura M, Takahashi K, Suzuki K, et al. The proportion of consolidation to ground-glass opacity on high resolution CT is a good predictor for distinguishing the population of non-invasive peripheral adenocarcinoma. Lung Cancer. 2003;42:303–10.

18

Diffusion-weighted MR imaging of locally advanced breast carcinoma: the optimal time window of predicting the early response to neoadjuvant chemotherapy

Li Yuan[1,2], Jian-Jun Li[2], Chang-Qing Li[2], Cheng-Gong Yan[1], Ze-Long Cheng[1], Yuan-Kui Wu[1], Peng Hao[1], Bing-Quan Lin[1] and Yi-Kai Xu[1]*

Abstract

Background: It is very difficult to predict the early response to NAC only on the basis of change in tumor size. ADC value derived from DWI promises to be a valuable parameter for evaluating the early response to treatment. This study aims to establish the optimal time window of predicting the early response to neoadjuvant chemotherapy (NAC) for different subtypes of locally advanced breast carcinoma using diffusion-weighted imaging (DWI).

Methods: We conducted an institutional review board-approved prospective clinical study of 142 patients with locally advanced breast carcinoma. All patients underwent conventional MR and DW examinations prior to treatment and after first, second, third, fourth, sixth and eighth cycle of NAC. The response to NAC was classified into a pathologic complete response (pCR) and a non-pCR group. DWI parameters were compared between two groups, and the optimal time window for predicting tumor response was established for each chemotherapy regimen.

Results: For all the genomic subtypes, there were significant differences in baseline ADC value between pCR and non-pCR group ($p < 0.05$). The time point prior to treatment could be considered as the ideal time point regardless of genomic subtype. In the group that started with taxanes or anthracyclines, for Luminal A or Luminal B subtype, postT1 could be used as the ideal time point during chemotherapy; for Basal-like or HER2-enriched subtype, postT2 as the ideal time point during chemotherapy. In the group that started with taxanes and anthracyclines, for HER2-enriched, Luminal B or Basal-like subtype, postT1 could be used as the ideal time point during chemotherapy; for Luminal A subtype, postT2 as the ideal time point during chemotherapy.

Conclusions: The time point prior to treatment can be considered as the optimal time point regardless of genomic subtype. For each chemotherapy regimen, the optimal time point during chemotherapy varies across different genomic subtypes.

Keywords: Breast carcinoma, Magnetic resonance imaging (MRI), Diffusion-weighted imaging (DWI), Neoadjuvant chemotherapy (NAC), Therapeutic response

* Correspondence: xuyikai1997@126.com
[1]Department of Medical Imaging Center, Nanfang Hospital, Southern Medical University, #1838 Guangzhou Avenue North, Guangzhou City 510515, Guangdong Province, China
Full list of author information is available at the end of the article

Background

Neoadjuvant chemotherapy (NAC) has become a standard treatment for locally advanced breast carcinoma. The major clinical benefit of NAC, compared with adjuvant therapy, is the downstaging of large tumor and increased rate of breast-conserving surgery [1, 2]. However, some cases are not sensitive to NAC, and have no significant decrease or even enlarge in tumor size after treatment. Therefore, treatment efficacy should be predicted as early as possible, on which clinicians can tailor the therapeutic strategy and prevent unnecessary treatment, and thus improve the outcome of tumor [3]. At present, the assessment of the size or volume of residual tumor using conventional MRI is an important basis for the prediction of tumor response. But many tumors don't have a distinct decrease in size until several weeks or months after chemotherapy because of relatively slow tumor shrinkage, therefore, it is very difficult to predict the response to NAC only on the basis of change in tumor size [4].

Diffusion-weighted imaging (DWI) is a functional MRI technique that can reflect the subtle change in extra-cellular water diffusion within the tumor area [5]. Several previous studies [6, 7] have demonstrated that ADC value derived from DWI can be used as a valuable parameter for evaluating the early response to treatment because it is convenient and needn't require an intravenous injection of an exogenous contrast media [8]. The exploration of the optimal time window of DWI examination is very useful for predicting the response to NAC as early as possible. If ADC value derived from DWI prior to treatment can be used for discriminating pCR and non-pCR group, the baseline time point can be considered as the optimal time point, on which treatment regimen can be adjusted or tailored appropriately before chemotherapy. However, if baseline ADC value does not work, the exploration of the ideal time point during the chemotherapy is also necessary in order to make the best use of DWI in predicting tumor response, especially for the patients who are resistant to NAC. However, there has been no study on the optimal time window for predicting the early response to NAC using DWI.

Methods

In the present study, we aimed to systematically analyze the dynamic change in ADC value before and after chemotherapy initiated in order to establish the optimal time widow for predicting the response to NAC for different subtypes of locally advanced breast carcinoma.

Study design and population

This is a prospective observational clinical single-center study. Our study received approval from institutional ethics committee and written informed consent from all patients. Between January 2013 and April 2016, 155 patients with locally advanced breast carcinoma were recruited to this study.

Inclusion criteria were as follows: ① All patients had histologically proven breast carcinoma. The clinical stage stayed at II or III (requirement for breast conserving surgery). The axillary lymph node metastases were suspected or determined on the basis of imaging studies (ultrasonography and MRI), physical examination or/and fine-needle aspiration biopsy. ② The patients would complete a full course of NAC and subsequently undergo breast-conserving surgery. ③ There was no contraindication to MR examination. ④ The patients were younger than 70 years old.

Exclusion criteria consisted of ① unable to complete the full course of NAC, ② failure to complete all the follow-up MR examinations on schedule, ③ existence of obvious artifacts on DW images.

Neoadjuvant chemotherapy and classification for response to treatment

All the patients were treated with 4 to 8 cycles according to their regimen protocols and physical situation. A flow chart of the study design depicting number of patient and time-points they were measured/examined was seen on the Fig. 1. There were two types of NAC regimens administered in 3-week long cycle as follows: (1) Taxane-based with anthracyclines delivered in four, six or eight cycles. (2) Anthracycline/taxane-based consisting of four+four cycles, where anthracycline treatment and cyclophosphamide were followed by taxanes (CA-T), or vice versa (T-CA) [9, 10]. In some patients with Her2/Neu-positive lesions, trastuzumab was used in combination with NAC regimen (but not concurrently). According to the chemotherapy regimens, the patients were classified into three groups including the group started with taxanes, started with anthracyclines and started with taxanes and anthracyclines..

The tumor size of the lesion before or after treatment was measured and compared by two radiologists in consensus. Tumor size was defined as the largest diameter of the lesion measured with electronic calipers on the largest cross section of the tumor. After surgery, an experienced pathologist blindly assessed all specimen slices. According to Miller and Payne grading system [11], the pathologic response to NAC was classified into five grades as follows: grade 1, there were some changes of individual malignant tumor cells, but no reduction in overall cellularity; grade 2, there was a minor loss of invasive tumor cells(< 30%), but overall cellularity was still high; grade 3: there was a considerable reduction in tumor cells(30%~ 90%); grade 4: there was a marked disappearance of invasive tumor cells(> 90%) such that only small clusters or widely dispersed cells could be

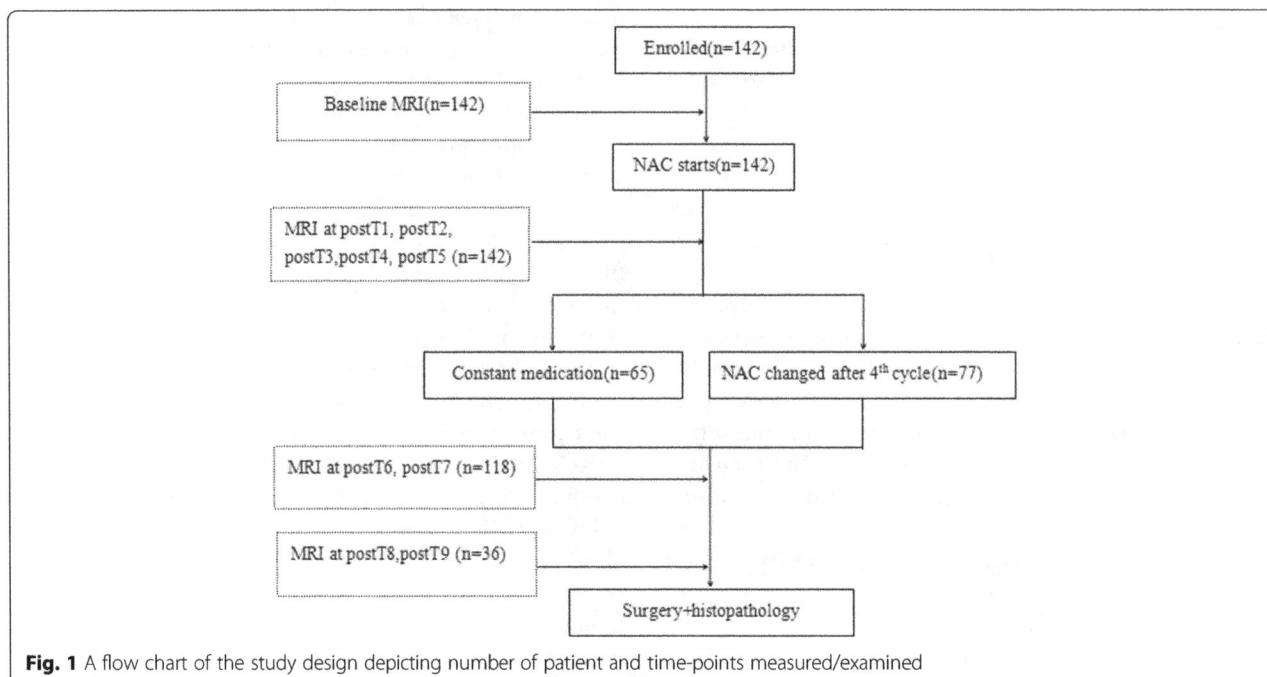

Fig. 1 A flow chart of the study design depicting number of patient and time-points measured/examined

detected; grade 5: there was no invasive tumor cell identifiable in the sections from the site of the previous tumor, only a little ductal carcinoma in situ or tumor stroma remained. All the patients were divided into pCR and non-pCR group. Grade 1 to 4 was regarded as non-pCR group, and grade 5 as pCR group.

MR technique and image analysis

MR examination was performed on a 3.0 T scanner (Discovery MR 750, GE Healthcare, USA) with an 8-channel phased-array breast coil. The time points of MR examinations were seen on the Fig. 1. The time points included before chemotherapy (baseline), 21 days (postT1, after 1 cycle), 42 days (postT2, after 2 cycles), 63 days (postT3, after 3 cycles), 84 days (postT4, after 4 cycles), 126 days (postT5, after 6 cycles) and 168 days (postT6, after 8 cycles) after chemotherapy initiated.

Conventional sequences included axial fat-suppression T2WI, axial fat-suppression T1WI and axial multi-phase dynamic contrast-enhanced (DCE) sequence. The parameters for axial fat-suppression T2WI were as follows: TR/TE: 4787/85.0 ms; FOV: 30x30cm; matrix size: 256×256; section thickness: 5 mm; inter-slice gap: 1 mm; number of excitation (NEX): 2. The parameters for axial fat-suppression T1WI were as follows: TR/TE: 640/1.7 ms; FOV: 32x32cm; matrix size:256×256; section thickness: 5 mm; inter-slice gap: 1 mm; NEX: 1. For DCE-MRI sequence, transverse 3D Vibrant-Flex was scanned before and repeated 8 times after intravenous administration of 0.1 mmol/kg Gd-DTPA (Magnevist; Bayer, Berlin, Germany) at 2 mL/s (followed by a flush

of 20-mL saline solution) via a power injector with a 15-s timing delay. Axial diffusion-weighted MR images were acquired using a single shot echo-planar imaging (SS-EPI) sequence. The parameters were as follows: four b values: 0, 300, 600 and 1000s/mm^2; TR/ TE: 2400/ 62 ms; field of view (FOV): 300x250mm; matrix size: 128×160; section thickness: 4 mm; inter-slice gap: 1 mm; receiver bandwidth: 250 kHz; parallel imaging (ASSET) factor: 2; scanning duration: 1 min and 58 s.

The original data were transferred to GE AW 4.6 post-processing work station. ADC images were produced automatically with software (MADC Function tools, GE Healthcare, USA). The whole volume of interest (VOI) was isolated using manual segmentation by two radiologists with more than 7 years' experience on breast MRI diagnosis. T2WI and DCE-MR images were used as the references to determine the extents of lesion on the corresponding ADC maps. The radiologists manually contoured the edge of target lesions slice by slice with the help of DCE-MR images using the segment tool. The VOI encompassed the profiles of mass as much as possible and avoided recognizable necrotic, hemorrhagic and cystic areas. Two radiologists were blinded to each other's results to allow measurement of inter-observer variability. Eventually, the measurements of all parameters for each VOI were recorded.

Pathologic analysis

After the surgery, sections were cut and stained with hematoxylin and eosin (HE) according to standard histologic protocols. Positivity for the HER-2 protein was evaluated according to the criteria of the Hercep Test. HER-2 membrane staining intensity and pattern were evaluated using the 0 to 3+ scale, and 3+ (uniformly intense membrane staining in at least 30% of tumor cells) was regarded as positive [12]. The percentage of nuclei with immunoreactivity to estrogen receptor(ER), progesterone receptor (PR) and Ki-67 was classified as continuous data from 0 to 100%. ER-positive and PR-positive cases showed staining in at least 10% of the tumor cell nuclei. Ki-67 was defined as low if ≤20% Ki-67 was detected and as high if > 20% Ki-67 was detected [13]. Lesions were classified into four subtypes according to immuno-cytochemical characteristics: Luminal A (ER+ and/or PR+, plus HER2-, and low-expression of Ki-67), Luminal B (ER+ and/or PR+, plus HER2+, and high-expression of Ki-67), HER2-enriched (ER- and PR-, plus HER2+) and Basal-like(ER- /HER2-) [12, 13]. Percentage of stroma was determined according to the criteria established by Mesker et al. [14]. Visual fields were scored only where both stroma and tumor were present and where tumor cells were seen on all the slides of the microscopic image field. Percentage of stroma was classified into stroma-rich (≤50% tumor percentage) and stroma-poor group (> 50% tumor percentage). Three stromal components, including collagen, fibroblasts and lymphocytes, were evaluated. The presence of a central fibrotic focus was defined as a characteristic tumor stroma with scarlike features or a radiating fibrosclerotic core surrounded by invasive carcinoma cells [15]. MVD was determined from the CD34 immunohistochemical-staining slides. A single countable vessel was defined as any positively stained endothelial cell or cell cluster separate from adjacent microvessels or tumor cells. The vessels containing erythrocytes in the lumen were excluded. Five high power fields were counted, and the average was determined [16].

Statistical analysis

Statistical analyses were performed using statistical software (SPSS, version 22.0; IBM Corp., Armonk, NY, USA). Inter-observer agreement on measurement of ADC value was analyzed using Bland-Altman method [17], and the mean difference, standard deviation (SD), 95% limits of agreement and intraclass correlation coefficient (ICC) were calculated. The distribution of DWI parameter was determined using Kolmogorov–Smirnov test. In this study, ADC values and △ADC for the subgroups didn't fit a normal distribution. Consequently, the multiple comparisons of parameters between pCR and non-pCR group or among different time points were performed using Mann-Whiney U test or Friedman test. A level of p value < 0.05 was regarded as statistically significant.

The correlations between DWI parameters and histological response to neoadjuvant chemotherapy were analyzed using Spearman correlation test. The potency of DWI parameters for discriminating pCR and non-pCR

was assessed using a receiver operating characteristic (ROC) analysis. The resulting threshold value was used to calculate the sensitivity and specificity.

Results

Patient characteristics

Of 155 patients, 13 patients were excluded because of no completion of the full course of chemotherapy ($n = 2$), failure to undergo follow-up MR examinations on schedule ($n = 3$), image distortions (n = 2), no surgery after NAC (n = 2), surgery before completion of chemotherapy ($n = 2$), distant metastasis ($n = 1$), and lack of proper pathological result ($n = 1$). Eventually, 142 patients were included into this study. According to pathological findings, 40 cases were regarded as pCR, and 102 cases as non-pCR.

The demographic, clinical and pathological characteristics for pCR and non-pCR group were summarized in Table 1. The table showed that there were no differences in mean age, menopausal status, histologic type, cycles of NAC and surgery method between pCR and non-pCR group($p < 0.05$). There was a higher percentage of tumors staged at III in non-pCR than in pCR group ($p = 0.03$); there was a difference in constituent ratio of genomic subtype between pCR and non-pCR group ($p = 0.04$). Luminal A subtype had the lowest pCR rate (20%, 5/25), and Basal-like subtype had the highest pCR rate (32.5%, 13/40).

Inter-observer agreement on ADC measurement

The mean value, standard deviation (SD), mean difference, 95% limits of agreement for measurements and intra-class correlation (ICC) were summarized in Table 2. The statistical analyses showed that a good agreement between two observers was obtained in terms of ADC measurement at each time point.

Baseline measurement

For all the genomic subtype, there were significant differences in ADC value between pCR and non-pCR group($p < 0.05$). For Luminal A, Luminal B, Basal-like and HER2-enriched subtype, the areas under the curves (AUCs) of ROC for baseline ADC value in discriminating pCR and non-pCR were 0.556, 0.538, 0.534 and 0.601 respectively.

Measurement during chemotherapy for the group started with taxanes

The differences in ADC values between pCR and non-pCR group were found only at the minority of time points ($p < 0.05$), while the differences in △ADC between two groups were found at the majority of time points ($p < 0.05$). For Luminal A or Luminal B subtype, the difference in △ADC between pCR and non-pCR group achieved significance as early as postT1, and the

Table 1 The demographic and pathological characteristics for non-pCR and pCR group

Variables	pCR (n = 40)	non-pCR (n = 102)	P-value
Mean age (yrs)	47.3 ± 11.0	43.3 ± 10.0	0.10
Menopausal status			0.09
Premenopausal	23(57.5%)	58(56.9%)	
Postmenopausal	17(42.5%)	44(43.1%)	
Histologic type			0.06
IDC	29(72.5%)	80(78.4%)	
ILC	11(27.5%)	22(21.6%)	
Clinical stage			0.03
IIa	8(20.0%)	9(8.8%)	
IIb	11(27.5%)	10(9.8%)	
IIIa	12(30.0%)	30(29.4%)	
IIIb	4(10.0%)	27(26.5%)	
IIIc	5(12.5%)	26(25.5%)	
Axillary lymph node metastases			0.07
yes	17(42.5%)	32(31.4%)	
no	23(57.5%)	70(68.6%)	
Cycles of NAC			0.06
4 cycles	8(20.0%)	16(15.7%)	
6 cycles	23(57.5%)	59(57.8%)	
8 cycles	9(22.5%)	27(26.5%)	
Surgery			0.07
Breast-conserving surgery	15(37.5%)	36(35.3%)	
Modified radical mastectomy	25(62.5%)	66(64.7%)	
Genomic subtype			0.04
Luminal A	5(12.5%)	20(29.4%)	
Luminal B	14(35.0%)	30(33.3%)	
Basal-like	13(32.5%)	27(15.7%)	
HER2-enriched	8(20.0%)	25(23.5%)	

Note: pCR: pathologic complete response; IDC: invasive ductal carcinoma; ILC: invasive lobular carcinoma; NAC: neoadjuvant chemotherapy

correlation between △ADC and treatment efficacy achieved the highest level at postT1(Spearman coefficient:0.679, 0.618). For Basal-like or HER2-enriched subtype, the difference in △ADC between pCR and non-pCR group achieved significance as early as postT2, and the correlation between △ADC and treatment efficacy achieved the highest level at postT2 (Spearman coefficient:0.647, 0.629)(Table 3).

Measurement during chemotherapy for the group started with anthracyclines

The differences in ADC values between pCR and non-pCR group were found only at the minority of time points ($p < 0.05$), while the differences in △ADC between two groups were found at the majority of time points ($p < 0.05$). For Luminal A or Luminal B subtype, the difference in △ADC between pCR and non-pCR group achieved

significance as early as postT1, and the correlation between △ADC and treatment efficacy achieved the highest level at postT1(Spearman coefficient:0.647, 0.578). For Basal-like or HER2-enriched subtype, the difference in △ADC between pCR and non-pCR group achieved significance as early as postT2, and the correlation between △ADC and treatment efficacy achieved the highest level at postT2 (Spearman coefficient: 0.637, 0.646)(Table 4).

Measurement during chemotherapy for the group started with taxanes and anthracyclines

The differences in ADC values between pCR and non-pCR group were found only at the minority of time points ($p < 0.05$), while the differences in △ADC between two groups were found at the majority of time points ($p < 0.05$). For Luminal B, HER2-enriched or Basal-like subtype, the difference in △ADC between pCR and

Table 2 Inter-observer agreements on ADC measurement

ADC value (10^{-3} mm^2/s)	ADC value (10^{-3} mm^2/s)	Mean Difference	95% limits of agreement	ICC†
Base-line				
Observer 1	0.9021 ± 0.42	0.0151	−1.512, 1.474	0.9925–0.9974
Observer 2	0.9172 ± 0.37			
PostT1				
Observer 1	1.0784 ± 0.52	0.0113	−1.1203, 1.308	0.9782–0.9824
Observer 2	1.0671 ± 0.53			
PostT2				
Observer 1	1.2607 ± 0.67	0.0157	−1.1214, 1.312	0.9897–0.9568
Observer 2	1.2764 ± 0.70			
PostT3				
Observer 1	1.3645 ± 0.71	0.0104	−1.1124,1.212	0.9901–0.9969
Observer 2	1.3745 ± 0.72			
PostT4				
Observer 1	1.4753 ± 0.74	0.0036	−1.1313, 1.239	0.9912–0.9981
Observer 2	1.4789 ± 0.79			
PostT5				
Observer 1	1.5286 ± 0.88	0.0087	−1.1412,1.3129	0.9899–0.9965
Observer 2	1.5373 ± 0.94			
PostT6				
Observer 1	1.5541 ± 0.89	0.0112	−1.1423,1.3278	0.9798–0.9908
Observer 2	1.5653 ± 0.90			

Note: Data are mean ± standard deviations; †: ICC = intra-class correlation coefficient

non-pCR group achieved significance as early as postT1, and the correlation between △ADC and treatment efficacy achieved the highest level at postT1(Spearman coefficient:0.667, 0.628, 0.609). For Luminal A subtype, the difference in △ADC between pCR and non-pCR group achieved significance as early as postT2, and the correlation between △ADC and treatment efficacy achieved the highest level at postT2 (Spearman coefficient: 0.656)(Table 5).

The optimal time window of predicting response to chemotherapy

According to the results mentioned above, baseline time point could be considered as the optimal time point regardless of genomic subtype. In the group that started with started with taxanes or anthracyclines, for Luminal A or Luminal B subtype, postT1 could be used as the ideal time point during chemotherapy(Fig. 2). For Basal-like or HER2-enriched subtype, postT2 as the ideal

Table 3 The correlations between ADC/△ADC value and final tumor response to NAC started with taxanes

Items	Luminal A	Luminal B	HER2-enriched	Basal-like
The time point when there was a significant correlation between ADC and tumor response	baseline(−0.324)	baseline($r = -0.346$)	baseline(−0.324)	baseline(−0.378)
	postT1(0.348)	postT1($r = 0.396$)	postT2(0.431)	postT2(0.397)
	postT4(0.357)	postT3($r = 0.323$)	postT5(0.368)	postT4(0.334)
	postT6(0.334)	postT6($r = 0.335$)	postT6(0.412)	postT6(0.345)
The time point when there was a significant correlation between △ADC and tumor response	postT1(0.679)	postT1(0.618)	postT2(0.629)	posT2(0.647)
	postT2(0.548)	postT2(0.478)	postT3(0.545)	postT3(0.521)
	postT3(0.538)	postT4(0.556)	postT4(0.526)	postT4(0.506)
	postT4(0.593)	postT5(0.538)	postT5(0.534)	postT5(0.547)
	postT5(0.556)	postT6(0.512)	postT6(0.498)	postT6(0.456)

Note: The data in the parentheses are presented as Spearman coefficient

Table 4 The correlations between ADC/△ADC value and final tumor response to NAC started with anthracyclines

Items	Luminal A	Luminal B	HER2-enriched	Basal-like
The time point when there was a significant correlation between ADC and tumor response	baseline(−0.326)	baseline($r = -0.348$)	baseline(−0.332)	baseline(−0.313)
	postT1(0.357)	postT1($r = 0.391$)	postT2(0.423)	postT2(0.358)
	postT4(0.335)	postT3($r = 0.347$)	postT5(0.368)	postT4(0.347)
	postT6(0.329)	postT6($r = 0.348$)	postT6(0.389)	postT6(0.349)
The time point when there was a significant correlation between △ADC and tumor response	postT1(0.647)	postT1(0.578)	postT2(0.646)	posT2(0.637)
	postT2(0.526)	postT2(0.487)	postT3(0.543)	postT3(0.549)
	postT3(0.538)	postT4(0.532)	postT4(0.527)	postT4(0.536)
	postT4(0.587)	postT5(0.522)	postT5(0.524)	postT5(0.546)
	postT5(0.554)	postT6(0.487)	postT6(0.498)	postT6(0.495)

Note: The data in the parentheses are presented as Spearman coefficient

time point during chemotherapy (Fig. 3). In the group that started with taxanes and anthracyclines, for HER2, Luminal B or Basal-like subtype, postT1 could be used as the ideal time point during the chemotherapy; for Luminal A subtype, postT2 as the ideal time point during the chemotherapy.

The prediction performance of imaging parameters during chemotherapy

For all the subtypes, the AUC of ROC for △ADC from baseline to the ideal time point during chemotherapy was higher than that of ADC value at each time point($p < 0.05$)(Table 6). In the group that started with taxanes, the highest AUC of ROC for △ADC (=0.865) was seen in Luminal B subtype, the cut-off value was 0.5746×10^{-3} mm^2/s, which yielded a sensitivity of 89.4% and a specificity of 83.4%. In the group that started with anthracyclines, the highest AUC of ROC for △ADC (=0.845) was seen in Luminal A subtype, and the cut-off value was 0.5589×10^{-3} mm^2/s, which yielded a sensitivity of 87.3% and a specificity of 73.4%. In the group that started with anthracyclines and taxanes, the highest AUC of ROC for △ADC (=0.879) was seen in Basal-like subtype, and

the cut-off value was 0.5854×10^{-3} mm^2/s, which yielded a sensitivity of 89.9% and a specificity of 82.6%.

Comparison of pathologic/histologic characteristics of tumor between pCR and non-pCR group

The pathologic/histologic characteristics of tumor for pCR and non-pCR group were summarized in Table 7. Microvessel density (MVD) was higher in pCR than in non-pCR group ($p = 0.04$). There was a higher percentage of stroma-poor tumors in pCR than in non-pCR group ($p = 0.03$). There was no difference in dominant cell type between two groups ($p = 0.07$). There was a higher percentage of central fibrosis in non-pCR than in pCR group ($p = 0.04$).

Discussion

To our best knowledge, this is the first clinical study on exploration of the optimal time window of predicting the response to NAC for locally advanced breast carcinoma in light of DWI, which provides an important guidance for the appropriate adjustment of treatment regimens as early as possible in those patients who don't have a satisfactory response to chemotherapy.

Table 5 The correlations between ADC/△ADC value and final tumor response to NAC started with taxanes and anthracyclines

Items	Luminal A	Luminal B	HER2-enriched	Basal-like
The time point when there was a significant correlation between ADC and tumor response	baseline(−0.326)	baseline($r = -0.367$)	baseline(−0.368)	baseline(−0.349)
	postT1(0.358)	postT1($r = 0.387$)	postT2(0.425)	postT2(0.393)
	postT4(0.351)	postT3($r = 0.345$)	postT5(0.398)	postT4(0.326)
	postT6(0.329)	postT6($r = 0.331$)	postT6(0.367)	postT6(0.319)
The time point when there was a significant correlation between △ADC and tumor response	postT2(0.656)	postT1(0.667)	postT1(0.628)	posT1(0.609)
	postT3(0.556)	postT2(0.469)	postT3(0.541)	postT3(0.546)
	postT4(0.539)	postT4(0.534)	postT4(0.529)	postT4(0.529)
	postT5(0.587)	postT5(0.529)	postT5(0.518)	postT5(0.538)
	postT6(0.531)	postT6(0.486)	postT6(0.492)	postT6(0.476)

Note: The data in the parentheses are presented as Spearman coefficient

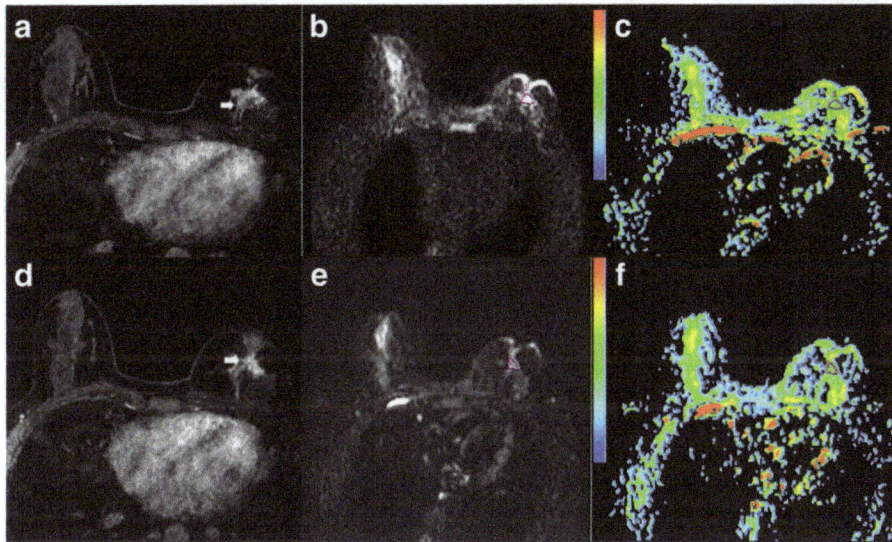

Fig. 2 DCE-MR images of a patient who suffered from breast carcinoma and received the chemotherapy started with taxanes, DWI and ADC images in pCR group. Red color represent high ADC value, green color represent mediate ADC value, and blue color represent low ADC value. **a, d** DCE-MR images at baseline and postT1, There was an irregular mass in the left breast and confirmed to be breast carcinoma with Luminal A subtype. After one cycle of NAC, the tumor didn't have no significant decrease in diameter. **b, e** DW images at baseline and postT1, The images showed how the whole volume of interest (VOI) was placed within the tumor area manually. **c, f** ADC maps at baseline and postT1, ADC values were 0.8162×10^{-3} mm^2/s at baseline and 1.4756×10^{-3} mm^2/s at postT1, ADC value varied significantly as early as postT1

The main advantage of DWI is that this technique can be used to quantitatively measure extra-cellular water diffusion within the tumor area, on which the dynamic change of tumor micro-environment is monitored. However, DWI has some technical limitations, such as ghosting, insufficient fat suppression and insufficient signal noise ratio (SNR) [18]. In order to improve the imaging quality or maximally reduce the imaging artifact, the following measures were taken. First, all the patients were instructed to keep gentle breathing during MR

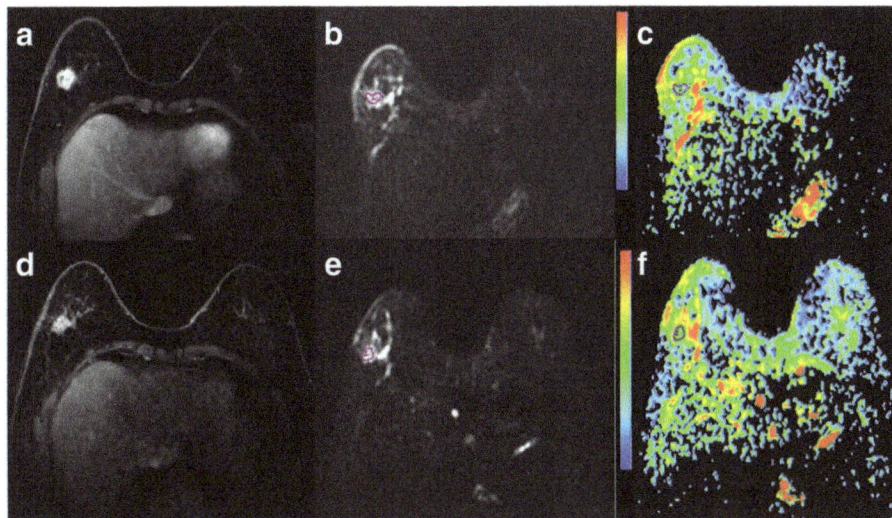

Fig. 3 DCE-MR images of a patient who suffered from breast carcinoma and received the chemotherapy started with anthracyclines, DWI and ADC images in non-pCR group. Red color represent high ADC value, green color represent mediate ADC value, and blue color represent low ADC value. **a, d** DCE-MR images at baseline and postT2, There was an irregular mass in the right breast and confirmed to be breast carcinoma with Basal-like subtype. After two cycles of NAC, the tumor size didn't have no significant decrease in diameter. **b, e** DW images at baseline and postT2, The images showed how the whole volume of interest (VOI) was placed within the tumor area manually. **c, f** ADC maps at baseline and postT2, ADC values were 0.9345×10^{-3} mm^2/s at baseline and 1.3320×10^{-3} mm^2/s at postT2, ADC value varied significantly as early as postT2

Table 6 Area under the curve from the ROC analysis of pCR prediction using different MRI measures

AUC	ADC at baseline	ADC at the ideal time point during chemotherapy	ΔADC from baseline to the ideal time point during chemotherapy
Started with taxanes			
Luminal A	0.556(0.513~0.612)	0.598(0.546~0.636)	0.678(0.598~0.749)
Luminal B	0.558(0.525~0.623)	0.602(0.567~0.645)	0.865(0.748~0.930)
Basal-like	0.543(0.503~0.605)	0.589(0.558~0.649)	0.723(0.614~0.843)
HER2-enriched	0.537(0.521~0.619)	0.593(0.549~0.638)	0.745(0.678~0.832)
Started with anthracyclines			
Luminal A	0.545(0.521~0.598)	0.587(0.529~0.620)	0.845(0.769~0.920)
Luminal B	0.598(0.534~0.628)	0.612(0.528~0.656)	0.723(0.678~0.789)
Basal-like	0.612(0.567~0.654)	0.621(0.557~0.678)	0.756(0.698~0.845)
HER2-enriched	0.578(0.543~0.626)	0.614(0.551~0.636)	0.734(0.658~0.798)
Started with anthracyclines and taxanes			
Luminal A	0.534(0.509~0.589)	0.567(0.546~0.600)	0.738(0.645~0.798)
Luminal B	0.545(0.502~0.620)	0.587(0.538~0.621)	0.756(0.655~0.809)
Basal-like	0.578(0.527~0.600)	0.602(0.567~0.629)	0.879(0.789~0.923)
HER2-enriched	0.602(0.526~0.645)	0.623(0.569~0.667)	0.783(0.698~0.823)

Note: The data in the parentheses were 95% confidence intervals

examination. Second, 3.0 T MR scanner was used in order to improve SNR of images, while 3.0 T MR scanner also has some disadvantages, such as increased magnetic susceptibility artifact and eddy current related distortion [19]. Therefore, we used the narrow FOV and volume homogenization block matching the size of the unilateral breast in order to improve the homogeneity of the local magnetic field. Rosenkrantz et al. [19] demonstrated that ADC reproducibility was moderate at both 1.5 T and 3.0 T, and there was no significant difference in measurement of ADC value between 1.5 T and 3.0 T. Therefore, field strength may have no significant influence on the quantitative measurement of ADC value.

Table 7 The difference in pathological/histological characteristics between pCR and non-pCR group

Parameters	pCR	Non-pCR	P-value
Microvessel density[a]	35.1 ± 6.67	22.6 ± 6.14	0.04
Percentage of stroma(n)			0.03
Stroma-rich	13(32.5%)	60(58.8%)	
Stroma-poor	27(67.5%)	42(41.2%)	
Dominant cell type(n)			0.07
Fibroblast	13(32.5%)	40(39.2%)	
Collegan	20(50.0%)	42(41.2%)	
Lymphocyte	7(17.5%)	20(19.6%)	
Central fibrosis(n)			0.04
Absent	25(62.5%)	40(39.2%)	
Present	15(37.5%)	62(60.8%)	

Note: [a]Data are mean values±standard deviations; pCR: pathologic complete response

There exists a controversy on the value of baseline ADC in predicting the response to NAC for breast carcinoma. Some studies [20, 21] didn't find a significant correlation between baseline ADC and pathologic response to chemotherapy, while other studies [22, 23] suggested that breast cancer with lower baseline ADC value had better treatment efficacy. This study showed that, for all the subtypes, baseline ADC value was significantly lower in pCR than in non-pCR group. According to several previous studies [24–26], the possible explanation is that, for non-PCR group, there are more necrosis and greater destruction of normal vasculature, which results in higher ADC value because of free diffusion or an increase of diffusing molecules. Because that the differences in baseline ADC value between pCR and non-pCR group were found for all the subtypes, the time point prior to treatment may be considered as the ideal time point of DWI examination, which allows the clinician to predict the response to NAC before treatment and thus to adjust the regimens appropriately as early as possible. However, according to ROC analysis, the predicting performance of baseline ADC value is greatly lower than that of ADC or ΔADC during the chemotherapy for each genomic subtype. Therefore, it is not adequate to evaluate tumor response only on the basis of baseline ADC value.

This study showed that, compared with ADC, ΔADC was a more sensitive parameter for predicting the response to NAC. According to our results, the differences in ADC value between two groups were found only at the minority of time points, while the difference in ΔADC between two groups were found at the majority of time points. Similarly, Iwasa et al. [6] investigated the feasibility of DWI in evaluating the early response to NAC for breast carcinoma, and found that ADC value didn't correlate with response rate, but △ADC had a significant correlation with response rate. Therefore, △ADC is more valuable and accurate in predicting the early response to NAC. More specifically, a significant △ADC indicates the chemo-sensitivity, while a minute △ADC indicates a less satisfactory response or even no response.

In order to avoid the influence on the ADC measurement by different chemotherapy regimens, the optimal time window of DWI examination during the chemotherapy was explored for each chemotherapy regimen. This study found that the optimal time window for the prediction of tumor response varied across different subtypes for every chemotherapy regimen. For example, in the group that started with taxanes or anthracyclines, for Luminal A or Luminal B subtype, postT1 could be used as the ideal time point during chemotherapy. For Basal-like or HER2-enriched subtype, postT2 could be considered as the ideal time point during chemotherapy. The differences in the optimal time window across four genomic subtypes might be due to high heterogeneity of breast carcinoma. For example, successful chemotherapy causes cytotoxic tumor cell death, which results in a decrease in the proportion of immature microvessel density, but the degree of decrease in microvascular structures varies across different subtypes [27–29]. Bedair et al. [30] compared the potency of ADC value at different time points in predicting the early response to NAC for breast cancer, and found that the difference in percentage increase of ADC value between responders and non-responders achieved a significance after 3 cycles of chemotherapy. Bedair et al. selected only three time points (before start of chemotherapy, after completion of three cycles and at the end of chemotherapy), while our study selected seven time points before, during and after chemotherapy. Consequently, we believe that the optimal time window established by us is more reasonable and accurate.

O'Flynn et al. [31] investigated the value of △ADC in predicting pathologic response to chemotherapy for all the subtypes, and found that the area under ROC curve of △ADC from pre-treatment to after two cycles of chemotherapy for predicting responders was 0.69, which is lower than the result acquired by us. For example, in the group that started with taxanes, for Luminal B subtype, the AUC of ROC for △ADC in discriminating pCR and non-pCR was 0.865. The discrepancy between two studies may be due to the difference in patient constitution, MR device, method of imaging analysis or selection of time points. Especially, the selection of different time points may be the most important reason. It was worthwhile to note that the sensitivity and specificity at the cut-off value for each subtype were not so excellent, therefore, it is still a challenge that these cut-off values are used to discriminate pCR from non-pCR in clinical settings. Nevertheless, the results acquired by us provide useful information on the prediction of pathologic response to NAC, on which individual chemotherapy regimens can be adjusted or optimized more rapidly, and allows patients to receive the most appropriate treatment.

To better understand the value of DWI parameters in predicting the response to NAC, we also investigated the value of some pathologic characteristics in predicting the response to NAC. This study showed that MVD, tumor stroma ratio and central fibrosis were important factors for predicting the response to NAC. The tumors that had high MVD, tumor stroma ratio or little central fibrosis were prone to be sensitive to NAC, which was similar to several previous studies [32, 33]. However, it is worthwhile to note that these histologic/pathologic characteristics of tumor are obtained after surgery following the completion of NAC, and not enough to represent the status of histologic/pathologic characteristics during the course of chemotherapy.

Minarikova et al. [3] explored the predictive value of multiple imaging parameters that acquired from DWI and DCE-MRI at different time points during chemotherapy in breast cancer, and found that the measurement of tumor size served as a better predictor than ADC values. In contrast, ADC can reflect the micro-environment of tumor after chemotherapy, and could be used as an important supplement to mid-therapy diameter changes. Therefore, the combination of multi-parametric MRI can improve the accuracy and reliability of prediction of response to NAC. In the future, it is necessary to make the further study to explore the optimal MRI acquisition and evaluation method, as well as the ideal time point of predicting the response to NAC using DCE-MRI combined with DWI.

There are several limitations to this study. First, not all the patients received MR examination after 4 cycles of NAC, which might result in evaluation bias at the time points after 4 cycles. Second, according to our results, the time point prior to treatment could be used as the ideal time point of DWI examination, but the potency of ADC value at this time point was greatly lower that of ADC value or △ADC during chemotherapy for each subtype, therefore, the ideal time point during chemotherapy was explored, which was an important supplement to the time point prior to treatment. Finally, our study was limited by the small sample size with differing rates of pCR within the tumor subtypes, and further studies with a large number of patients are needed to confirm our preliminary results.

Conclusions

In summary, the time point prior to treatment can be considered as the optimal time point regardless of genomic subtype. For each chemotherapy regimen, the optimal time point during chemotherapy varies across different genomic subtypes during chemotherapy. Compared with ADC value at each time point, △ADC is a more reliable sensitive parameter for predicting tumor response. The results acquired by us provide useful information on the prediction of pathologic response to NAC, which promises to serve as a useful guidance for the adjustment of individual treatment regimens more rapidly.

Abbreviations

△ADC: Change in ADC; ADC: Apparent diffusion coefficient; AUC: Area under the curve; DCE: Dynamic contrast enhanced; DWI: Diffusion-weighted imaging; FOV: Field of view; HE: Hematoxylin and eosin; MRI: Magnetic resonance imaging; MVD: Microvessel density; pCR: Pathological complete response; ROC: Receiver operating characteristic; ROI: Region of interest; TR/TE: Repetition time/time to echo; VOI: Volume of interest

Acknowledgements
Not applicable

Funding

We have no financial and personal relationships with other people or organizations that inappropriately influence our works. There is no professional or other personal interest of any nature or kind in any product, service and/or company.

Authors' contributions

YL, XYK and YCG conceived of the present idea. XYK supervised the project. CLZ, WYK and HP acquired, analyzed and interpreted the patient data. YL and LBQ were major contributors in writing the manuscript. LJJ and LCQ gave technical support and conceptual advice. All authors read and revised the manuscript critically, approving the final manuscript.

Competing interests

The authors declare that they have no competing interests.

Author details

[1]Department of Medical Imaging Center, Nanfang Hospital, Southern Medical University, #1838 Guangzhou Avenue North, Guangzhou City 510515, Guangdong Province, China. [2]Department of Radiology, Hainan General Hospital, Haikou 570311, Hainan Province, China.

References

1. Tate SC, Andre V, Enas N, Ribba B, Gueorguieva I. Early change in tumour size predicts overall survival in patients with first-line metastatic breast cancer. Eur J Cancer. 2016;66:95–103.

2. Mistry KA, Thakur MH, Kembhavi SA. The effect of chemotherapy on the mammographic appearance of breast cancer and correlation with histopathology. Br J Radiol. 2016;89:20150479.

3. Minarikova L, Bogner W, Pinker K, Valkovič L, Zaric O, Bago-Horvath Z, Bartsch R, Helbich TH, Trattnig S, Gruber S. Investigating the prediction value of multiparametric magnetic resonance imaging at 3 T in response to neoadjuvant chemotherapy in breast cancer. Eur Radiol. 2017;27:1901–11.

4. Murata Y, Kubota K, Hamada N, Miyatake K, Tadokoro M, Nakatani K, Ue H, Tsuzuki K, Nishioka A, Iguchi M, Maeda H, Ogawa Y. Diffusion-weighted magnetic resonance imaging for assessment after neoadjuvant chemotherapy in breast cancer, based on morphological concepts. Oncol Lett. 2010;1:293–8.

5. Leong KM, Lau P, Ramadan S. Utilisation of MR spectroscopy and diffusion weighted imaging in predicting and monitoring of breast cancer response to chemotherapy. Radiat Oncol. 2015;59:268–77.

6. Iwasa H, Kubota K, Hamada N, Nogami M, Nishioka A. Early prediction of response to neoadjuvant chemotherapy in patients with breast cancer using diffusion-weighted imaging and gray-scale ultrasonography. Oncol Rep. 2014;31:1555–60.

7. Richard R, Thomassin I, Chapellier M, Scemama A, de Cremoux P, Varna M, Giacchetti S, Espié M, de Kerviler E, de Bazelaire C. Diffusion-weighted MRI in pretreatment prediction of response to neoadjuvant chemotherapy in patients with breast cancer. Eur Radiol. 2013;23:2420–31.

8. King AD, Thoeny HC. Functional MRI for the prediction of treatment response in head and neck squamous cell carcinoma: potential and limitations. Cancer Imaging. 2016;16:23.

9. Kaufmann M, von Minckwitz G, Mamounas E, Cameron D, Carey LA, Cristofanilli M, Denkert C, Eiermann W, Gnant M, Harris JR, Karn T, Liedtke C, Mauri D. Recommendations from an international consensus conference on the current status and future of neoadjuvant systemic therapy in primary breast cancer. Ann Surg Oncol. 2012;19:1508–16.

10. Rubovszky G, Horváth Z. Recent advances in the neoadjuvant treatment of breast cancer. J Breast Cancer. 2017;20:119–31.

11. Ogston KN, Miller ID, Payne S, Hutcheon AW, Sarkar TK, Smith I, Schofield A, Heys SD. A new histological grading system to assess response of breast cancers to primary chemotherapy: prognostic significance and survival. Breast. 2003;12:320–7.

12. Liu Y, Huang X, Bi R, Yang W, Shao Z. Similar prognoses for invasive micropapillary breast carcinoma and pure invasive ductal carcinoma: a retrospectively matched cohort study in China. PLoS One. 2014;9:e106564.

13. Che S, Zhao X, Ou Y, Li J, Wang M, Wu B, Zhou C. Role of the intravoxel incoherent motion diffusion weighted imaging in the pre-treatment prediction and early response monitoring to neoadjuvant chemotherapy in locally advanced breast cancer. Medicine (Baltimore). 2016;95:e2420.

14. Mesker WE, Junggeburt JM, Szuhai K. The carcinoma-stromal ratio of colon carcinoma is an independent factor for survival compared to lymph node status and tumor stage. Cell Oncol. 2007;29:387–98.

15. Ko ES, Han BK, Kim RB, Cho EY, Ahn S, Nam SJ, Ko EY, Shin JH, Hahn SY. Apparent diffusion coefficient in estrogen receptor-positive invasive ductal breast carcinoma: correlations with tumor-stroma ratio. Radiology. 2014;271:30–7.

16. Kim SH, Lee HS, Kang BJ, Song BJ, Kim HB, Lee H, Jin MS, Lee A. Dynamic contrast-enhanced MRI perfusion parameters as imaging biomarkers of angiogenesis. PLoS One. 2016;11:e0168632.

17. Bland JM, Altman DG. Statistical methods for assessing agreement between two methods of clinical measurements. Lancet. 1986;1:307–10.

18. Cui Y, Dyvorne H, Besa C, Cooper N, Taouli B IVIM. Diffusion-weighted imaging of the liver at 3.0T: comparison with 1.5T. Eur J Radiol Open. 2015;2:123–8.

19. Rosenkrantz AB, Oei M, Babb JS, Niver BE, Taouli B. Diffusion-weighted imaging of the abdomen at 3.0 Tesla: image quality and apparent diffusion coefficient reproducibility compared with 1.5 Tesla. J Magn Reson Imaging. 2011;33:128–35.

20. Yalcin B. Overview on locally advanced breast cancer: defining, epidemiology, and overview on neoadjuvant therapy. Exp Oncol. 2013;35:250–2.

21. Bufi E, Belli P, Costantini M, Di Matteo M, Bonatesta A, Franceschini G, Terribile D, Mulé A, Nardone L, Bonomo L. Role of the apparent diffusion coefficient in the prediction of response to neoadjuvant chemotherapy in patients with locally advanced breast cancer. Clin Breast Cancer. 2015;15:370–80.

22. Hahn SY, Ko EY, Han BK, Shin JH, Ko ES. Role of diffusion-weighted imaging as an adjunct to contrast-enhanced breast MRI in evaluating residual breast cancer following neoadjuvant chemotherapy. Eur J Radiol. 2014;83:283–8.

23. Sharma U, Danishad KK, Seenu V, Jagannathan NR. Longitudinal study of the assessment by MRI and diffusion-weighted imaging of tumor response in patients with locally advanced breast cancer undergoing neoadjuvant chemotherapy. NMR Biomed. 2009;22:104–13.

24. Li X, Abramson RG, Arlinghaus LR, Kang H, Chakravarthy AB, Abramson VG, Farley J, Mayer IA, Kelley MC, Meszoely IM, Means-Powell J, Grau AM, Sanders M. Multi-parametric magnetic resonance imaging for predicting pathological response after the first cycle of neoadjuvant chemotherapy in breast cancer. Investig Radiol. 2015;50:195–204.

25. Liu Y, Sun HR, Bai RJ, Ye Z. Time-window of early detection of response to concurrent chemoradiation in cervical cancer by using diffusion-weighted MR imaging: a pilot study. Radiat Oncol. 2015;10:185–92.

26. Woodhams R, Kakita S, Hata H. Wabuchi K, Kuranami M, Gautam S, Hatabu H, Kan S. Mountford C. identification of residual breast carcinoma following neoadjuvant chemotherapy: diffusion weighted imaging–comparison with contrast-enhanced MR imaging and pathologic findings. Radiology. 2010; 254:357–66.

27. Eom HJ, Cha JH, Choi WJ, Chae EY, Shin HJ, Kim HH. Predictive value of DCE-MRI for early evaluation of pathological complete response to neoadjuvant chemotherapy in resectable primary breast cancer: a single-center prospective study. Breast. 2016;30:80–6.

28. Sun X, Yang L, Yan X, Sun Y, Zhao D, Ji Y, Wang K, Chen X, Shen B. DCE-MRI-derived parameters in evaluating abraxane-induced early vascular response and the effectiveness of its synergistic interaction with cisplatin. PLoS One. 2016;11:e0162601.

29. Bedair R, Priest AN, Patterson A, McLean MA, Graves MJ, Manavaki R, Gill AB, Abeyakoon O, Griffiths JR, Gilbert FJ. Assessment of early treatment response to neoadjuvant chemotherapy in breast cancer using non-mono-exponential diffusion models: a feasibility study comparing the baseline and mid-treatment MRI examinations. Eur Radiol. 2017;27:2726–36.

30. O'Flynn EA, Collins D, D'Arcy J, Schmidt M, de Souza NM. Multi-parametric MRI in the early prediction of response to neo-adjuvant chemotherapy in breast cancer: value of non-modelled parameters. Eur J Radiol. 2016;85:837–42.

31. Li Y, Wei X, Zhang S, Zhang J. Prognosis of invasive breast cancer after adjuvant therapy evaluated with VEGF microvessel density and microvascular imaging. Tumour Biol. 2015;36:8755–60.

32. Majidinia M, Yousefi B. Breast tumor stroma: a driving force in the development of resistance to therapies. Chem Biol Drug Des. 2017;89:309–18.

33. Tse GM, Chaiwun B, Wong KT, Yeung DK, Pang AL, Tang AP, Cheung HS. Magnetic resonance imaging of breast lesions--a pathologic correlation. Breast Cancer Res Treat. 2007;103:1–10.

19

The utility of measuring the apparent diffusion coefficient for peritumoral zone in assessing infiltration depth of endometrial cancer

Lei Deng[1†], Qiu-ping Wang[1†], Rui Yan[2], Xiao-yi Duan[3], Lu Bai[1], Nan Yu[4], You-min Guo[1] and Quan-xin Yang[1*]

Abstract

Background: The invasion depth of endometrial cancer is one of the most important prognosis factors. The aim of the current study was to investigate the diagnostic value of the apparent diffusion coefficient (ADC) of the peritumoral zone for assessing the infiltration depth of endometrial cancer.

Methods: An institutional review board approved this prospective study, and all study participants provided informed consent. A total of 58 patients (mean age 54 ± 8.3 years, range 34–69 years) with endometrial cancer were prospectively enrolled. Two radiologists assessed all preoperative magnetic resonance images with T1, T2, and diffusion-weighted imaging, and determined the location of the deepest invasion of the tumor. The peritumoral zone was defined as a 5-mm-thick zone surrounding and adjacent to the cancerous endometrium. The mean ADC (ADCm) values of the tumor and the peritumoral zone were measured. Sensitivity, specificity, positive and negative predictive values, and the area under the receiver operating characteristic curve (Az) were calculated for visual inspection, and an ADC cutoff value for the peri-endometrial zone was determined for predicting the myometrial invasion depth.

Results: The ADCm values of tumors and peritumoral zones were 0.83×10^{-3} mm^2/sec and 1.06×10^{-3} mm^2/sec, respectively. There was no significant difference between the ADCm values of the tumors in the superficial and deep myometrial invasion groups ($P > 0.05$). However, the ADCm value at the peritumoral zone in the deep myometrial invasion group (1.23×10^{-3} mm^2/sec) significantly differed from that in the superficial myometrial invasion group (0.99×10^{-3} mm^2/sec) ($p = 0.005$). In assessments of deep myometrial invasion, the sensitivity, specificity, negative predictive value, and positive predictive value were 0.58, 0.93, 0.84, and 0.77, respectively, for the ADCm cutoff value of the peritumoral zone, and 0.71, 0.80, 0.87, and 0.60. respectively, for visual inspection. The accuracy of myometrial invasion depth assessment using the ADCm cutoff value and visual inspection were 83 and 78%, respectively. The Az for both was 0.76.

Conclusion: ADCm at the peritumoral zone can predict deep myometrial invasion of endometrial cancer. This value can therefore enhance confidence in preoperative endometrial cancer evaluation, and when tailoring surgical approaches.

Keywords: Diagnostic imaging, Diffusion, Endometrial carcinoma, Endometrial neoplasm, Magnetic resonance imaging

* Correspondence: quanxy6285@163.com
†Lei Deng and Qiu-ping Wang contributed equally to this work.
[1]Department of Radiology, the First Affiliated Hospital, Xi'an Jiaotong University Xi'an, #277, Yanta West Road, Xi'an 710061, Shaanxi, China
Full list of author information is available at the end of the article

Background

Endometrial cancer is the sixth most common malignant disorder in women worldwide [1]. Its prognosis depends on multiple factors,with the depth of myometrial invasion being one of most important [2]. This depth may be used as a surrogate marker to determine possible lymphovascular space invasion and the risk of lymph node metastases [3, 4]. The prevalence of lymph node metastases increases from 3% with superficial myometrial invasion to 46% with deep myometrial invasion [5], and the recurrence risk was reportedly intermediate to moderately high in patients with deep myometrial invasion [6]. Therefore, accurate preoperative delineation of the myometrial invasiveness of endometrial cancer is essential.

Magnetic resonance imaging (MRI) is recommended for the management and preoperative staging of endometrial cancer [7]. Recently, diffusion-weighted (DW) imaging has been introduced to better evaluate tissue composition in gynecologic tumors [8]. DW images can qualitatively analyze the myometrial invasion depth of endometrial cancer [9, 10], especially in combination with T2WI [11]. Apparent diffusion coefficient (ADC) values allow normal endometrium or benign lesions to be differentiated from endometrial carcinoma [12, 13]; however, they could not quantitatively diagnose the myometrial infiltration depth of endometrial cancer [13, 14]. According to FIGO 2009, a tumor that invades ≥50% of the myometrium is defined as deep myometrium infiltration of endometrial cancer [15], whereas superficial myometrial invasion is defined as tumor invasion < 50% of the myometrium invasion depth. The integration of the junctional zone is very important for the assessment of myometrium infiltration depth [16]. However, in the presence of pitfalls such as a loss of junctional zone definition, poor tumor to myometrium contrast, myometrial compression by polypoid tumor, leiomyomas, and adenomyosis, morphologic inspection are challenging for the accurate assessment of myometrial invasion depth [17]. As the previously studies reported, in a normal uterus, the ADC value of junctional zone was the lowest among the three layers and the highest in the outer myometrium [18, 19]. The most important prognostic factor is the variation of invasion depth with different degrees of integration of the junctional zone, as mentioned above. Hence, a change in diffusion may also be present in the peritumoral zone of endometrial cancer.

The purpose of this study was to explore the diagnostic value of the ADC value of the peritumoral zone for predicting the myometrial invasion depth of endometrial cancer in comparison with the ADC value of the tumor.

Methods

Study population

Our institutional review board approved this prospective study, and all study participants provided informed consent.

All patients were histopathologically confirmed to have primary untreated endometrial cancer via fractional dilatation and curettage or biopsy. Patients were excluded if they had (a) any contraindications for MRI (such as a cardiac pacemaker or defibrillator, insulin pump, aneurysm clip, implanted neural stimulator, cochlear implant, or metal shrapnel or bullet); (b) pelvic or hip metal prostheses; (c) not provided informed consent; (d) any contraindications for surgery; or (e) unavailable postoperative histological reports.

Between April 2012 and January 2014, based on surgery and pathology, a total of 58 consecutive patients (mean age 54 ± 8.3 years, range 34–69 years) were enrolled. All the patients underwent pelvic MRI as part of their initial staging before surgery.

Imaging protocol

The MRI was performed with a 3.0-T MRI unit (Signa HDx 3.0 T, GE Medical Systems, GE Healthcare, Waukesha, Wis, USA) with an 8US TORSOPA coil. All subjects had fasted for 6 h and were trained to hold their breaths at the end of expiration before scanning. For all examinations, patients were placed in the supine position and had a partially filled bladder. T1-weighted, T2-weighted, and DW images of the pelvis were acquired. Fast spin-echo T2-weighted images were initially obtained in the sagittal, axial, and coronal planes with the following parameters: repetition time (TR)/echo time (TE) 3680–6240 ms/85–89 ms, field of view 30–35 cm, number of acquired signals 2, section thickness 5 mm, and bandwidth 35.71–83.33 KHz. Following this sequence, axial fast spin-echo T1-weighted images were acquired with the following parameters: number of acquired signals 2, section thickness 5 mm, and bandwidth 50 KHz.

Axial oblique DW imaging (oblique to the corpus) of the pelvis was performed using the single-shot echo-planar technique with fat suppression (TR/TE 5000 ms/67.6 ms, matrix 128 × 128, field of view 35 × 35 cm, number of acquired signals 4, section thickness 5 mm, and b values 0 and 1000 s/mm^2). The array spatial sensitivity encoding technique was used as the parallel imaging technique during DW image scanning. The ADC map of each DW image was produced with a GE Advantage Windows (AW) 4.4 Workstation.

Imaging analysis

All MR sequences were randomized in order and viewed by two radiologists with 10 and 8 years of experience in gynecologic radiology, who were blinded to the histopathological findings and patients' names, but were aware that the patients had been diagnosed with endometrial cancer. Disagreements were resolved by consensus. For visual inspection, the readers evaluated the standard anatomic sequences (T1-and T2-weighted imaging) as well as the DW images for the depth of myometrial invasion, which was scored as 'superficial' if the tumor invaded up to 50% of the myometrial thickness and 'deep' if the tumor extended beyond 50% of the myometrium thickness. Tumor maximal diameter (as tumor size) [20–22] was calculated on multiple sequences, and the largest value was recorded. Quantitative analysis of DW images was performed using ADC maps which were generated on the scanner console using the $b = 1000$ s/mm^2 and $b = 0$ s/mm^2 images. Regions of interest (ROIs) were applied to tumors and peritumoral zones. The peritumoral zone was defined as a 5-mm-thick zone surrounding and adjacent to the cancerous endometrium [23]. The radiologists reviewed the T2 and DW images and determined the location of the deepest invasion of the tumor. An elliptical ROI (mean area, 20mm^2) was then drawn along the deepest invasion margin of the lesion for measuring the ADC of the peritumoral zone. The pictorial illustration of ROI placement on peritumoral zone is depicted in Fig. 1. For measuring the ADC of the tumor, ROIs were applied to the tumor that contained the largest endometrial cancerous area, avoiding artifacts from the neoplastic/non-neoplastic interface and visible lesions or vascular structures in the myometrium. The ROI setting was on the cross-section of the T2-weighted image obtained via echo planar imaging ($b = 0$ s/mm^2), and it was manually copied to the corresponding ADC map, whereupon ADC values were automatically calculated (Fig. 2). For quality control, the placements of ROIs were determined by the two radiologists. Disagreements were resolved by consensus. The measurement was repeated three times and the interval between the measurements was 1 week. The final data recorded was ADCm (mean ADC) value averaged from the three measurements by the two radiologists.

Histopathological analysis

All endometrial cancer patients underwent a total abdominal hysterectomy and bilateral salpingo-oophorectomy, including 20 patients who underwent pelvic lymphadenectomy simultaneously. After resection, the uterus was cut into 5 mm-thick axial sections for evaluation of myometrial invasion depth, which was performed the same way as the MRI interpretation. A pathologist with 15 years of experience in gynecologic disease who was blinded to the imaging results assessed FIGO stage, histological type, tumor grade (G1, well differentiated; G2, moderately differentiated; and G3, poorly differentiated), and depth of myometrial invasion (superficial myometrial invasion, the tumor invades < 50% of the myometrium; deep myometrial invasion, the tumor invades ≥50% of the myometrium).

Statistical analysis

The ADCm values of the superficial and deep myometrial invasion of the tumor or peritumoral zone were compared using the independent sample *t*-test; two-tailed *p* values of < 0.05 were considered statistically significant. The cutoff ADCm value of the peritumoral zone in endometrial cancer was obtained by drawing a receiver operating characteristic (ROC) curve. In order to maximize both of sensitivity and specificity, we applied the Youden's index (Youden's index = Sensitivity+Specificity-1). We chose the point closest to the upper left corner of the curve as a cutoff, where the Youden's index was maximal. The cutoff ADCm value and visual inspection were used as the diagnostic indexes to evaluate deep myometrial invasion. The sensitivity, specificity, positive predictive value (PPV), and negative predictive value (NPV) of the ADCm cutoff and visual inspection were calculated and represented with 95% confidence intervals. All statistical analyses were performed by IBM SPSS

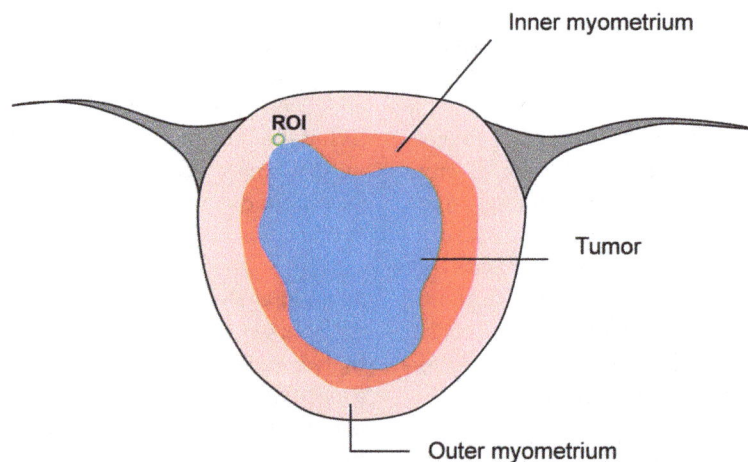

Fig. 1 The pictorial illustration of ROI placement on peritumoral zone of endometrial cancer. The tumor area is in blue, and the inner & outer myometrium is in red&pink. An elliptical region of interest (ROI) was drawn along the margin of deepest invasion of the tumor (i.e., peritumoral zone)

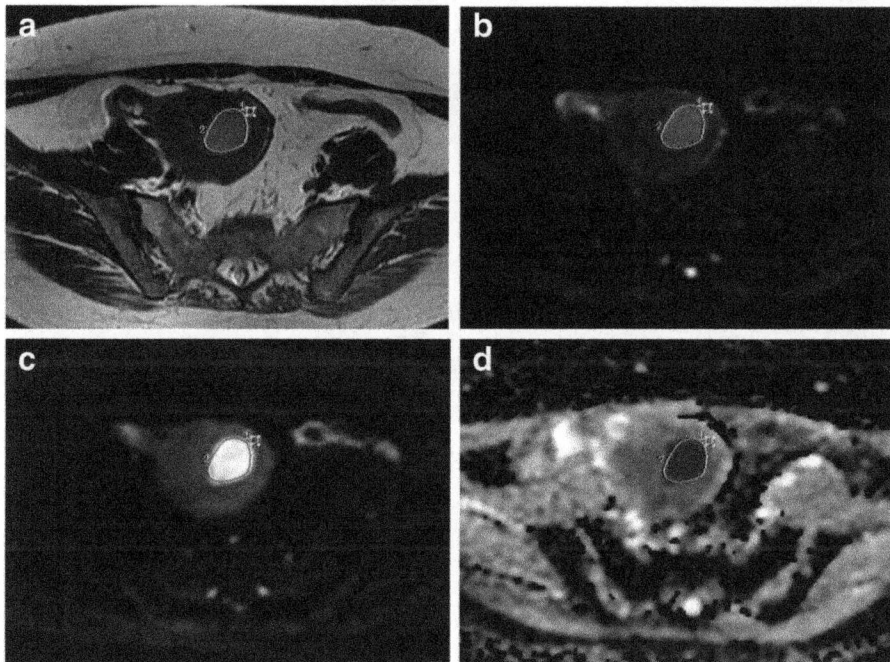

Fig. 2 Endometrial adenocarcinoma with superficial myometrial invasion in a 43-year-old woman. An elliptical region of interest (ROI) was placed on peritumoral zone (ROI$_1$ with green color), which was assessed subjectively on a cross-section of the T2-weighted image obtained by echo planar imaging ($b = 0$ s/mm^2). In addition, a freehand ROI (ROI$_2$ with pink color) was placed on the tumor which contained the largest endometrial cancerous area, avoiding artifacts from the neoplastic/non- neoplastic interface and visible lesions or vascular structures in the myometrium. **a** T2-weighted image; **b** diffusion-weighted magnetic resonance image ($b = 0$ s/ mm^2); **c** diffusion-weighted magnetic resonance image ($b = 1000$ s/mm^2); **d** apparent diffusion coefficient map

statistical software, version 19.0. The ROC curve was drawn using Stata/SE 12.0 for windows. The pictorial illustration of the ROI placement was drawn by FREEHAND, version 11.0.2.

Results

Histopathological findings

The intervals between MRI examination and surgery were 0–21 days (mean 4 days). Of the 58 patients with endometrial cancer, postoperative histological assessment revealed endometrioid adenocarcinoma in 43, adenosquamous carcinoma in 11, mixed endometrioid/serous papillary carcinoma in 2, and mixed endometrioid/mucinous papillary carcinoma in 2. The tumor was confined to the endometrium or involved the inner half of the myometrium (superficial myometrial invasion) in 41 cases, and involved the outer half of the myometrium (deep myometrial invasion) in the remaining 17 cases. The relevant histopathological findings are shown in Table 1.

Quantitative analysis

Of the 58 endometrial cancers, the mean tumor size was 3.9 ± 1.9 cm. The ADCm values of tumor and the peritumoral zone were $(0.83 \pm 0.11) \times 10^{-3}$ mm^2/sec and $(1.06 \pm 0.22) \times 10^{-3}$ mm^2/sec, respectively. There was no significant difference between the ADCm values of tumor in the

superficial and deep myometrial invasion groups (superficial invasion, 0.84×10^{-3} mm^2/sec and deep invasion, 0.82×10^{-3} mm^2/sec; $p > 0.05$). The ADCm value at the peritumoral zone of the deep myometrial invasion and that of the superficial myometrial invasion were 1.23×10^{-3} mm^2/sec and 0.99×10^{-3} mm^2/sec, respectively, which was a significant difference ($p = 0.005$) (Table 2 and Fig. 3).

Table 1 Patients' surgical and pathological findings

	Variable	Data
Myometrial invasion	superficial	41
	deep	17
	endometrioid	43
Histological type	adenosquamous	11
	mixed endometrioid/mucinous papillary	2
	mixed endometrioid/serous papillary	2
Histological grade	1	13
	2	36
	3	9

FIGO International federation of gynecology and obstetrics

Table 2 Apparent diffusion coefficient values for different depth of myometrial invasion ($\times 10^{-3}$ mm^2/sec)

	Peritumoral zone		Tumor	
	ADC	p	ADC	p
Superficial	0.99 ± 0.15	0.005*	0.84 ± 0.10	> 0.05
Deep	1.23 ± 0.27		0.82 ± 0.14	

ADC Apparent diffusion coefficient
*p < 0.05 was considered a statistically significant difference

Diagnostic performance of the ADC cutoff value of the peritumoral zone and the visual inspection

The diagnostic performances of the two methods for assessing deep myometrial involvement are summarized in Table 3. The ADC cutoff value of the peritumoral zone for assessing deep myometrial invasion was 1.17×10^{-3} mm^2/sec. An additional figure file shows this in more detail [see Additional file 1]. For assessing deep myometrial invasion of endometrial cancer, the specificity for the ADCm cutoff value of the peritumoral zone (0.93) was higher than for visual inspection (0.80), as were the PPVs (ADCm, 0.77; vs. visual inspection, 0.60). The areas under the ROC curve (Az) were 0.76 for both methods, but the diagnostic accuracy for the ADCm cutoff value (83%) was higher than for visual inspection. The ROC curves are depicted in Fig. 4.

Discussion

Our results suggested that the ADCm of a tumor could not differentiate deep myometrial invasion from superficial myometrial invasion in endometrial cancer, which is concordant with previous researches [13, 14]. However, the ADCm of the peritumoral zone in the deep myometrial invasion group differed significantly from that of the superficial myometrial invasion group, and was therefore potentially useful for ruling out deep myometrial invasion. Moreover, it was more accurate than visual inspection for assessing deep myometrial invasion, and so could be used as a quantitative MRI tool for helping assess deep myometrial invasion of endometrial cancer.

DW imaging is a functional technique that provides information about water mobility, tissue cellularity, and the integrity of the cellular membrane. In biological tissues, water mobility, i.e., Brownian motion, is restricted via interaction with cell membranes and macromolecules at a microscopic level. In addition to providing essential qualitative information regarding the diffusivity of water molecules in a given tissue, DW imaging enables quantitative information to be obtained with the use of ADC maps [24]. Calculating the ADC can provide quantitative analysis of Brownian motion. The higher the signal of a region in a DW image, the lower the ADC values are, indicating thicker tissues with more densely populated cells [25].

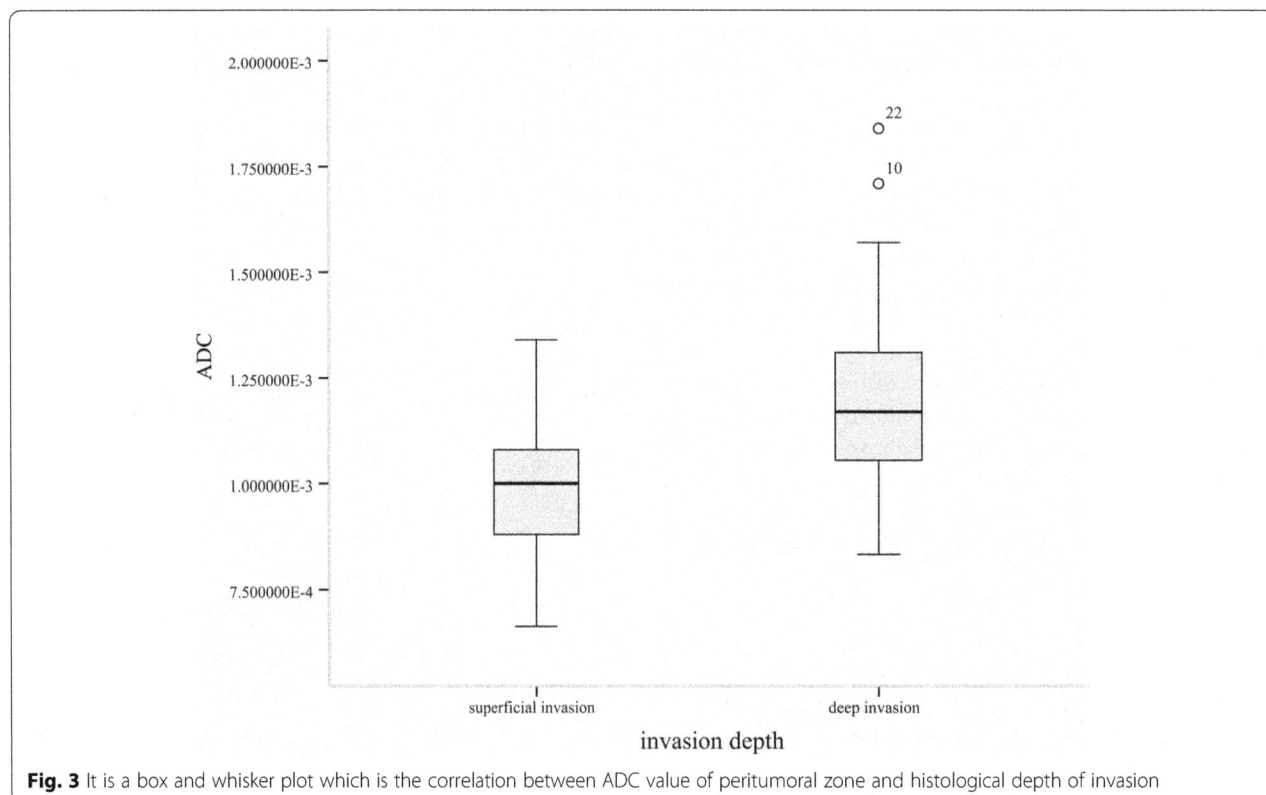

Fig. 3 It is a box and whisker plot which is the correlation between ADC value of peritumoral zone and histological depth of invasion

Table 3 Diagnostic performance of deep myometrial invasion assessment by ADC cutoff value and visual inspection of peritumoral zone

Method	Findings				Acc	Az	Sensitivity (95% CI)	Specificity (95% CI)	NPV (95% CI)	PPV (95% CI)
	TP	FP	FN	TN						
ADC cutoff	10	3	7	38	0.83	0.76	0.59	0.93	0.84	0.77
							(0.33–0.81)	(0.79–0.98)	(0.70–0.93)	(0.46–0.94)
Visual inspection	12	8	5	33	0.78	0.76	0.71	0.80	0.87	0.60
							(0.44–0.89)	(0.65–0.91)	(0.71–0.95)	(0.36–0.80)

Data are means and numbers in parentheses are 95% confidence intervals

ADC Apparent diffusion coefficient, *Az* Area under the receiver operating characteristic curve, *Acc* Accuracy, *NPV* Negative predictive value, *PPV* Positive predictive value, *CI* Confidence interval, *TP* True-positive, *FP* False-positive, *FN* False-negative, *TN* True-negative

In this study, the peritumoral zone was defined as a 5-mm-thick zone surrounding and adjacent to the cancerous endometrium. In patients with normal endometrium, it is the junctional zone of the uterus. Three distinct layers can be visualized via T2-weighted MRI in a normal uterus: a high signal intensity layer corresponding to the endometrial stripe, an inner low signal intensity layer that is adjacent to the basal endometrium (the junctional zone or subendometrial layer), and an outer medium signal intensity subserosal zone or outer myometrium [26]. The junctional zone has increased nuclear area, decreased extracellular matrix, and lower water content in comparison with the outer myometrium. In addition, junctional zone myocytes are thought to express different extracellular matrix components [27, 28]. These features not only shorten the T2 but also restrict diffusion, which gives rise to a low signal zone on the ADC map and the lowest ADC value of this region in the normal uterus [18]. Previous studies showed that in the normal uterus, the ADC value of the junctional zone was the lowest among the three layers and that of the outer myometrium was the highest [18, 19]. In deep myometrium infiltration of endometrial cancer, the tumor invades ≥50% of the myometrium and thus appears as a complete disruption of the junctional zone. When this happens, the peritumoral zone actually includes a majority of the outer myometrium and a small amount of cancerous tissue, which is indicated by a higher signal zone on T2-weighted imaging and ADC maps in comparison with the normal junctional zone. In contrast, in superficial myometrial invasion (< 50% of myometrium invasion depth), the peritumoral zone consists of partial junctional zone, partial outer myometrium, and a small amount of cancerous tissue which exhibit a lower signal in comparison with deep myometrial invasion on T2-weighted imaging and ADC maps. Accordingly, there should be a restricted diffusion difference between deep and superficial myometrial invasion. This was confirmed by our result showing that the ADCm of peritumoral zone of deep myometrial invasion (1.23×10^{-3} mm²/sec) was significantly greater than that of superficial myometrial invasion (0.99×10^{-3} mm²/sec) ($p = 0.005$). Thus, the ADCm value of the peritumoral zone may provide useful information for differentiating deep myometrial invasion from superficial myometrial invasion in endometrial cancer.

In the current study, in endometrial cancer patients, the ADCm values of the tumor exhibiting deep myometrial invasion and superficial myometrial invasion did not differ significantly. This finding is concordant with results previously reported by Lin et al. [14] and Rechichi et al. [13]. A possible explanation for this finding is that cellular density

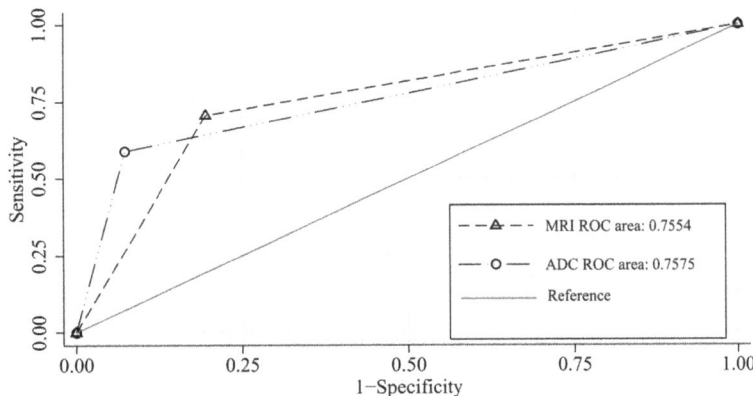

Fig. 4 Az values of the two methods obtained from ROC

and medium interstice are the main factors affecting Brownian motion. A tissue with high cellular density and medium interstice, such as neoplastic tissue, corresponds to high signal in DW imaging. Conversely, tissue with lower signal in DW imaging (i.e., normal issue) corresponds to a region with a higher ADC value [24]. Notably however, other important features of tumor cells such as nuclear atypia cannot be assessed by DW imaging [29]. That is, the ADC value alone is not sufficient for ascertaining the invasiveness of a tumor.

The current study had some limitations. One was the small size of the deep myometrial invasion group. The deep infiltration group included 17 patients (29.3% of the entire study group), which might have biased the sensitivity, specificity, PPV, and NPV of the two assessment methods such that they did not reach statistical significance. Moreover, the study lacked objective assessments to determine the location of the deepest myometrial invasion where an ROI should be set.

Conclusion

The ADC value obtained at the peritumoral zone can predict deep myometrial invasion of endometrial cancer. This value could therefore enhance confidence in the preoperative evaluation of endometrial cancer, and be useful when tailoring the surgical approach.

Abbreviations

ADC: Apparent diffusion coefficient; ADCm: Mean apparent diffusion coefficient; DW: Diffusion-weighted; FIGO: Federation of Gynecology and Obstetrics; MRI: Magnetic resonance imaging; NPV: Negative predictive value; PPV: Positive predictive value; ROC: Receiver operating characteristic; ROI: Region of interest; TE: Echo time; TR: Repetition time

Acknowledgements

We would like to thank Editage (www.editage.cn) for English language editing, and Mr. Tao Song for the pictorial illustration.

Funding

Not applicable.

Authors' contributions

LD, LB and RY made substantial contributions to conception and design, acquisition of data, analysis and interpretation of data; NY, X-yD and Q-pW were involved in drafting the manuscript. Q-xY and Y-mG gave final approval of the version to be published. Q-xY agreed to be accountable for all aspects of the work in ensuring that questions related to the accuracy or integrity of any part of the work are appropriately investigated and resolved. All authors read and approved the final manuscript.

Competing interests

The authors declare that they have no competing interests.

Author details

[1]Department of Radiology, the First Affiliated Hospital, Xi'an Jiaotong University Xi'an, #277, Yanta West Road, Xi'an 710061, Shaanxi, China. [2]Department of Radiology, the Northwest Women and Children Hospital, #1616, Yanxiang Road, Xi'an 710054, Shaanxi, China. [3]Department of Nuclear Medicine, the First Affiliated Hospital, Xi'an Jiaotong University Xi'an, #277, Yanta West Road, Xi'an 710061, Shaanxi, China. [4]Department of Radiology, The Affiliated Hospital of Shaanxi University of traditional Chinese Medicine, #2. Wei Yang West Road, Xian Yang 712000, Shaanxi, China.

References

1.   Siegel R, Ma J, Zou Z, Jemal A. Cancer statistics, 2014. CA Cancer J Clin. 2014;64(1):9–29.
2.   Burke WM, Orr J, Leitao M, Salom E, Gehrig P, Olawaiye AB, Brewer M, Boruta D, Villella J, Herzog T, et al. Endometrial cancer: a review and current management strategies: part I. Gynecol Oncol. 2014;134(2):385–92.
3.   Rockall AG, Meroni R, Sohaib SA, Reynolds K, Alexander-Sefre F, Shepherd JH, Jacobs I, Reznek RH. Evaluation of endometrial carcinoma on magnetic resonance imaging. Int J Gynecol Cancer. 2007;17(1):188–96.
4.   Larson DM, Connor GP, Broste SK, Krawisz BR, Johnson KK. Prognostic significance of gross myometrial invasion with endometrial cancer. Obstet Gynecol. 1996;88(3):394–8.
5.   Berman ML, Ballon SC, Lagasse LD, Watring WG. Prognosis and treatment of endometrial cancer. Am J Obstet Gynecol. 1980;136(5):679–88.
6.   Morice P, Leary A, Creutzberg C, Abu-Rustum N, Darai E. Endometrial cancer. Lancet. 2015;
7.   Hardesty. Use of preoperative MR imaging in the Management of Endometrial Carcinoma Cost Analysis. Radiology. 2000;215(1)
8.   Thoeny HC, Forstner R, De Keyzer F. Genitourinary applications of diffusion-weighted MR imaging in the pelvis. Radiology. 2012;263(2):326–42.
9.   Gallego JC, Porta A, Pardo MC, Fernandez C. Evaluation of myometrial invasion in endometrial cancer: comparison of diffusion-weighted magnetic resonance and intraoperative frozen sections. Abdom Imaging. 2014;39(5): 1021–6.
10. Das SK, Niu XK, Wang JL, Zeng LC, Wang WX, Bhetuwal A, Yang HF. Usefulness of DWI in preoperative assessment of deep myometrial invasion in patients with endometrial carcinoma: a systematic review and meta-analysis. Cancer Imaging. 2014;14(1):32.
11. Deng L, Wang Q-p, Chen X, Duan X-y, Wang W, Guo Y-m. The combination of diffusion- and T2-weighted imaging in predicting deep myometrial invasion of endometrial Cancer: a systematic review and meta-analysis. J Comput Assist Tomogr. 2015;39(5):661–73.
12. Fujii S, Matsusue E, Kigawa J, Sato S, Kanasaki Y, Nakanishi J, Sugihara S, Kaminou T, Terakawa N, Ogawa T. Diagnostic accuracy of the apparent diffusion coefficient in differentiating benign from malignant uterine endometrial cavity lesions: initial results. Eur Radiol. 2008;18(2):384–9.
13. Rechichi G, Galimberti S, Signorelli M, Franzesi CT, Perego P, Valsecchi MG, Sironi S. Endometrial cancer: correlation of apparent diffusion coefficient with tumor grade, depth of myometrial invasion, and presence of lymph node metastases. AJR Am J Roentgenol. 2011;197(1):256–62.
14. Lin G, Ng KK, Chang CJ, Wang JJ, Ho KC, Yen TC, Wu TI, Wang CC, Chen YR, Huang YT, et al. Myometrial invasion in endometrial cancer: diagnostic accuracy of diffusion-weighted 3.0-T MR imaging–initial experience. Radiology. 2009;250(3):784–92.
15. Pecorelli S. Revised FIGO staging for carcinoma of the vulva, cervix, and endometrium. Int J Gynaecol Obstet. 2009;105(2):103–4.
16. Beddy P, O'Neill AC, Yamamoto AK, Addley HC, Reinhold C, Sala E. FIGO staging system for endometrial cancer: added benefits of MR imaging. Radiographics. 2012;32(1):241–54.
17. Sala E, Rockall A, Kubik-Huch RA. Advances in magnetic resonance imaging of endometrial cancer. Eur Radiol. 2011;21(3):468–73.
18. Kuang F, Ren J, Huan Y, Chen Z, Zhong Q. Apparent diffusion coefficients of normal uterus in premenopausal women with 3.0-T magnetic resonance imaging. J Comput Assist Tomogr. 2012;36(1):54–9.
19. Kilickesmez O, Bayramoglu S, Inci E, Cimilli T, Kayhan A. Quantitative diffusion-weighted magnetic resonance imaging of normal and diseased uterine zones. Acta Radiol (Stockholm, Sweden: 1987). 2009;50(3):340–7.

20. Bourgioti C, Chatoupis K, Tzavara C, Antoniou A, Rodolakis A, Moulopoulos LA. Predictive ability of maximal tumor diameter on MRI for high-risk endometrial cancer. Abdom Radiol (NY). 2016;41(12):2484–95.

21. Yang Y, Zhao L, Wang Z, Tang J, Geng J, Hong N, Wang J, Wei L. Clinical value of transvaginal ultrasound, MRI and hysteroscopy in the assessment of endometrial cancer lesion size. Zhonghua fu chan ke za zhi. 2016;51(1):36–9.

22. Berretta R, Patrelli TS, Migliavacca C, Rolla M, Franchi L, Monica M, Modena AB, Gizzo S. Assessment of tumor size as a useful marker for the surgical staging of endometrial cancer. Oncol Rep. 2014;31(5):2407–12.

23. McLaughlin RL, Newitt DC, Wilmes LJ, Jones EF, Wisner DJ, Kornak J, Proctor E, Joe BN, Hylton NM. High resolution in vivo characterization of apparent diffusion coefficient at the tumor-stromal boundary of breast carcinomas: a pilot study to assess treatment response using proximity-dependent diffusion-weighted imaging. J Magn Reson Imaging. 2014;39(5):1308–13.

24. Colagrande S, Pallotta S, Vanzulli A, Napolitano M, Villari N. The diffusion parameter in magnetic resonance: physics, techniques, and semeiotics. La Radiologia Medica. 2005;109(1–2):1–16.

25. Manenti G, Di Roma M, Mancino S, Bartolucci D, Palmieri G, Mastrangeli R, Miano R, Squillaci E, Simonetti G. Malignant renal neoplasms: correlation between ADC values and cellularity in diffusion weighted magnetic resonance imaging at 3 T. La Radiologia Medica. 2008;113(2):199–213.

26. Fusi L, Cloke B, Brosens JJ. The uterine junctional zone. Best Pract Res Clin Obstet Gynaecol. 2006;20(4):479–91.

27. McCarthy S, Scott G, Majumdar S, Shapiro B, Thompson S, Lange R, Gore J. Uterine junctional zone: MR study of water content and relaxation properties. Radiology. 1989;171(1):241–3.

28. Scoutt LM, Flynn SD, Luthringer DJ, McCauley TR, McCarthy SM. Junctional zone of the uterus: correlation of MR imaging and histologic examination of hysterectomy specimens. Radiology. 1991;179(2):403–7.

29. Whittaker CS, Coady A, Culver L, Rustin G, Padwick M, Padhani AR. Diffusion-weighted MR imaging of female pelvic tumors: a pictorial review. Radiographics. 2009;29(3):759–74. discussion 774-758

20

Accuracy of F-18 FDG PET/CT with optimal cut-offs of maximum standardized uptake value according to size for diagnosis of regional lymph node metastasis in patients with rectal cancer

Sung Uk Bae[1], Kyoung Sook Won[2], Bong-Il Song[2], Woon Kyung Jeong[1], Seong Kyu Baek[1] and Hae Won Kim[2]* ⓘD

Abstract

Background: The low sensitivity of F-18 fluorodeoxyglucose (FDG) positron emission tomography/computed tomography (PET/CT) for the evaluation of metastatic lymph nodes (LNs) is mainly due to the partial volume effect in patients with rectal cancer. This retrospective study evaluated the diagnostic accuracy of F-18 FDG PET/CT with optimal cut-off values of the maximum standardized uptake value (SUV_{max}), according to LN size, for the evaluation of regional LN in rectal cancer patients.

Methods: This study included 176 patients with rectal cancer who underwent F-18 FDG PET/CT for initial staging. Patients were classified based on the long-axis diameter of the regional LN on CT images as small (≤ 7 mm; $n = 118$) and large (> 7 mm; $n = 58$) LN groups. The optimal cut-off value of SUV_{max} was determined for each group, using receiver operating characteristic curve analysis. Areas under the curve (AUC) were compared by C-statistics using two methods: the cut-off value of SUV_{max} optimized according to LN size, and a fixed SUV_{max} cut-off value of 2.5.

Results: The optimal cut-off values of SUV_{max} for the small and large LN groups were 1.1, and 2.1, respectively. The sensitivity, specificity, and accuracy of F-18 FDG PET/CT using the optimal cut-off values were 90.6, 70.9, and 76.3% in the small LN group, and 68.6, 78.3, and 72.4% in the large LN group. The sensitivity, specificity, and accuracy of F-18 FDG PET/CT using the fixed cut-off value were 18.8, 100, and 78.0% in the small LN group, and 51.4, 87.0, and 65.5% in the large LN group. The AUC was significantly higher using the optimal cut-off values than the fixed cut-off value (0.808 vs. 0.594, $p = 0.005$) in the small LN group, but not in the large LN group (0.734 vs. 0.692, $p = 0.429$).

Conclusions: Application of the lower cut-off value of SUV_{max} improves the diagnostic performance of F-18 FDG PET/CT for the evaluation of small regional LNs in patients with rectal cancer.

Keywords: Rectal cancer, Lymph node metastasis, Maximum standardized uptake value, Partial volume effect, F-18 FDG, PET/CT

* Correspondence: hwkim.nm@gmail.com
[2]Department of Nuclear Medicine, Keimyung University Dongsan Medical Center, 56 Dalseong-ro, Jung-gu, Daegu 41931, Republic of Korea
Full list of author information is available at the end of the article

Background

Globally, colorectal cancer is the second most common cancer in women and the third most common cancer in men [1]. In Korea, the rectum was the most common site of cancer among both men and women in 1999 and again in 2009 [2]. Lymph node (LN) metastasis is one of the most important prognostic factors for patients with rectal cancer [3]. Additionally, LN metastasis plays a primary role in the determination of the operability and the extent of LN dissection. Survival is directly related to the presence of residual metastatic LNs after the primary operation. The accurate diagnosis of LN metastasis in initial staging may improve the prognosis and allow the early use of second-line therapy in patients with rectal cancer [4].

Conventional computed tomography (CT) and magnetic resonance imaging (MRI) have been commonly used for LN staging in patients with rectal cancer. However, both CT and MRI are limited by low sensitivity in the evaluation of small metastatic LNs [5–8]. Recently, F-18 fluorodeoxyglucose (FDG) positron emission tomography/computed tomography (PET/CT) has been proven to be useful for the preoperative staging of rectal cancer by revealing metabolic information of the lesion [9–11]. However, F-18 FDG PET/CT has also shown low sensitivity for the detection of LN metastasis [12, 13]. The low sensitivity of F-18 FDG PET/CT in the evaluation of metastatic LNs is mainly due to the partial volume effect, which spills out of the radioactivity into the background of small lesions < 10 mm in size, leading to underestimation of the true standardized uptake value (SUV) [14–16].

Several methods have been developed to correct the partial volume effect, and have significantly improved the diagnostic accuracy of metastatic LNs [17, 18]. However, there have been several limitations of the clinical use of partial volume correction due to the complexity of the method. Any method to consider size differences of LNs on F-18 FDG PET/CT images must be practical. Previous studies of an F-18 FDG PET/CT quantitative approach used a fixed cut-off of the maximum standardized uptake value (SUV_{max}) in the diagnosis of LN metastasis, without considering the size differences of the LNs. Application of optimal SUV_{max} cut-off values according to LN size may improve the sensitivity of F-18 FDG PET/CT and may be practically useful for evaluation of the regional LNs in patients with rectal cancer. Thus, the aim of this study was to evaluate the diagnostic accuracy of F-18 FDG PET/CT using optimal SUV_{max} cut-off values according to LN size to evaluate regional LNs in patients with rectal cancer.

Subjects and methods

Study population

We retrospectively analyzed the medical records of patients who underwent preoperative F-18 FDG PET/CT followed by curative operations for rectal cancer at our institution between January 2009 and August 2016. We excluded patients who underwent preoperative chemoradiation therapy and those with an interval of > 4 weeks between F-18 FDG PET/CT and surgery. A retrospective cross-sectional analysis was performed to review the surgical and pathological findings and the F-18 FDG PET/CT results. Patients were classified based on the long-axis diameter of the regional LN on CT images as small (≤ 7 mm; $n = 118$) and large (> 7 mm; $n = 58$) LN groups. The reference value for long-axis diameter was determined as 7 mm, because the partial volume effect is significant when the target of interest is smaller than 2 times of the PET/CT system's full-width at half-maximum (FWHM) (< 8 mm) [18], and the long-axis diameter range on multiple detector CT has been reported as 7–10 mm for the diagnosis of metastatic regional LN [19, 20]. This study was approved by the Institutional Review Board of our institution.

Histopathologic examination

All surgeries were performed by qualified, experienced colorectal surgeons. Mesorectal excisions were performed in all patients; extended LN dissections were only performed if metastatic LNs were detected in frozen biopsies. All resected LNs underwent histopathologic exams for pathologic confirmation while labeling the exact location. The sensitivity, specificity, and accuracy of F-18 FDG PET/CT were calculated using the histopathologic result as the gold standard. A true positive was defined as a match between the location of the metastatic LN on pathologic examination and the location of the positive LN on an F-18 FDG PET/ CT image.

F-18 FDG petPET/CT

Two different F-18 FDG PET/CT systems were used (Discovery STE 16, GE Healthcare, Milwaukee, WI, USA; and Biograph mCT 64, Siemens Healthcare, Knoxville, TN, USA). The patients were required to fast for > 6 h before the scan, and the blood glucose level was measured to confirm that the level was < 180 mg/dL before injecting the F-18 FDG. In patients with diabetes, administration of antihyperglycemic drugs was stopped 12 h before the scan. Patients received intravenous administration of 4.0 MBq/kg (Biograph mCT) and 7.0 MBq/kg (Discovery STE) F-18 FDG according to the PET/CT system. Patients were encouraged to rest during the F-18 FDG uptake period. Images were acquired

60 min after F-18 FDG administration. A non-contrast CT scan was obtained for attenuation correction and localization. Immediately after the CT scan, PET images were acquired from the base of the skull or top of the brain to the proximal thigh. The Discovery STE-16 PET/CT scanner acquired images with a slice thickness of 3.75 mm simultaneously for a longitudinal field of view (FOV) of 780 mm. The transaxial FOV was 70 cm, and the matrix size was 128×128. Spatial resolution in air was 4.29 mm FWHM. The PET images were reconstructed from CT data for attenuation correction using the OSEM iterative algorithm with 20 subsets and two iterations. The Biograph mCT-64 PET/CT scanner acquired images with a slice thickness of 3 mm simultaneously for a longitudinal FOV of 500 mm. The transaxial FOV was 58.8 cm, and the matrix size was 256×256. Spatial resolution in air was 4 mm FWHM. The PET images were reconstructed from CT data for attenuation correction using the TrueX algorithm and an all-pass filter with 21 subsets and two iterations.

An experienced nuclear physician blinded to the histopathologic and colonoscopic results reviewed the F-18 FDG PET/CT images on a workstation (Advantage Workstation version 4.3; GE Healthcare). The locations of the regional LNs were recorded as the perirectal, superior rectal, inferior mesenteric, or internal iliac areas. Suspicious lymph nodes less than 3 mm were ignored because they cannot be differentiated from vascular structures or other nonspecific soft tissue densities. The ROIs (long-axis diameter range, 3–17 mm) were drawn in consensus around the regional LNs, and the SUV_{max} was measured using each dedicated PET workstation (ADW version 4.3 for Discovery STE-16 and syngo MI for Biograph mCT-64). The optimal SUV_{max} cut-off values were determined using receiver operating characteristic curve (ROC) analysis for the small and large LN groups. When the measured SUV_{max} exceeded the optimal cut-off value or 2.5, the LN was considered positive. In addition, subgroup analyses were performed according to the PET/CT scanner (PET A and B), T stage (early and advanced T stages), and F-18 FDG uptake of the primary tumor (low and high tumor SUV_{max}). Patients who were examined using the Discovery STE-16 PET/CT scanner were classified into the PET A group and patients who were examined using the Biograph mCT-64 PET/CT scanner were classified into the PET B group. Patients with T1 or T2 stage were classified into the early T stage group and patients with T3 or T4 stage were classified into the advanced T stage group. Patients with SUV_{max} of the primary tumor lower than 13.0, which was the median value of SUV_{max}, were classified into the low tumor SUV_{max} group and patients with SUV_{max} of the primary tumor higher than 13.0 were classified into the high tumor SUV_{max} group. The optimal SUV_{max} cut-off values were determined for each subgroup.

Statistical analyses

The optimal cut-off values of the SUV_{max} in each group and each subgroup were calculated using ROC analysis. The sensitivities, specificities, and accuracies of PET/CT using the optimal SUV_{max} cut-off values according to LN size, and a fixed SUV_{max} cut-off value of 2.5, were calculated for each group, each subgroup, and for all patients together. The areas under the curve (AUCs) of the optimal and fixed SUV_{max} cut-off values were compared using C-statistics. A p-value < 0.05 was considered significant.

Results

Patient characteristics

Of 296 patients who underwent preoperative F-18 FDG PET/CT and follow-up curative surgery for rectal cancer, 120 patients were excluded from this study according to the exclusion criteria (Fig. 1). A total of 176 patients were included. Table 1 summarizes the patient characteristics. Patients were classified into the small ($n = 118$) or large ($n = 58$) LN groups. Regional LN metastasis was confirmed pathologically in 32 patients (27.1%) in the small LN group, and 35 patients (60.3%) in the large LN group.

The SUV_{max} of large LNs was significantly higher than that of small LNs in the overall patient analysis (3.2 vs. 1.2, $p < 0.001$). There was no significant difference in the SUV_{max} of small and large LNs between the PET A and B groups (1.2 vs. 1.2, $p = 0.964$ and 2.6 vs. 3.7, $p = 210$). The SUV_{max} of the small LN in the advanced T stage group was significantly higher than that in the early T stage group (1.5 vs. 1.0, $p < 0.001$), but the SUV_{max} of large LN was not significantly different between these two groups (3.6 vs. 2.0, $p = 0.110$). The SUV_{max} of the small LN in the high tumor SUV_{max} group was significantly higher than that in the low tumor SUV_{max} group (1.0 vs. 1.4, $p < 0.016$), but the SUV_{max} of large LN was not significantly different between these two groups (3.6 vs. 2.5, $p = 0.230$).

Accuracy of F-18 FDG PET/CT

The optimal cut-off values of SUV_{max} for the diagnosis of regional LN metastasis were 1.1 in the small LN group, and 2.1 in the large LN group. The sensitivity, specificity, accuracy, and AUC using the optimal SUV_{max} cut-off values were 90.6, 70.9, 76.3%, and 0.808 in the small LN group, and 68.6, 78.3, 72.4%, and 0.734 in the large LN group, respectively (Table 2). Using the fixed SUV_{max} cut-off value of 2.5, the corresponding values were 18.8, 100, 78.0%, and 0.594 in the small LN group,

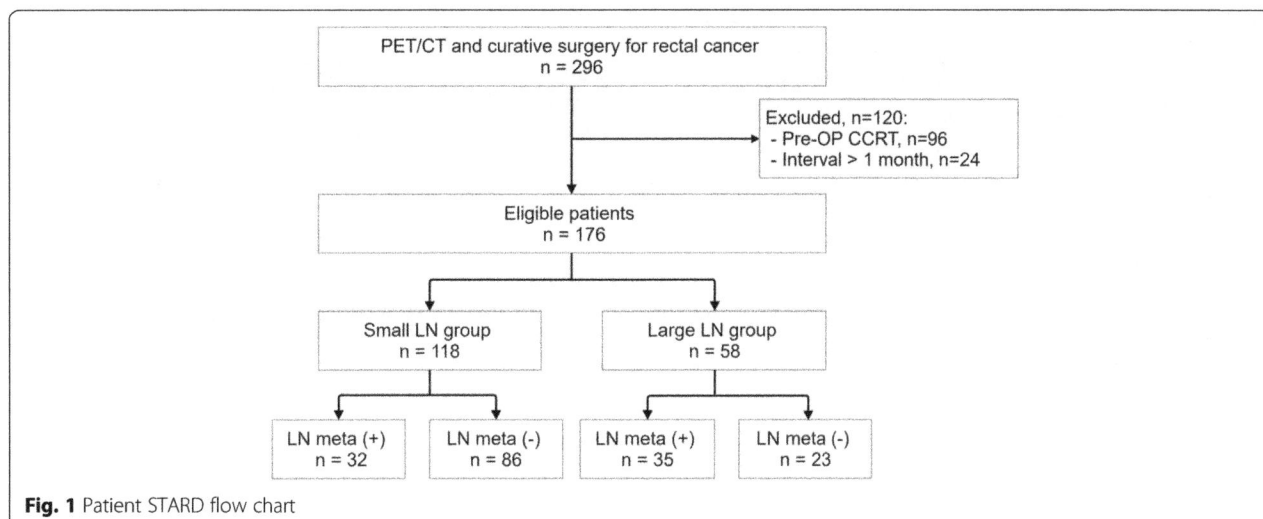

Fig. 1 Patient STARD flow chart

and 51.4, 87.0, 65.5%, and 0.692 in the large LN group, respectively. The AUCs of PET/CT using the optimal cut-off values were significantly higher than those using the fixed cut-off value of 2.5 in the small LN group ($p = 0.005$). Figure 2 shows a representative

Table 1 Patient characteristics

Characteristics[a]	Overall ($n = 176$)	Group[b]	
		Small LN[c] ($n = 118$)	Large LN ($n = 58$)
Age, years	66.7 (10.4)	67.4 (9.3)	65.3 (12.4)
Male, %	56.8	61	48.3
AJCC[d] Stage, n			
I	69	59	10
II	38	27	11
III	69	32	37
IV	0	0	0
LN diameter, mm	6.2 (3.0)	4.6 (1.7)	9.4 (2.5)
SUV$_{max}$ of LN	1.8 (2.2)	1.2 (0.7)	3.2 (3.2)
PET/CT scanner, n			
Discovery STE-16	79	54	25
Biograph mCT-64	97	64	33
T stage, n			
T1–2	81	68	13
T3–4	95	50	45
SUV$_{max}$ of primary tumor, n			
High SUV$_{max}$ (< 13.0)	84	64	20
Low SUV$_{max}$ (> 13.0)	92	54	38

[a]All values are presented as means (SD)
[b]Patients were categorized by the long-axis diameter of the regional LN, as follows: small LN, ≤ 7 mm; large LN, > 7 mm
[c]LN lymph node
[d]AJCC American Joint Committee on Cancer

case of regional LN metastasis that was predicted by using the optimal SUV$_{max}$ cut-off values, but not by the fixed SUV$_{max}$ cut-off value of 2.5. There was no significant difference in the AUC between the two methods in the large LN group ($p = 0.429$).

In overall patients, the sensitivity, specificity, accuracy, and AUC of F-18 FDG PET/CT, using the optimal cut-off values, were 76.1, 74.3, 75.0%, and 0.752, respectively whereas on using the fixed cut-off value, the sensitivity, specificity, accuracy, and AUC were 35.8, 97.2, 73.9%, and 0.665, respectively. The AUC of PET/CT using the optimal cut-off value was higher than that using the fixed cut-off value of 2.5 in all patients, but not statistically significant ($p = 0.071$).

Subgroup analysis was performed according to the PET/CT scanner. In the PET A group, the optimal cut-off values of SUV$_{max}$ were 1.1 for small LN and 2.1 for large LN. In the PET B group, the optimal cut-off values of SUV$_{max}$ were 1.0 for small LN and 1.9 for large LN. Table 3 shows the sensitivity, specificity, accuracy, and AUC in the PET A and B groups. In the small LN of the PET A group, the AUC using the optimal cut-off value was significantly higher than that using the fixed cut-off value of 2.5 ($p = 0.047$). There were no significant differences in the AUCs between PET/CT using the optimal and fixed cut-off values in the large LN of the PET A group ($p = 0.866$), as well as small and large LNs of the PET B group ($p = 0.110$ and $p = 0.162$). Subgroup analysis according to the T stage revealed that the optimal cut-off values were 0.9 for small LN and 1.8 for large LN in the early T stage group and 1.1 for small LN and 2.1 for large LN in the advanced T stage group. There were no significant differences in the AUCs between PET/CT using the optimal and fixed cut-off values in the small and large LNs of the early and advanced T stage groups ($p = 0.188$, $p = 1.000$, $p = 0.231$

Table 2 Comparison of the diagnostic values between PET/CT using the cut-off values of SUV$_{max}$ optimized according to the lymph node (LN) size and the fixed SUV$_{max}$ cut-off value of 2.5

Group	Cut-off values	Sensitivity (%)	Specificity (%)	PPV[a] (%)	NPV[b] (%)	Accuracy (%)	AUC[c]	p
Overall	2.5	35.8	97.2	88.9	71.1	73.9	0.665	0.071
	Opt[d]	76.1	74.3	64.6	83.5	75	0.752	
Small LN	2.5	18.8	100	100	76.8	78	0.594	0.005
	1.1	90.6	70.9	53.7	95.3	76.3	0.808	
Large LN	2.5	51.4	87	85.7	54.1	65.5	0.692	0.429
	2.1	68.6	78.3	82.8	62.1	72.4	0.734	

[a]*PPV* positive predictive value
[b]*NPV* negative predictive value
[c]*AUC* area under the curve
[d]*Opt* optimal cut-off values of SUV$_{max}$ (1.1 in the small LN group and 2.1 in the large LN group)

and $p = 0.822$). Additional file 1: Table S1 shows the sensitivity, specificity, accuracy, and AUC in the early and advanced T stage groups. Subgroup analysis according to the SUV$_{max}$ of the primary tumor revealed that the optimal cut-off values were 1.0 for small LN and 1.3 for large LN in the low tumor SUV$_{max}$ group, and 1.1 for small LN and 2.1 for large LN in the high tumor SUV$_{max}$ group. There were no significant differences in the AUCs between PET/CT using the optimal and fixed cut-off values in the small and large LNs of the low and high tumor SUV$_{max}$ groups ($p = 0.070$, $p = 0.908$, $p = 0.177$ and $p = 0.491$). Additional file 2: Table S2 shows the sensitivity, specificity, accuracy, and AUC in the low and high tumor SUV$_{max}$ groups.

Discussion

The present study revealed improved diagnostic performance of F-18 FDG PET/CT in the evaluation of metastatic LNs in patients with rectal cancer using the optimal SUV$_{max}$ cut-off values according to the size of the LN. Application of a lower SUV$_{max}$ cut-off value to evaluate a small LN increased the sensitivity of PET/CT in the detection of metastatic LNs in patients with rectal cancer. The AUCs of the PET/CT with optimal SUV$_{max}$ cut-off values were significantly higher than those with a fixed cut-off value of 2.5 in the small LN group. These results suggest that F-18 FDG PET/CT can diagnose LN metastasis as accurately in small LNs as in large LNs if a lower SUV$_{max}$ cut-off value is applied. Although the concept of this hypothesis is widely known, the present study proved it practically in sufficient number of patients with rectal cancer.

LN metastasis in rectal cancer is directly correlated with prognosis. The 5-year survival rate is > 95% in rectal cancer patients without LN metastasis, but decreases to 50~ 70% in patients with LN metastasis [3]. Additionally, the LN stage of rectal cancer is one of the most important determining factors for adjuvant chemotherapy and extended LN dissection [21, 22]. The procedure of choice for rectal cancer patients with a clinical stage of N0 or N1 is total mesorectal excision, which is surgical excision of the mesorectal fat, including all LNs. In more

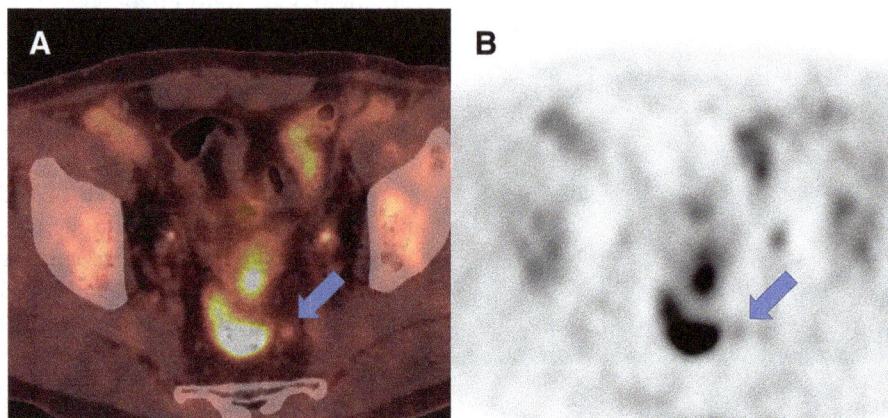

Fig. 2 A representative case of regional LN metastasis predicted by optimal SUV$_{max}$ cut-off values, but not by the fixed SUV$_{max}$ cut-off value of 2.5. (**a**) A mildly hypermetabolic lymph node (arrow) was observed in the left perirectal region. The long-axis diameter of the LN was 6 mm, and the patient was classified into the small LN group according to the size criteria. (**b**) The SUV$_{max}$ of the LN was 1.8, and exceeded the optimal SUV$_{max}$ cut-off value of 1.1. Histopathologic examination revealed that the lesion was a metastatic LN

Table 3 Comparison of diagnostic values between PET/CT using the optimized cut-off values and the fixed cut-off value of 2.5 in patients imaged by PET A and B

Groups	Cut-off values	Sensitivity (%)	Specificity (%)	PPV[a] (%)	NPV[b] (%)	Accuracy (%)	AUC[c]	p
PET A								
Overall	2.5	36.7	98.0	91.7	71.6	74.7	0.673	0.169
	Opt	76.7	77.6	67.6	84.4	77.2	0.771	
Small LN	2.5	18.8	100.0	100.0	74.5	75.9	0.594	0.047
	1.1	87.5	73.7	58.3	93.3	77.8	0.806	
Large LN	2.5	57.1	90.9	88.9	62.5	72.0	0.740	0.866
	2.1	78.6	72.7	78.6	72.7	76.0	0.756	
PET B								
Overall	2.5	35.1	96.7	86.7	70.7	73.2	0.659	0.520
	Opt	75.7	65.0	57.1	81.3	69.1	0.703	
Small LN	2.5	18.8	100.0	100.0	78.7	79.7	0.594	0.110
	1.0	93.8	60.4	44.1	96.7	68.8	0.771	
Large LN	2.5	47.6	83.3	83.3	47.6	60.6	0.655	0.162
	1.9	61.9	83.3	86.7	55.6	69.7	0.726	

[a]*PPV* positive predictive value
[b]*NPV* negative predictive value
[c]*AUC* area under the curve
[d]*Opt* optimal cut-off values of SUV_{max}

advanced cancers with a clinical stage of N2, preoperative concurrent chemoradiotherapy is recommended. Extended LN dissection is required in patients with suspected metastatic LNs in the lateral pelvic region [23–25]. Application of the optimal SUV_{max} cut-off values according to the LN size allows determination of treatment strategies and improves the prognosis of patients with rectal cancer by improving the accuracy of the diagnosis of LN metastasis with F-18 FDG PET/CT.

F-18 FDG PET/CT is beneficial in the preoperative staging of rectal cancer, though it showed low sensitivity and accuracy in the diagnosis of LN metastasis [12, 13]. There is no definite evidence supporting F-18 FDG PET/CT as the routine clinical application in the evaluation of LN metastasis, though F-18 FDG PET/CT could be used to supplement the possibility of suspected metastatic LNs detected by other imaging modalities. For a quantitative approach to the diagnosis of LN metastasis on F-18 FDG PET/CT images, a fixed cut-off value of SUV_{max} of 2.5 has been commonly used to diagnose metastatic LNs [5, 12]. However, the sensitivity (38~65%) of F-18 FDG PET/CT in the diagnosis of LN metastasis were low compared to those of CT and MRI [13]. In accordance with previous studies, the corresponding values using a fixed SUV_{max} cut-off value of 2.5 in the present study were comparably low. However, there was significant improvement in the sensitivity of PET/CT when using an SUV_{max} cut-off value optimized according to LN size.

The primary cause of the low sensitivity of F-18 FDG PET/CT in the diagnosis of LN metastasis is the partial volume effect [14–16], which causes the underestimation of radioactivity concentration in structures with less than two to three times the spatial resolution of PET (4~5 mm). Due to the partial volume effect, the quantitative evaluation of LN metastasis has not been a routine practice in the interpretation of F-18 FDG PET/CT images. Due to the partial volume effect, lower optimal SUV_{max} cut-off values were determined for the evaluation of small LNs than for the large LNs. Several techniques have been developed to calibrate the partial volume effect. In addition, many studies revealed significant improvement in the diagnostic performance of F-18 FDG PET/CT for the determination of small lesions after partial volume correction [17, 18]. However, partial volume correction methods are generally too complex to be clinically applicable, and most require additional equipment or applications. Therefore, we applied the optimal SUV_{max} cut-off values according to LN size to compensate for the partial volume effect, which resulted in significant improvement in the AUC. This approach could be a more rapid and simpler method for calibration of the partial volume effect.

CT and MRI have conventionally been used to evaluate LN metastasis in rectal cancer by evaluating the size and shape of the LN [5, 6]. A diameter of 5~10 mm has been applied as the threshold to diagnose metastatic LNs, but many studies have revealed the limitations of using size criteria alone for LN staging in rectal cancer.

Approximately 60% of metastatic LNs are < 5 mm in diameter [26]. Therefore, evaluating the shape of the LN can also be useful in diagnosis. In most metastatic LNs, the loss of the fatty hilum and kidney bean-shaped structure can be detected. A recent meta-analysis study including 12 CT studies reported that the pooled sensitivity and specificity of CT for LN metastasis were 71% and 67%, respectively [27]. Another meta-analysis study including 21 MRI studies reported that the pooled sensitivity and specificity of MRI for LN metastasis were 77 and 71%, respectively [28]. In the present study, F-18 FDG PET/CT using a fixed SUV_{max} cut-off value of 2.5 showed low sensitivity (35.8%) and high specificity (97.2%), whereas F-18 FDG PET/CT using SUV_{max} cut-off values optimized according to size showed high sensitivity (76.1%) and high specificity (74.3%). The diagnostic value of the present study is considered to be comparable to those of previous CT or MRI studies. However, direct comparison of diagnostic value is limited between the present study and previous CT or MRI studies, because there are heterogeneities between studies including differences in protocols, radiologists' experience, approach to image interpretation, and methodologic quality. Further studies with comparison of diagnostic value between F-18 FDG PET/CT, CT, and MRI in the same patient population could provide important information in selecting diagnostic modalities for preoperative staging of rectal cancer.

The limitation of the present study was the use of two different scanners (Discovery STE-16, GE Healthcare; and Biograph mCT-64, Siemens Healthcare), which could not be avoided owing to the retrospective study design. The difference in the resolution and administered dose of F-18 FDG, according to the two different scanners, could have caused differences in the SUV_{max} and could have affected some of the results of the present study. However, previous studies have shown that the difference in the SUV_{max} of the same lesion between two different scanners is < 0.05 [29]. In the present study, there were no significant differences in the SUV_{max} of small and large LNs between the two scanners. Furthermore, the difference between the optimal cut-off values of the two scanners was only 0.1 for small LNs. Although the effect of using two different scanners on the results of the present study would be negligible, further prospective studies involving the use of one PET/CT scanner and a large population are needed for more valid optimal cut-off values.

Conclusions

Application of the lower cut-off value of SUV_{max} increases the sensitivity of F-18 FDG PET/CT for evaluation of the small regional LNs in patients with rectal cancer. F-18 FDG PET/CT using the optimized SUV_{max}

cut-off values according to the LN size has the potential to show improved diagnostic performance for the detection of regional LN metastasis in patients with rectal cancer. Further prospective studies involving the use of one PET/CT scanner and a large population are needed.

Abbreviations

AUC: areas under the curve; CT: conventional computed tomography; FDG: fluorodeoxyglucose; LN: lymph node; MRI: magnetic resonance imaging; PET/CT: positron emission tomography/computed tomography; ROC: receiver operating characteristic curve; SUV: standardized uptake value; SUV_{max}: maximum standardized uptake value

Funding

This study was supported by a National Research Foundation of Korea (NRF) grant funded by the Korea Government (MSIP) (no. 2014R1A5A2010008 and no. 2017R1C1B5017721).

Authors' contributions

HWK and SUB participated in the design of the study, and drafted the manuscript. SUB, WKJ and SKB collected the patients'data. BWK and BS processed the figures, helped draft the manuscript, and performed a critical revision of the manuscript. KSW and SUB conceived and designed the study and supervised the project. All authors read and approved the final version of the manuscript.

Competing interests

The authors declare that they have no competing interests

Author details

[1]Department of Surgery, Keimyung University Dongsan Medical Center, Daegu, Republic of Korea. [2]Department of Nuclear Medicine, Keimyung University Dongsan Medical Center, 56 Dalseong-ro, Jung-gu, Daegu 41931, Republic of Korea.

References

1. Shaukat A, Church TR. Colorectal-cancer incidence and mortality after screening. N Engl J Med. 2013;369(24):2355.
2. Shin A, Kim KZ, Jung KW, Park S, Won YJ, Kim J, et al. Increasing trend of colorectal cancer incidence in Korea, 1999-2009. Cancer Res Treat. 2012;44(4):219–26.
3. Zhou L, Wang JZ, Wang JT, Wu YJ, Chen H, Wang WB, et al. Correlation analysis of MR/CT on colorectal cancer lymph node metastasis characteristics and prognosis. Eur Rev Med Pharmacol Sci. 2017;21(6):1219–25.
4. Glynne-Jones R, Wyrwicz L, Tiret E, Brown G, Rodel C, Cervantes A, et al. Rectal cancer: ESMO Clinical Practice Guidelines for diagnosis, treatment and follow-up. Ann Oncol. 2017;28(suppl_4):iv22–40.
5. Tateishi U, Maeda T, Morimoto T, Miyake M, Arai Y, Kim EE. Non-enhanced CT versus contrast-enhanced CT in integrated PET/CT studies for nodal staging of rectal cancer. Eur J Nucl Med Mol Imaging. 2007;34(10):1627–34.
6. Bipat S, Glas AS, Slors FJ, Zwinderman AH, Bossuyt PM, Stoker J. Rectal cancer: local staging and assessment of lymph node involvement with endoluminal US, CT, and MR imaging--a meta-analysis. Radiology. 2004;232(3):773–83.

7. Kim NK, Kim MJ, Yun SH, Sohn SK, Min JS. Comparative study of transrectal ultrasonography, pelvic computerized tomography, and magnetic resonance imaging in preoperative staging of rectal cancer. Dis Colon Rectum. 1999;42(6):770–5.

8. Park IJ, Kim HC, Yu CS, Ryu MH, Chang HM, Kim JH, et al. Efficacy of PET/CT in the accurate evaluation of primary colorectal carcinoma. Eur J Surg Oncol. 2006;32(9):941–7.

9. Kijima S, Sasaki T, Nagata K, Utano K, Lefor AT, Sugimoto H. Preoperative evaluation of colorectal cancer using CT colonography, MRI, and PET/CT. World J Gastroenterol. 2014;20(45):16964–75.

10. Abdel-Nabi H, Doerr RJ, Lamonica DM, Cronin VR, Galantowicz PJ, Carbone GM, et al. Staging of primary colorectal carcinomas with fluorine-18 fluorodeoxyglucose whole-body PET: correlation with histopathologic and CT findings. Radiology. 1998;206(3):755–60.

11. Kantorova I, Lipska L, Belohlavek O, Visokai V, Trubac M, Schneiderova M. Routine (18)F-FDG PET preoperative staging of colorectal cancer: comparison with conventional staging and its impact on treatment decision making. J Nucl Med. 2003;44(11):1784–8.

12. Tsunoda Y, Ito M, Fujii H, Kuwano H, Saito N. Preoperative diagnosis of lymph node metastases of colorectal cancer by FDG-PET/CT. Jpn J Clin Oncol. 2008;38(5):347–53.

13. Brush J, Boyd K, Chappell F, Crawford F, Dozier M, Fenwick E, et al. The value of FDG positron emission tomography/computerised tomography (PET/CT) in pre-operative staging of colorectal cancer: a systematic review and economic evaluation. Health Technol Assess. 2011;15(35):1–192. iii-iv

14. Rahmim A, Qi J, Sossi V. Resolution modeling in PET imaging: theory, practice, benefits, and pitfalls. Med Phys. 2013;40(6):064301.

15. Soret M, Bacharach SL, Buvat I. Partial-volume effect in PET tumor imaging. J Nucl Med. 2007;48(6):932–45.

16. Steinert HC, Hauser M, Allemann F, Engel H, Berthold T, von Schulthess GK, et al. Non-small cell lung cancer: nodal staging with FDG PET versus CT with correlative lymph node mapping and sampling. Radiology. 1997;202(2):441–6.

17. Boussion N, Cheze Le rest C, Hatt M, Visvikis D. Incorporation of wavelet-based denoising in iterative deconvolution for partial volume correction in whole-body PET imaging. Eur J Nucl Med Mol Imaging. 2009;36(7):1064–75.

18. Bettinardi V, Castiglioni I, De Bernardi E, Gilardi M. PET quantification: strategies for partial volume correction. Clin Transl Imaging. 2014;2(3):199–218.

19. Inoue Y, Saigusa S, Hiro J, Toiyama Y, Araki T, Tanaka K, et al. Clinical significance of enlarged lateral pelvic lymph nodes before and after preoperative chemoradiotherapy for rectal cancer. Mol Clin Oncol. 2016;4(6):994–1002.

20. Rollven E, Abraham-Nordling M, Holm T, Blomqvist L. Assessment and diagnostic accuracy of lymph node status to predict stage III colon cancer using computed tomography. Cancer Imaging. 2017;17(1):3.

21. Choi PW, Kim HC, Kim AY, Jung SH, Yu CS, Kim JC. Extensive lymphadenectomy in colorectal cancer with isolated Para-aortic lymph node metastasis below the level of renal vessels. J Surg Oncol. 2010;101(1):66–71.

22. Song SH, Park SY, Park JS, Kim HJ, Yang CS, Choi GS. Laparoscopic Para-aortic lymph node dissection for patients with primary colorectal cancer and clinically suspected Para-aortic lymph nodes. Ann Surg Treat Res. 2016;90(1):29–35.

23. Akasu T, Sugihara K, Moriya Y. Male urinary and sexual functions after mesorectal excision alone or in combination with extended lateral pelvic lymph node dissection for rectal cancer. Ann Surg Oncol. 2009;16(10):2779–86.

24. Kim DJ, Chung JJ, Yu JS, Cho ES, Kim JH. Evaluation of lateral pelvic nodes in patients with advanced rectal cancer. AJR Am J Roentgenol. 2014;202(6):1245–55.

25. Yano H, Saito Y, Takeshita E, Miyake O, Ishizuka N. Prediction of lateral pelvic node involvement in low rectal cancer by conventional computed tomography. Br J Surg. 2007;94(8):1014–9.

26. Brown G, Richards CJ, Bourne MW, Newcombe RG, Radcliffe AG, Dallimore NS, et al. Morphologic predictors of lymph node status in rectal cancer with use of high-spatial-resolution MR imaging with histopathologic comparison. Radiology. 2003;227(2):371–7.

27. Nerad E, Lahaye MJ, Maas M, Nelemans P, Bakers FC, Beets GL, et al. Diagnostic accuracy of CT for local staging of Colon Cancer: a systematic review and meta-analysis. Am J Roentgenol. 2016;207(5):984–95.

28. Al-Sukhni E, Milot L, Fruitman M, Beyene J, Victor JC, Schmocker S, et al. Diagnostic accuracy of MRI for assessment of T category, lymph node metastases, and circumferential resection margin involvement in patients with rectal cancer: a systematic review and meta-analysis. Ann Surg Oncol. 2012;19(7):2212–23.

29. Sunderland JJ, Christian PE. Quantitative PET/CT scanner performance characterization based upon the society of nuclear medicine and molecular imaging clinical trials network oncology clinical simulator phantom. J Nucl Med. 2015;56(1):145–52.

21

The differentiation of pancreatic neuroendocrine carcinoma from pancreatic ductal adenocarcinoma: the values of CT imaging features and texture analysis

Chuangen Guo[1], Xiaoling Zhuge[2], Qidong Wang[1], Wenbo Xiao[1], Zhonglan Wang[3], Zhongqiu Wang[3], Zhan Feng[1*] and Xiao Chen[3*]

Abstract

Background: Imaging findings for pancreatic neuroendocrine carcinoma (PNEC) and pancreatic ductal adenocarcinoma (PDAC) often overlap. The aim of this study was to demonstrate the value of computed tomography (CT) imaging features and texture analysis to differentiate PNEC from PDAC.

Methods: Twenty-eight patients with pathologically-proved PDAC and 14 patients with PNEC were included in this study. CT imaging findings, including tumor boundary, size, enhancement degree, duct dilatation and parenchymal atrophy were used to compare PDAC and PNEC. CT texture features were extracted from CT images at the arterial and portal phases.

Results: More PNEC than PDAC had well-defined margins (57.1% vs 25.0%, $p = 0.04$). Parenchymal atrophy was more common in PDAC than in PNEC (67.9% vs 28.1%, $p = 0.02$). CT attenuation values (HU) and contrast ratios of PNEC inthe arterial and portal phases were higher than those of PDAC ($p < 0.05$ or 0.01). Entropy was lower and uniformity was higher in PNEC compare to PDAC at the arterial phase ($p < 0.05$). Contrast ratio showed the highest area under curve (AUC) for differentiating PNEC from PDAC (AUC = 0.98–0.99). Entropy and uniformity also showed an acceptable AUC (0.71–0.72).

Conclusions: Our data indicate that CT imaging features, including tumor margin, enhanced degree and parenchymal atrophy, as well as texture parameters can aid in the differentiation of PNEC from PDAC.

Keywords: Pancreatic neuroendocrine carcinoma, Pancreatic ductal adenocarcinoma., Computed tomography., Texture analysis.

Background

Pancreatic neuroendocrine carcinoma (PNEC) is a rare tumor that accounts for 2–3% of pancreatic neuroendocrine neoplasms (PNENs) [1, 2]. Recently, several studies reported that PNEC usually showed hypovascular pattern in contrast-enhanced computed tomography (CT) or magnetic resonance imaging (MRI) [3–6]. In addition, ill-defined borders and lymph node invasion are also common in PNEC. These key imaging features are also critical imaging findings in pancreatic ductal adenocarcinoma (PDAC). Overlaps in imaging findings between PNEC and PDAC have been reported previously [7]. In a prior study, we found that 57% of PNEC was misdiagnosed as PDAC [6].

The treatment strategies and prognosis of PNEC and PDACs are substantially different. For PNEC, surgical therapy is available if curative resection is possible even in cases with limited metastases [8, 9]. In addition, several reports indicate that therapy with sunitinib or everolimus is also helpful for PNEC [10, 11]. Usually, the prognosis of

* Correspondence: gerxyuan@zju.edu.cn; chxwin@163.com
[1]Department of Radiology, the First Affiliated Hospital, College of Medicine Zhejiang University, 79 Qingchun road, Hangzhou 310003, China
[3]Department of Radiology, the Affiliated Hospital of Nanjing University of Chinese Medicine, 155 Hanzhong road, Nanjing 210029, China
Full list of author information is available at the end of the article

PNEC is better than PDAC. Therefore, correctly identifying PNEC and PDAC is an important prerequistite treatment.

Previous several studies have shown that CT and MRI are useful for differential diagnosis of hypovascular pancreatic tumors [6, 12]. Recently, texture analysis that extracts, analyzes, and interprets quantitative imaging features has been widely used to diagnose, characterize and improve tumor staging and therapy response assessment in cancer field [13]. Canellas et al. [14] indicated that CT texture analysis and CT features are predictive for PNENs aggressiveness. However, to the best of our knowledge, no studies have examined differences in texture parameters between PNEC and PDAC. The aim of our study was to investigate the utility of CT imaging findings and CT texture features in identifying PNEC from PDACs.

Material and methods

Study population

We used medical records to identify 21 patients with surgically or biopsy-proven PNEC diagnosed between January 2012 to July 2017 accordance with the WHO 2010 classification for PNENs. Seven patients were excluded because they did not receive a preoperative CT examination or lacked dynamic contrast-enhanced CT images. We also searched the medical record from January 2017 to July 2017 and identified 78 patients with surgically or biopsy-proven PDAC. Twelve patients who did not receive CT examination or lacked dynamic contrast-enhanced CT images, while six patients whose tumor presented as dominantly cystic were also excluded. Among the remaining 60 subjects, we randomly selected 28 patients in a proportion of 1: 2 with respect to PNEC. Ultimately, a total of 28 PDAC patients and 14 PNEC patients were included in this study. Histological diagnose of PNEC were based on the following criteria: PNEC G3, > 20 mitoses per 10 HPF, Ki-67 index > 20%. This retrospective study was approved by institutional review board of the Affiliated Hospital of College of Medicine Zhejiang University and the need for formal consent of patients was waived.

CT protocol

All CT imaging was performed using the same multidetector CT system (Brilliance 128, Philips Healthcare, Best, The Netherlands) following to a standardized protocol. Three phase images (conventional, arterial and portal venous) were obtained from each patient. The CT scanning parameters were as the following: tube voltage of 120 kV; slice thickness of 3 mm; beam collimation, 128×0.625 mm; and automatic tube current modulation. Contrast-enhanced CT images were obtained after intravenous administration of iohexol (300 mg/mL, Bayer Health Care Pharmaceuticals, Germany) at a rate of 3.0 mL/s via a power injector (1.5 ml/kg), followed by a 20-mL bolus of sodium chloride. The enhanced images were obtained at the arterial phase (30–35 s) and the portal phase (55–60s).

Image analysis

The images were reviewed by two abdominal radiologists with more than six years of clinical experience. They were blind to the pathologic data. The following imaging parameters were recorded based on the unenhanced images: tumor location, size, tumor margins (well-circumscribed or ill-defined border), pancreatic duct dilatation, parenchymal atrophy (absent or present), and lymph node invasion or local invasion (confirmed by histological examination). The definition of tumor margin was obtained from a previous study [15]. Well-circumscribed was defined as smooth margins without spiculation or with less than 80% infiltration, and pancreatic duct dilation was defined as a main pancreatic duct diameter ≥ 4 mm. Quantitative data, including tumor attenuation on unenhanced CT scan, contrast ratio at arterial phase (AER) [Hounsfield Unit (HU) values of tumor/HU values of normal parenchyma measured in the arterial phase], and contrast ratio at portal venous phase (PER) (HU values of tumor/HU values of normal parenchyma measured in the portal phase), were also measured. For AER and PER measurements, the regions of interest (ROIs) were set at the solid components, avoiding necrotic or cystic components.

Texture analysis

The images obtained at the arterial phase and portal phase were used for texture analysis. ROIs were manually drawn in every visualized tumor images in consensus by two abdominal radiologists. The necrotic components were excluded from ROIs. One of them performed the texture analysis by using Matlab2014b (MathWorks, Natick, MA, USA). The regions outside the ROI were set with the average value ofthe pixels inside the ROI in order to reduce the impact of nontarget regions. Texture data from the whole tumor was obtained. We used the filtration-histogram approach and Laplacian-of-Gaussian band-pass filters (sigma values of 0.5, 1.5 and 2.5). The texture parameters under different filters, including kurtosis, skewness, entropy and uniformity, were analyzed. The mathematical expression and means of those parameters have been described in a previous report [14].

Statistical analysis

Data were managed and analyzed with SPSS 16.0 (SPSS Inc., Chicago, IL, USA). Quantitative data were displayed as means ± standard deviations and qualitative data were expressed as numbers (percentage). We used the χ^2 text or Fisher exact test for categorical

Table 1 Patient characteristics and CT imaging findings

Characteristics	PDAC(n = 28)	PNEC(n = 14)	P values
Age(years)	62.6 ± 9.7 (42–75)	56.4 ± 11.6 (25–71)	< 0.05
Gender			0.31
Male	17 (60.7%)	11 (78.6%)	
Female	11 (39.3%)	3 (21.4%)	
Size(cm)	3.56 ± 1.45	5.10 ± 4.42	0.09
Location			0.18
Head or neck	19 (67.9%)	6 (42.9%)	
Body or tail	9 (22.1%)	8 (57.1%)	
Margin			0.04
Well-defined	7 (25.0%)	8 (57.1%)	
Indistinct	21 (75.0%)	6 (42.9%)	
CT attenuation value(HU)			
Un-enhanced phase	33.8 ± 4.76	37.8 ± 5.86	0.23
Arterial phase	44.2 ± 8.56	64.6 ± 10.37	< 0.01
Portal phase	52.3 ± 7.49	64.9 ± 11.06	0.01
Parenchymal atrophy	19 (67.9%)	4 (28.6%)	0.02
Pancreatic duct dilatation	16 (71.4%)	7 (50.0%)	0.19
Positive lymph nodes or local invasion	14 (50.0%)	3 (21.4%)	0.10

PDAC pancreatic ductal adenocarcinomas; *PNEC* pancreatic neuroendocrine carcinoma
CT computed tomography

variables and the Mann-Whitney U test for continuous variables. Receiver operating characteristics (ROC) curve analysis was performed and the area under the curve (AUC), sensitivity, and specificity was calculated to ascertain diagnostic ability. Interobserver agreements in ROIs were assessed with Conger's kappa test. P values < 0.05 were considered statistically significant.

Result

The characteristics of subjects are listed in Table 1. The age of patients with PNEC was lower than that of patients with PDAC($p < 0.05$). CT images of PNEC and PDAC were provided in Fig. 1. Both two lesions showed hypovascular pattern on contrast-enhanced images. No significant differences were found in gender, size, tumor

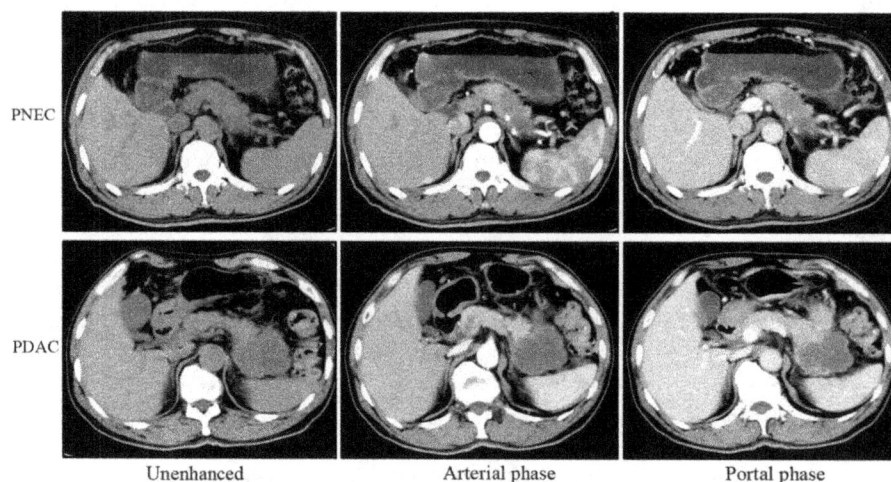

Fig. 1 The computed tomography imaging findings in a 66-year-old woman with pancreatic neuroendocrine carcinoma (PNEC, white arrow) and a 62-year-old man with pancreatic ductal adenocarcinoma (PDAC, black arrow). Unenhanced and contrast-enhanced CT images at the arterial phase and portal phase showed ill-defined, hypovascular mass

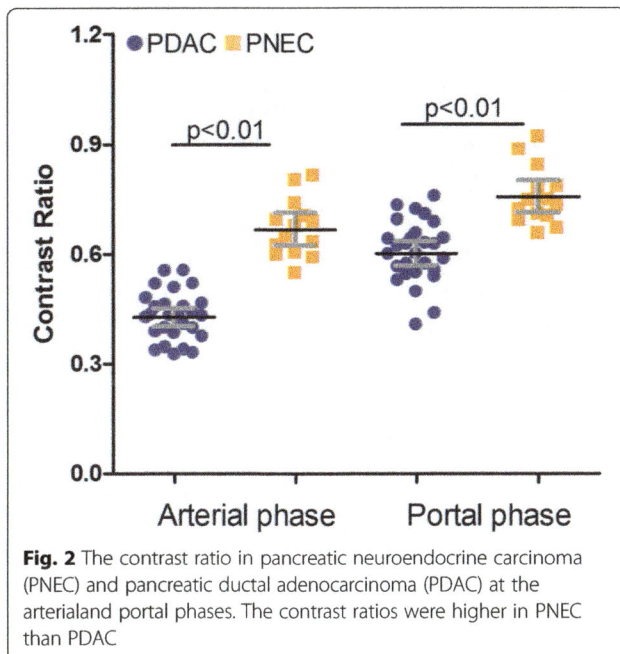

Fig. 2 The contrast ratio in pancreatic neuroendocrine carcinoma (PNEC) and pancreatic ductal adenocarcinoma (PDAC) at the arterialand portal phases. The contrast ratios were higher in PNEC than PDAC

location, and pancreatic duct dilatation between those two lesions. More PNEC showed well-defined margin than the PDAC (57.1% vs 25.0%, $p = 0.04$). Parenchymal atrophy was more common in PDAC than PNEC (67.9% vs 28.1%, $p = 0.02$). Positive lymph nodes or local invasion was more common in PDAC, but no significant differences were observed. The CT attenuation values (HU) of PNEC at arterial and portal phase were higher than those of PDAC ($p < 0.05$ or 0.01). Similar results were observed in contrast ratio (Fig. 2).

Next, we examined the CT texture in PDAC and PNEC. The Kappa value for ROIs was 0.82. No significant differences were observed in kurtosis and skewness between PNEC and PDAC. Compared to PDAC at the portal phase, PNEC had lower entropy and higher uniformity ($p < 0.05$) (Fig. 3). However, no differences were observed at the arterial phase.

The sensitivity and specificity of the different imaging features for differentiating PNEC from PDAC ranged from 0.47–1.00 and 0.57–1.00 (Table 2, Fig. 4). AER and PER showed the higher AUC compared with other markers. For other imaging features, the AUC were 0.66–0.70. The sensitivity and specificity of the texture features (entropy and uniformity) for PNEC identification (vs. PDAC) ranged from 0.74–0.79 and 0.65–0.70 at the portal phase. The AUC were 0.71–0.72 at portal phase.

Discussion

PNEC is a rare pancreatic neuroendocrine neoplasm that is often misdiagnosed as PDAC on qualitative imaging. In the present study, we showed that quantitative imaging analysis, such as contrast ratio at arterial phase and portal phases, can differentiate PNEC from PDAC with good sensitivity and specificity. In addition, our data indicate that texture features (including entropy and uniformity) can also assist in differentiating PNEC and PDAC.

PNEC and PDAC have similar imaging findings, including hypovascular pattern on contrast-enhanced imaging and local or distal metastases. Despite this fact, only a few studies have examined the differentiation between hypovascular PNENs and PDAC. Jeon et al. [12] indicated that the MR enhancement pattern at portal phase or delayed phase was useful in differentiating between hypovascular PNENs from PDAC. They also showed that well-defined margin and lower frequencies of ductal dilatation were more common in hypovascular PNENs than PDAC. In the present study, we also showed that similar enhancement pattern in the portal phase (PER), and tumor margins were helpful in differentiating PNEC from PDAC. However, no differences were observed in ductal dilatation. PNETs G1/G2 with hypovascular enhancement may have been included in their study. In our current study, we only included PNEC G3. However, we previously found that contrast ratio at arterial phase and portal phase in MRI can potentially

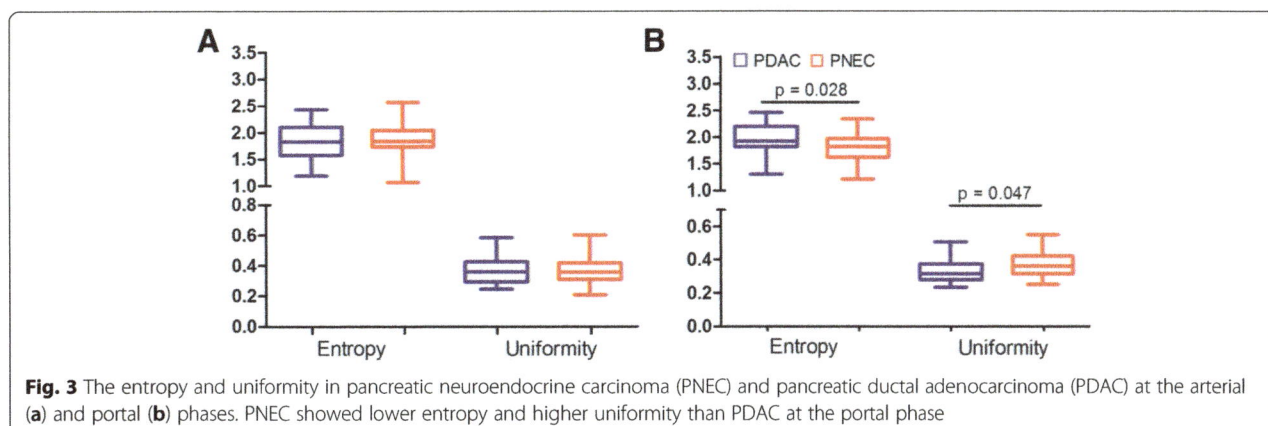

Fig. 3 The entropy and uniformity in pancreatic neuroendocrine carcinoma (PNEC) and pancreatic ductal adenocarcinoma (PDAC) at the arterial (**a**) and portal (**b**) phases. PNEC showed lower entropy and higher uniformity than PDAC at the portal phase

Table 2 Diagnostic performance of CT features and texture features for differentiating PNEC from PDAC

	Variables	AUC	Sensitivity (95% CI)	Specificity (95% CI)	Cutoff point
CT features	AER	0.99	1.0 (0.77–1.0)	0.93 (0.66–1.00)	0.56
	PER	0.98	0.93 (0.66–1.0)	1.00 (0.77–1.00)	0.63
	Size	0.67	0.47 (0.28–0.69)	1.00 (0.72–1.00)	2.73
	Margins	0.66	0.75 (0.55–0.89)	0.57 (0.29–0.82)	
	Parenchymal atrophy	0.70	0.68 (0.48–0.84)	0.71 (0.42–0.92)	
Texture features at portal phase	F3 uniformity	0.72	0.79 (0.54–0.94)	0.65 (0.41–0.85)	0.34
	F3 entropy	0.71	0.74 (0.49–0.91)	0.70 (0.46–0.88)	1.89

f1-f3 denote sigma values of 0.5, 1.5 and 2.5, respectively. *CI* confidence interval; *AER* enhancement ratio at arterial phase; *PER* enhancement ratio at portal phase; *AUC* area under the curve

differentiate the two tumors [6]. Our data based on CT imaging are consistent with the previous findings. Those results demonstrated that quantitative imaging analysis is useful in differentiating PNEC and PDAC.

Interestingly, studies are finding that imaging texture analysis has great potential to improve cancer detection, staging, treatment and prognosis evaluation [13]. Several studies have demonstrated that texture features are valuable to grade PNENs [14–17]. However, the value of texture analysis in differentiating PNEC and PDAC is not well-understood. In our study, we found that PNEC had higher uniformity and lower entropy compared with PDAC on contrast-enhance images at portal phase. Entropy is a measure of randomness in the intensity of images. Entropy and uniformity reflect texture complexity and homogeneity in the tumors, respectively. Entropy is valuable in distinguishing malignant tumors from benign lesions [18]. Shindo et al. [19] showed that the entropy of ADC values in PDAC was higher than PNETs, which was consistent with our findings. Abundant fibrous stroma is typical histopathological features of PDAC. PNEC usually present more cellularity and a lower fibrous stroma [12]. Therefore, the complexity of enhancement in PDAC may be higher than that in PNEC.

Consequently, low uniformity and high entropy are observed in PDAC. Although the ROC analysis showed that the diagnostic performance of texture parameters in differentiating PNEC from PDAC were not better than traditional quantitative indexes (i.e., AER and PER), texture analysis may be an important supplementary analysis for radiologists.

Our study has several following limitations. First, the sample size for PNEC is small due to the rarity of PNEC. Second, selection bias is unavoidable because our study is a retrospective study with single institution design. Third, scan parameters (e.g., slice thickness and reconstruction algorithm) may affect the texture analysis. Finally, since this was an exploratory study, only a few texture parameters were analyzed.

Conclusions

Our data show that CT imaging features, including tumor margin, parenchymal atrophy, and contrast ratio at arterial phase and portal phase, are valuable in differentiating PNEC from PDAC. In addition, our data also indicate that assessing texture parameters – including entropy and uniformity –is a promising future direction for improving differentiation.

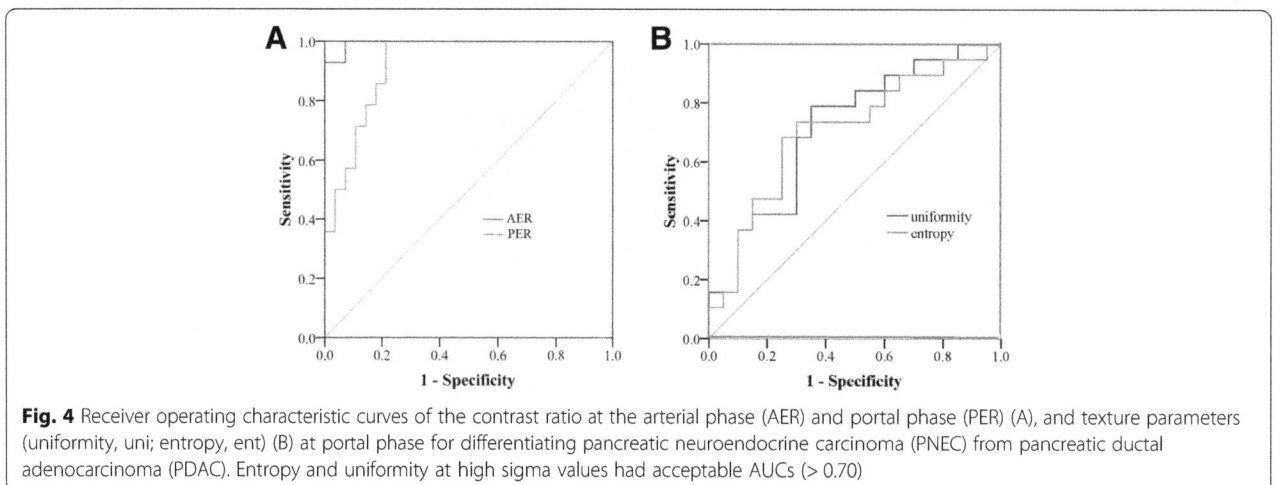

Fig. 4 Receiver operating characteristic curves of the contrast ratio at the arterial phase (AER) and portal phase (PER) (A), and texture parameters (uniformity, uni; entropy, ent) (B) at portal phase for differentiating pancreatic neuroendocrine carcinoma (PNEC) from pancreatic ductal adenocarcinoma (PDAC). Entropy and uniformity at high sigma values had acceptable AUCs (> 0.70)

Abbreviations
(AER: Contrast ratio at arterial phase; AUC: The area under the curve; CT: Computed tomography; HU: Hounsfield Unit; PDAC: Pancreatic ductal adenocarcinoma; PER: Contrast ratio at portal venous phase; PNEC: Neuroendocrine carcinoma; ROC: Receiver operating characteristics; ROI: Regions of interest

Funding
This study was supported by the Zhejiang Medical Science and Technology Project (2017KY331) and Primary Research & Development Plan of Jiangsu Province (BE2017772).

Authors' contributions
GC and XC: designed the study; CG, XZ, ZF, ZW and XC: conducted the experiments; CG, WX, QW, ZF, ZW and XC: analyzed the data; XC and ZW: advised study and revised the draft; CG and XC: wrote the draft. All authors read and approved the final manuscript.

Competing interest
The authors declare that they have no competing interests.

Author details
[1]Department of Radiology, the First Affiliated Hospital, College of Medicine Zhejiang University, 79 Qingchun road, Hangzhou 310003, China. [2]Department of Laboratory Medicine, the First Affiliated Hospital, College of Medicine Zhejiang University, 79 Qingchun road, Hangzhou 310003, China. [3]Department of Radiology, the Affiliated Hospital of Nanjing University of Chinese Medicine, 155 Hanzhong road, Nanjing 210029, China.

References
1. Lewis RB, Lattin GE, Paal E. Pancreatic Endocrine Tumors: Radiologic-Clinicopathologic correlation. Radiographics. 2010;30(6):1445–64.
2. Kim JH, Eun HW, Kim YJ, Han JK, Choi BI. Staging accuracy of MR for pancreatic neuroendocrine tumor and imaging findings according to the tumor grade. Abdom Imaging. 2013;38(5):1106–14.
3. Cappelli C, Boggi U, Mazzeo S, Cervelli R, Campani D, Funel N, et al. Contrast enhancement pattern on multidetector CT predicts malignancy in pancreatic endocrine tumours. Eur Radiol. 2015;25(3):751–9.
4. Kim DW, Kim HJ, Kim KW, Byun JH, Song KB, Kim JH, et al. Neuroendocrine neoplasms of the pancreas at dynamic enhanced CT: comparison between grade 3 neuroendocrine carcinoma and grade 1/2 neuroendocrine tumour. Eur Radiol. 2015;25(5):1375–83.
5. Lotfalizadeh E, Ronot M, Wagner M, Cros J, Couvelard A, Vullierme MP, et al. Prediction of pancreatic neuroendocrine tumour grade with MR imaging features: added value of diffusion-weighted imaging. Eur Radiol. 2017;27(4): 1748–59.
6. Guo C, Chen X, Wang Z, Xiao W, Wang Q, Sun K, et al. Differentiation of pancreatic neuroendocrine carcinoma from pancreatic ductal adenocarcinoma using magnetic resonance imaging: the value of contrast-enhanced and diffusion weighted imaging. Oncotarget. 2017; 8(26):42962–73.
7. Gandhi NS, Feldman MK, Le O, Morris-Stiff G. Imaging mimics of pancreatic ductal adenocarcinoma. Abdom Radiol (NY). 2018;43(2):273–84.
8. Lee L, Igarashi H, Fujimori N, Hijioka M, Kawabe K, Oda Y, et al. Long-term outcomes and prognostic factors in 78 Japanese patients with advanced pancreatic neuroendocrine neoplasms: a single-center retrospective study. Jpn J Clin Oncol. 2015;45(12):1131–8.
9. Ito T, Hijioka S, Masui T, Kasajima A, Nakamoto Y, Kobayashi N, et al. Advances in the diagnosis and treatment of pancreatic neuroendocrine neoplasms in Japan. J Gastroenterol. 2017;52(1):9–18.
10. Gilabert M, Rho YS, Kavan P. Targeted therapies provide treatment options for poorly differentiated pancreatic neuroendocrine carcinomas. Oncology. 2017;92(3):170–2.
11. Liu DJ, Fu XL, Liu W, Zheng LY, Zhang JF, Huo YM, et al. Clinicopathological, treatment, and prognosis study of 43 gastric neuroendocrine carcinomas. World J Gastroenterol. 2017;23(3):516–24.
12. Jeon SK, Lee JM, Joo I, Lee ES, Park HJ, Jang JY, et al. Nonhypervascular pancreatic neuroendocrine tumors: differential diagnosis from pancreatic ductal adenocarcinomas at MR imaging-retrospective cross-sectional study. Radiology. 2017;284(1):77–87.
13. Lubner MG, Smith AD, Sandrasegaran K, Sahani DV, Pickhardt PJ. CT texture analysis: definitions, applications, biologic correlates, and challenges. Radiographics. 2017;37(5):1483–503.
14. Canellas R, Burk KS, Parakh A, Sahani DV. Prediction of pancreatic neuroendocrine tumor grade based on ct features and texture analysis. AJR Am J Roentgenol. 2018;210(2):341–6.
15. Pereira JA, Rosado E, Bali M, Metens T, Chao SL. Pancreatic neuroendocrine tumors: correlation between histogram analysis of apparent diffusion coefficient maps and tumor grade. Abdom Imaging. 2015;40(8):3122–8.
16. Choi TW, Kim JH, Yu MH, Park SJ, Han JK. Pancreatic neuroendocrine tumor: prediction of the tumor grade using CT findings and computerized texture analysis. Acta Radiol. 2018;59(4):383–92.
17. De Robertis R, Maris B, Cardobi N, Tinazzi Martini P, Gobbo S, Capelli P, et al. Can histogram analysis of MR images predict aggressiveness in pancreatic neuroendocrine tumors? Eur Radiol. 2018;28(6):2582–91.
18. Hodgdon T, McInnes MD, Schieda N, Flood TA, Lamb L, Thornhill RE. Can quantitative CT texture analysis be used to differentiate fat-poor renal angiomyolipoma from renal cell carcinoma on unenhanced ct images? Radiology. 2015;276(3):787–96.
19. Shindo T, Fukukura Y, Umanodan T, Takumi K, Hakamada H, Nakajo M, et al. Histogram analysis of apparent diffusion coefficient in differentiating pancreatic adenocarcinoma and neuroendocrine tumor. Medicine. 2016; 95(4):e2574.

22

Renal cell carcinoma with venous extension: prediction of inferior vena cava wall invasion by MRI

Lisa C. Adams[1][*][†], Bernhard Ralla[2][†], Yi-Na Y. Bender[1], Keno Bressem[1], Bernd Hamm[1], Jonas Busch[1], Florian Fuller[3][†] and Marcus R. Makowski[1][†]

Abstract

Background: Renal cell carcinoma (RCC) are accompanied by inferior vena cava (IVC) thrombus in up to 10% of the cases, with surgical resection remaining the only curative option. In case of IVC wall invasion, the operative procedure is more challenging and may even require IVC resection. This study aims to determine the diagnostic performance of contrast-enhanced magnetic resonance imaging (MRI) for the assessment of wall invasion by IVC thrombus in patients with RCC, validated with intraoperative findings.

Methods: Data were collected on 81 patients with RCC and IVC thrombus, who received a radical nephrectomy and vena cava thrombectomy between February 2008 and November 2017. Forty eight patients met the inclusion criteria. Sensitivity and specificity as well as the positive and negative predictive values were calculated for preoperative MRI, based on the assessments of the two readers for visual wall invasion. Furthermore, a logistic regression model was used to determine if there was an association between intraoperative wall adherence and IVC diameter.

Results: Complete occlusion of the IVC lumen or vessel breach could reliably assess IVC wall invasion with a sensitivity of 92.3% (95%-CI: 0.75–0.99) and a specificity of 86.4% (95%-CI: 0.65–0.97) (Fisher-test: p-value< 0.001). The positive predictive value (PPV) was 88.9% (95%-CI: 0.71–0.98) and the negative predictive value reached 90.5% (95%-CI: 0.70–0.99). There was an excellent interobserver agreement for determining IVC wall invasion with a kappa coefficient of 0.90 (95%CI: 0.79–1.00).

Conclusions: The present study indicates that standard preoperative MR imaging can be used to reliably assess IVC wall invasion, evaluating morphologic features such as the complete occlusion of the IVC lumen or vessel breach. Increases in IVC diameter are associated with a higher probability of IVC wall invasion.

Keywords: Renal cell carcinoma, Inferior vena cava thrombus, Magnetic resonance imaging, Preoperative planning, Sensitivity and specificity

Background

Renal cell carcinoma (RCC) represent approximately 2–3% of all tumors and show a propensity for vascular growth with up to 10% of patients developing an inferior vena cava (IVC) thrombus [1, 2]. IVC wall invasion is a negative prognostic factor [3], whereby positive renal or caval vein margins are associated with worse survival outcomes [4, 5]. To date, surgical resection remains the only curative option, offering a 5-year-survival of up to 40–65%

* Correspondence: Lisa.adams@charite.de
[†]Equal contributors
[1]Department of Radiology, Charité, Charitéplatz 1, 10117 Berlin, Germany
Full list of author information is available at the end of the article

for RCC with intravascular growth, which is reduced in cases with IVC wall invasion [6–8].

In case of IVC wall invasion, surgery is more challenging, because it may necessitate segmental resection or even prosthetic replacement to prevent postoperative recurrence or venous insufficiency [9, 10]. The need for segmental resection or prosthetic replacement is typically determined intraoperatively. Therefore, the ability to predict IVC invasion preoperatively would be a clear advantage in terms of preoperative planning and a priori patient information.

High quality diagnostic imaging is a cornerstone of preoperative planning and management. With regard to the presence and extent of IVC invasion, MR is a powerful and accurate tool and is suggested to be more reliable than computed tomography (CT) [11]. However, data on the prediction of venous wall invasion by preoperative imaging are sparse. There have been only a limited number of studies - most of them with older generation MR scanners and a small number of patients - investigating the ability of CT or MRI to assess the extent of wall invasion and vena caval tumor extension [7, 9, 12–14]. While breach of the vessel wall with tumor signal on both sides of the vessel wall has been demonstrated to be a reliable sign of IVC wall invasion [9, 15], contact of the IVC thrombus with the vessel wall could not be established as a reliable predictor so far.

Methods

In the present study, we aimed to evaluate the accuracy of preoperative standard MRI for determining or ruling out wall invasion of the IVC, based on morphologic features such as vessel wall contact or vessel wall breach, with imaging findings being validated with intraoperative results. Furthermore, we sought to test for the potential association between wall invasion and IVC diameter or thrombus enhancement.

Study design and population

This retrospective study was approved by the Institutional Review Board. Between February 2008 and November 2017, 81 patients with histologically proven RCC and IVC thrombus received a radical nephrectomy and vena cava thrombectomy with an intraoperative assessment of IVC wall invasion. Of these patients, 48 patients obtained a preoperative MRI examination with a clinical routine protocol at a 1.5 T unit and could be included in our analysis, aiming to validate in vivo findings of IVC wall invasion with intraoperative findings.

The patient sample consisted of a total of 48 patients (10 women and 38 men, aged 38–79, mean 64.9 ± 9.8). The median time between the preoperative imaging and the date of surgery was 16.1 (± 13.3) days. With regard to the composition of the thrombus, there were 8 patients with bland thrombus (0 cases IVC wall invasion), 19 patients with tumor thrombus (16 cases with wall invasion) and 21 patients with mixed content (10 cases with wall invasion), whereby mixed content refers to a coexistence of bland thrombus and tumor thrombus. Circumferential cavectomy with prosthetic replacement of the IVC was performed in only 3 of the 48 patients (6.3%), whereas the other patients received a reconfiguration with continuous suturing. In the 3 cases with circumferential cavectomy, IVC tumor invasion was histologically confirmed. In 9 of the 48 patients (18.8%) with level IV thrombi, a cardiopulmonary bypass had to be used. During histological examination, 40 of the patients were revealed to have a clear cell RCC, seven patients showed papillary carcinomas and one patients had

an undifferentiated renal carcinoma, which could not be clearly classified. An overview of the patients' characteristics is provided by Table 1.

Imaging protocol

The MRI examinations from our hospital were performed on 1.5 T units (Aera/Avanto/Symphony/Sonata, Siemens Medical Solutions, Erlangen, Germany) with dedicated body-phased-array coils. All patients underwent a clinical routine imaging of the kidneys at 1.5 T, which included transverse, coronal and sagittal T2 half Fourier single-shot turbo spin echo sequences (HASTE), unenhanced axial 3D gradient echo pulse T1-weighted (FLASH) images, a T1- FLASH angiography, obtained prior to and after the intravenous administration of contrast agents, and a fat saturated volumetric interpolated breath-hold examination (VIBE) T1 3D sequence (see Table 2 for tabulated magnetic resonance imaging parameters).

Level of IVC extent, tumor thrombus enhancement and IVC diameter

Level of IVC extent was stratified following the classification of tumor thrombus level according to the Mayo

Table 1 Characteristics of the Study Population

Number of patients	48
Number of men/women	38/10
Mean age at surgery (range; SD)	64.9 (38–79; 9.8)
Involvement of the right kidney (number)	37
Thrombus level (number, %)	
I	9 (18.8)
II	17 (35.4)
III	13 (27.1)
IV	9 (18.8)
Fuhrman grade (number, %)	
1	2 (4.3)
2	19 (40.4)
3	18 (38.3)
4	8 (17.0)
TNM classification (number, %)	
T1	1 (2.1)
T2	1 (2.1)
T3a	15 (31.2)
T3b	22 (45.8)
T3c	7 (14.6)
T4	2 (4.2)
Number of clear cell carcinoma (%)	40 (83.3)
Number of papillary carcinoma (%)	7 (14.6)
Presence of preoperative metastases (number, %)	16 (33.3)

Table 2 Tabulated imaging parameters of the magnetic resonance sequences

Type of acquisition	T2 HASTE[a] axial	T2 HASTE[a] coronal	T2 TSE[b] axial (PACE)[b]	T1 FLASH[c]	Angiography T1 FLASH[c]	T1 VIBE[d]
Repetition time, TR (ms)	800	800	2430	186	2.88	4.74
Echo time, TE (ms)	94	89	79	4.76	0.98	2.38
Field of view (FOV)	340 × 340	400 × 400	340 × 340	340 × 340	500 × 500	373 × 373
Matrix size	320 × 320	320 × 320	320 × 320	320 × 320	512 × 512	320 × 320
Slice thickness (mm)	5	5	4	4	1.4	3
Pixel bandwidth (Hz/pixel)	300	422	260	260	440	400
Acquisition mode	2D	2D	2D	2D	3D	3D
Flip angle (°)	180	170	180	70	25	10
Voxel size	1.3 × 1.1 × 4.0	1.7 × 1.3 × 5.0	1.5 × 1.1 × 4.0	1.4 × 1.1 × 4.0	1.6 × 1.0 × 1.4	1.7 × 1.2 × 3.0

[a]Half Fourier Single-shot Turbo-spin Echo sequence
[b]Turbo Spin Echo with Prospective Acquisition Correction
[c]Fast low-angle shot magnetic resonance imaging
[d]Volumetric Interpolated Breath-hold Examination

staging system [16]: Level I refers to thrombi that extend into the IVC to no more than 2 cm above the renal vein. Level II represents IVC thrombi extending into into the IVC to more than 2 cm above the renal vein but not to the hepatic vein, whereby Levels I and II make up for approximately 50% of the thrombi. Level III IVC thrombi are defined as extending above the hepatic veins, but below the diaphragm, making up for about 40%. Level IV IVC thrombi extend above the diaphragm or into the right atrium and represent approximately 10% [17]. IVC thrombus levels for all patients were assessed at two time points, first, during preoperative imaging, and second by exploration during surgery.

With regard to the composition of IVC thrombus, an image-based differentiation was performed for bland thrombus, which was diagnosed, when there was no thrombus enhancement, tumor thrombus, which was assumed when the signal intensity was similar to that of the RCC and mixed content, which included both features and could e.g. also refer to a tumor thrombus covered by clot.

The maximum IVC diameters were measured on an axial section in two directions, which were perpendicular to each other.

Image analysis

All of the images were analyzed by use of PACS workstations (Centricity Radiology; GE Healthcare). All MRI images were evaluated by two radiologists blinded to the surgical and pathological findings and to the observations of the other in randomized order and in two different reading sessions, which were separated by a period of 2 weeks. IVC thrombi were analyzed based on the following properties: upper extent (infrahepatic, intrahepatic, infra-diaphragmatic or supra-diaphragmatic), thrombus enhancement, IVC diameter and wall invasion. If the IVC thrombus could clearly be delineated from the vessel wall and if there was no thickening or altered signal of the low-intensity vessel wall, invasion was

assumed to be absent. If there was a contact of the IVC thrombus with or even a visual breach of the IVC wall, IVC wall invasion was assumed to be present. More specifically, contact to the vessel wall referred to a loss of delineation between thrombus and vessel wall with complete occlusion of the vessel and blood signal loss in the affected area. Consequently, a diagnosis of wall invasion was made, when the tumor showed contact with the vessel wall or, if there was a breach or extension through the vessel wall [9]. Agreement between the two observers was also assessed. Finally, imaging findings were validated with intraoperative findings.

Intraoperative evaluation and procedure

Intraoperatively, wall invasion was reported, if the IVC thrombus showed any adherence to the IVC wall. Absence of IVC wall invasion was confirmed, if the caval thrombus could be easily removed.

If the IVC does not show any signs of advanced invasion intraoperatively and there is no evidence of the resection compromising the IVC lumen, the standard operative procedure at our institution involves a combination of thrombectomy with subsequent cavorrhaphy, using continuous polypropylene suturing. If there is advanced tumorous invasion with a breach of the vessel wall IVC resection, either segmental or circumferential, become necessary.

Statistical analysis

Statistical analysis was performed with "R" Statistical Software (Version 3.2.2, R Development Core Team, 2015). Variables were expressed as means ± standard deviations. Sensitivity and specificity as well as the positive and negative predictive values were calculated based on the assessments of the two readers for visual wall invasion. In case of a differing assessment, the opposite of the reference standard (intraoperative finding) was assumed in order to avoid an overestimation of the diagnostic performance. Cohen's kappa coefficient was used to measure interobserver agreement for categorical variables (invasion/no invasion). The intraclass coefficient (ICC) was used to assess interobserver and intermodality reliability for continuous data. Interobserver and intermodality reliability was considered poor for ICC/kappa values less than 0.40, fair for values from 0.40–0.59, good for values from 0.60–0.74 and excellent for values above 0.75. Furthermore, a logistic regression model was used to determine if there was an association between intraoperative wall adherence and IVC diameter. Fisher's exact test was used to assess if thrombus enhancement showed a significant association with IVC wall invasion. A p-value < 0.05 was considered statistically significant.

Results

All of the 48 patients underwent extended nephrectomy and thrombectomy, with the information available from surgery being used to confirm IVC wall invasion.

Validation with intraoperative findings

We found that contact of the IVC thrombus to or breach of the vessel wall could reliably diagnose wall invasion in preoperative MRI imaging with a sensitivity of 92.3% (95%-CI: 0.75–0.99) and a specificity of 86.4% (95%-CI: 0.65–0.97) (Fisher test: p-value < 0.001). The positive predictive value (PPV) was 88.9% (95%-CI: 0.71–0.98) and the negative predictive value reached 90.5% (95%-CI: 0.70–0.99) (refer to Table 3).

There were 26 cases of wall invasion, of which 24 were correctly identified based on contrast-enhanced MRI (see Figs. 1 and 2 for case examples). The two patients with IVC invasion, who were considered to have a non-adherent thrombus based on MRI, were revealed to have very small areas of adherence (less than 1 cm) intraoperatively. In one of these cases, the assessment of the observers differed. Of the 22 cases, where intraoperative findings revealed no presence of wall invasion, 19 could be correctly identified with MRI (see Fig. 3 for case example). In the three cases, where MRI could not identify absence of wall invasion, this was mostly due to respiratory motion artifacts on the axial images, with the observers' evaluation differing in two of the cases.

Table 3 Diagnostic performance of MRI with surgery as the reference standard

	Observer 1	Observer 2	Observer 1 and 2 combined
Sensitivity	0.92 (0.75–0.99)	0.96 (0.80–1.0)	0.92 (0.75–0.99)
Specificity	0.95 (0.77–1.0)	0.86 (0.65–0.97)	0.86 (0.65–0.97)
Negative predictive value	0.91 (0.72–0.99)	0.95 (0.75–1.0)	0.91 (0.70–0.99)
Positive predictive value	0.96 (0.80–1.0)	0.89 (0.72–0.98)	0.89 (0.71–0.98)

Point estimates and 95% confidence intervals are indicated in brackets

Interobserver agreement for IVC wall invasion

There was an excellent interobserver agreement for determining IVC wall invasion with a kappa coefficient of 0.95 (95%CI: 0.85–0.98). In three cases, the two observers assessed the presence or absence of invasion differently, whereby the opposite of the reference standard (findings at surgery) was chosen in order to avoid an overestimation of the diagnostic performance (see Table 4).

Regarding IVC diameter measurements, there was also an excellent interobserver agreement with an ICC coefficient of 0.90 (95%CI: 0.79–1.00).

Association between IVC diameter and probability of IVC invasion

Furthermore, we found that increases in IVC diameter were associated with a higher probability of IVC wall invasion, with the β-coefficient for the IVC diameter being 0.41 (standard error +/− 0.13). This influence also reached significance level ($p = 0.015$). Patients with IVC wall invasion showed a mean diameter of 42.96 mm ± 8.54 mm, while patients without wall invasion had a mean diameter 34.00 mm ± 7.25 mm. This difference was also significant ($p = 0.0.001$).

By contrast, intraoperative IVC wall invasion was not significantly related to the extent or level of IVC extent ($p > 0.05$).

Assessment of IVC wall invasion based on MR enhancement

A clear differentiation between invasive and noninvasive IVC thrombus based on MR enhancement patterns proved to be unfeasible, as enhancement was observed in 14 out of the 22 cases without IVC invasion, indicating a high number of false positives. However, none of the non-enhancing IVC thrombi showed signs of invasion, inferring a good estimate of the false negatives. Therefore, the association between enhancement and IVC invasion was significant (Fisher test: $p = 0.001$). This matches the finding of a significant association between the composition of the IVC thrombus (if it was a bland thrombus/venous clot, a tumor thrombus or an association of both) and enhancement. While no enhancement could be observed in patients with bland tumor thrombus, there was enhancement in patients with tumor thrombus and mixed content.

Discussion

This study suggests that preoperative MR imaging enables a reliable determination of IVC wall invasion in patients with RCC. More specifically, complete occlusion of the IVC lumen and breach of the vessel wall are indicators of IVC invasion with a high sensitivity and specificity. Furthermore, increases in IVC diameter were associated with a higher probability of IVC wall invasion.

IVC wall invasion has recently been recognized as an independent prognostic factor for the survival of patients

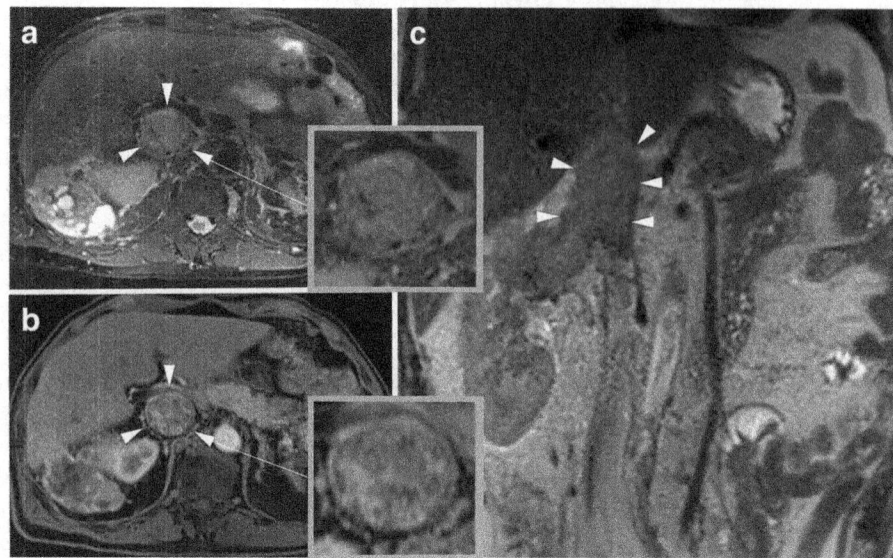

Fig. 1 Images in a 55-year old man with a clear cell renal cell carcinoma (RCC) and an inferior vena cava (IVC) tumor thrombus with wall invasion. The RCC extends from the right kidney into the suprahepatic IVC. **a** axial fat-saturated T2-weighted image. **b** T1-weighted contrast-enhanced 3D GRE (VIBE) image (arterial phase) and (**c**), coronal T2-weighted HASTE image for anatomic reference. Note that the thrombus completely obstructs the lumen of the IVC and shows direct contact with the vessel wall (**a**, **c**). The contrast-enhanced image (**b**) demonstrates a heterogeneous enhancement of the tumor thrombus, and contact to, but no breach of the vessel wall, which makes IVC wall invasion likely. During extended nephrectomy, this thrombus was partly adherent the IVC and after extraction of the IVC thrombus, continuous suturing became necessary. VIBE = Volumetric interpolated breath-hold examination

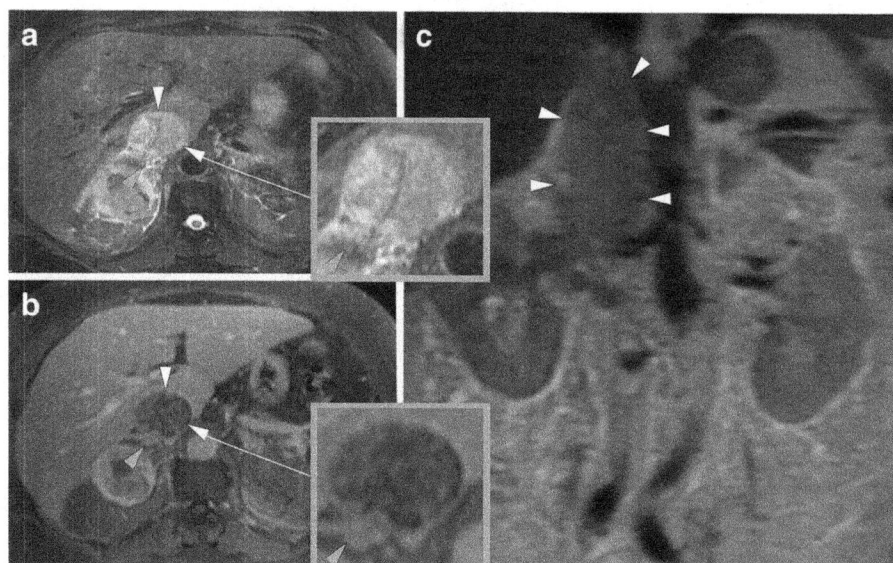

Fig. 2 Images in a 69-year old woman with a clear cell renal cell carcinoma (RCC) and an inferior vena cava (IVC) tumor thrombus with wall invasion. The RCC extends from the right kidney into the IVC and extends into the right atrium. **a** axial fat-saturated T2-weighted image. **b** T1-weighted contrast-enhanced 3D GRE (VIBE) image contrast enhanced 3D GRE image (arterial phase) and (**c**), coronal T2-weighted HASTE image for anatomic reference. Note that the thrombus completely obstructs the lumen of the IVC, but also seems to breach the vessel wall (**a**, **c**). The contrast-enhanced image (**b**) demonstrates a heterogeneous enhancement of the tumor thrombus and a clear breach of the vessel wall (gray arrowhead), which is highly suggestive of IVC wall invasion. During extended nephrectomy, this thrombus showed strong adherence to the IVC wall and during extraction, circumferential cavectomy with vascular reconstruction became necessary. VIBE = Volumetric interpolated breath-hold examination

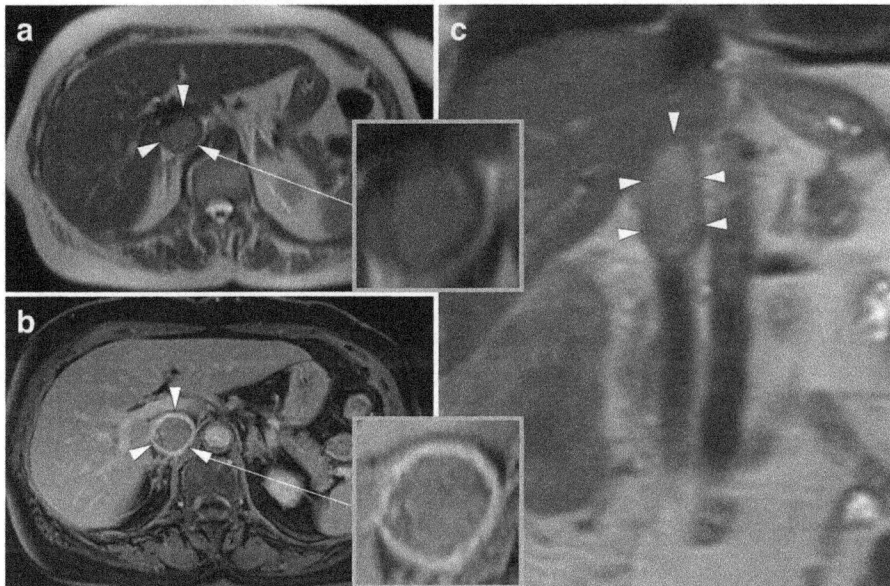

Fig. 3 Images in a 79-year old woman with a clear cell renal cell carcinoma (RCC) and bland inferior vena cava (IVC) thrombus without wall invasion. The RCC extends from the right kidney into the infrahepatic IVC. **a** axial T2-weighted HASTE image. **b** T1-weighted contrast-enhanced 3D GRE (VIBE) image and (**c**), the coronal T2-weighted HASTE image for anatomic reference. Note that the thrombus is floating in the IVC and that there is no complete obstruction of the caval lumen (**a, c**). The contrast-enhanced image (**b**) demonstrates that there is no enhancement of the tumor thrombus, contact to or breach of the vessel wall, so that IVC wall invasion appears unlikely. During extended nephrectomy, this thrombus could be easily removed from the IVC without necessitating segmental resection. HASTE = Half-Fourier-acquired singe-shot turbo spin echo, VIBE = Volumetric interpolated breath-hold examination

with IVC thrombi [16, 18–20]. During surgery, IVC wall invasion requires a very challenging reconstruction beyond standard cavorrhaphy, that might include segmental resection or prosthetic replacement. However, there has been limited data with only a handful of studies and - apart from the study by Psutka et al. - with small sample sizes [9, 12, 14, 21, 22]. With regard to MR imaging, the number of studies is even more limited, as Psutka et al., for example, chose a cross-sectional approach including both MRI and CT images, with CT having a comparably lower diagnostic performance, and using a combination of multiple radiographic parameters to predict IVC invasion [14]. By contrast, we propose a purely MR-based approach with focus on the direct detection of IVC wall invasion with clearly defined morphologic parameters.

In line with our results, previous studies found tumor signal on both sides of the vessel wall to be one of the most reliable indicators of vessel breach and of IVC wall invasion [9, 12, 21]. Furthermore, Myneni et al. proposed to use the low signal intensity line of the normal vessel wall on gradient echo (GRE) and T1-weighted images as a minor criterion for vessel wall invasion [13].

In addition, contrast enhancement of the thrombus or venous wall has been suggested as a criterion for distinguishing tumor thrombus from bland thrombus and for narrowing the diagnosis to wall invasion, the theory being that the neo-vascular bed of the tumor thrombus would adhere to the venous wall, whereas the bland thrombus would not [9, 12]. In the present study, thrombus enhancement was not reliable for excluding caval wall invasion, as enhancement was observed in more than 60% of the cases, where no wall invasion was found intraoperatively. However, it proved to be reliable

Table 4 Wall invasion by inferior vena cava thrombus on MRI versus invasion determined at surgery

Observer 1 MRI	Surgery	
	Wall invasion	Absence of wall invasion
Wall invasion	24	1
Absence of wall invasion	2	21
Observer 2 MRI	Surgery	
	Wall invasion	Absence of wall invasion
Wall invasion	25	3
Absence of wall invasion	1	19
Observers 1 + 2 MRI	Surgery	
	Wall invasion	Absence of wall invasion
Wall invasion	24	3
Absence of wall invasion	2	19

In three cases, the two observers assessed the presence or absence of invasion differently. In case of a differing assessment, the opposite of the reference standard (intraoperative finding) was assumed in order to avoid an overestimation of the diagnostic performance. This combined assessment (observers 1 + 2) is shown below for excluding invasion in cases, where no IVC enhancement was observed.

Furthermore, previous studies demonstrated an association between IVC diameters and wall invasion [14, 23]. Psutka et al. considered 24 mm or more on the level of the renal vein ostium to be a probable indicator of advanced IVC invasion [14, 23]. In the present study, probability of IVC wall invasion also was higher with increasing IVC diameters, which appears logical, as bigger thrombi show a higher propensity for invasion.

The presence of IVC wall invasion has also been incorporated into the American Joint Committee on Cancer (AJCC) cancer staging criteria for RCC, changing a stage T3b to a stage T3c [24].

Previous research suggested a superior diagnostic accuracy of MRI in detecting the upper extent of IVC thrombus due to its intrinsic contrast superiority [25]. However, in more recent studies, the diagnostic performance of CT and MRI in staging the level of IVC thrombus has been regarded to be similar [26–29]. However, to our knowledge there has not been a systematic comparison between multidetector CT and MRI concerning the detection of IVC wall invasion yet.

Even though it has to be acknowledged, that the preoperative assessment of IVC invasion cannot replace the value of surgical exploration, morphologic MR features may be used to predict the risk for complicated inferior vena cava resection in a reproducible manner, which is also supported by the strong interobserver agreement we found. In clinical practice, surgeons can use the additional information to optimize their preoperative planning, e.g. in consultation with the vascular surgeons or scheduling of the most experienced surgeons. The derived information is especially important in patients, in whom reconstruction of the IVC beyond cavorrhaphy is probable, to determine the need for specific operative resources (e.g. cardiopulmonary bypass) in advance and also to individually improve prior patient information [15]. Intraoperatively, the a priori assessment of wall invasion can be a helpful adjunct to additional examinations such as duplex ultrasound or transesophageal echocardiography, which can be used to further characterize the mobility, consistency and the exact extension of the thrombus [14].

Recent studies have focused on diffusion weighted imaging (DWI) as an emerging technique for quantitative readouts, with the apparent diffusions coefficient (ADC) values representing tumor cellularity [30]. DWI has shown promise in preoperative cancer staging, e.g. for endometrial, cervical, bladder, rectal or gastric cancer [31–34]. Especially the introduction of reduced field-of-view (FOV) techniques has enabled an improved tumor delineation with higher spatial resolution, decreased partial volume averaging and less susceptibility distortion [35]. Future studies on the preoperative evaluation of IVC invasion could, therefore, include reduced FOV DWI sequences to investigate whether additional information on thrombus composition may be gained. Furthermore, functional imaging, such as dynamic contrast enhanced (DCE) MRI, may improve assessment of thrombus and wall enhancement through the quantification of contrast-enhancement characteristics and the evaluation of microcirculation parameters. During DCE imaging, several contrast enhancement parameters can be used to better differentiate tumor tissue. Previous research suggested, that especially the early postcontrast phase could be relevant for tumor detection [36]. By contrast, there were also studies suggesting, that there was limited additional value for diagnosis of clinically relevant cancer [37]. Two notable disadvantages of the semi-quantitative parameters derived from DCE imaging is their direct estimation from the signal intensity measurements without physiological or empirical correlation and also their dependence on experimental factors such as sequence parameters or contrast dose, especially limiting their comparability and reproducibility between different sites [38].

In the present study, patients did not receive dynamic imaging, but only an early postcontrast phase. In everyday clinical practice, the time required for extensive examination protocols can be limited. Therefore, the objective of the present study was to test the performance and feasibility of a relatively short standard protocol for the preoperative evaluation of inferior vena cava wall invasion.

Regarding the results of the present study for MRI, the high sensitivity (92.3%) indicates, that the presence of IVC invasion is rarely underestimated and the high negative predictive value (90.5%) suggests, that if the IVC thrombus does not show any contact with the vessel wall, an IVC wall invasion can be reliably excluded. The comparably lower specificity shows, that a visual contact of the IVC thrombus with the vessel wall does not always correspond to IVC wall invasion, but still in more than 85% of the cases.

The excellent interobserver agreement for the assessment indicates the feasibility of using MR features for assessing IVC thrombus invasion in clinical practice. Complete occlusion of the IVC lumen or breach of the vessel wall may be used to predict the presence of IVC wall invasion and thus of complicated surgery.

This study has some limitations. Firstly, different MRI scanners were included over a relatively long period of time, resulting in a potential variability across scanners and imaging sessions, where the same scanner is used. Secondly, due to its retrospective design, a potential selection bias cannot be excluded. Thirdly, as intraoperative findings were used as the reference standard for wall invasion, presence of microscopic invasion cannot be excluded. Fourthly, as the present study is single center, external validation of the applied MR features is warranted. Furthermore, the addition of DWI or DCE imaging to the protocol might have further improved the preoperative assessment of IVC thrombus. Finally, MR imaging is contraindicated in some patients, e.g. patients with pacemakers, metallic foreign bodies or with severe claustrophobia.

Conclusions

This study indicates that standard preoperative MR imaging can be used to reliably assess IVC wall invasion, evaluating morphologic features such as the complete occlusion of the IVC lumen or vessel breach. The excellent interobserver agreement suggests an adequate reproducibility of the preoperative assessment in clinical practice. In future, MR morphologic features might be used to refine preoperative planning and improve prior patient information.

Abbreviations
CT: Computed tomography; GRE: Gradient-echo; ICC: Intraclass coefficient; IVC: Inferior vena cava; MRI: Magnetic resonance imaging; RCC: Renal cell carcinoma

Acknowledgements
LCA and BR are grateful for their participation in the BIH Charité - Junior Clinician Scientist Program funded by the Charité - Universitaetsmedizin Berlin and the Berlin Institute of Health. JB is participant in the BIH – Twinning Grant Program funded by the Charité - Universitaetsmedizin Berlin and the Berlin Institute of Health. MRM is grateful for the financial support from the Deutsche Forschungsgemeinschaft (DFG, 5943/31/41).

Funding
BH has received research grants for the Department of Radiology, Charité – Universitätsmedizin Berlin from the following companies: 1. Abbott, 2. Actelion Pharmaceuticals, 3. Bayer Schering Pharma, 4. Bayer Vital, 5. BRACCO Group, 6. Bristol-Myers Squibb, 7. Charite research organisation GmbH, 8. Deutsche Krebshilfe, 9. Dt. Stiftung für Herzforschung, 10. Essex Pharma, 11. EU Programmes, 12. Fibrex Medical Inc., 13. Focused Ultrasound Surgery Foundation, 14. Fraunhofer Gesellschaft, 15. Guerbet, 16. INC Research, 17. InSightec Ud., 18. IPSEN Pharma, 19. Kendlel MorphoSys AG, 20. Lilly GmbH, 21. Lundbeck GmbH, 22. MeVis Medical Solutions AG, 23. Nexus Oncology, 24. Novartis, 25. Parexel Clinical Research Organisation Service, 26. Perceptive, 27. Pfizer GmbH, 28. Philipps, 29. Sanofis-Aventis S.A, 30. Siemens, 31. Spectranetics GmbH, 32. Terumo Medical Corporation, 33. TNS Healthcare GMbH, 34. Toshiba, 35. UCB Pharma, 36. Wyeth Pharma, 37. Zukunftsfond Berlin (TSB), 38. Amgen, 39. AO Foundation, 40. BARD, 41. BBraun, 42. Boehring Ingelheimer, 43. Brainsgate, 44. PPD (Clinical Research Organisation), 45. CELLACT Pharma, 46. Celgene, 47. CeloNova BioSciences, 48. Covance, 49. DC Deviees, Ine. USA, 50. Ganymed, 51. Gilead Sciences, 52. Glaxo Smith Kline, 53. ICON (Clinical Research Organisation), 54. Jansen, 55. LUX Bioseienees, 56. MedPass, 57. Merek, 58. Mologen, 59. Nuvisan, 60. Pluristem, 61. Quintiles, 62. Roehe, 63. Sehumaeher GmbH (Sponsoring eines Workshops), 64. Seattle Genetics, 65. Symphogen, 66. TauRx Therapeuties Ud., 67. Accovion, 68. AIO: Arbeitsgemeinschaft Internistische Onkologie, 69. ASR Advanced sleep research, 70. Astellas, 71. Theradex, 72. Galena Biopharma, 73. Chiltern, 74. PRAint, 75. Inspiremd, 76. Medronic, 77. Respicardia, 78. Silena Therapeutics, 79. Spectrum Pharmaceuticals, 80. St. Jude., 81. TEVA, 82. Theorem, 83. Abbvie, 84. Aesculap, 85. Biotronik, 86. Inventivhealth, 87. ISA Therapeutics, 88. LYSARC, 89. MSD, 90. novocure, 91. Ockham oncology, 92. Premier-research, 93. Psi-cro, 94. Tetec-ag, 94. Tetec-ag, 95. Winicker-norimed, 96. Achaogen Inc., 97. ADIR, 98. AstraZenaca AB, 99. Demira Inc., 100.Euroscreen S.A., 101. Galmed Research and Development Ltd., 102. GETNE, 103. Guidant Europe NV, 104. Holaira Inc., 105. Immunomedics Inc., 106. Innate Pharma, 107. Isis Pharmaceuticals, 108. Kantar Health GmbH, 109. MedImmune Inc., 110. Medpace Germany GmbH (CRO), 111. Merrimack Pharmaceuticals Inc., 112. Millenium Pharmaceuticals Inc., 113. Orion Corporation Orion Pharma, 114. Pharmacyclics Inc., 115. PIQUR Therapeutics Ltd., 116. Pulmonx International Sárl, 117. Servier (CRO), 118. SGS Life Science Services (CRO), 119. Treshold Pharmaceuticals Inc. MRM received financial support from the Deutsche Forschungsgemeinschaft (DFG, 5943/31/41/91). LCA and BR are participants in the BIH Charité - Junior Clinician Scientist Program funded by the Charité - Universitaetsmedizin Berlin and the Berlin Institute of Health. JB is participant in the BIH – Twinning Grant Program funded by the Charité - Universitaetsmedizin Berlin and the Berlin Institute of Health.

Authors' contributions
MRM, LCA, FF and BR conceived of the present idea. MRM supervised the project. LCA, YB and KB acquired, analyzed and interpreted the patient data regarding wall invasion by IVC thrombus (MRI versus surgical findings). LCA was a major contributor in writing the manuscript. BH, MRM, JB and FF gave technical support and conceptual advice. All authors read and revised the manuscript critically, approving the final manuscript.

Competing interests
The authors declare that they have no competing interests.

Author details
[1]Department of Radiology, Charité, Charitéplatz 1, 10117 Berlin, Germany.
[2]Department of Urology, Charité, Charitéplatz 1, 10117 Berlin, Germany.
[3]Department of Urology, Charité, Hindenburgdamm 30, 12200 Berlin, Germany.

References
1. Ljungberg B, Bensalah K, Canfield S, Dabestani S, Hofmann F, Hora M, Kuczyk MA, Lam T, Marconi L, Merseburger AS, et al. EAU guidelines on renal cell carcinoma: 2014 update. Eur Urol. 2015;67:913–24.
2. Blute ML, Leibovich BC, Lohse CM, Cheville JC, Zincke H. The Mayo Clinic experience with surgical management, complications and outcome for patients with renal cell carcinoma and venous tumour thrombus. BJU Int. 2004;94:33–41.
3. Wagner B, Patard JJ, Mejean A, Bensalah K, Verhoest G, Zigeuner R, Ficarra V, Tostain J, Mulders P, Chautard D, et al. Prognostic value of renal vein and inferior vena cava involvement in renal cell carcinoma. Eur Urol. 2009;55:452–9.
4. Hatcher PA, Anderson EE, Paulson DF, Carson CC, Robertson JE. Surgical management and prognosis of renal cell carcinoma invading the vena cava. J Urol. 1991;145:20–3. discussion 23-24.
5. Rodriguez Faba O, Linares E, Tilki D, Capitanio U, Evans CP, Montorsi F, Martinez-Salamanca JI, Libertino J, Gontero P, Palou J. Impact of Microscopic Wall invasion of the renal vein or inferior vena cava on Cancer-specific survival in patients with renal cell carcinoma and tumor Thrombus: a multi-institutional analysis from the international renal cell carcinoma-venous Thrombus consortium. Eur Urol Focus. 2017. https://doi.org/10.1016/j.euf.2017.01.009.
6. Lambert EH, Pierorazio PM, Shabsigh A, Olsson CA, Benson MC, McKiernan JM. Prognostic risk stratification and clinical outcomes in patients undergoing surgical treatment for renal cell carcinoma with vascular tumor thrombus. Urology. 2007;69:1054–8.
7. Roubidoux MA, Dunnick NR, Sostman HD, Leder RA. Renal carcinoma: detection of venous extension with gradient-echo MR imaging. Radiology. 1992;182:269–72.
8. Manassero F, Mogorovich A, Di Paola G, Valent F, Perrone V, Signori S, Boggi U, Selli C. Renal cell carcinoma with caval involvement: contemporary strategies of surgical treatment. Urol Oncol. 2011;29:745–50.
9. Aslam Sohaib SA, Teh J, Nargund VH, Lumley JS, Hendry WF, Reznek RH. Assessment of tumor invasion of the vena caval wall in renal cell carcinoma cases by magnetic resonance imaging. J Urol. 2002;167:1271–5.

10. Zini L, Destrieux-Garnier L, Leroy X, Villers A, Haulon S, Lemaitre L, Koussa M. Renal vein ostium wall invasion of renal cell carcinoma with an inferior vena cava tumor thrombus: prediction by renal and vena caval vein diameters and prognostic significance. J Urol. 2008;179:450–4. discussion 454.

11. Kandpal H, Sharma R, Gamangatti S, Srivastava DN, Vashisht S. Imaging the inferior vena cava: a road less traveled. Radiographics. 2008;28:669–89.

12. Oto A, Herts BR, Remer EM, Novick AC. Inferior vena cava tumor thrombus in renal cell carcinoma: staging by MR imaging and impact on surgical treatment. AJR Am J Roentgenol. 1998;171:1619–24.

13. Myneni L, Hricak H, Carroll PR. Magnetic resonance imaging of renal carcinoma with extension into the vena cava: staging accuracy and recent advances. Br J Urol. 1991;68:571–8.

14. Psutka SP, Boorjian SA, Thompson RH, Schmit GD, Schmitz JJ, Bower TC, Stewart SB, Lohse CM, Cheville JC, Leibovich BC. Clinical and radiographic predictors of the need for inferior vena cava resection during nephrectomy for patients with renal cell carcinoma and caval tumour thrombus. BJU Int. 2015;116:388–96.

15. Psutka SP, Leibovich BC. Management of inferior vena cava tumor thrombus in locally advanced renal cell carcinoma. Ther Adv Urol. 2015;7:216–29.

16. Hatakeyama S, Yoneyama T, Hamano I, Murasawa H, Narita T, Oikawa M, Hagiwara K, Noro D, Tanaka T, Tanaka Y, et al. Prognostic benefit of surgical management in renal cell carcinoma patients with thrombus extending to the renal vein and inferior vena cava: 17-year experience at a single center. BMC Urol. 2013;13:47.

17. Neves RJ, Zincke H. Surgical treatment of renal cancer with vena cava extension. Br J Urol. 1987;59:390–5.

18. Chen X, Li S, Xu Z, Wang K, Fu D, Liu Q, Wang X, Wu B. Clinical and oncological outcomes in Chinese patients with renal cell carcinoma and venous tumor thrombus extension: single-center experience. World J Surg Oncol. 2015;13:14.

19. Cho MC, Kim JK, Moon KC, Kim HH, Kwak C. Prognostic factor for Korean patients with renal cell carcinoma and venous tumor thrombus extension: application of the new 2009 TNM staging system. Int Braz J Urol. 2013;39:353–63.

20. Whitson JM, Reese AC, Meng MV. Population based analysis of survival in patients with renal cell carcinoma and venous tumor thrombus. Urol Oncol. 2013;31:259–63.

21. Laissy JP, Menegazzo D, Debray MP, Toublanc M, Ravery V, Dumont E, Schouman-Claeys E. Renal carcinoma: diagnosis of venous invasion with Gd-enhanced MR venography. Eur Radiol. 2000;10:1138–43.

22. Vergho DC, Loeser A, Kocot A, Spahn M, Riedmiller H. Tumor thrombus of inferior vena cava in patients with renal cell carcinoma - clinical and oncological outcome of 50 patients after surgery. BMC Res Notes. 2012;5:5.

23. Gohji K, Yamashita C, Ueno K, Shimogaki H, Kamidono S. Preoperative computerized tomography detection of extensive invasion of the inferior vena cava by renal cell carcinoma: possible indication for resection with partial cardiopulmonary bypass and patch grafting. J Urol. 1994;152:1993–6. discussion 1997.

24. Edge SB, Compton CC. The American joint committee on Cancer: the 7th edition of the AJCC cancer staging manual and the future of TNM. Ann Surg Oncol. 2010;17:1471–4.

25. Hallscheidt PJ, Fink C, Haferkamp A, Bock M, Luburic A, Zuna I, Noeldge G, Kauffmann G. Preoperative staging of renal cell carcinoma with inferior vena cava thrombus using multidetector CT and MRI: prospective study with histopathological correlation. J Comput Assist Tomogr. 2005;29:64–8.

26. Guo HF, Song Y, Na YQ. Value of abdominal ultrasound scan, CT and MRI for diagnosing inferior vena cava tumour thrombus in renal cell carcinoma. Chin Med J. 2009;122:2299–302.

27. Gupta NP, Ansari MS, Khaitan A, Sivaramakrishna MS, Hemal AK, Dogra PN, Seth A. Impact of imaging and thrombus level in management of renal cell carcinoma extending to veins. Urol Int. 2004;72:129–34.

28. Cuevas C, Raske M, Bush WH, Takayama T, Maki JH, Kolokythas O, Meshberg E. Imaging primary and secondary tumor thrombus of the inferior vena cava: multi-detector computed tomography and magnetic resonance imaging. Curr Probl Diagn Radiol. 2006;35:90–101.

29. Lawrentschuk N, Gani J, Riordan R, Esler S, Bolton DM. Multidetector computed tomography vs magnetic resonance imaging for defining the upper limit of tumour thrombus in renal cell carcinoma: a study and review. BJU Int. 2005;96:291–5.

30. Takeuchi M, Matsuzaki K, Harada M. Carcinosarcoma of the uterus: MRI findings including diffusion-weighted imaging and MR spectroscopy. Acta Radiol. 2016;57:1277–84.

31. Huang YT, Chang CB, Yeh CJ, Lin G, Huang HJ, Wang CC, Lu KY, Ng KK, Yen TC, Lai CH. Diagnostic accuracy of 3.0T diffusion-weighted MRI for patients with uterine carcinosarcoma: assessment of tumor extent and lymphatic metastasis. J Magn Reson Imaging. 2018. https://doi.org/10.1002/jmri.25981.

32. Caivano R, Rabasco P, Lotumolo A, D'Antuono F, Zandolino A, Villonio A, Macarini L, Guglielmi G, Salvatore M, Cammarota A. Gastric cancer: the role of diffusion weighted imaging in the preoperative staging. Cancer Investig. 2014;32:184–90.

33. Delli Pizzi A, Cianci R, Genovesi D, Esposito G, Timpani M, Tavoletta A, Pulsone P, Basilico R, Gabrielli D, Rosa C, et al. Performance of diffusion-weighted magnetic resonance imaging at 3.0T for early assessment of tumor response in locally advanced rectal cancer treated with preoperative chemoradiation therapy. Abdom Radiol. 2018. https://doi.org/10.1007/s00261-018-1457-8.

34. Wang F, Wu LM, Hua XL, Zhao ZZ, Chen XX, Xu JR. Intravoxel incoherent motion diffusion-weighted imaging in assessing bladder cancer invasiveness and cell proliferation. J Magn Reson Imaging. 2018;47:1054–60.

35. Ota T, Hori M, Onishi H, Sakane M, Tsuboyama T, Tatsumi M, Nakamoto A, Kimura T, Narumi Y, Tomiyama N. Preoperative staging of endometrial cancer using reduced field-of-view diffusion-weighted imaging: a preliminary study. Eur Radiol. 2017;27:5225–35.

36. Ogura K, Maekawa S, Okubo K, Aoki Y, Okada T, Oda K, Watanabe Y, Tsukayama C, Arai Y. Dynamic endorectal magnetic resonance imaging for local staging and detection of neurovascular bundle involvement of prostate cancer: correlation with histopathologic results. Urology. 2001;57:721–6.

37. Luzurier A, Jouve De Guibert PH, Allera A, Feldman SF, Conort P, Simon JM, Mozer P, Comperat E, Boudghene F, Servois V, et al. Dynamic contrast-enhanced imaging in localizing local recurrence of prostate cancer after radiotherapy: limited added value for readers of varying level of experience. J Magn Reson Imaging. 2018. https://doi.org/10.1002/jmri.25991.

38. Mazaheri Y, Akin O, Hricak H. Dynamic contrast-enhanced magnetic resonance imaging of prostate cancer: a review of current methods and applications. World J Radiol. 2017;9:416–25.

23

Pain control for patients with hepatocellular carcinoma undergoing CT-guided percutaneous microwave ablation

Hong-Zhi Zhang[1], Jie Pan[1*], Jing Sun[1], Yu-Mei Li[1], Kang Zhou[1], Yang Li[1], Jin Cheng[1], Ying Wang[1], Dong-Lei Shi[1] and Shao-Hui Chen[2]

Abstract

Background: Hepatic percutaneous microwave ablation (MWA) is usually performed in patients under conscious sedation. Nonetheless, many patients reported pain during the procedure. The current study investigated the safety and effectiveness of analgesia given at personalized dosage during the MWA procedure.

Methods: A total of 100 patients with hepatocellular carcinomas (HCCs) were included in this study. These patients underwent CT-guided percutaneous MWA between February and October 2017. Patients were randomized into two groups: Experimental group (n = 50) and Control group (n = 50). Patients in the Control group were given 5 mg of morphine intravenously, followed by 10 mg of morphine injected subcutaneously 30 min before surgery. Patients in the Experimental group were given a personalized dosage of morphine during the procedure when the Visual Analogue Scale (VAS) was ≥4. Other clinical and treatment parameters were also analysed.

Results: A significantly less amount of morphine ($p < 0.001$) was used in the experimental group (7.18 ± 1.65 mg) than in the control group (17.40 ± 2.52 mg). No significant differences were found in the number of patients who needed to discontinue the surgery ($p = 0.242$). Other clinical parameters including heart rate, systolic and diastolic blood pressures at various time points were comparable. Importantly, a lower VAS was reported in the experimental group, indicating a lower pain intensity experienced by patients during the procedure.

Conclusion: The administration of personalized dosage of morphine to HCC patients undergoing percutaneous MWA is an effective and safe procedure for pain control.

Keywords: Microwave ablation, Hepatocellular carcinoma, Pain, Analgesia, Morphine

Introduction

Tumor ablation is defined as the direct application of chemical or thermal therapies to tumor to achieve substantial tumor destruction or eradication; and microwave ablation (MWA) has been recognized as an alternative treatment for patients with hepatocellular carcinoma (HCC). MWA may be used when the curative treatments of HCC (e.g. surgical resection or liver transplant) could not be performed. Studies reported that only 10–54% of all HCC patients were eligible for the curative surgical treatments [1–3]. Other clinical parameters including heart rate, and the difficulties with the surgical resection were related to the site, size, number of tumors, as well as the extrahepatic involvement and remaining liver function [4, 5]. MWA has become another choice to the treatment of HCC, providing effective and reproducible local tumor control and minimal morbidity [6, 7]. Additionally, MWA was a relatively low-risk and minimally invasive procedure for liver tumors [6, 7].

A conscious sedation and local anesthesia were usually sufficient for percutaneous CT-guided MWA, since the operation time of the MWA treatment was short, about 5 to 15 min [8]. However, many patients reported pain during and/or after the treatment [9, 10]. The risk of having at least moderate pain after the treatment may be

* Correspondence: markpan1968@163.com
[1]Department of Radiology, Peking Union Medical College Hospital, Peking Union Medical College, Chinese Academy of Medical Sciences, No. 1 Shuaifuyuan, Dongcheng District, Beijing 100730, China
Full list of author information is available at the end of the article

related to the ablation volume and time and post ablation increase in AST level [9]. The visceral pain caused by the thermal effects of the microwave could be severe, resulting in an uneven respiratory rate and increased surgical risk. For patients who are expected to have a long MWA procedure (e.g. 3 h or longer), a general anesthesia may be preferred.

As variations were seen in perceived pain and discomfort during the procedure, it is important to personalize the pain control strategy. An effective pain control strategy would allow a smooth operation. Conscious analgesic sedations, such as fentanyl, droperidol, midazolam, were used in a standard dose across patients [8, 11]. The current study investigated the outcome of pain control between patients using a standard versus personalized dose of morphine under local anesthesia. We also provided recommendations for the pain control strategy in HCC patients receiving MWA procedure.

Patients and methods

Patients

A total of 100 HCC patients receiving CT-guided MWA treatment between February and October 2017 were included in this study. All patients had a single lesion of HCC < 3 cm, and a single probe was used for the ablation. All patients had no cognitive and speech impairment, and no hearing or cerebrovascular diseases. The MWA was performed at 50–70 W for 5–6 min. The insertion of water-cooled microwave ablation needles (Nanjing Vision-China Medical Devices R&D Center, China) was performed under the guidance of real-time CT scans.

Medical information, including body weight, long-term drinking history, long-term use of analgesic drug history, history of allergies, hypertension and coronary heart disease were recorded. The number and diameter of HCC tumors were also recorded. This study has been approved by our institute's Ethics committees. All patients provided written informed consent.

Methods of analgesia

Patients were randomized into two groups: Experimental group ($n = 50$) and Control group ($n = 50$). The pain intensity was assessed for all patients before and during surgery using Visual Analogue Scale (VAS), ranging from '0' representing no pain to '10' representing worst pain imaginable [12]. Patients were given 8 mg intravenous injection of ondansetron hydrochloride and 5 mg of dexamethasone (Northeast Pharmaceutical Group Shenyang No. 1 Pharmaceutical. Co. Ltd., China) 30 min before surgery to prevent and alleviate nausea. During the surgery, injection of morphine or 2% lidocaine for skin puncture were used for anaesthesia.

Patients in the Control group were given 5 mg of morphine intravenously, followed by 10 mg of morphine injected subcutaneously 30 min before surgery. For patients in the Experimental group, the first dose of morphine was given at a dose calculated from the body weight at 0.1 mg/kg and was given subcutaneously during the procedure when the VAS was ≥4. If additional morphine was needed during the procedure, a fixed dose at 5 mg was given in both groups. Naloxone hydrochloride (0.4 mg) and simple respirator were prepared and given to patients only when needed. Patients were accompanied by a nurse during the procedure.

Evaluation

Vital signs including blood pressure, pulse rate, heart rate, and respiration rate were recorded before and after surgery. Oxygen saturation and the mental status were also recorded. During the surgery, the presence of nausea and vomiting and the number of times and doses of morphine used, were recorded. VAS evaluation was performed in post-initiation of ablation at 0.5 min, 1.5 min, 2.5 min, 3.5 min, 4.5 min, 5.5 min.

Statistical analyses

The SAS 9.3 was used for statistical analysis. Two-tailed test was used and $p < 0.05$ was considered as statistically significant. Categorical variables were presented in frequency (%); Chi-square test and Fisher's exact test were used for comparisons between groups. Continuous variables were presented as mean ± standard deviation; Student's t-test was used for analysis when the data were in normal distribution, or Wilcoxon rank-sum test was used. Two-way repeated measures ANOVA was used to compare intraoperative vital signs and pain score between two groups, and one-way repeated measures ANOVA was used for comparison within the group. The pre-operative vital signs and the pain score at 0.5 min of the ablation were used as baseline for comparison.

Results

The baseline clinical characteristics, including sex, age, weight, comorbidity, size and anatomical location of the lesions, were summarized in Table 1. There were no significant differences in these parameters between the control and experimental groups.

The ablation treatment parameters and morphine usage were compared between the two groups (Table 2). The average time used for the ablation procedure was similar between the groups (control group: 5.33 ± 0.62 min vs. experimental group: 5.41 ± 1.04 min, $p = 0.751$). Various outputs (50 W, 60 W, 70 W) were used for the ablation. All of the patients in the control groups used the 50 W probe, while most of the patients in the experimental group used the 50 W or 60 W probes, with one patient used the 70 W probes ($p < 0.001$). In the experimental group, morphine was injected at various time points when VAS was

Table 1 Comparison of baseline clinical characteristics between the two groups

Characteristics	Control Group n = 50	Experimental Group n = 50	p-value
Gender, n (%)			0.822
Male	13 (26.00)	14 (28.00)	
Female	37 (74.00)	36 (72.00)	
Hypertension, n (%)			0.106
Absent	41 (82.00)	34 (68.00)	
Present	9 (18.00)	16 (32.00)	
Coronary heart disease, n (%)			0.059
Absent	49 (98.00)	43 (86.00)	
Present	1 (2.00)	7 (14.00)	
Age (year), mean ± SD	60.3 ± 10.5	60.18 ± 11.71	0.896
Weight (kg), mean ± SD	68.48 ± 5.89	66.64 ± 10.57	0.286
Diameter of the largest lesion (cm)[a], mean ± SD	2.14 ± 0.96	2.08 ± 0.96	0.275
Distance between the lesion and liver surface (cm)[a], mean ± SD	2.78 ± 0.96	2.96 ± 1.16	0.343
Distance between the lesion and central hilar (cm)[a], mean ± SD	3.87 ± 1.23	4.07 ± 1.33	0.462

[a]Two missing cases in the control group (n = 48)

≥4 (6 patients at 0.5 min; 21 patients at 1.5 min; 12 patients at 2.5 min; 6 patients at 3.5 min); an average of 6.48 ± 1.01 mg of morphine was used for the first injection. Five patients (out of 50) had no morphine injection during the whole procedure (as the VAS was < 4). In the control group, 24 patients needed additional morphine injection during the procedure, while only 3 patients in the experimental group needed additional injection (p < 0.001). Overall, a significantly less amount of morphine (p < 0.001) was used in the experimental group (7.18 ± 1.65 mg) than in the control group (17.40 ± 2.52 mg). No

significant differences were found in the number of patients who needed to discontinue the surgery (p = 0.242).

We used VAS as a tool to assess the pain intensity of patients during the procedure (Table 3). Overall, both of the groups had a significantly lower VAS at various time points (1.5 min, 2.5 min, 3.5 min, 4.5 min, 5.5 min post-initiation of ablation) when compared to the baseline within the group at 0.5 min post-initiation of ablation (p < 0.001). When compared across the groups, a significantly lower VAS was found in the experimental group at various time points (0.5 min, 1.5 min, 2.5 min, 3.5 min, 4.5 min, 5.5 min post-initiation of ablation), indicating patients experienced a lower pain intensity during the whole treatment procedure.

Other clinical parameters including heart rate, systolic and diastolic blood pressures at various time points were also compared between the two groups, and no significant differences were found (Table 4, 5 and 6).

Discussion

Pain experienced during the ablation procedure is categorized in the side effect category, according to the guidelines for the standardization of terminology and reporting criteria for image-guided tumor ablation [13]. The intraoperative pain may affect the completion of a standardized treatment protocol. It has been reported that pain may be related to the side of the lesion and the amount of tissue necrosis [14], but the level of pain was unpredictable.

We found the administration of personalized dosage of morphine during the percutaneous CT-guided MWA treatment was an effective and safe procedure for pain control in HCC patients undergoing local anaesthesia. Local anaesthesia is commonly used for the tumor ablation procedure, since the operation time is usually short [8]. General anaesthesia may be indicated for patients with a low tolerance for pain, or patients with a history

Table 2 Comparison of treatment parameters and morphine usage between groups

Treatment parameters and Morphine usage	Control Group n = 50	Experimental Group n = 50	p-value
Ablation duration, mean ± SD	5.33 ± 0.62	5.41 ± 1.04	0.751
Ablation probes			< 0.001
50 W	50 (100.00)	28 (56.00)	
60 W	0 (0.00)	21 (42.00)	
70 W	0 (0.00)	1 (2.00)	
Dose level of morphine in the first administration, experimental group, (mg), mean ± SD	–	6.84 ± 1.01[a]	–
Number of patients needed additional morphine during surgery	24(48.00)	3 (6.67)	< 0.001
Total amount of morphine used (mg)	17.40 ± 2.52	7.18 ± 1.65[a]	< 0.001
Number of patients with surgery terminated	3 (6.00)	0 (0.00)	0.242

[a]Morphine was given to 45 patients in the Experimental group who reported VAS ≥ 4, and 5 patients had no morphine administrated during the whole procedure

Table 3 VAS evaluation of the two group of patients at various time points of the ablation

Time points Post initiation of ablation	Control Group n = 50	Experimental Group n = 50	p-value [a]
0.5 min	2.04 ± 1.97	1.02 ± 1.45	0.004
1.5 min	3.98 ± 1.95[c]	3.06 ± 1.27[b]	0.006
2.5 min	4.86 ± 1.7[c]	3.48 ± 1.30[b]	< 0.001
3.5 min	5.18 ± 1.62[c]	3.16 ± 1.20[b]	< 0.001
4.5 min	4.94 ± 1.64[c]	2.60 ± 1.09[b]	< 0.001
5.5 min	4.70 ± 1.46[c]	2.24 ± 0.85[b]	< 0.001
5 min after surgery	0.16 ± 0.55[c]	0.02 ± 0.14[b]	0.083
p-value	<0.001	<0.001	–

[a]Comparison between groups; [b]Comparison within groups; [c]Compared to 0.5 min of the Experimental Group and the p-values were < 0.05

of alcohol or drug abuse. However, the general anaesthesia would require a more extensive preoperative evaluation of patients, special technicians (e.g. anaesthetists) and equipment. Importantly, there is a higher risk for patients undergoing general anaesthesia. The pain control strategy discussed in this study may provide a way to expand the patient population that could receive CT-guided MWA under conscious sedation.

Our study found that patients in the experimental group received a significantly less amount of morphine when compared to the control group. Patients with thermal ablation of subcapsular or hilar lesions may require higher doses of analgesics [15]. In our study, patients' lesion locations with respect to central hilar and to the liver surface were comparable between groups, further suggesting the personalized dosage of morphine was at least equally effective. The reduced use of morphine

Table 4 Heart rate (mean ± SD, beats/ min) of the two groups of patients at various time points of the surgery

Time points Post initiation of ablation	Control Group	Experimental Group	p-value [a]
Before Surgery	70.56 ± 8.18	72.52 ± 10.37	0.437
Before initiation of ablation	71.84 ± 8.98[c]	74.06 ± 10.96[b]	0.271
0.5 min	72.88 ± 7.84[c]	74.64 ± 11.87[b]	0.384
1.5 min	74.58 ± 9.91[c]	74.48 ± 12.61	0.965
2.5 min	75.32 ± 10.57[c]	74.42 ± 12.3	0.696
3.5 min	76.52 ± 11.15[c]	73.37 ± 11.87	0.176
	77.33 ± 12.02[c]	73.79 ± 10.96	0.135
5.5 min	78.89 ± 12.29[c]	73.98 ± 9.69	0.044
5 min after surgery	73.22 ± 7.77[c]	71.86 ± 9.53	0.436
p-value	< 0.001	0.046	–

[a]Comparison between groups; [b]Comparison within groups; [c]Compared to Experimental Group before surgery, and the p-values were < 0.05

Table 5 Systolic blood pressures (mean ± SD, mmHg) of the two groups of patients at various time points of the surgery

Time points Post initiation of ablation	Control Group	Experimental Group	p-value [a]
Before Surgery	132.44 ± 11.83	135.22 ± 16.91	0.343
Before initiation of ablation	135.88 ± 12.41[c]	137.48 ± 18.27[d]	0.610
0.5 min	140.22 ± 13.58[c]	138.84 ± 20.07	0.688
1.5 min	142.94 ± 14.72[c]	142.4 ± 20.39[d]	0.880
2.5 min	144.36 ± 17.91[c]	143.84 ± 20.61[d]	0.893
3.5 min	146.02 ± 18.13[c]	145.16 ± 19.68[d]	0.822
4.5 min	146.06 ± 18.4[c]	144.63 ± 19.05[d]	0.708
5.5 min	147.05 ± 18.31[c]	142.21 ± 19.12[d]	0.235
5 min after surgery	136.50 ± 12.52[c]	138.34 ± 17.58	0.548
p-value	< 0.001	< 0.001	–

[a]Comparison between groups; [b]Comparison within groups; [c]Compared to Control Group before surgery, and the p-values were < 0.05. [d]Compared to Experimental Group before surgery, and the p-values were < 0.05

could help to reduce the side effects (e.g. nausea, vomiting, blood pressure, respiratory depression, etc.) [16]. In addition, this pain control strategy was safe. The vital signs and cases of surgery termination were comparable between the two groups.

The analgesic method used in the experimental group provided a satisfactory pain control. Conventionally, morphine was given before the insertion of needles [17]; depending on the tumor location, size, the position of the needle inserted, repeated scanning and adjustment of the needle angle may be needed, resulting further pain. Therefore, it is important to have a prompt administration of analgesia through a timely evaluation of pain during the procedure. In addition to the VAS,

Table 6 Diastolic blood pressures (mean ± SD, mmHg) of the two groups of patients at various time points of the surgery

Time points Post initiation of ablation	Control Group	Experimental Group	p-value [a]
Before Surgery	74.40 ± 8.65	72.50 ± 8.95	0.283
Before initiation of ablation	76.98 ± 8.22[c]	74.10 ± 10.74[d]	0.610
0.5 min	79.30 ± 9.25[c]	75.9 ± 9.76[d]	0.688
1.5 min	79.08 ± 10.20[c]	78.52 ± 10.46[d]	0.880
2.5 min	81.62 ± 11.83[c]	78.42 ± 9.94[d]	0.893
3.5 min	80.98 ± 12.03[c]	77.14 ± 9.39[d]	0.822
	82.15 ± 11.04[c]	78.27 ± 9.28[d]	0.708
5.5 min	82.11 ± 11.16[c]	76.00 ± 8.32[d]	0.235
5 min after surgery	76.74 ± 7.99	73.96 ± 7.92	0.548
p-value	< 0.001	< 0.001	–

[a]Comparison between groups; [b]Comparison within groups; [c]Compared to Control Group before surgery, and the p-values were < 0.05. [d]Compared to Experimental Group before surgery, and the p-values were < 0.05

other pain related parameters could be considered for assessing pain, such as the pain-related behaviours (facial expressions and postures), physiologic indicators (heart rate, blood pressure, respiratory rate).

The non-pharmacological methods of pain control, such as distraction, simple massage, and family support also helped to relive pain. A study reported that the non-pharmacological interventions used by ICU nurses complementary to pharmacological treatment could maximize the pain relief [18]. In our study, we also found that the support from nurses was important; it sometime helped to decrease the pain level perceived by patients.

Conclusion

We showed that the administration of personalized dosage of morphine to HCC patients undergoing percutaneous MWA is an effective and safe procedure for pain control.

Abbreviations
HCC: hepatocellular carcinoma; MWA: microwave ablation; VAS: Visual Analogue Scale

Acknowledgements
None.

Funding
No funding was received for this study.

Authors' contributions
HZZ and JP contributed to the conception and design of the study; JS, Y-M L, KZ contributed to the acquisition of data; YL and JC performed the experiments; YW, SHC and DLS contributed to the analysis of data; HZZ wrote the manuscript; All authors reviewed and approved the final version of the manuscript.

Competing interests
The authors declare that they have no competing interests.

Author details
[1]Department of Radiology, Peking Union Medical College Hospital, Peking Union Medical College, Chinese Academy of Medical Sciences, No. 1 Shuaifuyuan, Dongcheng District, Beijing 100730, China. [2]Department of Anesthesiology, Peking Union Medical College Hospital, Peking Union Medical College, Chinese Academy of Medical Sciences, Beijing, China.

References
1. Forner A, Llovet JM, Bruix J. Hepatocellular carcinoma. Lancet. 2012;379:1245–55.
2. Marin-Hargreaves G, Azoulay D, Bismuth H. Hepatocellular carcinoma: surgical indications and results. Crit Rev Oncol Hematol. 2003;47:13–27.
3. Takaki H, Yamakado K, Uraki J, Nakatsuka A, Fuke H, Yamamoto N, Shiraki K, Yamada T, Takeda K. Radiofrequency ablation combined with chemoembolization for the treatment of hepatocellular carcinomas larger than 5 cm. J Vasc Interv Radiol. 2009;20:217–24.
4. Cho YK, Kim JK, Kim WT, Chung JW. Hepatic resection versus radiofrequency ablation for very early stage hepatocellular carcinoma: a Markov model analysis. Hepatology. 2010;51:1284–90.
5. Khajanchee YS, Hammill CW, Cassera MA, Wolf RF, Hansen PD. Hepatic resection vs minimally invasive radiofrequency ablation for the treatment of colorectal liver metastases: a Markov analysis. Arch Surg. 2011;146:1416–23.
6. Iannitti DA, Martin RC, Simon CJ, Hope WW, Newcomb WL, McMasters KM, Dupuy D. Hepatic tumor ablation with clustered microwave antennae: the US phase II trial. HPB (Oxford). 2007;9:120–4.
7. Lu MD, Xu HX, Xie XY, Yin XY, Chen JW, Kuang M, Xu ZF, Liu GJ, Zheng YL. Percutaneous microwave and radiofrequency ablation for hepatocellular carcinoma: a retrospective comparative study. J Gastroenterol. 2005;40:1054–60.
8. Simon CJ, Dupuy DE, Mayo-Smith WW. Microwave ablation: principles and applications. Radiographics. 2005;25(Suppl 1):S69–83.
9. Andreano A, Galimberti S, Franza E, Knavel EM, Sironi S, Lee FT, Meloni MF. Percutaneous microwave ablation of hepatic tumors: prospective evaluation of postablation syndrome and postprocedural pain. J Vasc Interv Radiol. 2014;25:97–105 e101–102.
10. Kim KR, Thomas S. Complications of image-guided thermal ablation of liver and kidney neoplasms. Semin Intervent Radiol. 2014;31:138–48.
11. Xu HX, Xie XY, Lu MD, Chen JW, Yin XY, Xu ZF, Liu GJ. Ultrasound-guided percutaneous thermal ablation of hepatocellular carcinoma using microwave and radiofrequency ablation. Clin Radiol. 2004;59:53–61.
12. Williamson A, Hoggart B. Pain: a review of three commonly used pain rating scales. J Clin Nurs. 2005;14:798–804.
13. Goldberg SN, Grassi CJ, Cardella JF, Charboneau JW, Dodd GD 3rd, Dupuy DE, Gervais D, Gillams AR, Kane RA, Lee FT Jr, et al. Image-guided tumor ablation: standardization of terminology and reporting criteria. Radiology. 2005;235:728–39.
14. Poggi G, Tosoratti N, Montagna B, Picchi C. Microwave ablation of hepatocellular carcinoma. World J Hepatol. 2015;7:2578–89.
15. McGhana JP, Dodd GD 3rd. Radiofrequency ablation of the liver: current status. AJR Am J Roentgenol. 2001;176:3–16.
16. Rawal N. Analgesia for day-case surgery. Br J Anaesth. 2001;87:73–87.
17. Lee S, Rhim H, Kim YS, Choi D, Lee WJ, Lim HK, Shin B. Percutaneous radiofrequency ablation of hepatocellular carcinomas: factors related to intraprocedural and postprocedural pain. AJR Am J Roentgenol. 2009; 192:1064–70.
18. Gelinas C, Arbour C, Michaud C, Robar L, Cote J. Patients and ICU nurses' perspectives of non-pharmacological interventions for pain management. Nurs Crit Care. 2013;18:307–18.

24

Accurate FDG PET tumor segmentation using the peritumoral halo layer method: a study in patients with esophageal squamous cell carcinoma

Sungmin Jun[1], Jung Gu Park[2] and Youngduk Seo[3*]

Abstract

Background: In a previous study, FDG PET tumor segmentation (SegPHL) using the peritumoral halo layer (PHL) was more reliable than fixed threshold methods in patients with thyroid cancer. We performed this study to validate the reliability and accuracy of the PHL method in patients with esophageal squamous cell carcinomas (ESCCs), which can be larger and more heterogeneous than thyroid cancers.

Methods: A total of 121 ESCC patients (FDG avid = 85 (70.2%); FDG non-avid = 36 (29.8%)) were enrolled in this study. In FDG avid ESCCs, metabolic tumor length (ML) using SegPHL (ML_{PHL}), fixed SUV 2.5 threshold ($ML_{2.5}$), and fixed 40% of maximum SUV (SUVmax) ($ML_{40\%}$) were measured. Regression and Bland-Altman analyses were performed to evaluate associations between ML, endoscopic tumor length (EL), and pathologic tumor length (PL). A comparison test was performed to evaluate the absolute difference between ML and PL. Correlation with tumor threshold determined by the PHL method (PHL tumor threshold) and SUVmax was evaluated.

Results: ML_{PHL}, $ML_{2.5}$, and $ML_{40\%}$ correlated well with EL ($R^2 = 0.6464$, 0.5789, 0.3321, respectively; $p < 0.001$) and PL ($R^2 = 0.8778$, 0.8365, 0.6266, respectively; $p < 0.001$). However, $ML_{2.5}$ and $ML_{40\%}$ showed significant proportional error with regard to PL; there was no significant error between ML_{PHL} and PL. ML_{PHL} showed the smallest standard deviation on Bland-Altman analyses. The absolute differences between ML and PL were significantly smaller for ML_{PHL} and $ML_{40\%}$ than for $ML_{2.5}$ ($p < 0.0001$). The PHL tumor threshold showed an inverse correlation with SUVmax ($\sigma = -0.923$, $p < 0.0001$).

Conclusions: SegPHL was more accurate than fixed threshold methods in ESCC. The PHL tumor threshold was adjusted according to SUVmax of ESCC.

Keywords: Peritumoral halo layer, Tumor segmentation, FDG PET/CT, Esophageal cancer, Reliability test, Tumor length

Introduction

F-18 fluorodeoxyglucose (FDG) PET/CT is a noninvasive modality for staging and localization of various malignant tumors that have high glucose metabolism. FDG PET/CT can provide a variety of metabolic parameters, such as maximum standardized uptake value (SUVmax), metabolic tumor volume (MTV) [1, 2], total lesion glycolysis (TLG) [3], and metabolic tumor length (ML)

[4, 5]. Among these, SUVmax is the most commonly used FDG PET parameter because the measurement is easy and operator independent. Although SUVmax is a widely used parameter, it is a representation of the highest metabolic value of only one pixel within a metabolically active tumor. Thus, the total burden of the primary tumor cannot be evaluated by SUVmax.

MTV and TLG can provide volumetric metabolic information on malignant tumors. MTV is a measurement of the volume of a tumor with a high metabolism, while TLG is defined as the product of mean SUV and MTV [6]. A variety of methods have been used to measure and

---

* Correspondence: mdbabyduck@gmail.com
[3]Department of Nuclear Medicine, Busan Seongso Hospital, Suyeong-ro, Nam-gu, Busan 48453, Republic of Korea
Full list of author information is available at the end of the article

segment MTV. These include visual segmentation methods (SegVisual), where the region of interest is drawn manually [7, 8], fixed SUV threshold methods (SegSUV) [3, 6], fixed percentage of SUVmax threshold methods (Seg%) [3, 6], adaptive threshold methods (SegAdaptive) [6, 9], and gradient methods (SegGradient) [6, 10, 11]. Among these various segmentation approaches, SegSUV or Seg% is widely used to measure MTV because nearly all PET/CT workstations have an auto-segmentation program for fixed threshold methods. Accurate segmentation of MTV is also important for accurate measurement of TLG. Because TLG is a product of MTV and mean SUV (SUVmean), accurate MTV segmentation is essential for reliable TLG measurement. Furthermore, an accurate SUVmean estimate also requires accurate MTV segmentation. If segmented MTV is largely different from the true pathologic tumor volume, TLG will be inaccurate. ML is the length of the tumor on the PET image. The threshold determination for ML is similar to that for MTV [12].

SegAdaptive and SegGradient are known to be more accurate than SegSUV or Seg% [6, 10, 11]. The main principle of SegAdaptive is to adapt the percentage threshold of the phantom or tumor according to signal-to-background ratio [6, 9, 13]. Several optimal regression functions can be obtained by fitting various regression models [6, 9, 13, 14]. MTV using SegGradient is a method used to detect a large gradient change in radioactivity around the tumor. The large gradient change is located in the outmost peripheral portion of the tumor, and its location is used to define the tumor margin [11, 15, 16]. However, a specialized program and workstation, PET Edge® (MIM Software Inc., Cleveland, OH, USA), is needed to determine MTV using SegGradient.

Jun et al. [17] recently introduced a new method for MTV segmentation. They found a distinct layer between the tumor and background activity using a 10-step color scale with specific window level settings and named the distinct layer the "peritumoral halo layer (PHL)." Segmentation using the PHL method (SegPHL) was more reliable than MTV segmented by SegSUV or Seg%. Although SegPHL might be reliable, the previous study was performed in patients with a small and visually homogeneous type of tumor, namely papillary thyroid carcinoma [17]. Thus, further validation of large, heterogeneous tumors is needed to determine if SegPHL can be widely applied in clinical settings.

Our aim was to compare variously segmented MLs (i.e., ML segmented by SUV 2.5 ($ML_{2.5}$), 40% of SUVmax ($ML_{40\%}$), and PHL (ML_{PHL})) of esophageal squamous cell carcinoma (ESCC) with pathological tumor length (PL) and to identify whether SegPHL could be used to reliably define tumor margin in ESCC, which can be large and/or heterogeneous.

Methods

Subjects

This retrospective study was approved by the institutional review board of our hospital and performed in accordance with the Helsinki Declaration. Between January 2013 and June 2017, 137 consecutive patients who had undergone pretreatment FDG PET/CT were evaluated for this study. Patient selection, main parameters, and evaluations are represented graphically in Fig. 1. Among the 137 patients, 16 were excluded for the following reasons: (1) conglomerated hypermetabolic metastatic lymph nodes (LNs) closely adjacent to the main hypermetabolic ESCC ($n = 13$, 2) invasion of the gastric cardia ($n = 2$), and intense physiologic left ventricular FDG uptake of the heart that was closely adjacent to the ESCC ($n = 1$). A total of 121 patients were finally enrolled in this study.

Among the 121 patients, 58 underwent esophagectomy, 2 underwent endoscopic submucosal dissection (ESD), 29 underwent concurrent chemoradiation therapy (CCRT), 1 underwent radiation therapy, 10 underwent chemotherapy only, and 21 were lost to follow-up. Reasons for non-operative therapy are illustrated in Fig. 1. Of the total patients, 111 (91.7%) were men, and 10 (8.3%) were women. Tumor locations were the upper third of the esophagus in 18 (14.9%), mid third in 64 (52.9%), lower third in 31 (25.6%), upper and mid esophagus in 6 (5.0%), and mid and lower esophagus in 2 (1.7%). The median age of the 121 patients at the time of FDG PET/CT pretreatment was 63 years (range: 33–85 years). The time interval between FDG PET/CT and esophagectomy or ESD was less than 6 weeks (median = 7.5 days; range = 1–39 days).

Measurement of endoscopic length

Among the 121 enrolled patients, 116 underwent evaluation of esophagogastroduodenoscopy (EGD) at our hospital (Table 1). Endoscopic length (EL) was routinely measured and reported by the operator in centimeters. The distance from the incisors was recorded on the basis of markings on the endoscope shaft at the distal edge of the ESCC. Thereafter, the endoscope was drawn to the proximal edge of the ESCC. The distance from the incisors was again estimated. EL was defined as the difference in the distances of the proximal and distal edges from the incisors [18].

Acquisition of FDG PET/CT

Patients fasted for at least six hours before FDG injection (370–444 MBq). Serum glucose level was measured before FDG injection. Scanning was performed 50–70 min after injection of FDG using a Biograph Duo PET/CT scanner (Siemens Healthcare, Erlangen, Germany) or a Biograph 16 PET/CT scanner (Siemens Healthcare, Erlangen, Germany).

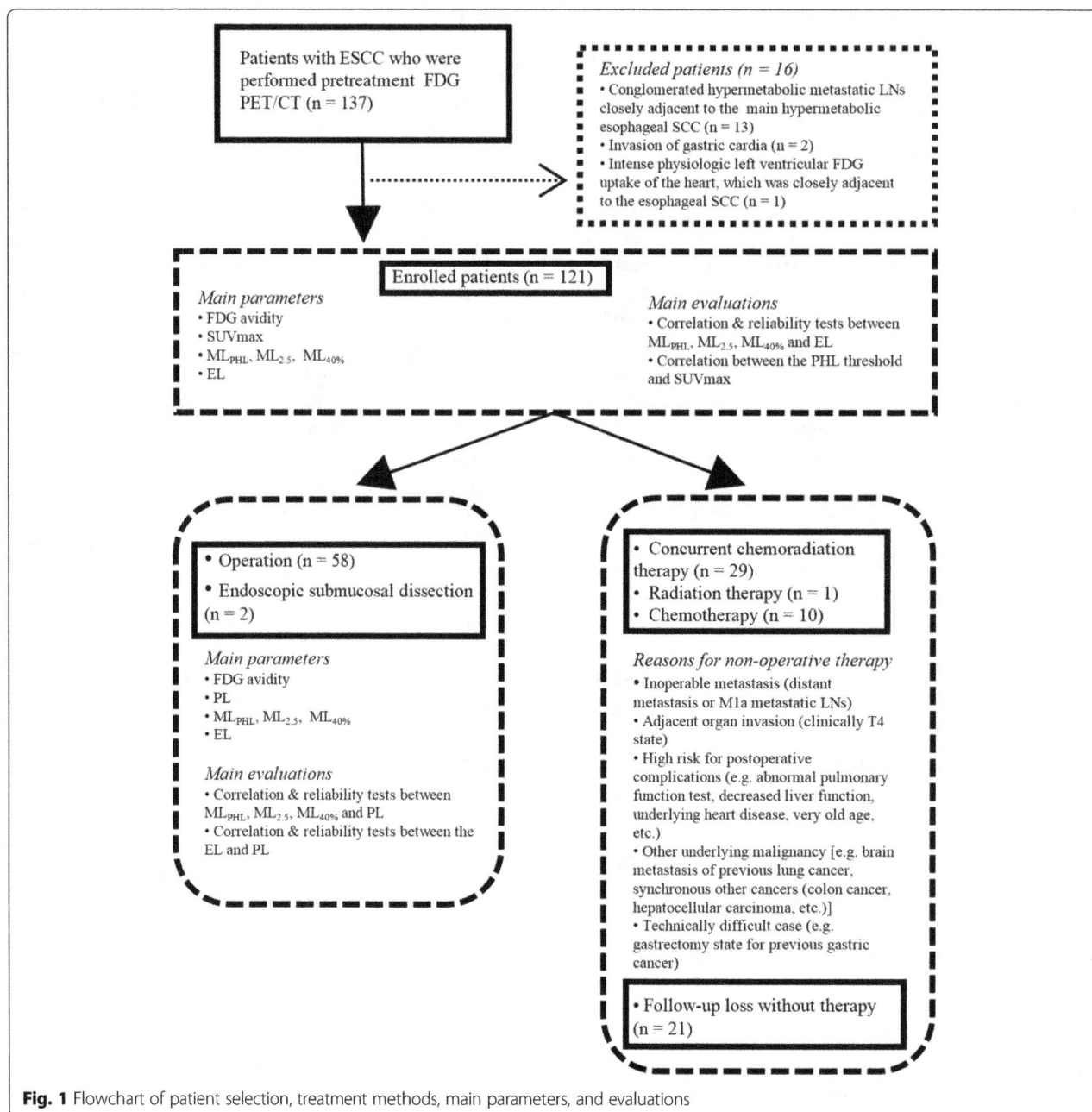

Fig. 1 Flowchart of patient selection, treatment methods, main parameters, and evaluations

Patients were asked to rest before acquisition of PET/CT images. Before the PET scan, a low-dose CT scan (5 mm slices) at an interval of 5 mm was performed for attenuation correction and anatomic co-registration. Intravenous contrast material was not used. PET images were acquired using an acquisition time of 3 min per table position, with an approximate 28% overlap. Images were obtained from the skull base to the proximal thigh with the patient in supine position. Images were reconstructed by a 3D row-action maximum-likelihood algorithm for iterative and ordered-subset expectation maximization using the Biograph system. PET images were corrected for attenuation using a CT-derived transmission map. Voxel size after reconstruction was 2.65 × 2.65 × 2.65 mm.

Identification of PHL and determination of tumor threshold on FDG PET/CT

All FDG PET/CT studies were reviewed on a workstation (Siemens Syngo.via, Siemens Healthcare, Erlangen, Germany). First, we evaluated FDG avidity of the primary ESCC. We considered ESCC to be FDG-avid if abnormal focal or ellipsoid tumoral hypermetabolic activity was visible in the esophagus. If there was no abnormal

Table 1 Comparison of demographics and characteristics of primary esophageal SCCs according to FDG avidity on PET/CT ($n = 121$)

	FDG-avid ($n = 85$)	FDG-non-avid ($n = 36$)	P value
Age (years)			0.5403
Median, range	63, 48–85	67, 33–81	
Sex (male/female)	79/6	32/4	0.4818
Tumor location			0.3251
Upper third	14	4	
Mid third	43	21	
Lower third	20	11	
Upper to mid	6	0	
Mid to lower	2	0	
Pretreatment endoscopy in our hospital (performed/not performed)	83 / 2	33 / 3	0.1553
Treatment methods			0.0405*
Operation	37	22	
Endoscopic submucosal dissection	0	1	
Concurrent chemoradiation therapy	25	4	
Radiation therapy alone	1	0	
Chemotherapy alone	9	1	
Follow-up loss without any therapy (follow-up loss/treatment in our hospital)	13 / 72	8 / 28	0.4321

*Statistically significant

FDG-avid lesion, we recorded the case as FDG-non-avid ESCC. We measured the SUVmax of FDG-avid ESCCs.

The PHL was identified, and the tumor threshold (PHL tumor threshold) was determined as described by Jun and colleagues for papillary thyroid cancer [17]. ESCCs, however, can be visually heterogeneous, unlike papillary thyroid carcinomas, which are almost always small and visually homogeneous. Therefore, the visual tumor pattern was also described in this section.

An example of identification of PHL and PHL tumor threshold is provided in Fig. 2. PET window level and color scale for PHL identification (PHL image settings) were set as follows:

1. PET contrast window level was set in SUV units (not Bq/mL or % units);

2. The top value of the window level was set slightly higher than the SUVmax of the ESCC (e.g., if the SUVmax was $13.00 \sim 13.09$, the top value was set to 13.1), and the bottom value was set to 0;

3. Color scale was changed to a 10-step color scale. We used the Spectrum 10 scale of our workstation.

After inputting these settings, the PHL and PHL tumor threshold were identified according to the following steps:

1. The view around the ESCC was magnified for accurate identification of the PHL.

2. The PHL was identified by an abrupt increase in layer thickness with minimal or mild distortion of the main tumor contour and was between tumoral uptake and background activity [17]. In the present study, the PHL was easy to determine by examining magnified MIP images.

3. The PHL tumor threshold was determined using PHL. Using the PHL imaging settings described above, each color layer represents 10% of the SUVmax. PHL was located between the tumor and the background. Thus, the outermost point of the tumor was the same as the innermost point of the PHL. If the PHL was located at 20–30% of SUVmax, the percentage SUVmax in the innermost portion of the PHL (i.e., PHL tumor threshold) was determined to be 30% (Fig. 2).

After this series of steps, tumoral uptake patterns were classified as visually homogeneous or visually heterogeneous [19]. Tumoral uptake of the ESCC comprised the hottest cores and regular or irregular tumor layers (not the PHL) (Fig. 3). In visually homogeneous ESCCs, the hottest core was located in the center of the ESCC and was surrounded by regular tumor layers (Fig. 3a). In contrast, in visually heterogeneous ESCCs, the hottest core or the hottest multiple cores were located in the eccentric portion of the tumor. In these heterogeneous tumors, several irregular inner layers were visible around the eccentric hottest core, and single or multiple regular outer layers of the tumor enveloped the hottest core and irregular inner layers (Figs. 3b, c). Regardless of visual tumor heterogeneity, the PHL was always located between tumoral uptake and background activity. Classification of visual tumor heterogeneity in our study was similar to that used by Tixier et al. [19] with the exception of the PHL image settings.

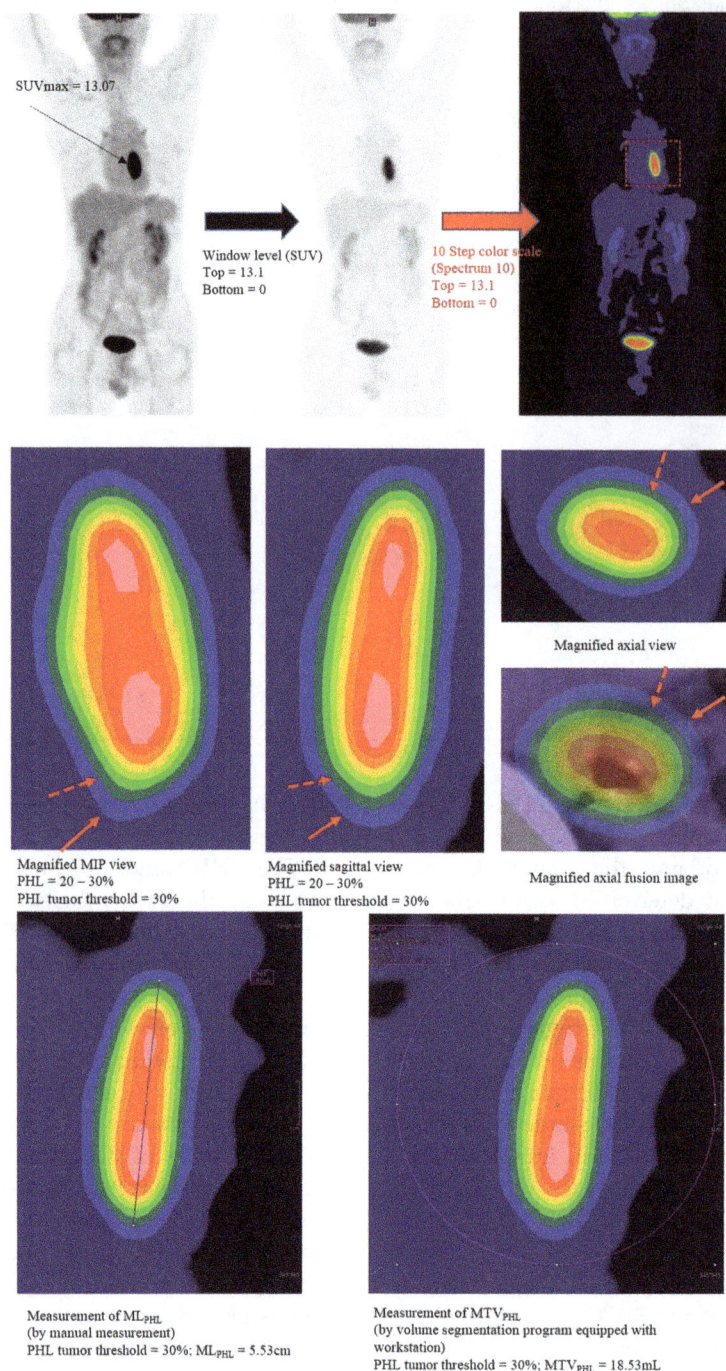

Fig. 2 Representative images to determine PHL tumor threshold and to measure ML$_{PHL}$ and MTV$_{PHL}$. Step 1 (upper): PHL image settings. A segmental hypermetabolic lesion (SUVmax = 13.07) is identified in the mid esophagus (upper left). The window level is set in SUV units. The top value is set to slightly higher than SUVmax (top value 13.1 > 13.07), and the bottom value is set to zero (upper middle). Thereafter, the color scale is changed to a 10-step color scale, which was Spectrum 10 in our study (upper right). A magnified view is used to determine background activity and PHL. Magnification of the ESCC (red dotted box) is performed. Step 2 (middle): Magnified view of the ESCC using PHL image settings (red dotted box in the upper right image). In this image, each layer represents 10% of SUVmax. The hottest core is > 90% of SUVmax. There are two hot cores in this ESCC. PHL is located between the tumor and the background activity. In this image, the background activity is the dark blue layer (10–20% of SUVmax), and the PHL is located at 20–30% of SUVmax (light blue layer; red arrows). Therefore, the PHL tumor threshold is 30% of SUVmax (i.e., the innermost portion of the PHL; red dotted arrow). Layer thickness increases abruptly in the PHL. Step 3 (lower): Measurement of ML$_{PHL}$ and MTV$_{PHL}$. After we determined PHL tumor threshold, we manually measured ML$_{PHL}$ using the ruler tool of the workstation (lower left). MTV$_{PHL}$ was measured by the auto-segmentation program after applying PHL tumor threshold (lower right; 30% of SUVmax in this ESCC)

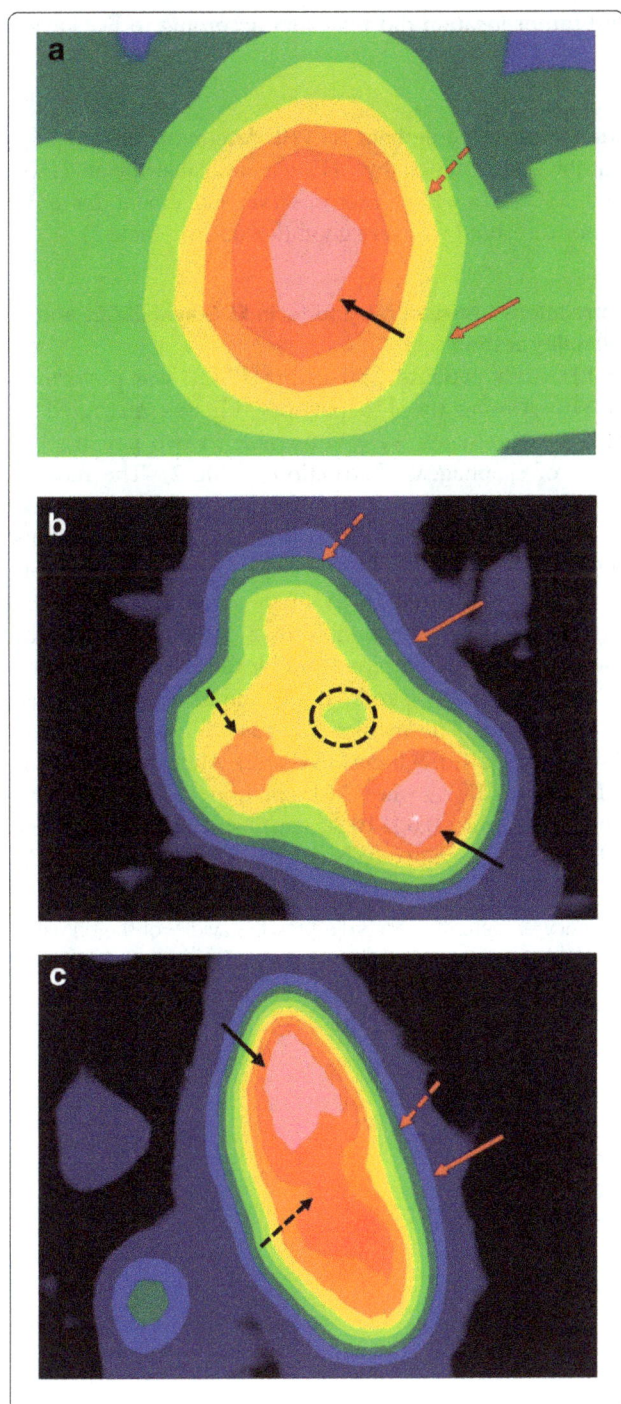

Fig. 3 Visual patterns of the tumors. **a** Visually homogeneous pattern. The hottest core (black arrow) was located in the center of the ESCC. There were no significant irregular layers in the tumor. PHL (50–60% of SUVmax; yellowish green layer) was located between the tumor and the background activity (red arrow). PHL tumor threshold (red dotted arrow) was determined to be 60% of SUVmax (i.e., the innermost portion of the PHL). **b** Visually heterogeneous pattern. The hottest core was eccentrically located in the ESCC, and a small cold defect was visible (small yellowish green portion in black dotted circle). An irregular layer was also present (black dotted arrow). PHL (20–30% of SUVmax; light blue layer) was located between the tumor and the background activity (red arrow). PHL tumor threshold (red dotted arrow) was determined to be 30% of SUVmax (i.e., the innermost portion of the PHL). **c** Visually heterogeneous pattern. The hottest core was eccentrically located in the ESCC (black arrow). A prominent irregular layer was present (black dotted arrow). PHL (20–30% of SUVmax; light blue layer) was located between the tumor and the background activity (red arrow). PHL tumor threshold (red dotted arrow) was determined to be 30% of SUVmax (i.e., the innermost portion of the PHL)

The locations of the PHL and visual tumor heterogeneity were determined by two nuclear medicine physicians who were blinded to pathologic tumor length (PL) and EL values. If the two physicians disagreed, the final decision was made by consensus.

Measurements of metabolic tumor length

After determination of PHL tumor threshold, we measured ML_{PHL}, $ML_{2.5}$, and $ML_{40\%}$ of the ESCC. A straight line was drawn using the ruler tool of our workstation in sagittal view (Fig. 2). ML_{PHL} and $ML_{40\%}$ were measured using the PHL tumor threshold and fixed at 40% of SUVmax on the PHL image setting. $ML_{2.5}$ was measured on SUV2.5 iso-contour images with a PET window bottom value of 2.50 SUV and a top value of 2.51 SUV. When SUVmax of the tumor was lower than 2.5, $ML_{2.5}$ was recorded as 0.

Evaluation of pathologic tumor length (pathologic reference standard)

PL measurements of ESCCs are performed routinely in our hospital. PL was measured by the following procedure. An incision was made along the longitudinal esophageal axis. Thereafter, the esophageal specimen with a straight alignment was set on a flat table. The specimen was sent for pathological examination after preservation in 10% neutral buffered formalin. The PL of the ESCC specimen was measured using a ruler and recorded.

Statistical analyses

Major parameters and analyses in our study are presented in Fig. 1. Demographic and tumor data according to FDG avidity of ESCC were compared using Fisher's exact test, chi-square test, or Mann-Whitney U test. Weighted

Kappa statistics were performed to evaluate inter-observer agreement between the two nuclear medicine physicians for PHL tumor threshold. Regression analyses were performed to evaluate the correlations between ML_{PHL}, $ML_{2.5}$, $ML_{40\%}$, EL, and PL. Bland-Altman plots and Pearson correlation coefficients were used to evaluate the reliability of ML, EL, and PL. Relationships between PHL tumor threshold and SUVmax were evaluated by Spearman's rank correlation. MedCalc® for Windows (MedCalc Software, Mariakerke, Belgium) was the statistical software package used for all statistical analyses.

Results

Clinical situation according to FDG avidity of ESCC

A total of 121 ESCC patients were enrolled in our study. Demographics and other characteristics of ESCCs according to FDG avidity are shown in Tables 1 and 2. There were 85 FDG avid ESCCs (visually homogeneous: $n = 48$; visually heterogeneous: $n = 37$) and 36 FDG non-avid ESCCs. FDG avidity of ESCCs was related to inoperability ($p = 0.0405$), EL ($p = 0.0042$), PL ($p = 0.0001$), presence of metastatic LNs on FDG PET/CT ($p = 0.0005$), presence of M1a metastatic LN or distant metastasis ($p = 0.0037$), and pathologic depth of invasion ($p < 0.0001$). The frequency of metastatic LNs on pathologic specimens tended to be higher in FDG avid ESCCs than in FDG non-avid ESCCs but without statistical significance ($p = 0.0941$). Age, sex,

and tumor location did not differ according to FDG avidity of ESCC.

Inter-observer agreement for PHL determination

Tumor segmentation by PHL was available for all FDG-avid ESCCs ($n = 85$). Inter-observer agreement for PHL tumor threshold was very good (k = 0.936) (Table 3).

Correlations between ML and EL in FDG-avid ESCCs and reliability testing

In 121 study patients, pretreatment EGD was performed in 116. Among the 116 patients, EL was measured in 114; measurements were impossible in two patients because of esophageal obstruction (Table 2). The median EL in the 114 patients was 3.0 cm (range 0.5–9.0 cm; interquartile range 2.0–5.0 cm). Among the 85 patients with FDG avid ESCC, EGD was performed for 83 (Table 1). EL was measured in 81 of those patients, while EL measurement was impossible in 2 patients because the endoscope could not pass through the ESCC. Therefore, MLs (ML_{PHL}, $ML_{2.5}$, and $ML_{40\%}$) and EL were compared in 81 patients. The median EL was 3.5 cm in FDG avid ESCCs (range 1.0–9.0 cm) (Table 2). Medians of ML_{PHL}, $ML_{2.5}$, and $ML_{40\%}$ were 3.81 cm (range 0.80–9.80 cm), 4.80 cm (range 0.00–10.30 cm), and 4.40 cm (range 1.88–9.39 cm), respectively. In the 85 FDG avid ESCCs,

Table 2 Comparison of endoscopic length, pathologic length, and frequency of metastasis according to FDG avidity of the primary ESCC

	FDG-avid ($n = 85$)	FDG-non-avid ($n = 36$)	P value
Endoscopic passage to distal portion of the tumor* (possible/impossible)	81/2	33/0	1.0000
Endoscopic length (cm)**			0.0042[†]
Median, range	3.5, 1.0–9.0	2.0, 0.5–9.0	
Pathologic length (cm)***			0.0001[†]
Median, range	3.5, 0.9–7.6	1.7, 0.15–6.0	
Metastatic LN on FDG PET/CT (yes/no)	40 / 45	5 / 31	0.0005[†]
M1a metastatic LN or distant metastasis on FDG PET/CT (yes/no)	21 / 64	1 / 35	0.0037[†]
Presence of metastatic LN on pathologic specimens**** (yes/no)	18 / 19	5 / 16	0.0941
Pathologic depth of invasion (T stage)***			< 0.0001[†]
Basement membrane (Tis)	0	3	
Mucosa (T1a)	2	9	
Submucosa (T1b)	11	11	
Muscularis propria (T2)	9	0	
Adventitia (T3)	15	0	
Invasion of adjacent structures (T4)	0	0	

*Pretreatment endoscopic evaluation was performed in 116 patients at our hospital
**Measurement of endoscopic length was impossible in 2 patients with total esophageal obstruction
***Measurement of pathologic length and depth of invasion was possible for 60 patients who were treated by surgery ($n = 58$) or ESD ($n = 2$). There was no T4 case in these patients
****Frequency test of pathologically confirmed metastatic LNs was performed for 58 operative patients
LN = lymph node; ESD = endoscopic submucosal dissection
[†]Statistically significant

Table 3 Inter-observer agreement test for determination of PHL tumor threshold

		Observer A							
	PHL tumor threshold	20%	30%	40%	50%	60%	70%	80%	90%
Observer B	20%	2							
	30%	1	40						
	40%		2	13					
	50%			2	6				
	60%				1	2	2		
	70%						5	1	
	80%						1	5	
	90%								2

$k = 0.936$

there was only 1 case where the SUVmax of the ESCC was lower than 2.5 and the $ML_{2.5}$ was zero.

ML_{PHL}, $ML_{2.5}$, and $ML_{40\%}$ were significantly correlated with EL (ML_{PHL}: $p < 0.001$, slope = 0.91, $R^2 = 0.6464$; $ML_{2.5}$: $p < 0.001$, slope = 0.96, $R^2 = 0.5789$; $ML_{40\%}$: $p < 0.001$, slope = 0.49, $R^2 = 0.3321$) (Figs. 4a-c). In Bland-Altman analyses (Fig. 4d-f), the biases between ML_{PHL}, $ML_{2.5}$, and $ML_{40\%}$ and EL were 0.1 cm (limits of agreement = $- 2.62 \sim 2.69$ cm; SD = 1.3532), 0.7 cm (limits of agreement = $- 2.53 \sim 3.89$ cm; SD = 1.6357), and 0.5 cm (limits of agreement = $- 2.87 \sim 3.83$; SD = 1.7096), respectively. Bias and standard deviation were smallest for ML_{PHL} and EL. There was significant proportional error between $ML_{2.5}$ and EL on the Bland-Altman plot ($r = 0.3458$, $p = 0.0016$). No significant error was found between ML_{PHL} or $ML_{40\%}$ and EL on the Bland-Altman plots (ML_{PHL}: $r = 0.2102$, $p = 0.0597$; $ML_{40\%}$: $r = - 0.2027$, $p = 0.0695$).

Comparisons between MLs, EL, and PL

Of the 121 study patients, PL measurements were performed in 60 (58 esophagectomy and 2 ESD patients) (Fig. 1). Among these 60 patients, 2 did not undergo EGD in our hospital. Correlation between EL and PL was assessed in 58 patients (56 esophagectomy and 2 ESD patients). EL was significantly correlated with PL ($R^2 = 0.5482$, slope = 0.77, $p < 0.001$) (Fig. 5a). In Bland-Altman analysis (Fig. 5e) of the 58 patients, the bias between EL and PL was 0.3 cm (limits of agreement = $- 2.29 \sim 2.90$ cm, SD = 1.3254 cm). There was no significant proportional error between EL and PL on the Bland-Altman plot ($r = 0.0629$, $p = 0.6390$).

Of the 85 patients with FDG avid ESCCs, esophagectomy was performed in 37 (Table 1). ML and PL were compared in these 37 patients. ML_{PHL}, $ML_{2.5}$, and $ML_{40\%}$ were significantly correlated with PL (ML_{PHL}: $R^2 = 0.8778$, slope = 1.03, $p < 0.001$; $ML_{2.5}$: $R^2 = 0.8365$, slope = 1.27, $p < 0.001$; $ML_{40\%}$: $R^2 = 0.6266$, slope = 0.61, $p < 0.001$) (Figs. 5b-d). In Bland-Altman analyses (Fig. 5f-h), the biases between ML_{PHL}, $ML_{2.5}$, and $ML_{40\%}$ and

PL were $- 0.32$ cm (limits of agreement = $- 1.67 \sim 1.03$ cm; SD = 0.6869 cm), 0.0 cm (limits of agreement = $- 2.13 \sim 2.23$ cm; SD = 1.1117 cm), and 0.3 cm (limits of agreement = $- 1.81 \sim 2.44$ cm; SD = 1.0847 cm), respectively. The biases of ML_{PHL}, $ML_{2.5}$, and $ML_{40\%}$ were less than 0.5 cm. However, ML_{PHL} showed the smallest SD in Bland-Altman analysis.

There was no significant proportional error between ML_{PHL} and PL ($r = 0.2902$, $p = 0.0815$). However, there were significant proportional errors between $ML_{2.5}$, $ML_{40\%}$, and PL on Bland-Altman plots ($ML_{2.5}$: $r = 0.6036$, $p = 0.0001$; $ML_{40\%}$: $r = - 0.4049$, $p = 0.0129$). The proportional error of $ML_{2.5}$ implied that the value of $ML_{2.5}$ was smaller when average length was small and/or larger when average length was large. In contrast, the proportional error implied that $ML_{40\%}$ was larger when average length was small and/or smaller when average length was large.

The absolute differences between MLs (i.e., ML_{PHL}, $ML_{2.5}$, and $ML_{40\%}$) and PL were calculated as absolute value of (MLs - PL). The absolute difference was significantly smaller for ML_{PHL} and $ML_{40\%}$ than for $ML_{2.5}$ (ML_{PHL}: median 0.40 cm, interquartile range 0.20 $\sim$ 0.66 cm; $ML_{2.5}$: median 1.37 cm, interquartile range 0.84 $\sim$ 2.40 cm; $ML_{40\%}$: median 0.38 cm. interquartile range 0.24 $\sim$ 0.90; Kruskal-Wallis test: $p < 0.0001$) (Fig. 6).

Effects of SUVmax on ML measurement

We evaluated the differences between MLs (i.e., ML_{PHL}, $ML_{2.5}$, $ML_{40\%}$) and PL according to SUVmax of ESCC. The difference between ML_{PHL} and PL was only weakly correlated with SUVmax (Spearman correlation: $\sigma = 0.372$, $p = 0.0254$). However, the difference between $ML_{2.5}$ and PL showed a strong positive correlation with SUVmax (Spearman correlation: $\sigma = 0.806$, $p < 0.0001$). In contrast to $ML_{2.5}$, the difference between $ML_{40\%}$ and PL was strongly negatively correlated with SUVmax (Spearman correlation: $\sigma = - 0.789$, $p < 0.0001$). These results suggested that ML_{PHL} was less affected by SUVmax of ESCC than were $ML_{2.5}$ and $ML_{40\%}$.

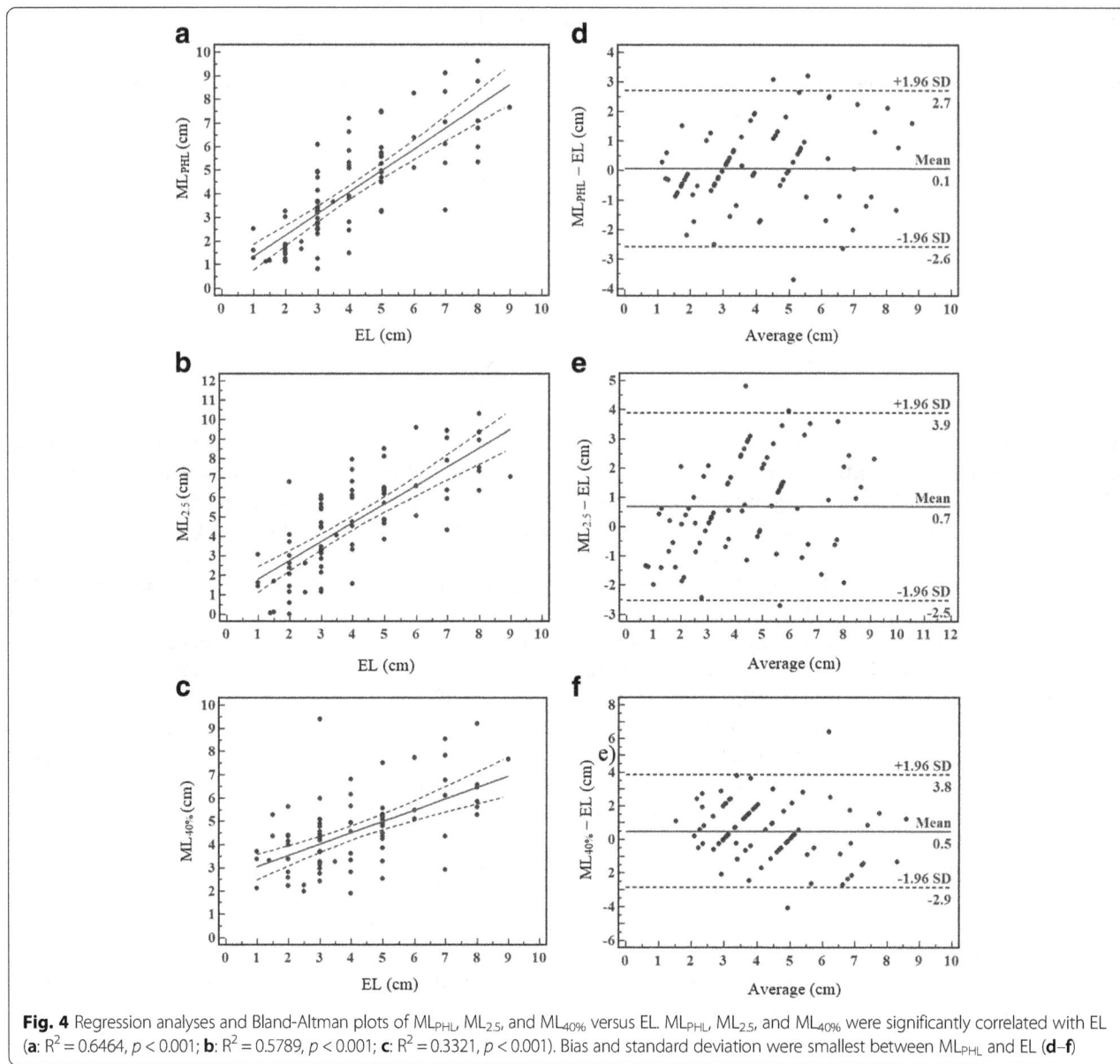

Fig. 4 Regression analyses and Bland-Altman plots of ML_{PHL}, $ML_{2.5}$, and $ML_{40\%}$ versus EL. ML_{PHL}, $ML_{2.5}$, and $ML_{40\%}$ were significantly correlated with EL (**a**: $R^2 = 0.6464$, $p < 0.001$; **b**: $R^2 = 0.5789$, $p < 0.001$; **c**: $R^2 = 0.3321$, $p < 0.001$). Bias and standard deviation were smallest between ML_{PHL} and EL (**d–f**)

Changes in PHL tumor threshold according to SUVmax

We evaluated the relationship between PHL tumor threshold and SUVmax in 85 FDG avid ESCCs as described in a previous study [17]. PHL tumor threshold (i.e., % SUVmax determined by the PHL method) showed a strong inverse correlation with SUVmax ($\sigma = -0.923$, $p < 0.0001$; Fig. 7a). SUV at the PHL tumor threshold (i.e., SUVmax × PHL tumor threshold) showed a strong positive correlation with SUVmax ($\sigma = 0.891$, $p < 0.0001$; Fig. 7b).

Discussion

The major finding of the current study is that SegPHL is more accurate and reliable for defining the tumor margin of ESCCs than are fixed threshold methods. In a previous study, Jun et al. [17] reported that SegPHL was

more reliable than fixed threshold methods for delineation of the margins of thyroid cancers. However, the thyroid cancers examined in that study were very small and visually homogeneous. They reported that PHL abruptly increased in layer thickness and was located between the tumor and the background. In the present study, we demonstrated that SegPHL was also accurate in ESCCs, which can be large and/or visually heterogeneous. ML_{PHL} was highly correlated with PL (Fig. 5), the bias and standard deviation of ML_{PHL} were small on the Bland-Altman plot (Fig. 5), and there were no serious proportional errors visible on the plot. The absolute difference between ML_{PHL} and PL was smaller than that of $ML_{2.5}$ and PL (Fig. 6). ML_{PHL} was less affected by SUVmax of the ESCC than were $ML_{2.5}$ and $ML_{40\%}$. The PHL

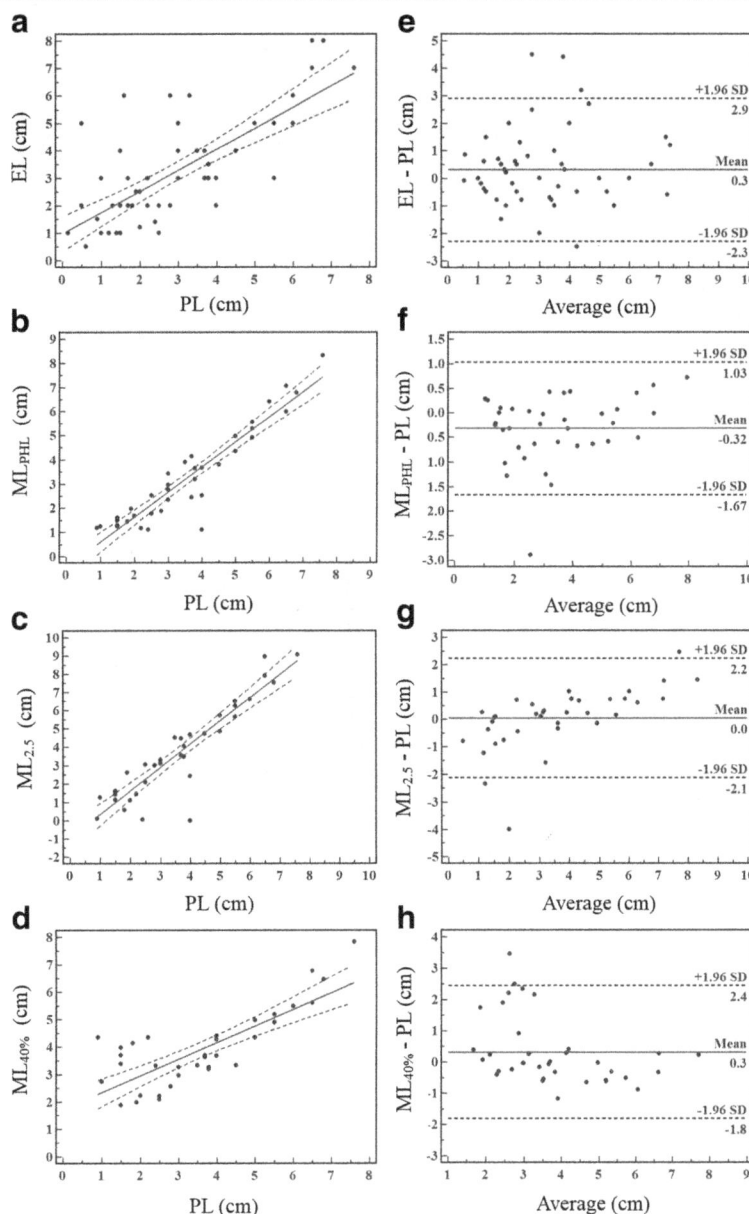

Fig. 5 Regression analyses and Bland-Altman plots of EL, ML_{PHL}, $ML_{2.5}$, and $ML_{40\%}$ versus PL. EL, ML_{PHL}, $ML_{2.5}$, and $ML_{40\%}$ were significantly correlated with PL (**a**: $R^2 = 0.5482$, $p < 0.001$; **b**: $R^2 = 0.8778$, $p < 0.001$; **c**: $R^2 = 8365$, $p < 0.001$; **d**: $R^2 = 0.6266$, $p < 0.001$). The standard deviation was smallest between ML_{PHL} and PL (**d–f**). There was significant proportional error between $ML_{2.5}$ or $ML_{40\%}$ and PL. However, no significant proportional error was found between ML_{PHL} and PL

tumor threshold (% of SUVmax) showed an inverse correlation with SUVmax (Fig. 7). The characteristics of the PHL were similar to those reported in a previous study [17]; PHL also showed an abrupt increase in layer thickness and was located between the tumor activity and the background. Furthermore, PHL tumor threshold changed according to SUVmax of the ESCC (Fig. 7), consistent with a previous PHL study [17].

The most widely used segmentation methods are Seg-SUV and Seg%. However, accurate tumor segmentation

with a fixed threshold is impossible with these methods because the optimal tumor threshold changes according to SUVmax or signal-to-background ratio [13, 20, 21]. The volume of a tumor with faint FDG uptake is highly overestimated by Seg%. In addition, MTV using Seg-SUV underestimates the MTV of a tumor with low metabolic activity and overestimates that of a tumor with high metabolic activity [6]. These shortcomings of Seg% and SegSUV were also found in our present study. The difference between $ML_{2.5}$ and PL was larger

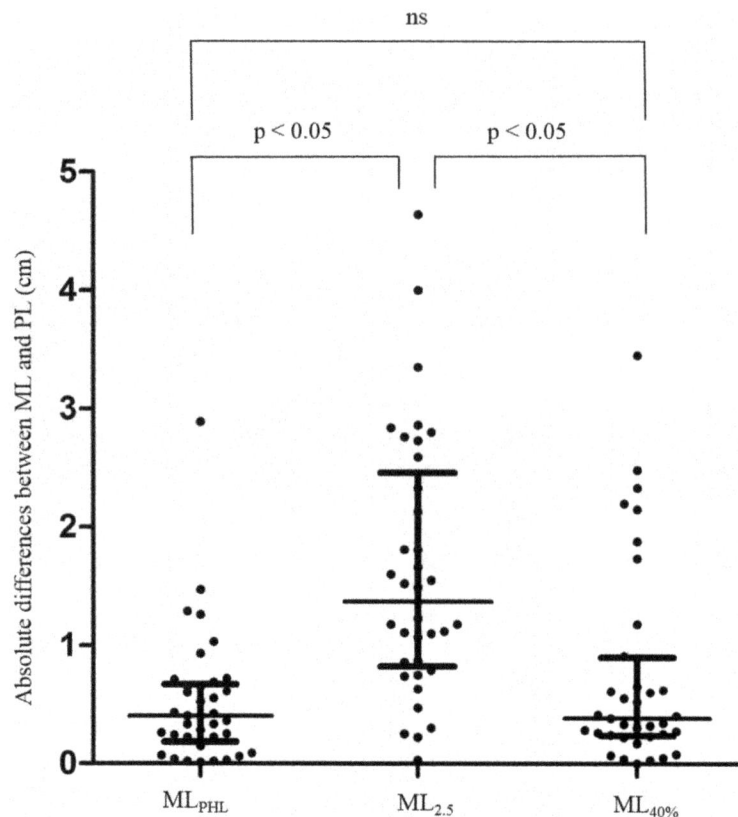

Fig. 6 Absolute differences between MLs and PL. Each dot represents an absolute difference between ML and PL. The middle horizontal bars represent medians, and the vertical bars represent interquartile ranges. Absolute differences between PL and ML were significantly smaller for ML$_{PHL}$ and ML$_{40\%}$ than for ML$_{2.5}$ (Kruskal-Wallis test: $p < 0.0001$, $p < 0.05$ by Dunn's post-hoc test)

when SUVmax was higher, and the difference between ML$_{40\%}$ and PL was larger when SUVmax was lower. However, ML$_{PHL}$ was less affected by SUVmax. The results of our study suggest that the PHL method could accurately segment FDG avid tumor regardless of SUVmax.

SegVisual has been reported to be more accurate than the fixed threshold method in some cases [7]. Although accurate tumor segmentation may be possible with visual tumor delineation, the SegVisual has several limitations. First, the reproducibility of SegVisual is low [22]. Second, visual tumor perception can be altered by the PET window level setting and the color scale [23–25]. Third, the process is quite slow, because no auto-segmentation program is used.

The SegPHL could be considered as a SegVisual because it involves the visual location of the background and the PHL. However, there are several major differences between SegPHL and SegVisual. First, inter-observer agreement for the SegPHL is very good (Table 3), unlike with SegVisual. This good agreement may be due to the use of specific PHL image settings (i.e., PET window level: top = SUVmax, bottom = 0; color scale = 10-step color scale).

Among our study population of 121 cases, PHL tumor threshold was concordant in 111 (91.7%). The second difference between SegPHL and SegVisual is that SegPHL uses commercial auto-segmentation programs to measure MTV$_{PHL}$ with a known, accurate PHL tumor threshold (i.e., % of SUVmax). Use of an auto-segmentation program allows more rapid measurement of MTV than is possible with SegVisual.

SegPHL may also be similar to SegGradient. The unique characteristics of PHL are location between the tumor and the background and abrupt increase in layer thickness compared to the inner layer without significant distortion of tumor shape [17]. In the gradient method, the tumor margin is considered the point at which a large gradient change occurs in the PET/CT image [11]. A previous study suggested that PHL was very similar to the large gradient change of SegGradient [17]. We also hypothesized that the location of the PHL would likely be very similar to that of the large gradient change of SegGradient. Furthermore, like SegGradient [11], SegPHL was more accurate than fixed threshold methods. The main differences between SegPHL and SegGradient are as follows. First, PHL tumor threshold is determined by visual

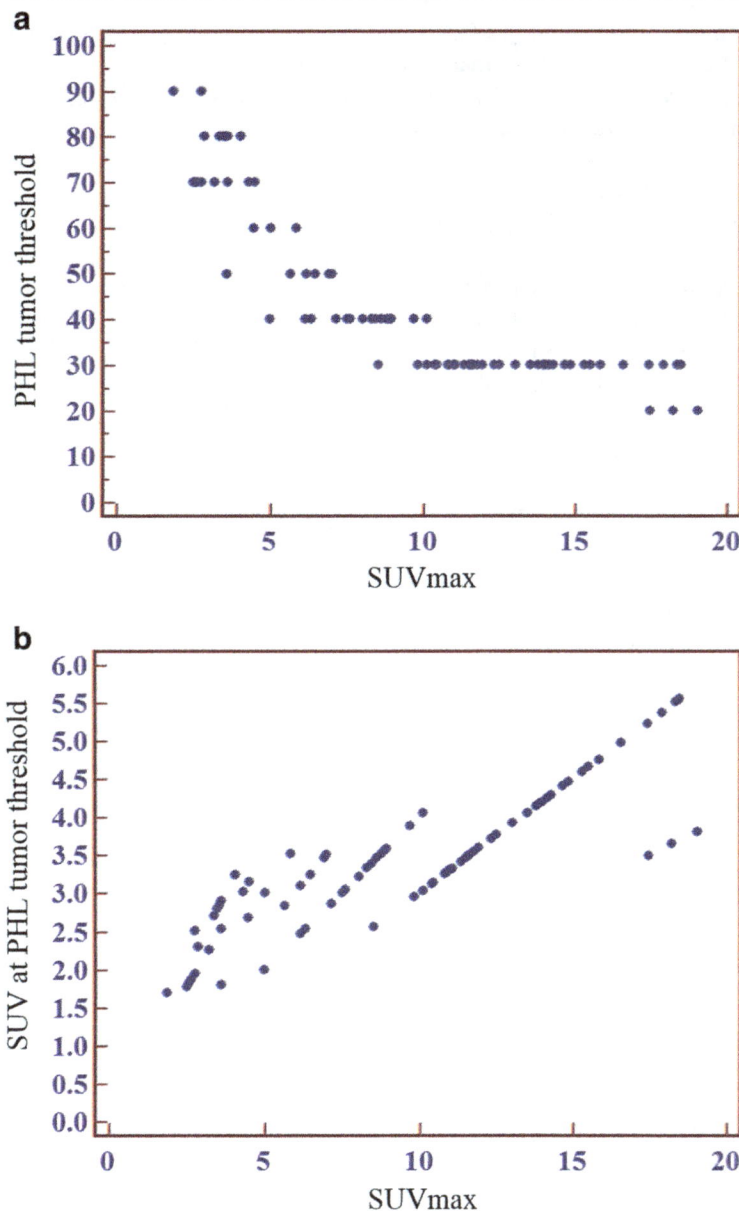

Fig. 7 Relationship between SUVmax and PHL tumor threshold. PHL tumor threshold (% of SUVmax) showed a strong inverse correlation with SUVmax (**a**: $\sigma = -0.923$, $p < 0.0001$). The SUV of PHL tumor threshold showed a strong positive correlation with SUVmax (**b**: $\sigma = 0.891$, $p < 0.0001$)

inspection of the tumor using PHL image settings. In contrast, SegGradient is determined using a special workstation. Second, an accurate percentage threshold can be determined by SegPHL (i.e., % of SUVmax). However, there is no way to determine an accurate % threshold of SegGradient. Third, although SegPHL is similar to Seg-Gradient, the exact point at which there is a large gradient change cannot be determined using SegPHL. In our study, we defined PHL tumor threshold as the starting point of the PHL (i.e., the innermost point of the PHL), as in Jun et al. [17]. However, the large gradient change of SegGra-dient could be located in the outermost point or in the

middle of the PHL. Another consideration is that the large gradient change of SegGradient might not be represented by a single % of SUVmax (i.e., the SUV of the large gradient change may differ in different parts of the tumor).

SegAdaptive is based on calibrated curves, where accurate % threshold changes as signal-to-background ratio changes [6, 13]. In this method, as the signal-to-background ratio increases, the accurate % threshold decreases [13]. Clinicians can choose an optimal regression equation to determine the accurate % threshold. Based on a phantom study, SegAdaptive is superior to fixed threshold methods [13, 26]. In our present study,

PHL tumor threshold showed a strong inverse correlation with SUVmax of ESCC ($\sigma = -0.923$, $p < 0.0001$; Fig. 7a), as reported for SegAdaptive in the phantom study. Similarly, Jun et al. [17] reported that PHL tumor threshold was inversely correlated with SUVmax of thyroid cancer.

Several studies have compared ML, MTV, PL, and pathologic tumor volume [12, 21, 27, 28]. The results of these reports suggest that there is no single optimal SUV or % of SUVmax threshold that can be used to define an accurate tumor margin [6]. In our present study, PHL tumor threshold (%) showed a significant inverse correlation with SUVmax of ESCC ($\sigma = -0.923$, $p < 0.0001$; Fig. 7a), and SUV of PHL tumor threshold had a significant positive correlation with SUVmax of ESCC ($\sigma = 0.891$, $p < 0.0001$; Fig. 7b). Our results are consistent with previous studies that compared ML, MTV, PL, and pathologic tumor volume [12, 21, 27] and with a previous PHL study of thyroid cancer [17]. The number of cases where ML was compared with PL was similar between our present study and other previous studies (Zhong et al. [12]: $n = 37$ in esophageal cancer; Borakati et al. [28]: $n = 21$ in esophageal cancer).

An accurate tumor segmentation method should satisfy the following conditions. First, the segmented ML has to have a high degree of correlation with PL. Second, the bias and standard deviation should be small on Bland-Altman plots. Third, no serious proportional errors should be found in Bland-Altman analysis. Fourth, the segmented ML should not be highly affected by SUVmax of ESCC. Fifth, the segmented ML should correlate strongly with EL. Among ML_{PHL}, $ML_{2.5}$, and $ML_{40\%}$, only ML_{PHL} satisfied these conditions. Although ESCCs in our present study were definitely larger and more visually heterogeneous than the thyroid cancers examined in a previous PHL study [17], SegPHL was the most accurate segmentation method among SegPHL, SegSUV, and Seg%. Therefore, we conclude that SegPHL is far more accurate than fixed threshold methods.

Our study had several limitations. First, the study design was a retrospective analysis. Thus, there might have been operator-dependent bias in the measurement of EL and PL. Second, comparison of MTV and pathologic tumor volume was impossible because a vertical incision along the esophagectomy specimen had to be performed to evaluate pathologic depth of invasion. The vertical incision process changed the ellipsoid tumor shape of the ESCC into a planar shape. Because a change in tumor shape could introduce serious bias, we only assessed the correlation between ML and PL. Third, PL was measured after formalin fixation, which could shrink the esophagectomy specimen.

Conclusion

In conclusion, SegPHL was more accurate than fixed threshold methods compared with PL. PHL tumor threshold was adjusted according to SUVmax of ESCC. We conclude that SegPHL might be used to accurately define the tumor margins of ESCCs.

Abbreviations

CCRT: concurrent chemoradiation therapy; EGD: esophagogastroduodenoscopy; EL: endoscopic tumor length; ESCC: esophageal squamous cell carcinoma; ESD: endoscopic submucosal dissection; FDG: F-18 fluorodeoxyglucose; ML: metabolic tumor length; $ML_{2.5}$: metabolic tumor length using SUV 2.5 threshold; $ML_{40\%}$: metabolic tumor length using fixed 40% of SUVmax threshold; ML_{PHL}: metabolic tumor length using the peritumoral halo layer method; MTV: metabolic tumor volume; PHL: peritumoral halo layer; PL: pathologic tumor length; Seg%: segmentation using fixed % of SUVmax; SegAdaptive: segmentation using the adaptive threshold method; SegGradient: segmentation using the gradient method; SegPHL: segmentation using the PHL method; SegSUV: segmentation using fixed SUV threshold; SegVisual: segmentation using visual delineation; SUV: standardized uptake value; SUVmax: maximum standardized uptake value; TLG: total lesion glycolysis

Acknowledgements

We would like to thank Dr. Hyo Sang Lee for statistical consultation and Dr. Bum Soo Kim for assisting with the review of FDG PET/CT images.

Funding

No funding was received.

Authors' contributions

SJ and YS wrote the manuscript and contributed to study conception. JP contributed to data collection and helped with image analyses. All authors read and approved the final manuscript.

Competing interests

The authors declare that they have no competing interests.

Author details

[1]Department of Nuclear Medicine, Kosin University Gospel Hospital, Kosin University College of Medicine, Busan 49297, South Korea. [2]Department of Radiology, Kosin University Gospel Hospital, Kosin University College of Medicine, Busan 49297, South Korea. [3]Department of Nuclear Medicine, Busan Seongso Hospital, Suyeong-ro, Nam-gu, Busan 48453, Republic of Korea.

References

1. Lemarignier C, Di Fiore F, Marre C, Hapdey S, Modzelewski R, Gouel P, et al. Pretreatment metabolic tumour volume is predictive of disease-free survival and overall survival in patients with oesophageal squamous cell carcinoma. Eur J Nucl Med Mol Imaging. 2014;41:2008–16. https://doi.org/10.1007/s00259-014-2839-y.
2. Surucu E, Demir Y, Sengoz T. The correlation between the metabolic tumor volume and hematological parameters in patients with esophageal cancer. Ann Nucl Med. 2015;29:906–10. https://doi.org/10.1007/s12149-015-1020-4.

3. Van de Wiele C, Kruse V, Smeets P, Sathekge M, Maes A. Predictive and prognostic value of metabolic tumour volume and total lesion glycolysis in solid tumours. Eur J Nucl Med Mol Imaging. 2013;40:290–301. https://doi.org/10.1007/s00259-012-2280-z.

4. Hollis AC, Quinn LM, Hodson J, Evans E, Plowright J, Begum R, et al. Prognostic significance of tumor length in patients receiving esophagectomy for esophageal cancer. J Surg Oncol. 2017;116:1114–22. https://doi.org/10.1002/jso.24789.

5. Roedl JB, Sahani DV, Colen RR, Fischman AJ, Mueller PR, Blake MA. Tumour length measured on PET-CT predicts the most appropriate stage-dependent therapeutic approach in oesophageal cancer. Eur Radiol. 2008;18:2833–40. https://doi.org/10.1007/s00330-008-1078-7.

6. Im HJ, Bradshaw T, Solaiyappan M, Cho SY. Current methods to define metabolic tumor volume in positron emission tomography: which one is better? Nucl Med Mol Imaging. 2018;52:5–15. https://doi.org/10.1007/s13139-017-0493-6.

7. Jeganathan R, McGuigan J, Campbell F, Lynch T. Does pre-operative estimation of oesophageal tumour metabolic length using 18F-fluorodeoxyglucose PET/CT images compare with surgical pathology length? Eur J Nucl Med Mol Imaging. 2011;38:656–62. https://doi.org/10.1007/s00259-010-1670-3.

8. Heron DE, Andrade RS, Flickinger J, Johnson J, Agarwala SS, Wu A, et al. Hybrid PET-CT simulation for radiation treatment planning in head-and-neck cancers: a brief technical report. Int J Radiat Oncol Biol Phys. 2004;60:1419–24. https://doi.org/10.1016/j.ijrobp.2004.05.037.

9. Doyeux K, Vauclin S, Hapdey S, Daouk J, Edet-Sanson A, Vera P, et al. Reproducibility of the adaptive thresholding calibration procedure for the delineation of 18F-FDG-PET-positive lesions. Nucl Med Commun. 2013;34:432–8. https://doi.org/10.1097/MNM.0b013e32835fe1f4.

10. Hatt M, Cheze-le Rest C, van Baardwijk A, Lambin P, Pradier O, Visvikis D. Impact of tumor size and tracer uptake heterogeneity in (18)F-FDG PET and CT non-small cell lung cancer tumor delineation. J Nucl Med. 2011;52:1690–7. https://doi.org/10.2967/jnumed.111.092767.

11. Sridhar P, Mercier G, Tan J, Truong MT, Daly B, Subramaniam RM. FDG PET metabolic tumor volume segmentation and pathologic volume of primary human solid tumors. AJR Am J Roentgenol. 2014;202:1114–9. https://doi.org/10.2214/AJR.13.11456.

12. Zhong X, Yu J, Zhang B, Mu D, Zhang W, Li D, et al. Using 18F-fluorodeoxyglucose positron emission tomography to estimate the length of gross tumor in patients with squamous cell carcinoma of the esophagus. Int J Radiat Oncol Biol Phys. 2009;73:136–41. https://doi.org/10.1016/j.ijrobp.2008.04.015.

13. Daisne JF, Sibomana M, Bol A, Doumont T, Lonneux M, Gregoire V. Tri-dimensional automatic segmentation of PET volumes based on measured source-to-background ratios: influence of reconstruction algorithms. Radiother Oncol. 2003;69:247–50.

14. Schaefer A, Kremp S, Hellwig D, Rube C, Kirsch CM, Nestle U. A contrast-oriented algorithm for FDG-PET-based delineation of tumour volumes for the radiotherapy of lung cancer: derivation from phantom measurements and validation in patient data. Eur J Nucl Med Mol Imaging. 2008;35:1989–99. https://doi.org/10.1007/s00259-008-0875-1.

15. Obara P, Liu H, Wroblewski K, Zhang CP, Hou P, Jiang Y, et al. Quantification of metabolic tumor activity and burden in patients with non-small-cell lung cancer: is manual adjustment of semiautomatic gradient-based measurements necessary? Nucl Med Commun. 2015;36:782–9. https://doi.org/10.1097/MNM.0000000000000317.

16. Murphy JD, Chisholm KM, Daly ME, Wiegner EA, Truong D, Iagaru A, et al. Correlation between metabolic tumor volume and pathologic tumor volume in squamous cell carcinoma of the oral cavity. Radiother Oncol. 2011;101:356–61. https://doi.org/10.1016/j.radonc.2011.05.040.

17. Jun S, Kim H, Nam HY. A new method for segmentation of FDG PET metabolic tumour volume using the peritumoural halo layer and a 10-step colour scale. A study in patients with papillary thyroid carcinoma. Nuklearmedizin. 2015;54:272–85. https://doi.org/10.3413/Nukmed-0749-15-06.

18. Bhutani MS, Barde CJ, Markert RJ, Gopalswamy N. Length of esophageal cancer and degree of luminal stenosis during upper endoscopy predict T stage by endoscopic ultrasound. Endoscopy. 2002;34:461–3. https://doi.org/10.1055/s-2002-31996.

19. Tixier F, Hatt M, Valla C, Fleury V, Lamour C, Ezzouhri S, et al. Visual versus quantitative assessment of intratumor 18F-FDG PET uptake heterogeneity: prognostic value in non-small cell lung cancer. J Nucl Med. 2014;55:1235–41. https://doi.org/10.2967/jnumed.113.133389.

20. Geets X, Lee JA, Bol A, Lonneux M, Gregoire V. A gradient-based method for segmenting FDG-PET images: methodology and validation. Eur J Nucl Med Mol Imaging. 2007;34:1427–38. https://doi.org/10.1007/s00259-006-0363-4.

21. Hyun SH, Choi JY, Shim YM, Kim K, Lee SJ, Cho YS, et al. Prognostic value of metabolic tumor volume measured by 18F-fluorodeoxyglucose positron emission tomography in patients with esophageal carcinoma. Ann Surg Oncol. 2010;17:115–22. https://doi.org/10.1245/s10434-009-0719-7.

22. Hatt M, Cheze-Le Rest C, Aboagye EO, Kenny LM, Rosso L, Turkheimer FE, et al. Reproducibility of 18F-FDG and 3'-deoxy-3'-18F-fluorothymidine PET tumor volume measurements. J Nucl Med. 2010;51:1368–76. https://doi.org/10.2967/jnumed.110.078501.

23. Schinagl DA, Span PN, Oyen WJ, Kaanders JH. Can FDG PET predict radiation treatment outcome in head and neck cancer? Results of a prospective study. Eur J Nucl Med Mol Imaging. 2011;38:1449–58. https://doi.org/10.1007/s00259-011-1789-x.

24. Lee JA. Segmentation of positron emission tomography images: some recommendations for target delineation in radiation oncology. Radiother Oncol. 2010;96:302–7. https://doi.org/10.1016/j.radonc.2010.07.003.

25. Njeh CF. Tumor delineation: the weakest link in the search for accuracy in radiotherapy. J Med Phys. 2008;33:136–40. https://doi.org/10.4103/0971-6203.44472.

26. Biehl KJ, Kong FM, Dehdashti F, Jin JY, Mutic S, El Naqa I, et al. 18F-FDG PET definition of gross tumor volume for radiotherapy of non-small cell lung cancer: is a single standardized uptake value threshold approach appropriate? J Nucl Med. 2006;47:1808–12.

27. Yu J, Li X, Xing L, Mu D, Fu Z, Sun X, et al. Comparison of tumor volumes as determined by pathologic examination and FDG-PET/CT images of non-small-cell lung cancer: a pilot study. Int J Radiat Oncol Biol Phys. 2009;75:1468–74. https://doi.org/10.1016/j.ijrobp.2009.01.019.

28. Borakati A, Razack A, Cawthorne C, Roy R, Usmani S, Ahmed N. A comparative study of quantitative assessment with fluorine-18-fluorodeoxyglucose positron-emission tomography and endoscopic ultrasound in oesophageal cancer. Nucl Med Commun. 2018;39:628–35. https://doi.org/10.1097/MNM.0000000000000844.

25

68Ga-PSMA PET/CT in prostate cancer patients – patterns of disease, benign findings and pitfalls

Zohar Keidar[1,2]* (ID), Ronit Gill[1], Elinor Goshen[3,4], Ora Israel[1,2], Tima Davidson[5], Maryna Morgulis[5], Natalia Pirmisashvili[1] and Simona Ben-Haim[6,7]

Abstract

Background: 68Ga-PSMA PET/CT has an important role in assessment of prostate cancer patients with biochemical recurrence and is evolving in staging high- and intermediate risk disease. The aim of present study was to describe the metastatic patterns and frequency of involved sites of prostate cancer and to assess the incidence of benign Ga68-PSMA avid PET/CT findings in a large patient population.

Methods: 68Ga-PSMA PET/CT studies performed in two tertiary medical centers over a period of 24 months were retrospectively reviewed. The incidence and location of pathological 68Ga-PSMA avid foci, suspicious to represent malignancy, as well as those of unexpected benign foci of increased 68Ga-PSMA activity were documented and analyzed.

Results: There were 445 68Ga-PSMA studies in 438 men (mean age 72.4, range 51–92 years) with prostate cancer referred for biochemical failure ($n = 270$, 61%), staging high-risk disease ($n = 112$, 25%), response assessment ($n = 30$, 7%), follow-up ($n = 22$, 5%) and suspected bone metastases (n = 11, 2%). 68Ga-PSMA avid disease sites were observed in 319 studies (72%), in 181 studies (67%) for biochemical recurrence, 94 studies for staging (84%) ($p < 0.05$), in 22 studies for response assessment (73%), 10 follow up studies (45%) and in five patients with suspected bone metastases (45%). 68Ga-PSMA avid lesions were most commonly detected in the prostate ($n = 193$, 43%), loco-regional spread ($n = 51$, 11%), abdomino-pelvic nodes ($n = 129$, 29%) and distant metastases ($n = 158$, 36%), including bone metastases ($n = 11$, 25%), distant lymphadenopathy ($n = 29$, 7%) and other organs ($n = 18$, 4%). Distant 68Ga-PSMA-avid metastases were commonly seen in patients with biochemical recurrence (14/21 lesions), but were not seen in patient referred for staging ($p < 0.013$). There were 96 non-malignant 68Ga-PSMA avid foci in 81 studies, most common in reactive lymph nodes ($n = 36$, 38%), nonmalignant bone lesions ($n = 21$, 22%), thyroid nodules ($n = 9$, 9%), ganglions (n = 9, 9%) and lung findings ($n = 8$, 8%).

Conclusion: The distribution of 68Ga-PSMA avid metastatic lesions is similar to data previously reported mainly from autopsy with comparable detection rates, indicating 68Ga-PSMA PET/CT is an accurate detection tool in patients with metastatic prostate cancer. If confirmed by further prospective studies 68Ga-PSMA PET/CT should be included in the guidelines to evaluate disease extent in these patients.

Keywords: Prostate cancer, 68Ga-PSMA, PET/CT

* Correspondence: zohar@keidar.net
[1]Department of Nuclear Medicine, Rambam Health Care Campus, Haifa, Israel
[2]The Bruce Rappaport Faculty of Medicine, Technion – Israel Institute of Technology, Haifa, Israel
Full list of author information is available at the end of the article

Introduction

Prostate cancer is the most common solid malignancy in men and the 3rd leading cause of cancer related death with estimated 161,360 new cases and 6730 estimated deaths in the United States in 2017 [1, 2]. The diagnosis of prostate cancer is obtained by biopsy after clinical, biochemical or imaging suspicion arises [2]. Staging is determined by histology and using imaging modalities, mainly CT and MRI. Patients are then stratified into three risk level groups according to their stage, PSA level and Gleason Score (GS). Metastatic prostate cancer has a recognizable pattern of spread, involving mainly regional lymph nodes (predominantly pelvic and para-aortic) and the skeleton (predominantly the spine) [3]. Additional extranodal metastatic sites occur in the lungs and liver [3, 4]. Treatment strategies of prostate cancer are based on the patient's risk group and include watchful waiting, hormonal therapy, radiotherapy, surgical intervention, chemotherapy or a combination of the above.

Prostate-specific membrane antigen (PSMA) is a type II transmembrane protein that acts as a glutamate carboxypeptidase enzyme [5, 6] and is a useful target for diagnostic and therapeutic applications in nuclear medicine because of its' high expression in prostate cancer cells. The physiologic biodistribution of radiolabeled PSMA, at present mainly using 68Ga, includes the salivary and lacrimal glands, the small intestine, liver and spleen. It can also be taken up, to a lesser extent, in normal prostate tissue [5, 6]. 68Ga-PSMA is a valuable tool in the assessment and management of advanced prostate cancer patients. However, a wide range of malignancies other than prostate cancer have also been reported to express PSMA as part of tumor neovasculature [7–9] with 68Ga-PSMA avidity described in cases of breast cancer [10], renal cell carcinoma [11], glioblastoma multiforme [12], hepatocellular carcinoma [13], differentiated thyroid cancer [14], colorectal carcinoma [15], non-small cell lung cancer [16] and follicular lymphoma [17]. PSMA uptake has been also reported in a large variety of benign lesions such as retroperitoneal schwannoma [18], desmoid tumor [19], Paget's disease of bone [20], sarcoidosis [21], sub-acute stroke [22] and bone fractures [23, 24]. Uptake in benign processes as well as in the celiac ganglia can mimic a lymph node metastasis [24, 25] and can therefore be pitfalls in clinical practice.

The aim of present study was to describe the metastatic patterns and frequency of involved sites of disease in prostate cancer and also to assess the incidence and outline the characteristics of benign Ga68-PSMA avid PET/CT findings in a large patient population.

Materials and methods

Study population

All 68Ga-PSMA PET/CT studies performed in two academic centers (RHCC and CSMC) over a 24-month period were retrospectively analyzed. In both centers the routine follow-up for patients with localized disease includes clinical follow-up every 3–6 months with PSA levels tested twice a year and digital rectal examination performed once a year. When PSA values increase, 68Ga-PSMA PET/CT is performed. In patients with metastatic disease, clinical follow-up is performed every 1–3 months including PSA levels and other blood tests. Bone scan and CT are performed every 3–6 months. 68Ga-PSMA PET/CT is performed when either radio ligand therapy using lutetium-177 PSMA or radiation therapy are considered. Patients' charts were extracted from the institutional database and were reviewed. The ethics committees of both centers approved this retrospective data analysis and patient consent has been waived. The following clinical data were retrieved and recorded: age, indication for 68Ga-PSMA PET/CT imaging, GS and PSA level at the time of diagnosis and at the time of the PET/CT study. Previous therapy administered prior to the PET/CT study was also recorded.

PET/CT acquisition and processing

PET and contrast enhanced CT (when not contraindicated) were acquired consecutively from head to the mid-thigh using a PET/CT system (Discovery 690, GE Healthcare, Milwaukee, US or Gemini XL, Philips Medical Systems, Cleveland, OH, US), approximately 60 min after the injection on average of 159 MBq (4.3 mCi) 68Ga-PSMA (range: 74 to 219.4 MBq, 2 to 5.9 mCi).

The following parameters were used for CT imaging: pitch 1.375:1, gantry rotation time 0.7 s, 120 kVp, automatically adjusted current in the range 100–650 mA, and a 2.5 mm slice thickness. A contrast enhanced CT scan was obtained 60 s after injection of 2 mL/kg of non-ionic contrast (Omnipaque 300; GE Healthcare). A PET scan followed in 3D acquisition mode for the same axial coverage. CT images were used for fusion with the PET data. PET images were reconstructed with CT attenuation correction using a 3D ordered subset expectation maximization (3D-OSEM) or a line of response row-action maximum-likelihood (LOR-RAMLA) algorithm.

Interpretation and analysis of PET/CT images

All studies were reviewed retrospectively with knowledge of the patient's clinical history and results of previous imaging studies. A team of two Nuclear Medicine physicians or a Nuclear Medicine Physician and a Radiologist interpreted the PET/CT studies in consensus. Any focal 68Ga-PSMA uptake higher than surrounding activity not associated with a known site of physiological uptake and with a corresponding morphological abnormality on CT was considered pathological and suspicious for malignancy. The fraction of 68Ga-PSMA PET/CT studies that were concluded as positive for malignancy was defined as "detectability rate". Any site of incidental 68Ga-PSMA uptake considered to represent non-malignant findings was separately documented. The incidence and location of pathological 68Ga-PSMA avid foci, suspicious to represent malignancy, as well as those of unexpected benign foci of increased 68Ga-PSMA activity were documented and analyzed. Findings were characterized as malignant or as benign based on clinical correlation and other imaging modalities, when available.

Statistical analysis

Differences between average PSA levels in the study groups were assessed using the parametric Mann-Whitney test. Difference in detectability rates as well as in disease distribution between patient groups, categorized according to referral indications, were assessed using the Chi square and Fisher tests. P value smaller then 0.05 was considered statistically significant.

Results

Four hundred and forty-five 68Ga-PSMA studies were performed in 438 men (mean age 72.4, range 51–92 years) with prostate cancer. Average GS was 7.5 (range 5–10). Average PSA level at diagnosis was 46.9 ng/mL (range 0–4000, median 11.0) and at the time of the PET/CT study 18.4 ng/mL (range 0.05–533, median 4.3). The indications for 68Ga-PSMA PET/CT included biochemical failure ($n = 270$, 61%), staging of high-risk disease ($n = 112$, 25%), assessment of response to anti-cancer therapy ($n = 30$, 7%), follow-up with no evidence of clinical, biochemical or imaging suspicious for recurrence on ($n = 22$, 5%) and suspected bone metastases on other imaging modalities performed as routine assessment ($n = 11$, 2%) (Table 1). Previous therapy, administered before PET/CT, is detailed in Table 1.

68Ga-PSMA avid sites of disease were detected in 319 studies (72%). Prostate gland involvement was detected in 193 studies (43%), loco-regional spread including seminal vesicles, bladder, rectum and adjacent fat tissue was seen in 51 studies (11%). Abdomino-pelvic nodal metastases were found in 129 studies (29%) and distant metastases including lymph nodes outside the abdomen and pelvis, bones and distant organs in 158 studies (36%) (Table 2). Radiotracer avidity (SUVmax) for different malignant sites is summarized in Table 2 and Fig. 1.

68Ga-PSMA avid bone metastases were diagnosed in 111 studies (25%) including oligometastases (up to three lesions, $n = 63$, 57%) and multiple metastases (more than three lesions, $n = 48$, 43%).

Fifty-five 68Ga-PSMA avid lymph node metastases outside the abdomen and pelvis were identified in 29 studies (7%), including the mediastinum ($n = 25$, 45%), the cervical, supra- and infra-clavicular regions ($n = 17$, 31%), the axillae ($n = 4$, 7%) and additional thoracic sites (retro-pectoral, internal mammary, retro-crural; $n = 9$, 16%).

Table 1 Patient Characteristics, $n = 445$

Parameter	Value
Age	72.4 years (51–92 years)
PSA	
At diagnosis	46.9 ng/ml (0–4000 ng/ml, median 11.0)
At time of 68Ga-PSMA PET/CT	18.4 ng/ml (0.05–533 ng/ml, median 4.3)
Gleason Score	
≤ 6	50 (11.4%)
7	128 (29%)
≥ 8	146 (33%)
Average	7.5
Therapy prior to 68Ga-PSMA PET/CT	
Radical Prostatectomy	150 (34%)
Radiotherapy/Brachytherapy	171 (38%)
Hormonal	206 (46%)
Chemotherapy	23 (5%)
Other	27 (6%)
No prior treatment	122 (28%)
Indication for PET/CT	270(61%)
Biochemical failure	112 (25%)
Staging –high risk	30 (7%)
Assess response to treatment	22 (5%)
Follow up	11 (2%)
Suspected bone metastases	

68Ga-PSMA avid metastases in other organs (21 lesions) were observed in 18 studies (4%). The distribution of these foci included the lungs ($n = 10$, 48%), liver ($n = 5$, 21%), brain ($n = 2$, 10%), pleura ($n = 2$, 10%), spleen ($n = 1$) and peritoneum ($n = 1$).

According to referral indications, none of the metastases in distant organs were found in patients evaluated at staging, whereas two thirds of these lesions occurred in patients who were investigated for biochemical failure (14/21, $p < 0.013$). 7 lesions were found in studies done for other indications (assess response to treatment, follow up and suspected bone metastases). There was no statistically significant difference between these groups in other sites of disease involvement including loco-regional spread (14% in staging vs. 10% in biochemical failure), abdomino-pelvic nodal metastases 32% vs. 30%), bone metastases (19% vs. 24%) and distant lymph nodes (4% vs. 7%).

The average PSA level in patients with disease limited to the prostate gland was 17.2 ng/mL compared to 28.9 ng/mL in patients with local or distant metastases ($p = 0.2$). The average PSA level in patients who were referred for staging of high risk disease was 29.9 ng/mL

Table 2 Distribution of 68Ga-PSMA avid sites of prostate cancer involvement

	No studies (%)	SUVmax (range)
$N = 319$	72%	
Prostate	193 (43%)	11.3 (2–61)
Loco-regional spread	51 (11%)	13 (2–78)
Abdomino-pelvic nodal metastases	129 (29%)	12 (1.4–100)
Distant metastases	158 (36%)	
Bone metastases	111 (25%)	12.5 (1.9–91)
Distant nodes	29 (7%)	11.3 (1.5–58)
Other[a]	18 (4%)	7.1 (1.8–14.6)

[a]68Ga-PSMA avid metastases in lungs ($n = 10$, 48%), liver ($n = 5$, 21%), brain ($n = 2$, 10%), pleura ($n = 2$, 10%), spleen ($n = 1$) and peritoneum ($n = 1$)

compared to 14.8 ng/mL in patients with biochemical failure ($p = 0.05$, borderline significant).

Detectability rates of active disease using 68Ga-PSMA were calculated for different PSA levels and according to study indications. The detection rate was 31% for PSA 0–0.99 ng/mL, 63% for 1–1.99 ng/mL, 74% for 2–3.99, 77% for 3–9.99 and 90% in patients with PSA higher than 10 ng/mL. In 270 studies performed for the assessment of biochemical failure there were 181 (67%) positive 68Ga-PSMA-PET/CT studies. In patients referred for staging of high risk disease 94 out of 112 studies (84%) were positive. The difference in detectability rates between these two patient groups was statistically significant ($p < 0.05$). Detectability rates of malignancy in the additional patient groups were of 73% ($n = 22$) in cases assessed for monitoring response to treatment, 45% in patients were referred for follow up ($n = 10$), and 45% in patients with suspected bone metastases ($n = 5$) (Fig. 2). Due to small patient numbers in these subgroups the level of statistical significance could not be calculated.

Ninety-six 68Ga-PSMA avid foci were categorized as non-malignant in 81 studies (18%). They were localized to benign reactive lymph nodes ($n = 36$, 38%, in the axilla, inguinal region and pulmonary hila), the skeleton ($n = 21$, 22%, including 7 fractures, 13 degenerative changes and one patient with diffuse bone uptake related to known anemia), the thyroid gland ($n = 9$, 9%, including 6 with focal uptake in thyroid nodules and 3 with diffuse thyroid uptake), lungs ($n = 8$, 8%, including 6 opacities representing inflammatory infiltrates and 2 lung nodules), ganglions ($n = 9$, 9%, including 7 in celiac ganglion, one in stellate ganglion and one in a trigeminal ganglion), gallbladder ($n = 5$, 5%, without any specific CT findings), stomach or gastro-esophageal region ($n = 4$, 4%), pancreas ($n = 2$, 2%) and one case each in an accessory spleen and a surgical scar. Radiotracer avidity (SUVmax) of the non-malignant sites is summarized in Table 3 and Fig. 3.

Discussion

68Ga-PSMA PET/CT has an important role in assessment of prostate cancer patients with biochemical recurrence [6, 26–31] and is evolving in staging high- and intermediate risk disease prior to surgery or radiotherapy [28, 32, 33].

In present study we have assessed the distribution of 68Ga-PSMA avid prostate cancer metastases in a large group of 445 patients from two tertiary medical centers referred mainly for biochemical recurrence (61% of patients) and staging of high grade disease (25%). The highest detectability rates of active disease were observed in these two groups of patients, 67% and 84% respectively. In a meta-analysis including 16 manuscripts and 1309 patients, the overall percentage of positive 68Ga-PSMA studies in biochemical recurrence was 76% (25), increasing from 42% in patients with PSA levels

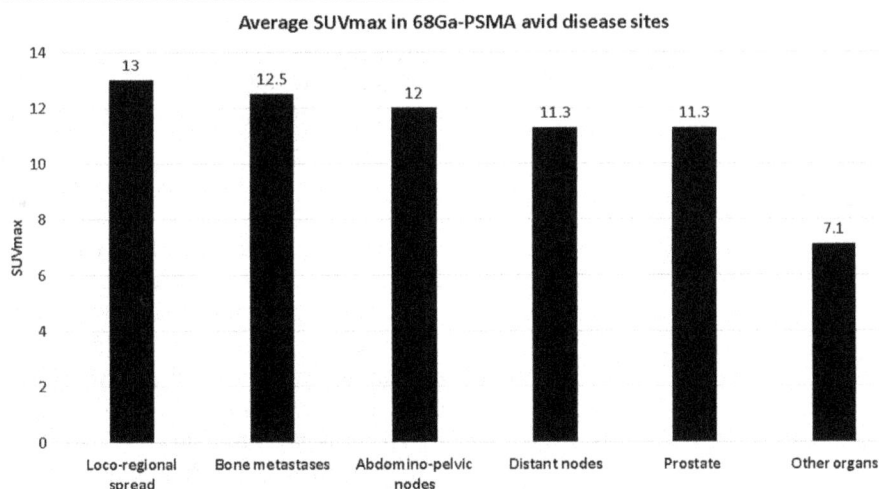

Fig. 1 Average SUVmax in 68Ga-PSMA-avid disease sites

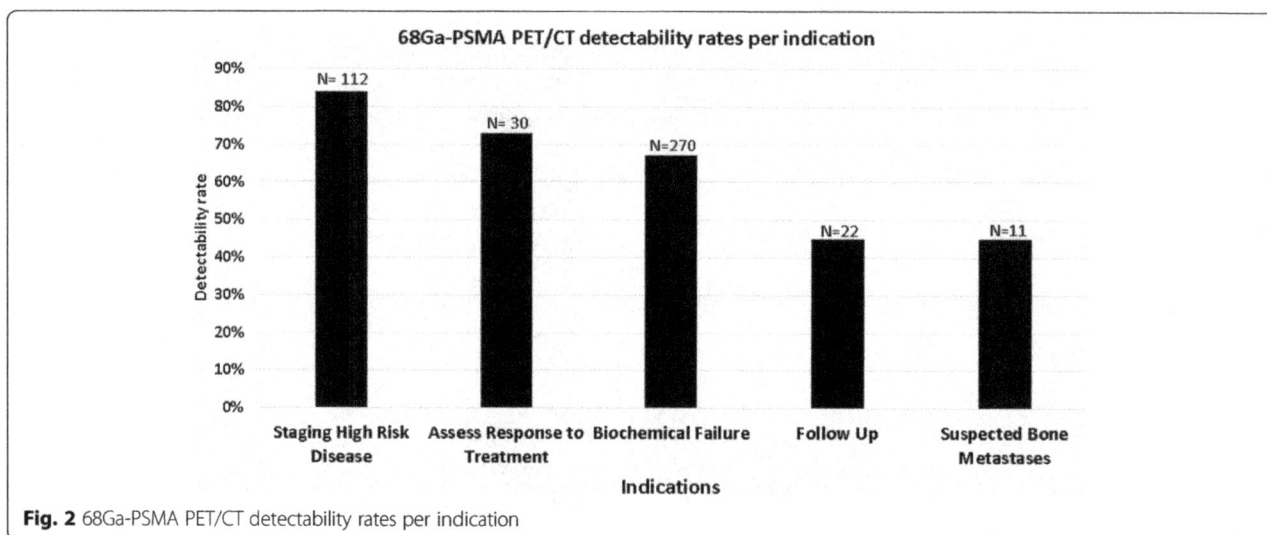

Fig. 2 68Ga-PSMA PET/CT detectability rates per indication

less than 0.2 to 95% when PSA was greater than 2 ng/mL (25). Detection rate of 67% in present study is comparable, taking into account the wide range of PSA values in the study population (0.05–533 ng/mL). In staging of high risk disease 93% of patients had intra-prostatic avidity whereas 68Ga-PSMA avid pelvic lymph node metastases were identified in 33.3% 4-20 mm in diameter. There were 66.7% false negative lymph nodes, measuring 1–10.8 mm in diameter (30). Another study in 51 patients with high risk disease reported sensitivity, specificity and accuracy of 53%, 86% and 76% in detecting lymph node metastases. Maximum length of tumor within the detected lymph node metastases was 5-30 mm,

compared to 0.2-8 mm for undetected involved lymph nodes [34]. In another study in 42 patients with intermediate to high risk prostate cancer 68Ga-PSMA PET/CT identified all 41 involved lymph nodes with a short axis diameter > 10 mm as well as 8/10 involved lymph nodes with a short axis diameter of 5-10 mm. There were no involved lymph nodes with short axis diameter < 5 mm [35]. In other studies, neither extrapelvic lymph node metastases nor visceral involvement was found [33, 34]. Similarly, in present study there were no distant 68Ga-PSMA avid metastases in patients referred for staging of high risk disease.

Although the present study population differs, the distribution of metastatic lesions bears some resemblance to data previously published mainly from autopsy [3]. Bubendorf et al. have assessed the metastatic spread of prostate cancer in an autopsy study of 1589 patients [3], about half of them with previously known prostate cancer and the rest with an occult tumor. Metastatic prostate cancer was diagnosed in 35% of patients. In patients with lymph node metastases paraaortic nodes (in 80%) and pelvic lymph node metastases (55%) were most common, followed by mediastinal (40%) and inguinal nodes (18%) with only rare involvement of other nodal sites. Bone metastases, predominantly in the spine, were present in 90% of patients with metastatic disease, 46% had lung metastases, 25% liver and 21% pleural metastases. Rare sites of metastatic disease included the adrenals in 13%, peritoneum in 7%, meninges in 6%, kidney and ureter/urethra 3% each, pericardium and spleen 2% each and brain, thyroid, bowel, pancreas and mesentery in 1% each (3). In present study overall 72% of patients who were referred for various indications, all with known prostate cancer had 68Ga-PSMA avid disease. The most common sites of 68Ga-PSMA avid metastases included abdomino-pelvic nodal metastases in 29%, skeletal metastases in 25%,

Table 3 Distribution of 68Ga-PSMA-avid non-malignant findings

N = 96	No (%)	SUVmax (range)
Benign lymph nodes	36 (38%)	2.5 (0.7–17.7)
Skeletal	21 (22%)	3 (1.4–5.5)
Fracture	7	
Degenerative	13	
Anemia	1	
Thyroid	9 (9%)	4 (2.3–9)
Focal (nodules)	6	
Diffuse	3	
Lungs	8 (8%)	2.6 (1.5–4.3)
Inflammatory infiltrates	6	
Nodules	2	
Ganglions	9 (9%)	4.1 (2.2–7.4)
Celiac	7	
Other[a]	2	
Gallbladder	5 (5%)	6.7 (5.8–8)
Stomach or GEJ	4 (4%)	3.2 (3–3.76)
Pancreas	2 (2%)	2.8 (2.7–2.9)
Accessory spleen	1	4.1
Surgical scar	1	3.3

[a]One stellate ganglion, one trigeminal ganglion

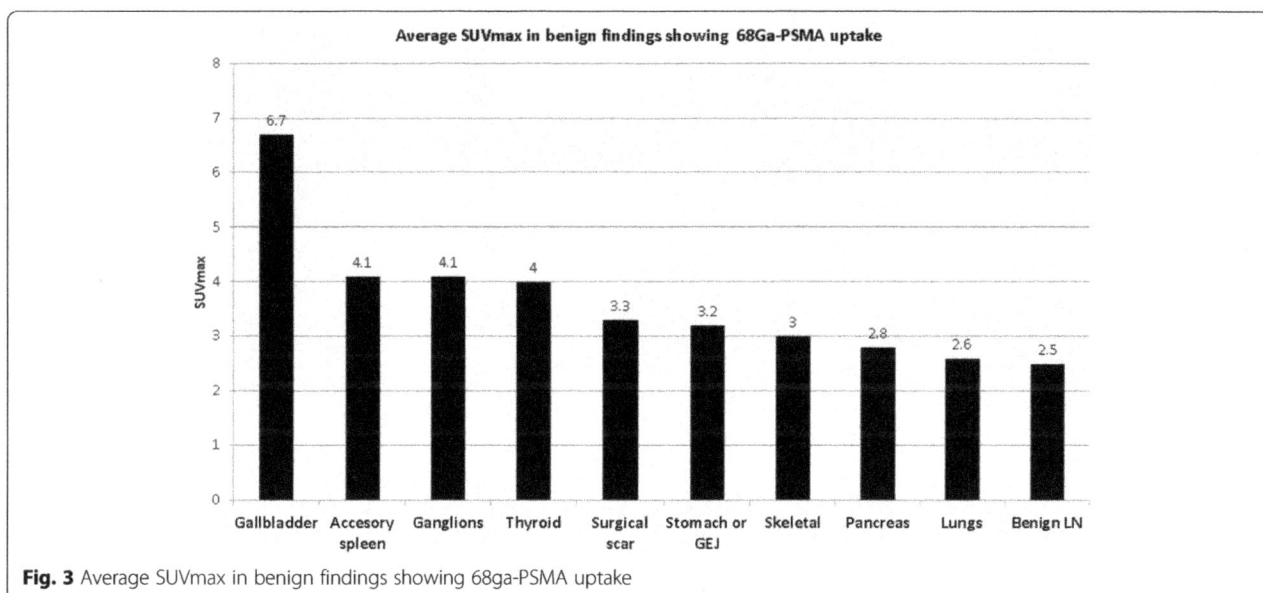

Fig. 3 Average SUVmax in benign findings showing 68ga-PSMA uptake

loco-regional spread in 11% and distant nodal metastases in 7% of cases. The most common distant nodal metastases were observed in the mediastinum, followed by cervical, supra- and infra-clavicular regions, with other nodal sites being less commonly involved. Other less common sites of 68Ga-PSMA avid metastases occurred in 4% of the studies, with almost half of them in the lungs, about 20% in the liver, and isolated cases of brain, pleura, spleen and peritoneal metastases. Interestingly, distant spread was most frequently seen in patients referred for the assessment of biochemical recurrence, but absent in patients referred for staging of high risk disease.

In present study 68Ga-PSMA avid bone metastases were diagnosed in 111 studies (25%). Focal 68Ga-PSMA uptake in the skeleton is usually considered to indicate the presence of bone metastases, unless it can be attributed to a corresponding skeletal lesion [18, 20, 23]. In current study, focal 68-Ga-PSMA uptake was also found in a variety of benign bone lesions. Caution and comparison with morphological findings on the CT component are therefore recommended prior to labeling, mainly solitary skeletal lesions, as metastatic. There is limited clinical evidence for the use of 68Ga-PSMA PET/CT in the evaluation of bone metastases in patients with prostate cancer. In a recent review of the published literature which included 31 case series and 6 case reports, 68Ga-PSMA PET/CT demonstrated higher diagnostic accuracy than bone scan in the initial staging and in biochemical recurrence, but not in patients with known metastatic prostate cancer [36].

Physiological distribution of 68Ga-PSMA as well as pitfalls and artifacts have been previously reported by several groups [5, 6, 10, 24, 25]. In the early days of using 68Ga-PSMA PET/CT, when the tracer was considered

specific for prostate cancer, pitfalls in the interpretation of 68Ga-PSMA PET/CT studies were described, most of them as case reports [5, 17, 18, 20, 21], as well as case reports of 68Ga-PSMA avidity in other tumors (9–15).

To provide an accurate interpretation of 68Ga-PSMA PET/CT studies it is therefore important to be knowledgeable of the physiologic distribution of the tracer, the pattern of disease spread, as well as of avidity related to potential benign pitfalls. In present study 96 benign foci of 68Ga-PSMA avidity were found in a subgroup of 81 patients. Following numerous case reports this is, to the best of our knowledge, the first study to assess the prevalence and degree of 68Ga-PSMA avidity of non-malignant findings in a large group of patients with prostate cancer. Benign lymph nodes were the most common site of non-malignant 68Ga-PSMA activity, representing 38% of foci, followed by skeletal uptake, mainly in degenerative changes and fractures, in 22%. Up to 10% of findings included focal or diffuse uptake in the thyroid, in lung lesions or ganglions. In present study the prevalence of celiac ganglion uptake was considerably lower (7%) compared to Krohn et al. who identified focal celiac ganglion activity in 76 of 85 patients (89%) [25]. Increased gallbladder uptake was seen in 5% of patients, compared to 10% previously reported in a series of 40 patients [5].

Although on average the intensity of 68Ga-PSMA uptake in non-malignant findings was significantly lower as compared to that of metastatic lesions, there is a wide range of SUVmax levels. While some of the metastatic lesions presented with SUVmax of 2 or less some of the benign 68Ga-PSMA avid findings showed an SUVmax above 6. Therefore, it is important to be aware of the possible non-malignant etiologies of tracer uptake of even moderate or high intensity.

While in present series no other 68Ga-PSMA avid malignant tumors were identified this tracer has been shown to accumulate in other cancers, specifically in the endothelial cells of tumoral and peri-tumoral capillaries, possibly related to angiogenesis [8, 11–17].

The major limitations of present study are its retrospective nature and the lack of histopathological correlative data, the latter compensated by clinical and imaging follow up. However, since this study includes a large patient cohort assessed in two tertiary centers who were referred for different indications present findings could be used as a basis in planning of prospective studies.

Conclusion

Present study shows 68Ga-PSMA avid sites of disease following the distribution pattern of prostate cancer involvement as previously described mainly in autopsy studies with comparable detection rates. 68Ga-PSMA PET/CT is therefore an accurate non-invasive tool. If current results will be confirmed by further prospective studies 68Ga-PSMA PET/CT should be included, in addition to MRI of the pelvis, in the recommendations and society guidelines to evaluate disease extent in patients with prostate cancer.

Abbreviations
CSMC: Chaim Sheba Medical Center; CT: Computed tomography; Ga: Gallium; GE: General Electrics; OSEM: Ordered Subsets Expectation-Maximization; GS: Gleason score; MRI: Magnetic resonance imaging; PET: Positron emission tomography; PSA: Prostate specific antigen; PSMA: Prostate specific membrane antigen; RHCC: Rambam Health Care Campus; SUV: Standardized Uptake Value

Acknowledgements
Not applicable.

Funding
This research did not receive any specific funding.

Authors' contributions
Guarantor of integrity of the entire study: ZK, SBH; study concepts and design: ZK, SBH; literature research: ZK, SBH, RG; data collection: SBH, RG, TD, NP,MM, EG; data analysis: RG, SBH; manuscript preparation: SBH, RG, ZK, manuscript editing: OI, SBH. All authors read and approved the final manuscript.

Competing interests
The authors declare that they have no competing interests.

Author details
[1]Department of Nuclear Medicine, Rambam Health Care Campus, Haifa, Israel. [2]The Bruce Rappaport Faculty of Medicine, Technion – Israel Institute of Technology, Haifa, Israel. [3]Department of Nuclear Medicine, Wolfson Medical Center, Holon, Israel. [4]Sackler School of Medicine, Tel Aviv University, Tel Aviv, Israel. [5]Department of Nuclear Medicine, Chaim Sheba Medical Center, Ramat Gan, Israel. [6]Department of Medical Biophysics and Nuclear Medicine, Hadassah University Hospital, Ein Kerem, Jerusalem, Israel. [7]University College London and UCL Hospitals, NHS Trust, London, UK.

References
1. Society AC. Cancer Facts&Figures: American cancer Societ- Atlanta; 2017.
2. Parker C, Gillessen S, Heidenreich A, Horwich A. Cancer of the prostate: ESMO clinical practice guidelines for diagnosis, treatment and follow-up. Ann Oncol. 2015;26(Suppl 5):v69–77.
3. Bubendorf L, Schopfer A, Wagner U, et al. Metastatic patterns of prostate cancer: an autopsy study of 1,589 patients. Hum Pathol. 2000;31(5):578–83.
4. Vinjamoori AH, Jagannathan JP, Shinagare AB, et al. Atypical metastases from prostate cancer: 10-year experience at a single institution. AJR Am J Roentgenol. 2012;199(2):367–72.
5. Demirci E, Sahin OE, Ocak M, Akovali B, Nematyazar J, Kabasakal L. Normal distribution pattern and physiological variants of 68Ga-PSMA-11 PET/CT imaging. Nucl Med Commun. 2016;37(11):1169–79.
6. Afshar-Oromieh A, Malcher A, Eder M, et al. PET imaging with a [68Ga] gallium-labelled PSMA ligand for the diagnosis of prostate cancer: biodistribution in humans and first evaluation of tumour lesions. Eur J Nucl Med Mol Imaging. 2013;40(4):486–95.
7. Fragomeni. PSMA-targeted Imaging: Beyond Prostate Cancer PET Center of Excellence Newsletter 2016;13(1).
8. Backhaus P, Noto B, Avramovic N, et al. Targeting PSMA by radioligands in non-prostate disease-current status and future perspectives. Eur J Nucl Med Mol Imaging. 2018;45(5):860–77.
9. Salas Fragomeni RA, Amir T, Sheikhbahaei S, Harvey SC, Javadi MS, Solnes LB, et al. Imaging of nonprostate cancers using PSMA-targeted radiotracers: rationale, current state of the field, and a Call to Arms. J Nucl Med. 2018; 59(6):871–7.
10. Sathekge M, Modiselle M, Vorster M, et al. (68) Ga-PSMA imaging of metastatic breast cancer. Eur J Nucl Med Mol Imaging. 2015;42(9):1482–3.
11. Demirci E, Ocak M, Kabasakal L, et al. (68) Ga-PSMA PET/CT imaging of metastatic clear cell renal cell carcinoma. Eur J Nucl Med Mol Imaging. 2014;41(7):1461–2.
12. Schwenck J, Tabatabai G, Skardelly M, et al. In vivo visualization of prostate-specific membrane antigen in glioblastoma. Eur J Nucl Med Mol Imaging. 2015;42(1):170–1.
13. Sasikumar A, Joy A, Nanabala R, Pillai MR, Thomas B, Vikraman KR. (68) Ga-PSMA PET/CT imaging in primary hepatocellular carcinoma. Eur J Nucl Med Mol Imaging. 2016;43(4):795–6.
14. Verburg FA, Krohn T, Heinzel A, Mottaghy FM, Behrendt FF. First evidence of PSMA expression in differentiated thyroid cancer using [(6)(8) Ga]PSMA-HBED-CC PET/CT. Eur J Nucl Med Mol Imaging. 2015;42(10):1622–3.
15. Huang YT, Fong W, Thomas P. Rectal Carcinoma on 68Ga-PSMA PET/CT. Clin Nucl Med. 2016;41(3):e167–8.
16. Shetty D, Loh H, Bui C, Mansberg R, Stevanovic A. Elevated 68Ga prostate-specific membrane antigen activity in metastatic non-small cell lung Cancer. Clin Nucl Med. 2016;41(5):414–6.
17. Kanthan GL, Coyle L, Kneebone A, Schembri GP, Hsiao E. Follicular lymphoma showing avid uptake on 68Ga PSMA-HBED-CC PET/CT. Clin Nucl Med. 2016;41(6):500–1.
18. Rischpler C, Maurer T, Schwaiger M, Eiber M. Intense PSMA-expression using (68) Ga-PSMA PET/CT in a paravertebral schwannoma mimicking prostate cancer metastasis. Eur J Nucl Med Mol Imaging. 2016;43(1): 193–4.
19. Kanthan GL, Hsiao E, Kneebone A, Eade T, Schembri GP. Desmoid tumor showing intense uptake on 68Ga PSMA-HBED-CC PET/CT. Clin Nucl Med. 2016;41(6):508–9.
20. Artigas C, Alexiou J, Garcia C, et al. Paget bone disease demonstrated on (68) Ga-PSMA ligand PET/CT. Eur J Nucl Med Mol Imaging. 2016;43(1):195–6.

21. Kobe C, Maintz D, Fischer T, Drzezga A, Chang DH. Prostate-Specific Membrane Antigen PET/CT in Splenic Sarcoidosis. Clin Nucl Med. 2015; 40(11):897–8.

22. Noto B, Vrachimis A, Schafers M, Stegger L, Rahbar K. Subacute stroke mimicking cerebral metastasis in 68Ga-PSMA-HBED-CC PET/CT. Clin Nucl Med. 2016;41(10):e449–51.

23. Gykiere P, Goethals L, Everaert H. Healing sacral fracture masquerading as metastatic bone disease on a 68Ga-PSMA PET/CT. Clin Nucl Med. 2016;41(7):e346–7.

24. Lambertini A, Castellucci P, Farolfi A, et al. Pictorial essay: normal variants, lesions, and pitfalls in 68Ga-PSMA PET imaging of prostate cancer. Clin Transl Imaging. 2018;6(3):239-47.

25. Krohn T, Verburg FA, Pufe T, et al. [(68) Ga]-PSMA-HBED uptake mimicking lymph node metastasis in coeliac ganglia: an important pitfall in clinical practice. Eur J Nucl Med Mol Imaging. 2015;42(2):210–4.

26. Eiber M, Maurer T, Souvatzoglou M, et al. Evaluation of hybrid (68) Ga-PSMA ligand PET/CT in 248 patients with biochemical recurrence after radical prostatectomy. J Nucl Med. 2015;56(5):668–74.

27. Perera M, Papa N, Christidis D, et al. Sensitivity, specificity, and predictors of positive (68) Ga-prostate-specific membrane antigen positron emission tomography in advanced prostate Cancer: a systematic review and meta-analysis. Eur Urol. 2016;70(6):926–37.

28. Roach PJ, Francis R, Emmett L, et al. The impact of (68) Ga-PSMA PET/CT on management intent in prostate Cancer: results of an Australian prospective multicenter study. J Nucl Med. 2018;59(1):82–8.

29. Vinsensia M, Chyoke PL. Hadaschik B, et al. (68) Ga-PSMA PET/CT and volumetric morphology of PET-positive lymph nodes stratified by tumor differentiation of prostate Cancer. J Nucl Med. 2017;58(12):1949–55.

30. Afaq A, Alahmed S, Chen SH, et al. Impact of (68) Ga-prostate-specific membrane antigen PET/CT on prostate Cancer management. J Nucl Med. 2018;59(1):89–92.

31. Calais J, Fendler WP, Eiber M, Gartmann J, Chu FI, Nickols NG, et al. Impact of (68) Ga-PSMA-11 PET/CT on the Management of Prostate Cancer Patients with biochemical recurrence. J Nucl Med. 2018;59(3):434–41.

32. Fendler WP, Schmidt DF, Wenter V, et al. 68Ga-PSMA PET/CT detects the location and extent of primary prostate Cancer. J Nucl Med. 2016;57(11):1720–5.

33. Budaus L, Leyh-Bannurah SR, Salomon G, et al. Initial experience of (68) Ga-PSMA PET/CT imaging in high-risk prostate Cancer patients prior to radical prostatectomy. Eur Urol. 2016;69(3):393–6.

34. Obek C, Doganca T, Demirci E, et al. The accuracy of (68) Ga-PSMA PET/CT in primary lymph node staging in high-risk prostate cancer. Eur J Nucl Med Mol Imaging. 2017;44(11):1806–12.

35. Zhang Q, Zang S, Zhang C, et al. Comparison of (68) Ga-PSMA-11 PET-CT with mpMRI for preoperative lymph node staging in patients with intermediate to high-risk prostate cancer. J Transl Med. 2017;15(1):230.

36. Zacho HD, Nielsen JB, Haberkorn U, Stenholt L, Petersen LJ. (68) Ga-PSMA PET/CT for the detection of bone metastases in prostate cancer: a systematic review of the published literature. Clin Physiol Funct Imaging. 2018;38(6):911-22.

26

Whole-body magnetic resonance imaging of Li-Fraumeni syndrome patients: observations from a two rounds screening of Brazilian patients

Daniele Paixão[1*], Marcos Duarte Guimarães[2], Kelvin César de Andrade[3,4], Amanda França Nóbrega[1], Rubens Chojniak[2] and Maria Isabel Achatz[5]

Abstract

Background: Li-Fraumeni syndrome (LFS) is an autosomal dominant disease that is associated with germline *TP53* mutations and it predisposes affected individuals to a high risk of developing multiple tumors. In Brazil, LFS is characterized by a different pattern of *TP53* variants, with the founder *TP53* p.R337H mutation being predominant. The adoption of screening strategies to diagnose LFS in its early stages is a major challenge due to the diverse spectrum of tumors that LFS patients can develop. The purpose of this study was to evaluate two rounds of whole-body magnetic resonance imaging (WB-MRI) which were conducted as a screening strategy for LFS patients.

Methods: Over a 4-year period, 59 LFS patients underwent two rounds of WB-MRI. Each MRI was characterized as positive or negative, and positive cases were further investigated to establish a diagnosis. The parameters used to evaluate the WB-MRI results included: positive rate, number of invasive investigations of positive results, and cancer detection rate.

Results: A total of 118 WB-MRI scans were performed. Positive results were associated with 11 patients (9.3%). Seven of these patients (11.8%) were identified in the first round of screening and 4 patients (6.7%) were identified in the second round of screening. Biopsies were performed in three cases (2.5%), two (3.4%) after the first round of screening and one (1.7%) after the second round of screening. The histopathological results confirmed a diagnosis of cancer for all three cases. There was no indication of unnecessary invasive procedures.

Conclusions: WB-MRI screening of LFS carriers diagnosed cancers in their early stages. When needed, positive results were further examined with non-invasive imaging techniques. False positive results were less frequent after the first round of WB-MRI screening.

Keywords: Li-Fraumeni syndrome, Whole-body MRI, Cancer screening, *TP53*, p.R337H mutation

Background

Li-Fraumeni syndrome (LFS) is a hereditary cancer predisposition syndrome that is associated with germline *TP53* mutations [1]. Those affected by this syndrome are at high risk of developing multiple tumors, both as children and as young adults. The spectrum of tumors that characterize LFS include premenopausal breast cancer, soft tissue sarcoma, osteosarcoma, adrenocortical carcinoma, and brain tumors [2–5]. However, other tumors associated with LFS have been reported as well, including leukemia, Wilms' tumor, lung, stomach, colorectal, pancreatic, prostate, and choroid plexus carcinomas [6–9].

In Brazil, there is a high prevalence of LFS due to a founder effect [10]. A germline arginine-to-histidine substitution at codon 337 (NC_000017.9: c.1010G > A; p.R337H) is present in 0.3% in the South/Southeastern Brazilian regions. It is estimated that penetrance of LFS associated with the p.R337H mutation is lower than that

* Correspondence: danipaixaop@gmail.com
[1]Department of Oncogenetics, A.C. Camargo Cancer Center, Professor Antonio Prudente Street, 211 – Liberdade, São Paulo, SP 01509-900, Brazil
Full list of author information is available at the end of the article

of other germline *TP53* mutations, with a cumulative lifetime risk of 50 to 60% [10–13].

Effective screening strategies for LFS patients represent a major challenge due to the wide spectrum of tumors and their variable ages at onset that characterize this syndrome. Previous studies have evaluated the use of ^{18}F-fluoro-deoxyglucose positron emission tomography/computed tomography (^{18}F-FDG-PET/CT) as a screening tool for LFS patients [14, 15]. However, since impaired p53 function may enhance the risk of radiation-induced primary tumors in these subjects, the use of this and other radiation-based imaging modalities is not recommended [16–18].

Whole-body magnetic resonance imaging (WB-MRI) is widely used in oncology and it has been proposed as a surveillance strategy for LFS patients [19–24]. This imaging method involves the acquisition of images of the entire body in one or more planes by using fast sequences, and high sensitivity and specificity have been reported for this method in the detection of a wide variety of malignant tumors [20–24]. For example, in a study by Villani et al. [19], a tumor surveillance protocol for both adult and children affected by LFS was proposed which included the use of WB-MRI for cancer screening. A total of 18 LFS patients carrying a *TP53* mutation were monitored for six years. Five malignant tumors were diagnosed in 7 out of 18 patients, including two choroid plexus carcinomas, two adrenocortical carcinomas, and one sarcoma. All of the tumors were diagnosed in asymptomatic patients and a 100% survival rate was reported at the end of the study. In comparison, the survival rate for patients who did not undergo surveillance during the same time period was 23%. These significant results led the National Comprehensive Cancer Network to propose that WB-MRI be included in its guidelines for the management and risk reduction of cancer in children and adults who harbor a *TP53* germline mutation [25].

In another study of WB-MRI conducted by Anupindi et al. [26], 24 children with cancer predisposition conditions, including LFS, paraganglioma-pheochomocytoma syndrome, and rhabdoid tumor syndrome, underwent a total of 50 WB-MRI screenings over five years. Abnormal findings were detected in 18% of the patients examined. Among these findings, a papillary thyroid carcinoma was confirmed to carry a *TP53* mutation. Thus, in this study, WB-MRI had 100% sensitivity and 94% specificity [26].

In 2017, Ballinger et al. [27] conducted a meta-analysis to estimate the performance and frequency of cancer detection by WB-MRI. A total of 578 patients with deleterious germline *TP53* mutations from 13 participating cohorts in six countries were coordinated through the Li-Fraumeni Exploration Research Consortium. Baseline WB-MRI screenings detected 225 lesions in 173 patients. Forty-two malignant neoplasms were identified in 39 individuals, and most of the them were early-stage neoplasms. The resulting cancer detection rate was 7%, although the false-positive rate was 43%. The false-negative rate was not estimated [27].

In 2017, Mai et al. [28] also evaluated a screening protocol that included WB-MRI for examining 116 patients of a National Cancer Institute (NCI) Li-Fraumeni cohort. In this baseline screening, cancers were detected in 6.9% of the cohort, and 34.5% of these lesions required further investigation. The false-positive rate was 29.6%.

Asdahl et al. [29] has cautioned against false positive results and cancer overdiagnosis in LFS screenings which may lead to psychological distress and unnecessary invasive procedures. However, for individuals with LFS, there is sufficient evidence to indicate that the benefits of screening outweighs its risks.

Considering this unique population that has a high frequency of LFS patients, the aim of this study was to evaluate the use of WB-MRI for early tumor detection in Brazilian LFS patients. Two rounds of WB-MRI screenings were performed and various radiological parameters were examined to evaluate this screening approach.

Methods
Patients
Between January 2013 and August 2017, LFS patients were recruited for this study from those undergoing follow-up in the Department of Oncogenetics at the A.C. Camargo Cancer Center (São Paulo, Brazil). It was confirmed that the enrolled patients carried a pathogenic germline mutation in the *TP53* gene. A subset of the enrolled patients had a previous history of cancer, yet none of the enrolled patients had evidence of current disease. Patients with a current malignancy or metastatic cancer, pregnant or lactating patients, patients who had surgery or received chemotherapy within the previous four months, and patients who refused to participate in the study were excluded.

Ethical issues
All patients signed a written informed consent after completing a consultation with a genetic counselor. This study was approved by the local Ethics Committee of the A.C. Camargo Cancer Center (protocol number 1832/13).

WB-MRI
WB-MRI was performed for 59 LFS patients over a 55-month period in the Nuclear Medicine Division of the Imaging Department, A.C. Camargo Cancer Center. Image acquisition included spin echo and turbo spin echo techniques with coverage tip to toe. Coronal T1-weighted images, short TI inversion recovery (STIR) images, and axial diffusion-weighted images were collected. A 1.5 T MRI

instrument (Signa Excite HD; GE Healthcare, Milwaukee, WI, USA) with a quadrature body coil and maximum power gradient of 33 mT/m and a pulse rate of 160 mT/m/s was used. Paramagnetic contrast reagent was not administered in any of the cases. The WB-MRI scanning time was 25–35 min. All images were interpreted by experienced radiologists using an Advantage Windows version 4.2–07 workstation (GE Healthcare). Functool (GE Healthcare) was used to analyze diffusion sequences.

The WB-MRI results were characterized as: (1) positive: defined as suspicious findings of malignancy or undetermined lesions present; or (2) negative: defined as probable benign lesions or an absence of lesions. Patients with positive WB-MRI results were referred to a specialist for clinical management and further follow-up imaging. We evaluated if there was indication of unnecessary invasive procedures in patients with positive results, i.e., biopsy or surgery performed with unconfirmed histopathological result of cancer.

Radiological parameters

The following radiological parameters were used to evaluate and interpret the WB-MRI results: (1) success rate was measured based on the number of exams performed without complication and without sedation/anesthesia; (2) positive rate was measured according to the number of positive WB-MRI results; (3) recall rate was measured based on the number of patients requiring further investigation after WB-MRI; and (4) cancer detection rate was measured based on the number of malignancies diagnosed by WB-MRI.

Results

A total of 118 WB-MRI scans were performed for 59 LFS patients (35 females, 24 males) from 23 families with a mean age of 38 years (range: 2–71) at the time of their initial WB-MRI examination. Among these patients, 50 (85%) carried the founder mutation, p.R337H, and 9 (15%) carried other germline TP53 mutations. A total of 27 (45%) patients had a prior history of cancer, with 12 previously receiving a diagnosis of multiple primary tumors (Additional file 1: Table S1). A second WB-MRI was performed for all of the patients after a minimum interval of 12 months.

The initial round of WB-MRI had a low positivity rate (11.8%), a low recall rate (11.8%), few invasive investigations

(3.4%), and a cancer detection rate of 3.4% (Table 1). The success rate for the execution of the initial WB-MRI screenings was high (95%). Only two pediatric patients and one adult patient who was claustrophobic required sedation. Positive results were obtained for seven patients, and further investigations with other imaging exams were performed to rule out suspected malignant lesions (Table 2). Two of these patients required biopsy and the histopathologic findings confirmed a diagnosis of cancer in both patients.

One of the positive patients was a 19-year-old female carrier of p.R337H (Y0102T000) with a previous history of multiple primary tumors. Her initial WB-MRI detected bilateral renal cortical alterations. An abdominal MRI further detected an enhanced solid lesion in the right kidney (Fig. 1a and b). Pathological findings confirmed papillary renal cell carcinoma (T1AN0M0, stage I). The second positive patient was a 29-year-old female carrier of p.R306X (Y0352T000). She was asymptomatic and had no previous history of cancer. Her initial WB-MRI screening detected a nodule in the left sacroiliac joint (Fig. 2a and b). A pelvic MRI further showed an enhanced solid expansive lesion present (Fig. 2c). Pathological findings confirmed the lesion to be grade 1 chondrosarcoma.

The positive rate and recall rate for the second round of WB-MRI screenings for all 59 patients were both 6.7%. The success rate was 100% and sedation/anesthesia was not needed for any of the screenings (Table 1). Four positive results were detected and further examinations were performed (Table 2). A biopsy was only performed for one patient and the histopathological results confirmed cancer. Meanwhile, the remaining three patients had their suspected lesions ruled as benign. Overall, the cancer detection rate for the second round of WB-MRI examinations was 1.7%, which is lower than the cancer rate in the first round of WB-MRI screenings. In addition, there was a lower indication of further investigation in the second round of WB-MRI examinations.

The confirmed positive finding in the second round of WB-MRI screenings involved a 61-year-old asymptomatic male carrier of p.R337H (Y0012T012) with a previous history of a thyroid cancer at the age of 54. An expansive lesion was detected in the proximal segment of the right humerus that was in contact with the short head of the biceps (Fig. 3a and b). This

Table 1 Summary of WB-MRI results according to various radiological parameters

Radiological parameters	1st WB-MRI, n = 59 % (n)	2st WB-MRI, n = 59 % (n)	Total, n = 118 % (n)
Positivity rate	11.8 (7)	6.7 (4)	9.3 (11)
Recall rate	11.8 (7)	6.7 (4)	9.3 (11)
Cancer detection rate	3.4 (2)	1.7 (1)	2.5 (3)
Success rate	95.0 (56)	100.0 (59)	98.0 (116)

Table 2 Further investigation of the positive cases identified in the first and second-round of WB-MRI screenings

Patient ID no.	M/F	Age (y)	TP53 mutation	WB-MRI findings	Further exams	Imaging diagnosis	Invasive exams	Cancer diagnosis
Y0012T044	F	40	p.R337H	Hyposignal area on T1, high signal focuses on STIR in left humeral head, nonspecific aspect.	Shoulder MRI	Vascular ectasia	No	No
Y0012T049	F	61	p.R337H	Rounded image in distal metaphyseal region of the right femur (2.2 cm) with hyposignal on T1 and hypersignal on STIR.	Leg MRI	Lobulated image in right femur compatible with enchondroma	No	No
Y0079T016	F	41	p.T125T	Sacral nodule (20 mm), nonspecific,	Lumbosacral spine CT	Enostoses	No	No
Y0099T001	F	34	p.R337H	Nodular area (17 mm) in the retroperitoneum, adjacent to pancreatic cephalic region.	Abdominal MRI	Unilocular pancreatic cyst	No	No
Y0102T000	F	17	p.R337H	Oval images in renal cortical, 16 mm in the lower pole of the right kidney and 20 mm in the upper pole of the left kidney.	Abdominal/ Pelvis MRI	Nodule with irregular borders and heterogeneous signal, predominantly high in T1 and intermediate in T2, with restrictions on diffusion sequence. Approximately, $23 \times 18 \times 18$ mm^3 in right kidney	Surgical resection	Renal cell carcinoma
Y0183T001	M	19	p.T125T	Image on the left lenticular nucleus, 8 mm.	Brain MRI	Cystic image in the left putamen, compatible with Virchow-Robin space	No	No
Y0352T000	F	29	p.R306X	Nodule 35×28 mm^2 at the left sacroiliac joint.	Pelvis MRI	Solid mass lesion $43 \times 34 \times 30$ mm^3, located in the posterior-inferior region of the left sacroiliac joint, with bone cortical irregularity in the sacral margin	Surgical resection	Grade 1 chondrosarcoma
Y0102T000	F	18	p.R337H	Nodule in the right adrenal gland with hypointense signal on T1, hyperintense signal on STIR, and diffusion sequence. Measures 15 mm, indeterminate aspect.	Abdominal MRI	Nodule in the right adrenal gland, non-aggressive features	No	No
Y0015T011	M	34	p.R337H	Images in humeral heads with hypointense signal on T1 and hyperintense signal on STIR, measuring up to 9 mm, suggestive of subchondral cysts.	Shoulder MRI, CT and scintigraphy	Radiolucent oval image in the scapular region with non-aggressive features, slight increase in bone metabolism, no change in blood flow, suggestive of cystic lesion or enchondroma	No	No
Y0012T012	M	61	p. R337H	Expansive lesion in the right humerus, measuring 48×34 mm^2, with isosignal to muscle on T1, hyperintense signal on STIR, and restriction on diffusion sequence.	Shoulder MRI	Expansive lesion in the right axillary region, next to the distal roots of the brachial plexus, measuring 32×22 mm^2, with hypointense signal on T1, hyperintense signal on STIR, suggestive of malignancy of neural sheath or soft tissue sarcoma	Biopsy (axilar lymph node)	High-grade sarcoma with muscle differen- tiation
Y0171T005	M	47	p. R337H	Subcutaneous nodule on the left shoulder.	Shoulder ultrasound	Echogenic nodule in the subcutaneous tissue of the left shoulder, measuring $65 \times 57 \times 12$ mm^3, characteristics of lipoma	No	No

finding suggested a malignancy of the neural sheath or a soft tissue sarcoma. Pathology subsequently confirmed the presence of a high-grade sarcoma with muscle differentiation.

Discussion

The adoption of a screening strategy for the early detection of tumors in LFS patients remains a challenge due to the wide spectrum of tumors that can develop.

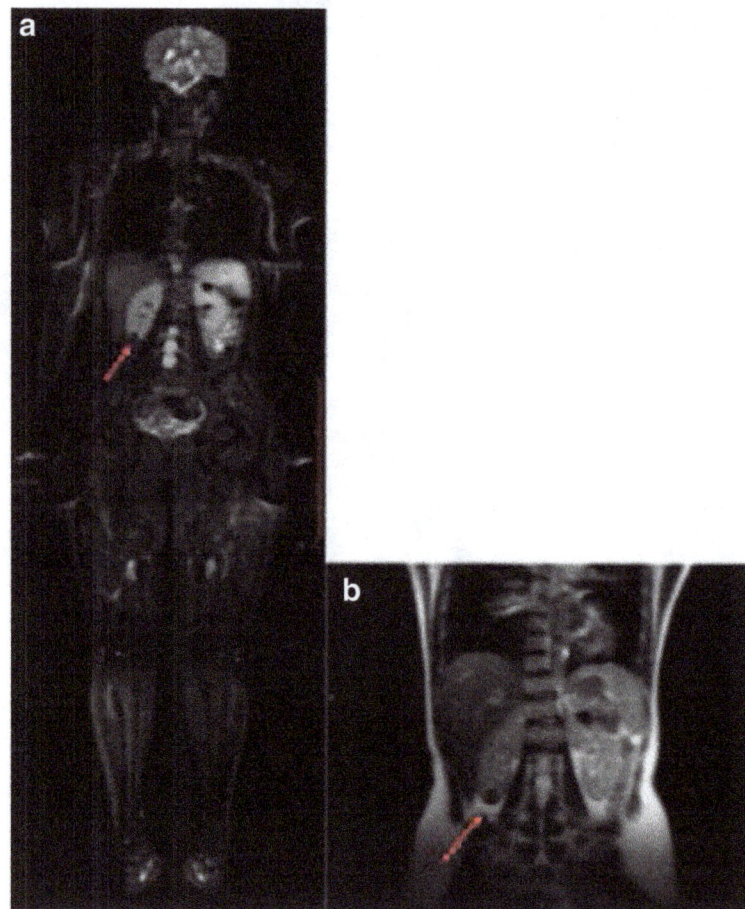

Fig. 1 Detection of a renal lesion by WB-MRI in LFS patient, Y0102T000. **a** STIR image of a 19-year-old with cortical oval kidney lesions in the right lower pole (16 mm) and in the left upper pole (20 mm) (indicated with arrows). **b** An abdominal MRI detected a complex nodule in the lower third of the right kidney, and it measured $23 \times 18 \times 18$ mm^3 (indicated with an arrow)

However, recent studies have shown that WB-MRI can be effective for the screening of patients with cancer predisposition syndromes, including LFS [19, 26].

WB-MRI with diffusion-weighted imaging has the advantage that it is a noninvasive technique that does not require exposure to ionizing radiation or paramagnetic contrast reagent. This is particularly relevant for LFS patients who are advised to avoid exposure to ionizing radiation due to their higher risk of developing radiation-induced primary tumors [14, 16–18]. In the present study, 118 WB-MRI screenings were performed for 59 carriers of germline *TP53* mutations. After two rounds of WB-MRI screenings, cancers were detected in two (4%) out of 50 carriers of the founder mutation, p.R337H, and one cancer (11%) was detected among 9 carriers of the other germline *TP53* mutations. For the three positive cases, biopsies were necessary and the histopathological results confirmed malignant lesions in each case: renal cell carcinoma, grade 1 chondrosarcoma, and soft tissue sarcoma. There was no indication of unnecessary invasive procedures. All of the lesions were also detected in their early stages of development in asymptomatic individuals. Consequently, surgical resection was the primary treatment with no additional need for chemotherapy or radiation treatment. Thus, WB-MRI screening in the present cohort was characterized by a high success rate, minimal need for sedation, and good tolerance and acceptance of the screening protocol.

It is important to note that one of the three diagnosed cancers were detected during the second round of WB-MRI screenings that were performed 12 months after the initial WB-MRI screenings. This result supports the relevance of annual examinations for LFS patients. These results are also consistent with previous observations that WB-MRI facilitates the early detection of malignant tumors [19, 26–28]. Low positivity and recall rates were observed, and further investigations of positive results predominantly involved radiological methods. Only a small proportion of the patients examined underwent an invasive exam with biopsies performed to confirm malignant tumors.

High false-positive rates in screening protocols have been shown to increase the potential for excessive subsequent

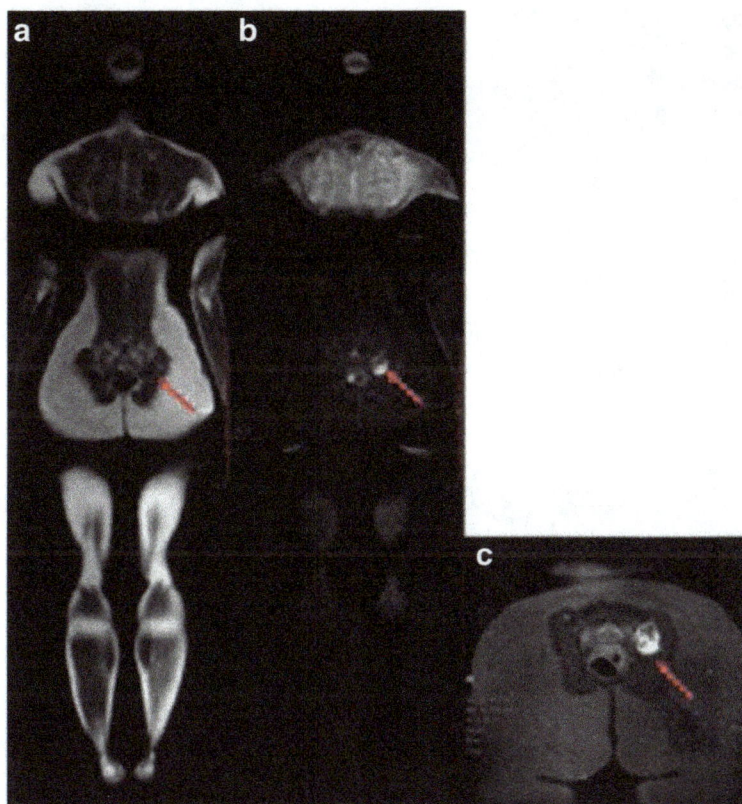

Fig. 2 Detection of a sacroiliac joint lesion by WB-MRI and pelvic MRI images of LFS patient, Y0352T000. A T1-weighted image (**a**) and a STIR image (**b**) were obtained with WB-MRI. **c** MRI of the sacroiliac region detected a solid expansive lesion in the posterior-inferior region of the left sacroiliac joint. Bone cortical irregularity was observed in the sacral margin and it was accompanied by bone edema (indicated with arrow)

investigations and unnecessary invasive procedures [29]. In the present study, a significantly lower positive rate was observed in the second round of WB-MRI screenings, thereby reducing the need for further investigations. This result was expected for a screening process and these data reinforce the findings of Ballinger et al. [27] that WB-MRI may be an integral part of a screening strategy for this high-risk population of patients.

It should be noted that there were limitations associated with the present study. For example, there was a high proportion of younger patients (< 40 y) included in the cohort examined, and the majority of the carriers examined harbored the p.R337H mutation. The latter has been characterized as having a reduced penetrance at younger ages compared to other classic mutations associated with LFS patients [10–13]. Among the 50 patients who carried the p.R337H mutation, the cancer detection rate was low. For example, it has been reported that approximately 15% of individuals carrying p.R337H develop cancer by the age of 30, whereas patients who carry other mutations in the TP53 gene present a risk of 50% up to the age of 35 years [5, 10, 30]. These observations may account

for the low rate of cancer detection that was observed in the present study.

Another limitation of the present study was that the WB-MRI results were not compared with other imaging modalities. However, to date, there is no gold standard that has been established for cancer screenings of LFS patients. Thus, it is not possible to evaluate the effectiveness of the exams performed.

A major challenge in the screening of LFS patients is the management of pediatric cases. A protocol proposed by Villani et al. [19] indicates specific tests for children with LFS, particularly for the detection of adrenocortical carcinomas, brain tumors, and hematological cancers, and the protocol recommends performing WB-MRI annually to detect sarcomas. There is still no consensus regarding the best age at which to start WB-MRI screenings, and its application to young children is challenging due to the need for sedation or general anesthesia, neither of which are without risks. Anupindi et al. [26] reported that 58% of pediatric patients required sedation for WB-MRI screenings, and complications from the procedure were documented in six patients. In the present study, use of sedation was necessary in two

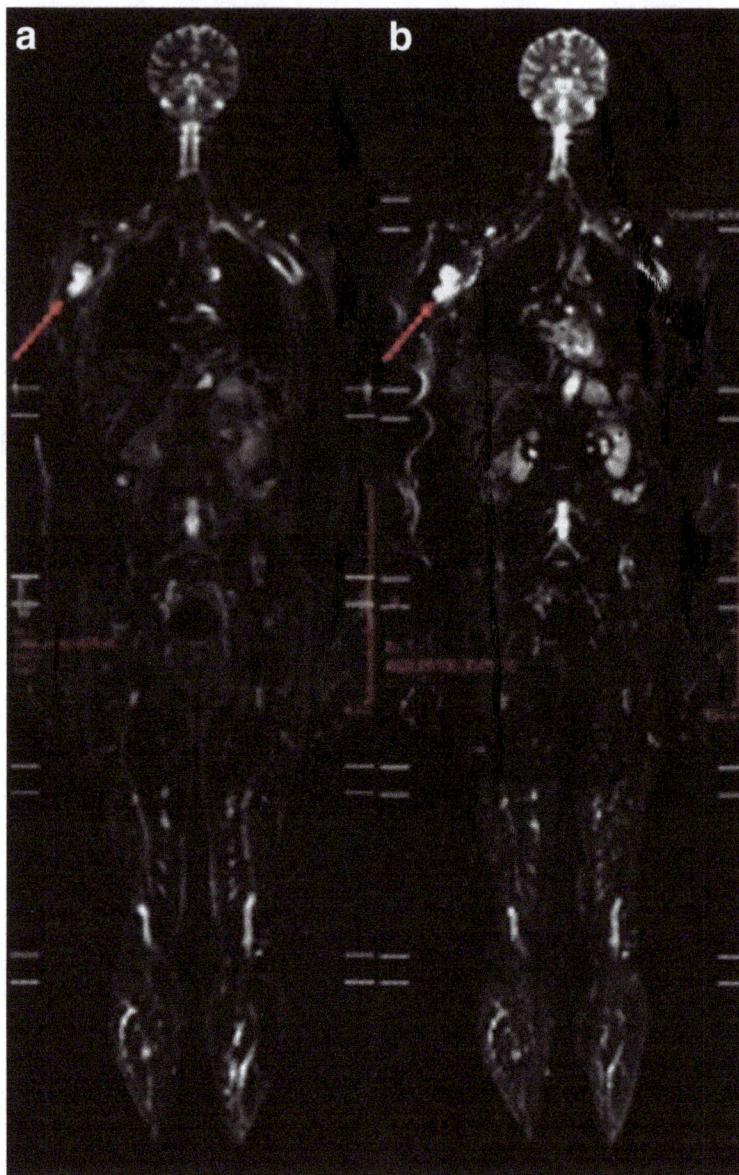

Fig. 3 WB-MRI of LFS patient, Y0012T012. A STIR image (**a**) and diffusion-weighted imaging (**b**) from WB-MRI. An expansive lesion (48 × 34 mm²) in contact with the short head of the biceps was detected in the proximal segment of the right humerus. The lesion exhibited a hyperintense signal on STIR and restriction on diffusion-weighted imaging scans (indicated with arrows)

pediatric cases involving a 2-year-old and a 3-year-old, and no further complications were observed. Thus, sedation for WB-MRI has generally been observed to be a safe procedure. However, the risk-benefit of WB-MRI with sedation/general anesthesia for children remains to be confirmed with further studies.

Conclusion

Despite the limitations associated with this study, a large cohort of LFS patients were evaluated with two rounds of WB-MRI screenings, including a large proportion of Brazilian LFS patients carrying the p.R337H mutation. Our results indicate that cancer screening based on WB-MRI facilitated the early detection of malignant neoplasms and it was characterized by lower recall rates and fewer follow-up invasive investigations. Furthermore, in the second round of screening, fewer positive results were observed. Therefore, we recommend that WB-MRI should be performed as a complementary method to other proposed tests for the surveillance of LFS patients, although longitudinal studies are still needed to better evaluate the effectiveness and long-term impact of WB-MRI on the survival of LFS patients.

Abbreviations
18F-FDG-PET/CT: 18F-fluorodeoxyglucose positron emission tomography/computed tomography; LFS: Li-Fraumeni syndrome; NCI: National Cancer Institute; STIR: Short TI inversion recovery; WB-MRI: Whole-body magnetic resonance imaging

Acknowledgements
We would like to acknowledge the LFS patients who participated in this study.

Funding
This research did not receive any specific grant from funding agencies in the public, commercial, or not-for-profit sectors.

Authors' contributions
RC, MIA, and DP designed the study. RC and MIA supervised the research. DP and MIA actively participated in genetic counseling consultations. DP acquired clinical data, with collaboration from AFN. RC and MDG analyzed the WB-MRI results. MDG and DP selected the WB-MRI images presented in this manuscript. RC, DP and MIA interpreted and discussed the results. DP, RC, MIA, and KCA wrote the manuscript. All of the authors approved and contributed to the final version of the manuscript.

Competing interests
The authors declare that they have no competing interest.

Author details
[1]Department of Oncogenetics, A.C. Camargo Cancer Center, Professor Antonio Prudente Street, 211 – Liberdade, São Paulo, SP 01509-900, Brazil. [2]Department of Imaging, A.C. Camargo Cancer Center, São Paulo, SP, Brazil. [3]Clinical Genetics Branch, Division of Epidemiology and Cancer Genetics, National Cancer Institutes, National Institutes of Health, Bethesda, MD, USA. [4]International Research Center, A.C. Camargo Cancer Center, São Paulo, SP, Brazil. [5]Centro de Oncologia, Hospital Sírio-Libanês, São Paulo, Brazil.

References
1. Merino D, Malkin D. p53 and hereditary cancer. Subcell Biochem. 2014; 85:1–16.
2. Li FP, Fraumeni JF Jr, Mulvihill JJ, et al. A cancer family syndrome in twenty-four kindreds. Cancer Res. 1988;48:5358–62.
3. Malkin D, Li FP, Strong LC, et al. Germline p53 mutations in a familial syndrome of breast cancer, sarcomas, and other neoplasms. Science. 1990;250:1233–8.
4. Srivastava S, Zou ZQ, Pirollo K, et al. Germ-line transmission of a mutated p53 gene in a cancer-prone family with li-Fraumeni syndrome. Nature. 1990;348:747–9.
5. Hisada M, Garber JE, Fung CY, et al. Multiple primary cancers in families with li-Fraumeni syndrome. J Natl Cancer Inst. 1998;90:606–11.
6. Hartley AL, Birch JM, Kelsey AM, et al. Are germ cell tumors part of the li-Fraumeni cancer family syndrome? Cancer Genet Cytogenet. 1989;42:221–6.
7. Garber JE, Burke EM, Lavally BL, et al. Choroid plexus tumors in the breast cancer-sarcoma syndrome. Cancer. 1990;66:2658–60.
8. Hartley AL, Birch JM, Tricker K, et al. Wilms' tumor in the Li-Fraumeni cancer family syndrome. Cancer Genet Cytogenet. 1993;67:133–5.
9. Varley JM, Evans DG, Birch JM. Li-Fraumeni syndrome - a molecular and clinical review. Br J Cancer. 1997;76:1–14.
10. Garritano S, Gemignani F, Palmero EI, et al. Detailed haplotype analysis at the TP53 locus in p.R337H mutation carriers in the population of Southern Brazil: evidence for a founder effect. Hum Mutat. 2010;31:143–50.
11. Achatz MI, Olivier M, Le Calvez F, et al. The TP53 mutation, R337H, is associated with li-Fraumeni and li-Fraumeni-like syndromes in Brazilian families. Cancer Lett. 2007;245(1–2):96–102.
12. Palmero EI, Schüler-Faccini L, Caleffi M, et al. Detection of R337H, a germline TP53 mutation predisposing to multiple cancers, in asymptomatic women participating in a breast cancer screening program in southern Brazil. Cancer Lett. 2008;261(1):21–5.
13. Custódio G, Parise GA, Kiesel Filho N, et al. Impact of neonatal screening and surveillance for the TP53 R337H mutation on early detection of childhood adrenocortical tumors. J Clin Oncol. 2013;31(20):2619–26.
14. Masciari S, Van den Abbeele AD, Diller LR, et al. F18-fluorodeoxyglucose-positron emission tomography/computed tomography screening in Li-Fraumeni syndrome. JAMA. 2008;299:1315–9.
15. Nogueira ST, Lima EN, Nóbrega AF, et al. 18F-FDG PET-CT for surveillance of Brazilian patients with Li-Fraumeni syndrome. Front Oncol. 2015;5:38.
16. Limacher JM, Frebourg T, Natarajan-Ame S, et al. Two metachronous tumors in the radiotherapy fields of a patient with Li-Fraumeni syndrome. Int J Cancer. 2001;96:238–42.
17. Strong LC. General keynote: hereditary cancer: lessons from Li-Fraumeni syndrome. Gynecol Oncol. 2003;88:S4–7. discussion S11–3
18. Bougeard G, Renaux-Petel M, Flaman JM, et al. Revisiting Li-Fraumeni syndrome from TP53 mutation carriers. J Clin Oncol. 2015;33(21):2345–52.
19. Villani A, Tabori U, Schiffman JD, et al. Biochemical and imaging surveillance in germline TP53 mutation carriers with Li-Fraumeni syndrome: a prospective observational study. Lancet Oncol. 2011;12:559–67.
20. Schick F. Whole-body MRI at high field: technical limits and clinical potential. Eur Radiol. 2005;15:946–59.
21. Ladd SC, Ladd ME. Perspectives for preventive screening with total body MRI. Eur Radiol. 2007;17:2889–97.
22. Ladd SC. Whole-body MRI as a screening tool? Eur J Radiol. 2009;70:452–62.
23. Schmidt G, Dinter D, Reiser MF, et al. The uses and limitations of whole-body magnetic resonance imaging. Dtsch Arztebl Int. 2010;107:383–9.
24. Canale S, Vilcot L, Ammari S, et al. Whole body MRI in paediatric oncology. Diagn Interv Imaging. 2014;95:541–50.
25. National Comprehensive Cancer Network. Genetic/familial high-risk assessment: breast and ovarian. Li-Fraumeni syndrome management. NCCN Clinical practice guidelines in oncology; Version 2. 2016. Available at: https://www.nccn.org/professionals/physician_gls/default.aspx#genetics_screening. Accessed 18 Apr 2016.
26. Anupindi SA, Bedoya MA, Lindell RB, et al. Diagnostic performance of whole-body MRI as a tool for Cancer screening in children with genetic Cancer-predisposing conditions. Am J Roentgenol. 2015;205(2):400–8.
27. Ballinger ML, Best A, Mai PL, et al. Baseline surveillance in Li-Fraumeni syndrome using whole-body magnetic resonance imaging: a meta-analysis. JAMA Oncol. 2017;3(12):1634–9.
28. Mai PL, Khincha PP, Loud JT, et al. Prevalence of cancer at baseline screeningin the National Cancer Institute Li-Fraumeni syndrome cohort. JAMA Oncol. 2017;3(12):1640–5.
29. Asdahl PH, Ojha RP, Hasle H. Cancer screening in Li-Fraumeni syndrome. [published online August 3, 2017]. JAMA Oncol. https://doi.org/10.1001/jamaoncol.2017.2459.
30. Gonzalez KD, Noltner KA, Buzin CH, et al. Beyond Li-Fraumeni syndrome: clinical characteristics of families with p53 germline mutations. J Clin Oncol. 2009;27:1250–6.

27

An international survey on hybrid imaging: do technology advances preempt our training and education efforts?

T. Beyer[1*], R. Hicks[2], C. Brun[3], G. Antoch[4] and L. S. Freudenberg[5]

Abstract

Background: Hybrid PET/CT and PET/MRI are increasingly important technologies in the evaluation of malignancy and require cooperation between radiologists and specialists in molecular imaging. The aim of our study was to probe the mindsets of radiological and nuclear medicine professionals in regard to current hybrid imaging practice and to assess relevant training aspirations and perceived shortfalls, particularly amongst young professionals. In this context, we initiated an international survey on "Hybrid Imaging Training".

Methods: An online survey was prepared on-line and launched on October-2, 2016. It was composed of 17 multiple-choice and open questions regarding the professional background, a perspective on hybrid imaging training efforts and lessons to be learned from disparate craft groups. The survey ran for 2 weeks. We report total responses per category and individual free-text responses.

Results: In total, 248 responses were collected with a mean age of all responders of (41 ± 11) y. Overall, 36% were within the target age range of (20–35) y. Across all responders, the majority (72%) commented on there being too few hybrid imaging experts in their country, whereas only 1% said that there were too many. Three quarters of the responders were in favour of a curriculum allowing sub-specialisation in hybrid imaging. With respect to reporting of hybrid imaging, confidence increased with age. The average rating across all responders on the level of cooperation among the two specialties suggested a low overall level of satisfaction. However, the survey feedback indicated the local (on-site) cooperation being somewhat better than the perceived cooperation between the relevant associations on a European level.

Conclusion: We consider these results to represent an appropriate cross-section of professional opinions of imaging experts across different demographic and hierarchical levels. Collectively they provide evidence supporting a need to address current shortfalls in developing hybrid imaging expertise through national educational plans, and, thus, contribute to helping improve patient care.

Keywords: Hybrid imaging, Training and education, Specialization, Conflict, Profession

Background

Over the centuries, there has been continuous improvement in the diagnosis and treatment of diseases. However, cardiovascular, cancerous and neurodegenerative diseases still pose a major challenge to healthcare systems today [1]. Patients suffering from any of these diseases expect an accurate diagnosis, which in almost all cases will be guided by non-invasive imaging procedures. These may include, for example, Computed Tomography (CT) and Magnetic Resonance Imaging (MRI) to assess the anatomy and morphological alterations of patients with great visual detail and spatial resolution [2], or Single Photon Emission Computed Tomography (SPECT) and Positron Emission Tomography (PET) that permit the assessment of metabolic and signaling pathways and their variants [3]. All of these imaging modalities represent exciting

* Correspondence: thomas.beyer@meduniwien.ac.at
[1]QIMP Group, Centre Medical Physics and Biomedical Engineering, Medical University Vienna, Währinger Str 18-20/4L, 1090 Vienna, Austria
Full list of author information is available at the end of the article

instrumentational and methodological approaches to diagnosing patients, and help us understand diseases better [4].

Stand-alone imaging modalities were first conceived in the 1950's and 1960's and have entered the market about a decade later. Today, there are ten thousand's of these imaging systems operational worldwide. While each modality has its merits it became clear that a combined use of "anatometabolic" imaging [5] had the potential to improve the diagnostic value of non-invasive imaging, and, thus, benefit patients and healthcare systems alike. As a consequence, we have witnessed the introduction of combined SPECT/CT [6], PET/CT [7] and PET/MR systems [8] in the first decade of the twenty-first century. Although the adoption of these hybrid imaging systems has varied widely over time and across regions, their clinical traction has grown and proven to yield a diagnostic benefit in a variety of clinical questions [9–11].

Whole-body PET/CT was introduced in 2001 with multiple generations and updates of PET/CT following suit; however, an international survey performed in 2011 demonstrated that the majority of PET/CT users still disregarded the diagnostic power of CT in a large fraction of patients [12]. Likewise, a survey performed in 2014 among international SPECT/CT users demonstrated that an overwhelming majority wanted to employ the SPECT/CT as a SPECT system with attenuation correction and coarse anatomical localization rather than assuming a closer integration of radiology-driven imaging perspectives [13]. When combined PET/MR imaging of humans was introduced a decade ago, an overwhelming number of studies focused (again) on attenuation correction [14] and a potential diagnostic equivalence of DIXON-type MR and low-dose CT images for the anatomical localization of the PET findings [15]. These are but a few examples that attest to a continuous hesitation towards a game-changing adoption of hybrid imaging and, in turn, to an ongoing debate about key responsibilities and ownership issues in hybrid imaging. This is particularly disconcerting in the field of cancer imaging since hybrid imaging techniques, such as [^{99m}Tc]MDP-SPECT/CT and [^{18}F]FDG-PET/CT, are widely used for the staging of common malignancies. With increasing availability of more specific tracers for various types of cancer, the penetration of these technologies into oncological imaging is likely to further increase [16]. An example of this is the use of [^{68}Ga]PSMA imaging for prostate cancer, which is likely to impact both PET/CT and PET/MRI imaging [17].

The territorial approaches towards the clinical adoption of "anatometabolic imaging" [5] originate to a large extent from perspectives of people and professionals whose experience and model of practice were developed prior to the availability of hybrid imaging [18]. However,

to date, we have no information about the mindset of "early" professionals in regard to combined imaging and their perceptions of relevant training requirements. This especially includes the new generation of young professionals who have been exposed only to a period of merging technologies and practices. Therefore, we have set out to probe the opinions on hybrid imaging of, in particular, the next generation of imaging specialists and to compare them to senior clinicians.

Methods

We have initiated an international survey, entitled "Hybrid Imaging Training" following the organization of the 3rd International Hybrid Imaging Course [19]. The survey consisted of 17 questions regarding the demographics and professional background of the responders (6), their confidence in dealing with hybrid imaging and their perspective on hybrid imaging training efforts (6), as well as lessons to be learned from disparate craft groups (5) (Table 1). In order to better understand variations in cross-specialty appreciation, we queried also what "nuclear medicine" could learn from "radiology", and vice versa (Table 1).

The survey was composed via Google Documents and a link was mailed to all participants of the 2016 and 2017 Asklepios ESOR (European School of Radiology) and ESHI (European Society for Hybrid Medical Imaging) Courses on Hybrid Imaging. Furthermore, it was advocated through the Aunt Minnie community on Oct-2, 2017, in addition to numerous individual mailings within the professional networks of the co-authors. Anonymized responses were received from Oct-2 to Oct-16, 2017 and tabulated for each question.

We report total responses per category; minimum, and maximum values (when applicable). The individual free-text responses were analysed using a content analysis that permits the inclusion of textual information and the systematic identification of properties, such as the frequencies of the most frequently used keywords by locating the most important structures of its communication content [20].

Results

In total, 248 eligible responses were collected. Of those, 149 and 164 eligible free text responses were received for the free text question on the cross-specialty learning experience for nuclear medicine and radiology, respectively.

Demographics

The mean age of all responders was (41 ± 11) years with 36% being of age 20-y to 35-y, and with 4% being older than 65-y. The majority of responders were male (65%). The highest number of responses (197/248) were collected from Europe (78%), followed by Africa (6%), Asia

Table 1 Hybrid Imaging Survey with 17 questions geared towards the probing the knowledge and attitude of young healthcare professionals in the context of clinical hybrid imaging

Demographics

Q1   Your age (y) and gender (m, f)

Q2   Your country of employment

Q3   Your place of work: radiology, nuc, joint common rad-nuc, nuc as part of rad, other

Q4   Who is the head of your department (if any): rad, nuc, physics, other ...?

Q5   Are you an MD w/ or w/o board certification (Nuc, Rad, Nuc/Rad, other)?

Q6   How many years of hybrid imaging experience do you have (y): SPECT/CT, PET/CT, PET/MR?

Training

Q7   In general, how confident do you feel when reporting hybrid imaging studies today (scale 1–10)?

Q8   What type of continuous education means (hybrid imaging) do you employ for yourself: literature, on-line courses/webinars, conferences, special courses (inter–/national), or fellowships (multiple choice, and each option ir–/regularly)?

Q9   In your country of employment, are there sufficient hybrid imaging experts (too few, too many, just right, don't know)?

Q10   Would you like a curriculum for a subspecialization for a certified, hybrid imaging expert (y, n, don't know)?

Q11   Would you like a joint curriculum (common trunk residency, or alike) for radiology and nuclear medicine (y/n)?

Q12   Are you aware of the Joint White Paper of ESR and EANM (https://www.ncbi.nlm.nih.gov/pubmed/17609961) (y/n)?

Cross-fertilization

Q13   From your perspective, how well do the European Society of Radiology (ESR) and the European Association of Nuclear Medicine (EANM) work together (scale 1–10)?

Q14   From your perspective, how well do your national Associations for Radiology and Nuclear Medicine work together (scale 1–10)?

Q15   From your personal experience, how well do radiologists and nuclear medicine specialists work together at your local hospital/institution/site (scale 1–10)?

Q16   What would you like to see happening in the next 5 years with regards to hybrid imaging (free text)?

Q17   In your opinion, what could radiology learn from nuclear medicine (free text) and what could nuclear medicine learn from radiology (free text)?

(6%), Middle East (4%), North Americas (4%) and South America (2%). Half of the responders work in Radiology departments (51%), 25% work in Nuclear Medicine departments, 17% in joint Radiology and Nuclear Medicine departments, and 7% in other institutions (Fig. 1a). Most departments, presumably including the joint departments, are run by a radiologist (62%), while one fourth is operated by a nuclear medicine physician (Fig. 1b). Across all responders, 18% were without any board certification, 36% and 18% were certified in radiology and nuclear medicine, respectively, while 15% were dual-certified. A third of the responders indicated that they had no experience with hybrid imaging, 22% said they had up to 4 years of experience with hybrid imaging and 22% indicated more than 10 years of experience.

Training

Report confidence increased with age (and experience) but less than half the responders (43%) indicated they were very confident (score 8–10 on a scale from 1 to 10) in reporting hybrid images. When being asked about their personal engagement in various education and training options, it became obvious that more accessible educational material increased its use (Fig. 2). When analyzing educational endeavours per age category, professionals without a board certification engage regularly in reviewing scientific literature (63%) and conference attendance (48%) with a comparatively low regular interest (27%) in webinars.

Across all responders, the majority (72%) commented on too few hybrid imaging experts being available in their country; 16% said there are just as many experts as needed, while 1% said there were too many. Responses were very similar if considering responders from Europe only (72%, 15% and 1%).

Three-quarters of the responders were in favour of a curriculum for a subspecialisation as a hybrid imaging expert (75% worldwide versus 73% in Europe). Most opponents were radiologists by training. Close to 90% of the responders were in favour of a joint curriculum along the suggested training options laid out in the previous White Paper developed jointly by the European Society of Radiology (ESR) and the European Association of Nuclear Medicine (EANM) [21].

Cross-fertilization

Figure 3a illustrates the average rating across all responders of the level of cooperation (1-very low, 10-very high) among the two specialties on a local, a national and a European basis showing that the overall level of satisfaction is low. The same observation was made across responses from European countries only (Fig. 3b). However, the survey feedback suggests the local (on-site) cooperation being somewhat better than the perception of cooperation between the relevant associations, EANM and ESR. To take this further, we analyzed the level of cooperation in Germany, where the cooperation of the national societies, the German Society of Nuclear Medicine - DGN and the German Society of Radiology - DRG, was perceived much better than that on the European level, with the same observation being made for the collaboration on a local level (Fig. 3c).

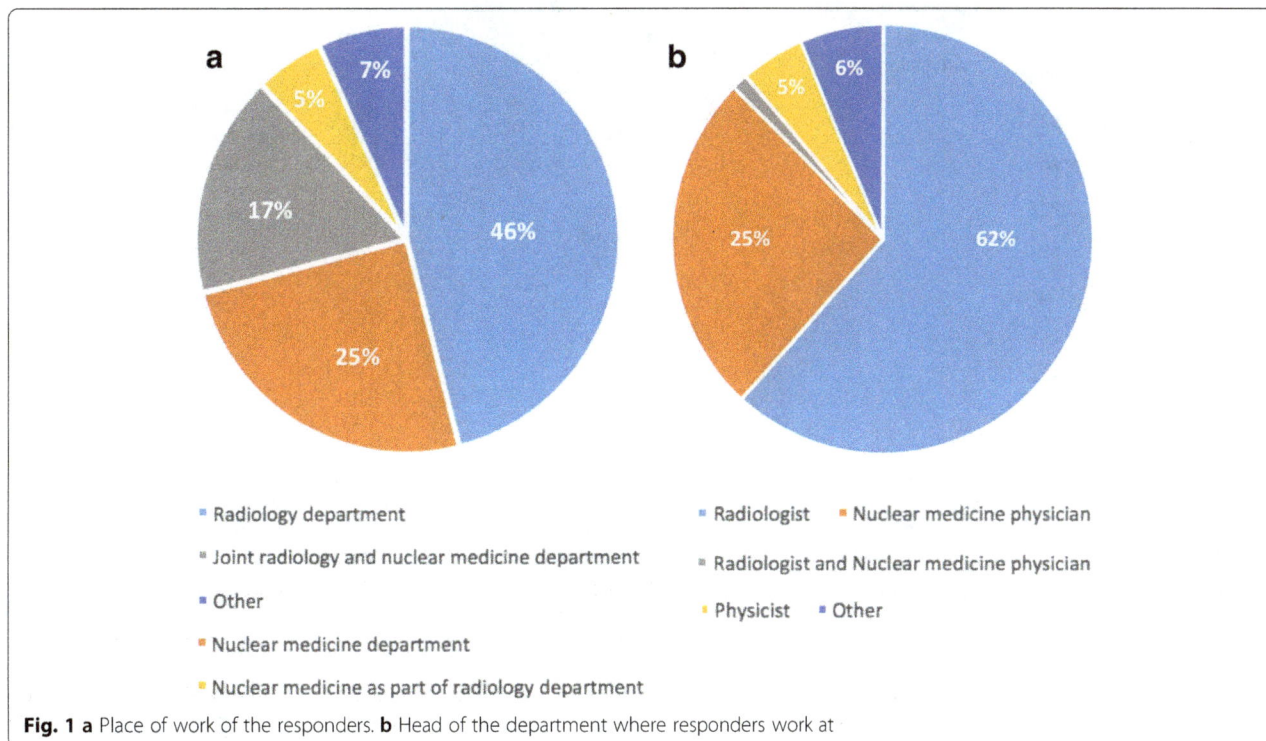

Fig. 1 **a** Place of work of the responders. **b** Head of the department where responders work at

a legend:
- Radiology department
- Joint radiology and nuclear medicine department
- Other
- Nuclear medicine department
- Nuclear medicine as part of radiology department

b legend:
- Radiologist
- Nuclear medicine physician
- Radiologist and Nuclear medicine physician
- Physicist
- Other

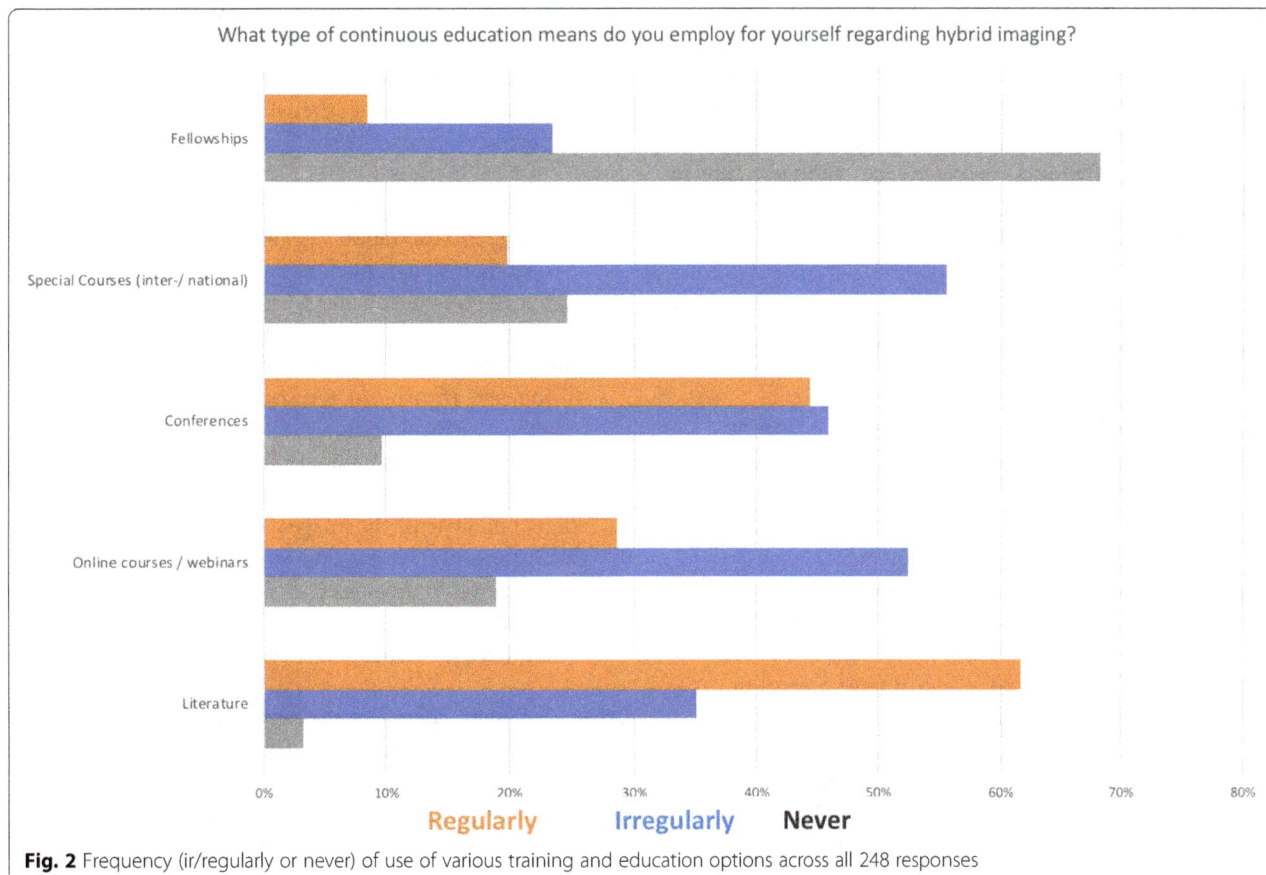

What type of continuous education means do you employ for yourself regarding hybrid imaging?

Regularly   Irregularly   Never

Fig. 2 Frequency (ir/regularly or never) of use of various training and education options across all 248 responses

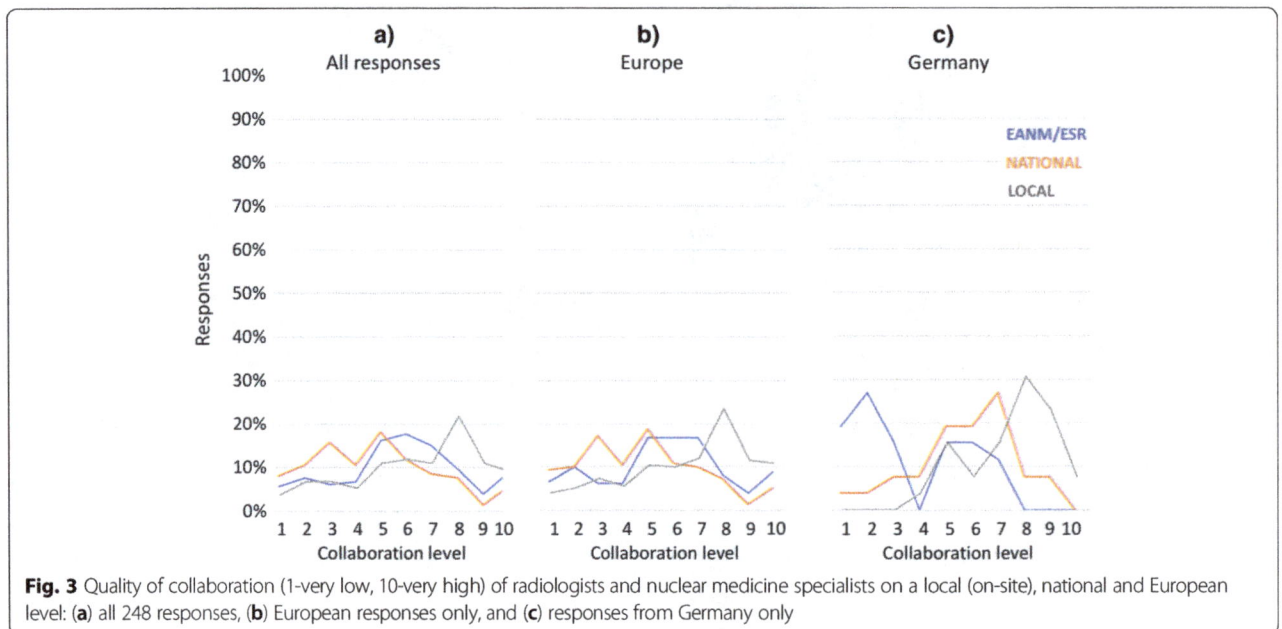

Fig. 3 Quality of collaboration (1-very low, 10-very high) of radiologists and nuclear medicine specialists on a local (on-site), national and European level: (**a**) all 248 responses, (**b**) European responses only, and (**c**) responses from Germany only

What can nuclear medicine learn from radiology?

The majority of the responders gave priority to "anatomy" (62%), followed by "competence in CT" (11%) and "competence in MRI" (12%), as well as knowledge of "comprehensive radiological imaging" (7%). Of note, many comments (> 20%) suggested that nuclear medicine should learn about "efficacy", "dynamics", "patient throughput and management", and "standardization". Responders also frequently suggested that nuclear medicine should learn "confidence" from their radiology counterparts. No differences between the younger (up to 35 years) and older participants (older than 35 years) were found. Some examples of individual responses included:

- "Nuclear medicine could learn precise localization of a lesion and structural changes in a disease" (from a 44-y/o male Austrian radiologist)
- "Dynamics. Radiology, particularly MRI, is a dynamic field and new techniques are currently being developed for clinical applications. Radiologists - I find - are more open to change and adapt quickly. Nucs can be a bit stiff to change." (from a 35-y/o female Canadian fellow in Radiology)
- "Patho-/anatomy, clinical integration and acceptance in clinical context, imaging technology, synoptical overviews as to what imaging method is best for which question." (from a 53-y/o male Swiss dual board certified medical doctor).

What radiology can learn from nuclear medicine?

Most responders stated that nuclear medicine teaching points for radiologists include "metabolic imaging" (49%) and the "knowledge of function, physiology and pathophysiology" (27%). Other important learning objectives included "radiopharmacy" (17%), quantification (6%), and knowledge of "comprehensive nuclear medicine imaging" (7%). Beyond that, many comments (> 25%) suggested that radiology should learn from nuclear medicine about "being physicians", "cooperation", "respect", "self-criticism", and "different way of thinking". No differences between the younger (up to 35 years) and older participants (older than 35 years) were found. Some specific responses were:

- "Nuclear Medicine imaging is a more physiologic way of image interpretation than an anatomic." (from a 41-y/o male Dutch nuclear medicine physician)
- "That life isn't black and white. Applied physiology. Therapeutic approach." (from a 48-y/o male German nuclear medicine physician)
- "Modesty." (from a 44-y/o male German dual board certified medical doctor)
- "Quality control: Nucs are used to reading images looking for potential artefacts in the image. [...] They don't blindly trust the images. They are aware of the limitations of their imaging modality and can interpret images even in the presence of some noise. They are I would say, well trained Support Vector Machines." (from a 35-y/o female Canadian fellow in radiology)

Other comments offered by the participants

Of note, 19 participants took the opportunity not only to answer both questions but to comment on the relationship between nuclear medicine and radiology. Some stress the obvious differences; others state that cooperation or common training are key. There were no distinguished differences between older and younger participants. Some specific comments were:

- "They [Nuclear Medicine and Radiology] are not separated. They complete each other in imaging diagnostic field." (from a 27-y/o female Albanian radiologist)
- "I think it's compatible and complementary." (from a 33-y/o female Polish fellow in radiology)
- "[One should] wash out the borders between radiology and nuclear medicine territories, rise up new specialisation - imaging experts with organ-specific sub-specialisations." (from a 37-y/o female Italian nuclear medicine physician)
- "Combination is the future solution." (from a 54-y/o female Swedish dual board certified medical doctor)
- "[Nuclear medicine] is a whole new discipline with a different way of thinking." (from a 64-y/o female Hungarian nuclear medicine physician)
- "My personal view is that I never learn anything more from NM specialist as the metabolic information is something as an additional quality of image as very well-known from multi-parametric imaging." (from a 47-y/o male Czech radiologist)

Discussion

The aim of this survey was to get an insight into current professional perspectives on the practice of hybrid imaging and any pertinent need for training and educational strategies for the international adoption of clinical hybrid imaging. Although this survey was geared towards collecting a global feedback, most of the responses (78%) collected were from Europe, thus, rendering this data more Eurocentric; similarly, most of the responders were male (65%). Hence, we assume that the heterogeneity of answers we described will be even more manifold.

Training

Taken together, the data above show that the majority of medical professionals in the domains of radiology and nuclear medicine want to engage in continuous education. Furthermore, there is a persistent interest and willingness in joint training programs. When being asked about their personal adoption of various education and training options (e.g., literature, on-line courses, attending conferences or special courses and fellowships), it became obvious that the more accessible are the educational offers, the more frequently they are being adopted; this refers to accessing literature while fellowships, for example, are rarely used. On-line courses and webinars are used infrequently, and there is room for more engagement by authorities and specialist's assemblies, particularly, In view of limited funds available.

Collaboration of nuclear medicine and radiology - theory (white paper)

Our survey indicated also that over half (54%) of responders were unaware of the joint ESR and EANM statement from 2007 [21, 22]. People who knew about this white paper were generally older than those who did not (46-y vs 38-y); likewise, they were mainly nuclear medicine specialists rather than radiologists (31% vs 19%). When being asked about a joint curriculum along the suggested training options laid out in the White Paper [21], 87% responded with "yes", with the fraction of proponents growing somewhat larger with professional age. Both responses are in line with the survey conducted among EANM and ESR members in 2010, when 77% and 85%, respectively, supported the idea of an interdisciplinary training programme [23].

Collaboration of nuclear medicine and radiology – Practice

The White Paper closed by stating "Both organizations [ESR and EANM] are committed to working together for the future benefit of both specialties" [21, 22]; our data indicate that a decade into hybrid imaging, this statement is perceived to have not yet materialized. The opinion trend surveyed here indicates a need for cooperation between the two specialties and a persistent wish for a strategy towards integrating hybrid imaging expertise into an interdisciplinary training [23–25], or into alternative forms of restructured training modules to account for multi-modality imaging [26].

As early adopters of hybrid imaging, we suggest embracing the numerous opportunities of hybrid imaging for the benefit of clinical patient management and healthcare systems. We should seize the opportunities of presenting high-sensitivity molecular information in judiciously tailored anatomical and morphological reference frames to engage referring clinicians in fostering personalized treatment plans, and to engage with other medical specialties in an attempt to merge knowledge about diseases for building models that help predict and assess disease of other patients in the future; big data can get bigger with hybrid images.

Our survey shows variations of the collaborations between the two specialties on local, national and international levels. Most participants consider the professional collaboration on a local level more positive than the collaboration between the National and European associations. In our view, this is an indicator that cooperation grows more complicated as soon as politics get involved. An interesting divergent finding is the considerably well-perceived cooperation of the Societies of Radiology and Nuclear Medicine in Germany (Fig. 3c). They have a long history of joint efforts towards the adoption of dual-modality imaging, given the national funding scheme for imaging system acquisitions put forward by the National Research Foundation (DFG), which forces the specialties to cooperate. Also, Germany has established a potential role model in negotiating joint training programs, as attested by the ongoing reviews of the national continuous educational procedures for radiology [27] and nuclear medicine [28].

Naturally, the engagement of local and national stakeholders takes time, but eventually helps build a sustainable framework for the continuous and efficient adoption of new imaging technologies without jeopardizing the core expertise of the adjoined specialties. Our survey indicates a wish of the daily users, including the next generation of "anatometabolic imagers", to extending similar collaborative efforts to the National and European level (Fig. 3a, b).

Beyond cooperation: What can we learn from each other?

The results of our content analysis above appear to reinforce the concept of "habitus" [29] as introduced by Pierre Bourdieau [30], who described the habitus as "a system of embodied dispositions, tendencies that organize the ways in which individuals perceive the social world around them and react to it. These dispositions are usually shared by people with similar background [...] and reflect the lived reality to which individuals are socialized, their individual experience and objective opportunities. Thus, the habitus represents the way group culture and personal history shape the body and the mind, and, as a result, shape social action in the present." Our survey (Table 1) suggests that the fundamental difference of a focus on physiology or anatomy led to different habitus' in the two specialist fields with respect to imaging, patient care, and self-perception. One participant even stated in short: "Nuclear medicine physicians are better physicians; radiologists are better imagers."

Perhaps this type of statement in the light of clinical hybrid imaging lends itself to the definition of a new mindset for hybrid imagers, which could be addressed from the start through a more intense collaboration, or, even better and more sustainable, a joint training and education path that helps bridge the differing mindsets of nuclear medicine physicians and radiologists, for they both do care about their patients. Such training path could start with the integration of radiologists and nuclear medicine physicians as members of a local multidisciplinary clinical team, pending the initiation of a new or the continuous expansion of existing communication platforms involving the two specialties. Further, both specialties could establish disease-centric fellowships that include subspecialty hybrid imaging training, such as a Cancer Imaging fellowship as to equip the younger generation with the tools and knowledge needed to demonstrate the impact that imaging can have on patient management and outcome (e.g., http://www.esor.org/cms/

website.php?id=/en/programmes/exchange_programmes_for_fellowships.htm). And finally, training efforts could be formalized in residency programmes, including a dedicated cancer imaging curriculum, such as that advocated by Howard and colleagues [31].

We appreciate that web-based surveys have drawbacks, such as lower response rates compared to other survey modes [32]. Nonetheless, we decided to benefit from the easy, rapid, and widespread distribution of Web-based questionnaires. Furthermore, Web-based surveys offer logistic advantages such as fast response collection and low costs [33]. As such, we consider these results a representative cross-section of professional opinions by imaging experts across different demographic and hierarchical levels that may help contribute to recognizing a need to better address needs for hybrid imaging expertise in national educational plans, and, thus, contribute to helping improve patient care. We hope this knowledge may help to refocus the discussions about the "homeland" of hybrid imaging from professional politics back to patient care. In short: hybrid imaging should be performed to the best possible diagnostic quality standards with the patient in mind - no more, no less.

Conclusion

Our international field study of hybrid imaging adopters indicates a persistent interest, particularly of the younger generation of imaging professionals, to offer training programmes to support the education and certification of hybrid imaging experts. Free text interviews yield valuable insights into the professional vanities of radiology and nuclear medicine experts, but can help define learning objectives in joint curricula. Cancer imaging is a field in which hybrid technologies already have an important role, and this is likely to expand. Therefore, the oncological imaging community could take a lead in improving training programmes and harmonising reporting methodology for the sake of a sustainable adoption of hybrid imaging techniques.

Authors' contributions

TB and LSF conceived the study and designed the questionnaire. CB implemented an e-Version of the survey and condensed the results. TB, LSF, CB and RH did engage in the data evaluation. All authors drafted, read and edited the manuscript and approved its final version.

Authors' information

TB is co-founder of cmi-experts Ltd. and recipient of research support from Siemens Healthineers, and reports no conflict of interest with this study.

Competing interests
The authors declare that they have no competing interests.

Author details
[1]QIMP Group, Centre Medical Physics and Biomedical Engineering, Medical University Vienna, Währinger Str 18-20/4L, 1090 Vienna, Austria. [2]The Sir Peter MacCallum Department of Oncology, the University of Melbourne, Melbourne 3000, Australia. [3]European Society for Hybrid Medical Imaging, Neutorgasse 10, 1010 Vienna, Austria. [4]Department of Diagnostic and Interventional Radiology, University Düsseldorf, Medical Faculty, Moorenstrasse 5, 40225 Düsseldorf, Germany. [5]ZRN Rheinland, Ueberseite 88, 41352 Korschenbroich, Germany.

References
1. http://www.who.int/mediacentre/factsheets/fs310/en/.
2. Brant W, Helms C. In: Brant W, Helms C, editors. Fundamentals of diagnostic radiology. Philadelphia: Lippincott Williams & Wilkins; 2007.
3. Valk PE, et al. Positron emission tomography. Basic science and clinical practice. London: Springer; 2003.
4. James ML, Gambhir SS. A molecular imaging primer: modalities, imaging agents, and applications. Physiol Rev. 2012;92(2):897–965.
5. Wahl RL, et al. "Anatometabolic" tumor imaging: fusion of FDG PET with CT or MRI to localize foci of increased activity. J Nucl Med. 1993;34:1190–7.
6. Patton JA, Delbeke D, Sandler MP. Image fusion using an integrated, dual-head coincidence camera with X-ray tube-based attenuation maps. J Nucl Med. 2000;41(8):1364–8.
7. Beyer T, et al. A combined PET/CT tomograph for clinical oncology. J Nucl Med. 2000;41(8):1369–79.
8. Schlemmer H, et al. Simultaneous MR/PET imaging of the human brain: feasibility study. Radiology. 2008;248(3):1028–35.
9. Bockisch A, et al. Hybrid imaging by SPECT/CT and PET/CT: proven outcomes in cancer imaging. Semin Nucl Med. 2009;39(4):276–89.
10. Beyer T, Veit-Haibach P. State-of-the-art SPECT/CT: technology, methodology and applications-defining a new role for an undervalued multimodality imaging technique. Eur J Nucl Med Mol Imaging. 2014;41(Suppl 1):S1–2.
11. Bailey D, et al. *Combined PET/MRI: Global Warming-Summary Report of the 6th International Workshop on PET/MRI, March 27–29*, 2017. Tübingen: Mol Imaging Biol; 2017.
12. Beyer T, Czernin J, Freudenberg L. Variations in clinical PET/CT operations: results from an international survey among active PET/CT users. J Nucl Med. 2011;52(2):303–10.
13. Wieder H, et al. Variations of clinical SPECT/CT operations: an international survey. Nuklearmedizin. 2012;51(4):154–60.
14. Wagenknecht G, et al. MRI for attenuation correction in PET: methods and challenges. MAGMA. 2013;26(1):99–113.
15. Eiber M, et al. Value of a Dixon-based MR/PET attenuation correction sequence for the localization and evaluation of PET-positive lesions. Eur J Nuc Med Mol Ima. 2011;38(9):1691–701.
16. Beyer T, et al. Nuclear medicine 2013: from status quo to status go. Eur J Nucl Med Mol Imaging. 2013;40(1):1794–6.
17. Afshar-Oromieh A, et al. Comparison of PET/CT and PET/MRI hybrid systems using a 68Ga-labelled PSMA ligand for the diagnosis of recurrent prostate cancer: initial experience. Eur J Nucl Med Mol Imaging. 2014;41(5):887–97.
18. Wagner H. Fused image tomography: where do we go from here? J Nucl Med. 1999;40(9):30N–1N.
19. http://www.esor.org/cms/website.php?id=/en/programmes/esor_courses_for_edir/hybrid_imaging.htm.
20. Krippendorff K. Content analysis. An introduction to its methodology. 3rd ed. Thousand Oaks: SAGE Publications; 2013. p. 456.
21. Delaloye AB, et al. White paper of the European Association of Nuclear Medicine (EANM) and the European Society of Radiology (ESR) on multimodality imaging. Eur J Nucl Med Mol Imaging. 2007;34(8):1147–51.
22. Gourtsoyiannis N, et al. White paper of the European Society of Radiology (ESR) and the European Association of Nuclear Medicine (EANM) on multimodality imaging. Eur Radiol. 2007;17(8):1926–30.
23. (ESR), E.A.o.N.M.E.E.S.o.R. Multimodality imaging training curriculum–parts II and III. Eur J Nuc Med Mol Ima. 2012;39(4):557–62.
24. Frey K, et al. ABNM position statement: nuclear medicine professional competency and scope of practice. J Nucl Med. 2011;52(6):994–7.
25. Delbeke D, et al. SNMMI/ABNM joint position statement on optimizing training in nuclear medicine in the era of hybrid imaging. J Nucl Med. 2012;53(9):1490–4.
26. Stegger L, et al. EANM-ESR white paper on multimodality imaging. Eur J Nuc Med Mol Ima. 2008;35(3):677–80.
27. http://www.bundesaerztekammer.de/aerztetag/beschlussprotokolle-ab-1996/113-daet-2010/top-iii/neue-bezeichnungen/58-nuklearmedizinische-diagnostik-in-der-radiologie/.
28. http://www.bundesaerztekammer.de/aerztetag/beschlussprotokolle-ab-1996/113-daet-2010/top-iii/neue-bezeichnungen/59-roentgendiagnostik-in-der-nuklearmedizin/.
29. https://en.wikipedia.org/wiki/Habitus_(sociology). Accessed 17 Apr 2018.
30. Bourdieu P, Loïc J. An invitation to reflexive sociology. Chicago: The University of Chicago Press; 1992.
31. Howard SA, et al. Cancer imaging training in the 21st century: an overview of where we are, and where we need to be. J Am Coll Radiol. 2015;12(7):714–20.
32. Manfreda K, et al. Web surveys versus other survey modes: a meta-analysis comparing response rates. Int J Market Res. 2008;50(1):79–104.
33. Cook C, Heath F, Thompson R. A meta-analysis of response rates in web- or internet-based surveys. Educ Psychol Meas. 2000;60(6):821–38.

28

Detection of gastric cancer and its histological type based on iodine concentration in spectral CT

Rui Li[1], Jing Li[2], Xiaopeng Wang[1], Pan Liang[1] and Jianbo Gao[1*]

Abstract

Background: Computed tomography (CT) imaging is the most common imaging modality for the diagnosis and staging of gastric cancer. The aim of this study is was to prospectively explore the ability of quantitative spectral CT parameters in the detection of gastric cancer and its histologic types.

Methods: A total of 87 gastric adenocarcinoma (43 poorly and 44 well-differentiated) patients and 36 patients with benign gastric wall lesions (25 inflammation and 11 normal), who underwent dual-phase enhanced spectral CT examination, were retrospectively enrolled in this study. Iodine concentration (IC) and normalized iodine concentration (nIC) during arterial phase (AP) and portal venous phase (PP) were measured thrice in each patient by two blinded radiologists. Moreover, intraclass correlation coefficient (ICC) was used to assess the interobserver reproducibility. Differences of IC and nIC values between gastric cancer and benign lesion groups were compared using Mann-Whitney U test. Furthermore, the gender, age, location, thickness and histological types of gastric adenocarcinoma were analyzed by Mann-Whitney U test or Kruskal-Wallis H test. Receiver operating characteristic (ROC) curves were used to evaluate the diagnostic efficacy of IC and nIC values, and the optimal cut-off value was calculated with Youden J.

Results: An excellent interobserver agreement (ICC > 0.6) was achieved for IC. Notably, the values of ICAP, ICPP, nICAP and nICPP were significantly higher in gastric cancer group ($Z = 5.870$, 3.894, 2.009 and 10.137, respectively; $P < 0.05$) than those in benign lesion group. Additionally, the values of ICAP, ICPP, nICAP and nICPP were significantly higher in poorly differentiated gastric adenocarcinoma group ($Z = 4.118$, 5.637, 6.729 and 2.950, respectively; $P < 0.005$) than those in well-differentiated gastric adenocarcinoma group. There were no statistically significant differences in the values of ICAP, ICPP, nICAP and nICPP between age, gender, tumor thickness and tumor location. Furthermore, the area under the curve (AUC) values of ICAP, nICAP, ICPP and nICPP were 0.745, 0.584, 0.662, and 0.932, respectively, for gastric cancer detection; while 0.756, 0.919, 0.851 and 0.684, respectively, in discriminating poorly differentiated gastric adenocarcinoma.

Conclusion: IC values exhibited great potential in the preoperative and non-invasive diagnosis of gastric cancer and its histological types. In particular, nICPP is more effective for the identification of gastric cancer, whereas nICAP is more effective in discriminating poorly differentiated gastric adenocarcinoma.

Keywords: Gastric, Adenocarcinoma, Spectral CT imaging, Iodine concentration, Histological degree

* Correspondence: gaojianbo_cancer@163.com
[1]Department of Radiology, the First Affiliated Hospital of Zhengzhou University, No. 1, East Jianshe Road, Zhengzhou 450052, Henan, China
Full list of author information is available at the end of the article

Background

Gastric cancer is the fifth most common cancer and the third leading cause of cancer-related deaths worldwide [1]. Gastric adenocarcinoma comprises 95% of all gastric cancers [2]. The incidence and mortality rates associated with gastric adenocarcinoma are both the highest among all malignant tumors of the digestive tract in China [3, 4], representing an emerging threat to human health. The mean survival time of patients with advanced gastric cancer is less than 1 year [5]. Therefore, early detection, diagnosis and treatment are advocated to improve the clinical outcomes and quality of life in patients with gastric cancer.

Histological grading has been considered a predictor of lymph node metastasis and poor survival in gastric cancer [6]. Hence, accurate assessment of histological types is crucial for individualizing patient management [7]. Gold standard for the diagnosis of gastric cancer and its histological types can be obtained through preoperative endoscopic biopsy in clinical practice. However, endoscopic biopsy is an invasive procedure, and may posses unavoidable sampling bias and incoincident with histological diagnosis during surgery [8]. As compared to invasive endoscopic biopsy, preoperative imaging technique offers many advantages as its non-invasive detection and histologic evaluation of tumors, as well as the assessment of regional or distant lymph node metastasis. Conventional contrast-enhanced CT imaging is the first-line imaging modality for the detection and staging of gastric cancer. Its combination with multiple planar reconstruction and virtual endoscopy has proven to be effective for the diagnosis of gastric wall invasion in patients with gastric cancer [9]. However, this technique relies solely on the morphological criteria, and lack of parameters for quantitative analysis.

Spectral CT provides material decomposition (MD) images that can quantitatively map the iodine concentration (IC) in the enhanced images of tissues. This IC value has been found to be strongly correlated with the actual IC in the phantom [10]. Preliminary studies have reported the use of IC value in differentiating benign from malignant lesions, evaluating tumor, node, and metastasis (TNM) staging and determining the efficacy of anticancer therapy [11–16]. However, to the best of our knowledge, only a few studies have employed IC value in discriminating the histological types of gastric adenocarcinoma [12, 17], and the results are inconsistent with respect to arterial phase (AP) and portal venous phase (PP). Indeed, the application of IC values for the discrimination of gastric cancer and its histological types is still in the exploratory stage.

Therefore, this study aimed to evaluate the diagnostic efficacy of IC values for the detection of gastric cancer and its histological type, and to investigate their correlations with clinical data.

Methods

Patients

Ethical approval was obtained from the institutional ethics review board, but the requirement of informed consent was waived due to the retrospective nature of the study. A total of 153 patients with gastric cancer and 45 patients with preoperative endoscopic biopsy-diagnosed benign gastric wall lesions (30 gastric inflammation and 15 normal gastric wall) who underwent spectral CT scans and surgical intervention were retrospectively enrolled from June 2013 to June 2016. Considering that the conditions of gastric wall beyond the sampling site are not accessible, the patients with gastric inflammation and normal gastric wall were grouped together. The exclusion criteria included pathologically-confirmed non-adenocarcinomas, history of preoperative therapy (such as radiotherapy and chemotherapy), severe artifacts on CT images, non-measurable lesions and incomplete clinical data. All the included patients completed the entire CT exam, and their gastric cavities were well distended on cross-sectional CT images without artifacts, and the gastric adenocarcinomas were clearly distinguished from normal gastric wall. Clinical data of patients, such as age, gender tumor thickness, tumor location and tumor differentiation were also documented.

CT scan protocol

After fasting for 8 h, patients were asked to consume 1000 mL of warm water and then injected with 20 mg of scopolamine (Specifications: 10 mg/mL; Hangzhou Minsheng Pharmaceutical Group Co., Ltd. Hangzhou, China) 10 min prior to examination. Patients were placed in the supine position, and scanned on GE Discovery CT750 HD scanner (GE Healthcare, Milwaukee, WI, USA) with gemstone spectral imaging (GSI) mode. Dual-energy CT images were acquired using a single x-ray source switches rapidly between 80 kVp and 140 kVp at less than 5 millisecond speed. The other acquisition parameters were as follows: 5 mm slice thickness, 40 mm detector coverage, 0.984 helical pitch, 630 mA tube current, 0.6 s rotation time, 512×512 matrix, and 40×40 cm field of view. AP and PP contrast-enhanced CT scans were performed with 40 and 70 s delays, respectively, after intravenous injection of 85–110 mL (1.5 mL per kg of body weight) iodinated contrast material (Ultravist 370, Bayer Schering Pharma, Berlin, Germany) at a rate of 3.0 ml/s through pump injector (Ulrich REF XD 2060-Touch, Ulrich Medical, Ulm, Germany). Contrast-enhanced CT images were reconstructed by using a standard kernel and 2.5 mm section thickness. The value of CT dose index volume (CTDIvol) for dual energy spectral mode in the abdomen was 23.84 mGy.

Image analysis

All data were transferred to GE AW 4.6 workstation (GE Healthcare, Milwaukee, WI, USA), and interpreted by two radiologists with 6 and 10 years of experience in gastrointestinal radiology. Data analysis was carried out independently using GSI Viewer software (GE Healthcare, Milwaukee, WI, USA) with a standard soft-tissue window (WL 40 and WW 400). Regions of interest (ROI) were drawn on the solid part of the tumor (about two-thirds of the area), with the exclusion of peripheral fat, visible vessel, calcification and cystic/necrotic areas. A circular ROI was placed into the aortic arch within the same CT slice, after the exclusion of calcified atherosclerotic plaque. Subsequently, the thickness of tumour was measured and recorded. In order to reduce the individual variation between patients, IC value was normalized by dividing the IC of lesion to that of aorta (nIC=IClesion/ICaorta) [12]. All IC values were repeatedly measured three times, and the average value was then calculated. Similarly, ROI of the three gastric regions (fundus, body and antrum) was measured for three times, and their average values were calculated.

Statistical analysis

All statistical analyses were performed with MedCalc v.9.2.0.0 (Frank Schoonjans, Broekstraat 52,B-9030 Mariakerke, Belgium). P values of less than 0.05 were considered statistically significant. Interobserver agreement for IC and nIC values was evaluated using intraclass correlation coefficient (ICC), which classified as poor (< 0.40), fair (0.40–0.59), good (0.60–0.74), or excellent (0.75–1.00). The values of IC and nIC at both AP and PP were expressed as median (P25, P75). Mann-Whitney U test was used to compare the IC values between cancer and benign gastric wall group, as well as the IC values among age, gender, tumor thickness and histological types. Kruskal-Wallis H test was used to compare the differences of IC and nIC values between different tumour sites, including funtus, body and antrum. Furthermore, ROC curves were used to evaluate the diagnostic values of IC and nIC in discriminating gastric cancer and its histological type.

Results
Clinical data

A total of 87 (57%) out of 153 gastric cancer patients and 36 (80%) out of 45 patients with benign gastric wall lesions were ultimately included in the study. Among the excluded patients, 18 of them were diagnosed as non-adenocarcinoma by surgical pathology, 12 patients with poor image quality (severe artifacts) evaluated by two radiologists in consensus, and 8 patients received preoperative therapy. A further 9 patients with benign gastric wall lesions and 28 gastric cancer patients were excluded from analysis due to the non-measurable lesions on enhanced CT images. Overall, clinical data of 87 gastric adenocarcinoma patients and 36 patients with

benign gastric wall lesions were used for final analyses. The clinical characteristics of all included patients are summarized in Table 1, while the images of gastric adenocarcinoma patients at different sites are shown in Fig. 1.

Interobserver agreement

The interobserver agreement of IC measurement between two readers was ranked from good to excellent. In particular, the values of ICAP, ICPP, nICAP and nICPP in were 0.664, 0.755, 0.913 and 0.980, respectively, in gastric cancer group and 0.694, 0.713, 0.897, 0.910, respectively, in benign gastric wall lesions group. The mean difference between the two observers was used for further analysis.

Comparison of IC and nIC values between benign gastric wall lesions and gastric cancer

As shown in Fig. 2 and Table 2, the values of ICAP, ICPP, nICAP and nICPP in benign gastric wall lesions group were 9.388 (7.497, 12.740) 100 μg/ml, 17.233 (14.448, 18.798) 100 μg/ml, 0.111 (0.076, 0.141) and 0.264 (0.068, 0.328), respectively. On the other hand, the values of ICAP, ICPP, nICAP and nICPP in gastric cancer group were 12.900 (11.508, 14.832) 100 μg/ml, 20.000 (18.623, 22.000) 100 μg/ml, 0.115 (0.105, 0.141)

Table 1 Clinical characteristics of 87 patients with gastric adenocarcinomas and 36 patients with benign gastric wall lesions

Characteristics	Statistics(mean, range)
Cancer peoples	87
Age (years)	55 (29–74)
Gender(M/F)	60/27
Tumor thickness (cm)	3.1 (1.0–8.9)
Tumor site	
Fundus	29 (33.3%)
Body	28 (32.3%)
Antrum	27 (31%)
Whole stomach	3 (3.4%)
Histological differentiation degree	
Highly differentiated adenocarcinoma	4 (4.6%)
Moderately differentiated adenocarcinoma	40 (46.0%)
Poorly differentiated adenocarcinoma	43 (49.4%)
Benign lesion peoples	36
Age (years)	53 (32–72)
Gender(M/F)	22/14
Gastric wall	
Inflammation	25(69%)
Normal	11(31%)

Abbreviations:*M* Male, *F* Female

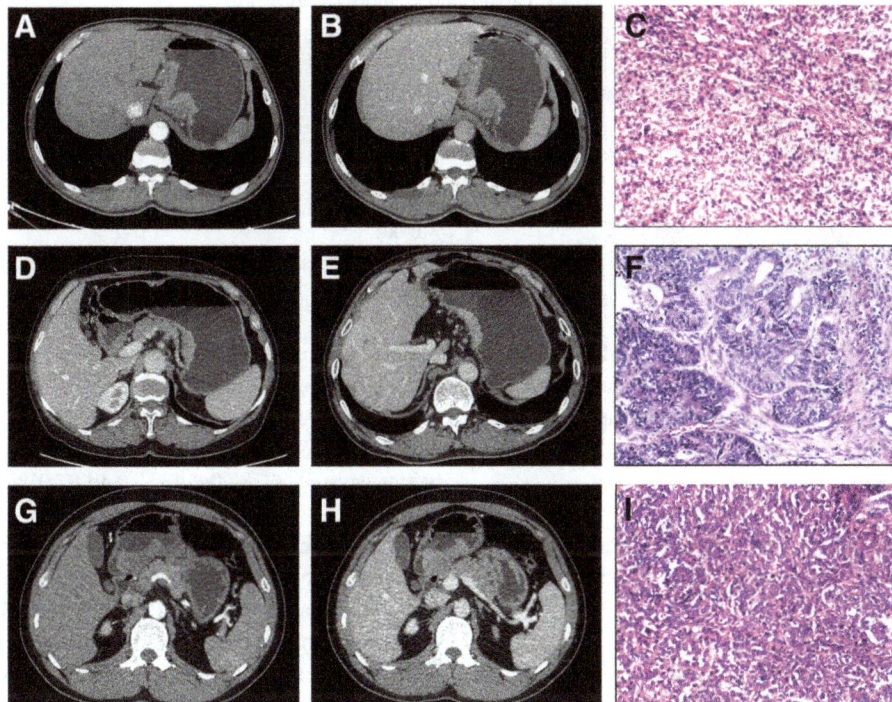

Fig. 1 Spectral CT images of patients with poorly and moderately differentiated gastric adenocarcinomas at different sites. **a** AP image shows moderate enhancement of fundal wall thickening in a 67-year-old male patient. The maximum thickness is 17.89 mm, and ICAP is 16.78 (100 μg/ml). **b** PP image demonstrates a ICPP value of 27.19 (100 μg/ml) in the same patient. c Photomicrograph of histological specimen indicates a poorly differentiated adenocarcinoma [hematoxylin and eosin (H&E) stain; original magnification × 100]. **d** AP image shows irregular wall thickening of the gastric body in a 41-year-old female patient. The maximum thickness is 14.24 mm, and ICAP is 14.46 (100 μg/ml). **e** PP image demonstrates a ICPP value of 24.57 (100 μg/ml) in the same patient. **f** Photomicrograph of histological specimen indicates a poorly differentiated adenocarcinoma. (H&E stain; original magnification × 100). **g** AP image shows antrum wall thickening with surface ulcers in a 56-year-old male patient. The maximum thickness is 20.32 mm and ICAP is 11.79 (100 μg/ml). **h** PP image demonstrates a ICPP value of 20.19 (100 μg/ml) in the same patient. **i** Photomicrograph of histological specimen indicates a moderately differentiated adenocarcinoma (H&E stain; original magnification × 100)

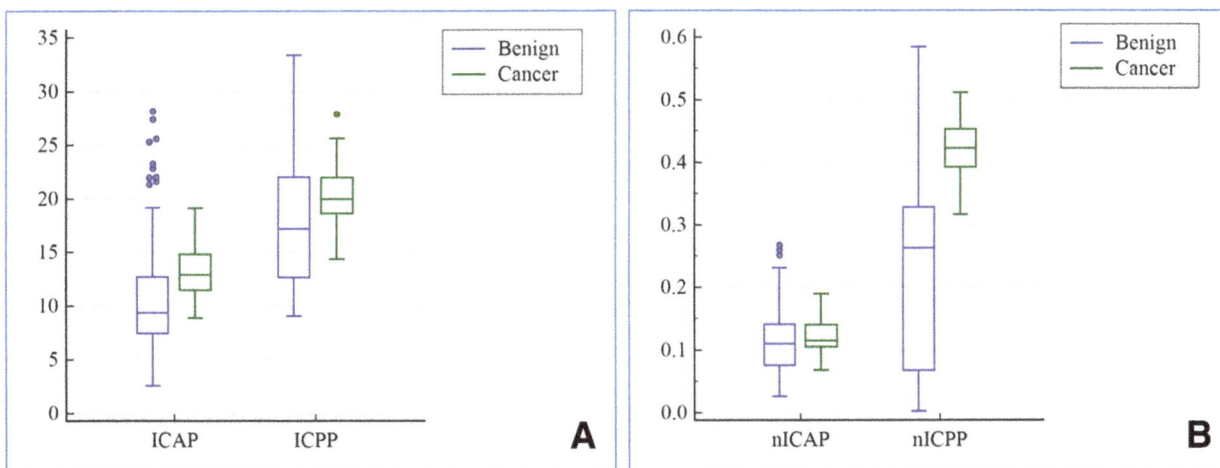

Fig. 2 Differences in IC and nIC values between between gastric cancer and benign lesion groups. Box-and-whisker plots (box: 25, 75%; centreline: medium; whisker: min, max) reveal that (**a**) ICAP, ICPP, (**b**) nICAP and nICPP of gastric adenocarcinoma group were significantly higher than benign gastric wall group, with $P < 0.0001$, $P = 0.0001$, $P = 0.0445$ and $P < 0.0001$, respectively

Table 2 Comparison of IC and nIC values between gastric cancer and benign lesion groups

Group	Number	ICAP(100 µg/ml)	ICPP(100 µg/ml)	nICAP	nICPP
Benign	108	9.388 (7.497, 12.740)	17.233 (14.448, 18.798)	0.111 (0.076, 0.141)	0.264 (0.068, 0.328)
Cancer	87	12.900 (11.508, 14.832)	20.000 (18.623, 22.000)	0.115 (0.105, 0.141)	0.423 (0.392, 0.453)
Z value		5.870	3.894	2.009	10.137
P value		< 0.0001	=0.0001	=0.0445	< 0.0001

Abbreviations: *ICAP* arterial phase iodine concentration, *ICPP* portal venous phase iodine concentration, *nICAP* normalized arterial phase iodine concentration, *nICPP* normalized portal venous phase iodine concentration

and 0.423 (0.392, 0.453), respectively. Notably, these values were significantly higher in gastric cancer group than those in benign gastric wall lesions group [$Z = 5.870$ (ICAP), 3.894 (ICPP), 2.009 (nICAP) and 10.137 (nICPP); $P < 0.005$].

Comparison of IC and nIC values between gender, age, thickness, location and histological types of gastric adenocarcinoma

As compared to female patients, the values of ICAP, ICPP, nICAP and nICPP were slightly higher in male patients (Table 3). However, none of these differences were statistically significant [$Z = 0.922$ (ICAP), 1.372 (ICPP), 1.636 (nICAP) and 1.449 (nICPP); $P > 0.05$]. All gastric cancer patients were divided into young (≤ 55 years old) and older (> 55 years old) groups according to the mean age of 55 years old. The values of ICAP, ICPP, nICAP and nICPP in young group were slightly higher than those in older group, but the differences were not statistically significant ($Z = 0.613$, 1.066, 1.935 and 0.583, respectively; $P > 0.05$). In addition, the patients were divided into small (≤ 3.1 cm) and large (> 3.1 cm) tumor groups according to the mean thickness of 3.1 cm. The values of ICAP, ICPP, nICAP and nICPP in small tumor group were slightly higher than those in large tumor group, but not significantly different ($Z = 1.083$, 0.706, 0.103 and 1.272, respectively; $P > 0.05$). Similarly, the values of ICAP, ICPP, nICAP and nICPP were not significantly different among the three tumor location groups (H values = 0.205, 4.221, 1.859 and 4.836, respectively; $P > 0.05$). Furthermore, the moderately and well-differentiated gastric adenocarcinoma groups were combined into a single group, due to the limited numbers of cases in well-differentiated tumor group ($n = 4$). As shown in Figure 3, the values of ICAP, ICPP, nICAP and nICPP were significantly higher in poorly differentiated group than those in well-differentiated group ($Z = 4.118$, 5.637, 6.729 and 2.950, respectively; $P < 0.05$).

Diagnostic accuracy of IC values in detecting gastric cancer

The AUC values of ICAP, nICAP, ICPP and nICPP for the gastric cancer detection were 0.745, 0.584, 0.662 and 0.923, respectively (Fig. 4 and Table 4). Of note, nICPP demonstrated the greatest ability in discriminating gastric cancer.

Besides, the optimal cut-off values of ICAP, nICAP, ICPP and nICPP were 10.343, 0.089, 14.913 and 0.364, respectively. The sensitivities of ICAP, nICAP, ICPP and nICPP were 95.40, 96.55, 98.85 and 91.95%, respectively; while the specificities were 58.33, 37.04, 43.52 and 87.96%, respectively.

Diagnostic accuracy of IC values in discriminating the histological types of gastric adenocarcinoma

The AUC values of ICAP, nICAP, ICPP, and nICPP in discriminating poorly and well-differentiated gastric adenocarcinoma were 0.756, 0.919, 0.851 and 0.684, respectively (Fig. 4 and Table 4). Of note, nICAP demonstrated the greatest ability in discriminating the histological types of gastric adenocarcinoma, whereas nICPP showed the lowest. The optimal cut-off values of ICAP, nICAP, ICPP and nICPP were 14.460, 0.125, 20.461 and 0.431, respectively. The sensitivities of ICAP, nICAP, ICPP, and nICPP were 53.49, 79.07, 69.77 and 60.47%, respectively; while the specificities were 93.18, 97.73, 90.91 and 79.55%, respectively.

Discussion

Spectral CT extends the capabilities of conventional CT, which uses a rapid kilovoltage switching technique to acquire monochromatic images of tissues, in a similar way to those obtained from a single X-ray source [18–20]. Subsequent elemental decomposition analysis can be performed to obtain iodinated contrast attenuation map, thereby allowing iodine density to be calculated [21, 22]. As a result, this can assist the radiologists to address diagnostic errors. Hence, the present study investigated the role of quantitative spectral CT parameters for the discrimination of gastric cancer and its histological types, and examined their correlations with clinical features. The major findings of this study were as follow: (1) IC values in gastric cancer were higher than benign gastric wall lesions, in which nICPP demonstrated the greatest diagnostic efficacy; (2) IC values in poorly differentiated gastric adenocarcinoma were higher than in well-differentiated caners, in which nICAP showed the highest diagnostic efficacy; and (3) IC values were not significantly different between age, gender, tumor thickness and tumor location.

Table 3 Comparison of IC and nIC values between gender, age, location, thickness and histological types of gastric adenocarcinoma

Clinical features	Number of cases	ICAP (100 μg/ml)	ICPP (100 μg/ml)	nICAP	nICPP
Gender					
Male	60	13.018 (11.511, 15,780)	20.464 (18.843, 22.570)	0.125 (0.108, 0.147)	0.431 (0.398, 0.462)
Female	27	12.893 (11.456, 14.385)	19.480 (18.635, 21.485)	0.117 (0.105, 0.136)	0.412 (0.389, 0.443)
Z value		0.922	1.372	1.636	1.449
P value		> 0.05	> 0.05	> 0.05	> 0.05
Age					
Young(≤55 y)	41	13.010 (11.483, 16.675)	20.460 (18.868, 22.570)	0.138 (0.108, 0.153)	0.430 (0.400, 0.455)
Older (> 55 y)	46	13.009 (11.450, 14.440)	19.480 (18.780, 22.000)	0.119 (0.107, 0.136)	0.421 (0.389, 0.463)
Z value		0.613	1.066	1.935	0.583
P value		> 0.05	> 0.05	> 0.05	> 0.05
Sites					
Fundus	29	12.900 (11.543, 16.675)	20.010 (18.742, 22.240)	0.119 (0.106, 0.147)	0.423 (0.394, 0.435)
Body	28	13.672 (11.465, 15.787)	21.835 (19.815, 23.040)	0.140 (0.115, 0.151)	0.642 (0.404. 0.486)
Antrum	27	13.674 (11.930, 15.735)	20.200 (19.253, 22.108)	0.127 (0.111,0.141)	0.430 (0.399, 0.472)
H value		0.205	4.221	1.859	4.836
P value		> 0.05	> 0.05	> 0.05	> 0.05
Thickness					
Small (≤3.1 cm)	38	13.205 (11.890, 15.780)	20.332 (19.022, 22.105)	0.128 (0.109, 0.142)	0.433 (0.393, 0.468)
Large (> 3.1 cm)	49	12.780 (11.111, 14.532)	19.815 (18.783, 22.570)	0.119 (0.107, 0.147)	0.417 (0.396, 0.433)
Z value		1.083	0.706	0.103	1.272
P value		> 0.05	> 0.05	> 0.05	> 0.05
Differentiation					
Poorly	43	14.530 (13.168, 15.670)	21.780 (20.030, 23.348)	0.141 (0.127, 0.155)	0.433 (0.411, 0.472)
Well-differentiated	44	11.880 (11.240, 13.120)	18.855 (17.270, 19.800)	0.106 (0.100, 0.113)	0.410 (0.391, 0.431)
Z value		4.118	5.637	6.729	2.950
P value		< 0.0001	< 0.0001	< 0.0001	=0.0032

Abbreviations: *ICAP* arterial phase iodine concentration, *ICPP* portal venous phase iodine concentration, *nICAP* normalized arterial phase iodine concentration, *nICPP* normalized portal venous phase iodine concentration

Iodine concentration reflects the vessel density and the blood volume in different tissue regions during a contrast-enhanced CT scan. Tang et al. [15] reported a high consistency between spectral CT-measured IC and actual IC, and thus it is a useful parameter to indicate the physiological function. The growth and progression of solid tumors depend upon the formation of new blood vessels, which is different from normal tissues or benign lesions. Several studies have reported that CT imaging is useful for distinguishing small hepatocellular carcinoma from other hepatic lesions [23, 24], small intrahepatic mass-forming cholangiocarcinoma from small liver abscess [25], malignant from benign pulmonary nodules [26], and gastric cancer from benign gastric mucosal lesions [11]. Indeed, the quantitative IC measurement is significantly higher in cancerous lesions compared to benign lesions, and its accuracy is greater than that of conventional CT. In addition, Liu et al. examined the patients with papillary thyroid cancer, and their results suggested that nIC measured during AP and PP are significantly higher in metastatic lymph nodes as compared to benign lesions [27]. Taken together, our results

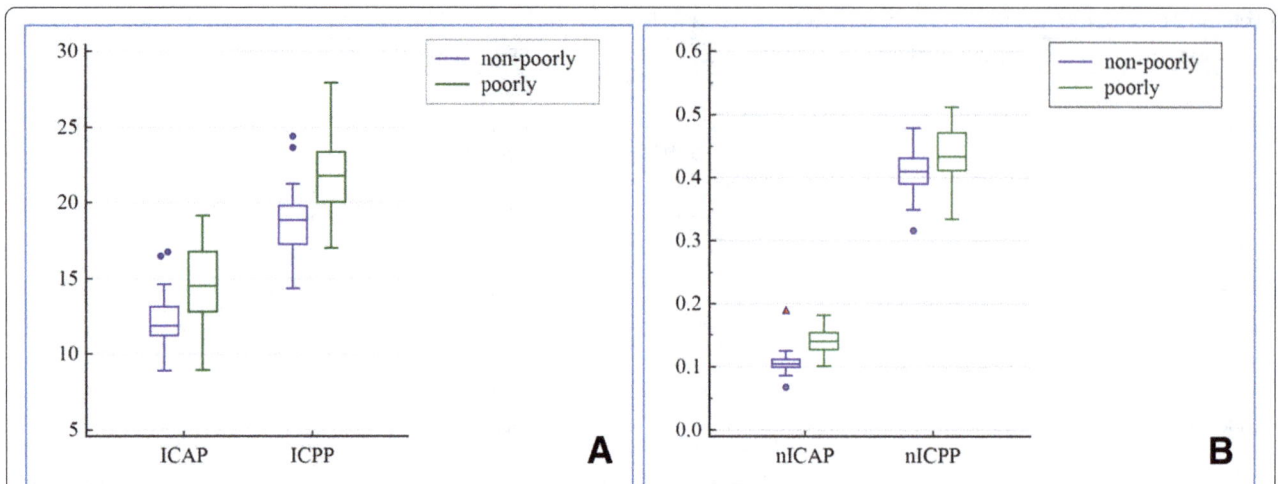

Fig. 3 Differences in IC and nIC values between poorly and well-differentiated gastric adenocarcinoma groups. Box-and-whisker plots (box: 25, 75%; centreline: medium; whisker: min, max) indicate that (**a**) ICAP, ICPP, (**b**) nICAP and nICPP of poorly differentiated gastric adenocarcinoma group were significantly higher than well-differentiated gastric adenocarcinoma group, with $P < 0.0001$, $P < 0.0001$, $P < 0.0001$ and $P = 0.0032$, respectively

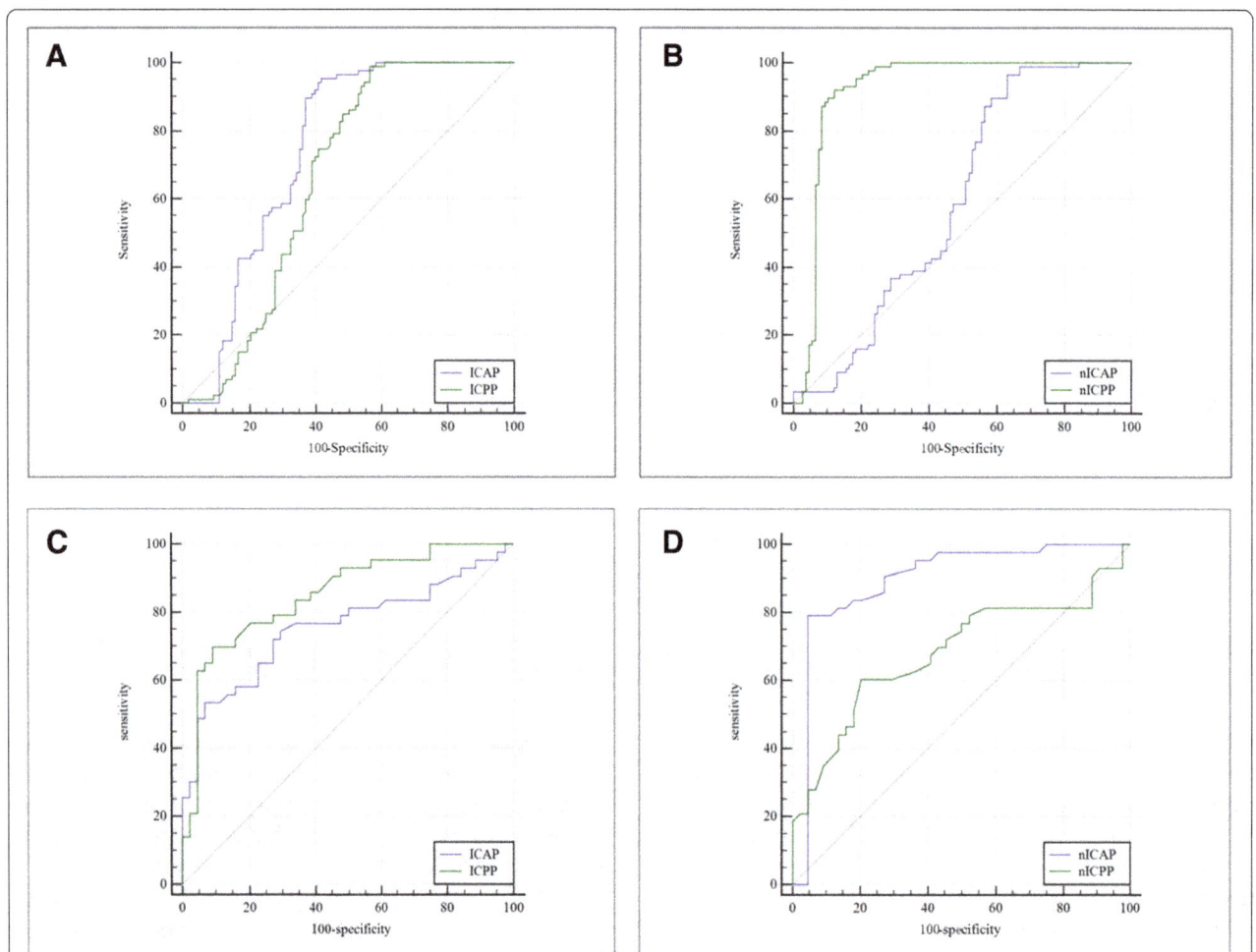

Fig. 4 ROC curves for ICAP, ICPP, nICAP and nICPP. The ROC curves of (**a**) ICAP, ICPP, (**b**) nICAP and nICPP between gastric cancer and benign gastric wall lesions groups. nICPP has the highest AUC value, followed by ICAP, ICPP and nICAP. The ROC curves of (**c**) ICAP, ICPP, (**d**) nICAP and nICPP between poorly and well-differentiated gastric adenocarcinoma groups. nICAP has the highest AUC value, followed by ICPP, ICAP and nICPP

Table 4 The ROC curves of IC and nIC values

ROC	ICAP	ICPP	nICAP	nICPP
Cancer				
AUC	0.745	0.662	0.584	0.923
sensitivity	95.40%	98.85%	96.55%	91.95%
specificity	58.33%	43.52%	37.04%	87.96%
Optimum cutoff values	10.343	14.913	0.089	0.364
Youden index	0.537	0.424	0.336	0.799
Poorly differentiated				
AUC	0.756	0.851	0.919	0.684
sensitivity	53.49%	69.77%	79.07%	60.47%
specificity	93.18%	90.91%	97.73%	79.55%
Optimum cutoff values	14.460	20.461	0.125	0.431
Youden index	0.467	0.607	0.768	0.400

Abbreviations: *ROC* Receiver operating characteristic curves, *AUC* area under the curve, *ICAP* arterial phase iodine concentration, *ICPP* portal venous phase iodine concentration, *nICAP* normalized arterial phase iodine concentration, *nICPP* normalized portal venous phase iodine concentration

are consistent with the aforementioned studies, in which the values of IC are higher in cancer than in benign lesions, due to the increased angiogenesis during tumor development, leading to their enhancement in CT scan [28].

The degree of tumor differentiation is a predictive and prognosis biomarker for patients with gastric cancer [29], which can be distinguished quantitatively by dual-energy spectral CT (DESCT). Pan et al. [12] evaluated the clinical usefulness of DESCT in the classification and staging of gastric cancer. Their findings indicated that monochromatic images obtained from DESCT can be used to improve the accuracy of preoperative staging, and quantitative IC measurement is helpful in distinguishing the poorly and well-differentiated gastric carcinoma, as well as the metastatic and non-metastatic lymph nodes. A similar pattern of results was obtained, where IC and nIC values were significantly lower in well-differentiated gastric cancer compared to poorly differentiated ones, which can be explained by the differences in tumor angiogenesis. Du et al. [30] have suggested that vascular endothelial growth factor (VEGF) expression and microvessel density (MVD) are closely correlated with histological degree, in which their levels are reduced in early stage gastric carcinoma compared to progressive carcinoma. Chang et al. [31] have reported that MVD is significantly associated with poorly differentiated gastric adenocarcinoma. Moreover, Hu et al. [32] demonstrated that the nIC value of three-phase enhanced CT scan is positively correlated with MVD. Additionally, Chen et al. reported that poorly differentiated gastric cancer exhibited higher MVD and nIC value, and a positive correlation between them [33]. A CT perfusion study on gastric cancer has revealed that the lower the degree of tumor differentiation, the higher the permeability surface area [34]. These findings indicate that poorly differentiated tumors may

increase vasopermeability and immature endothelial cells, thereby explaining the high values of IC and MVD in gastric patients with poorly differentiated adenocarcinoma.

nIC can minimize the effects of individual variability, such as contrast dose, injection rate and individual differences in circulation, and thereby it is more efficacy than IC. Both nICAP and nICPP were found to be significantly different between gastric cancer group and benign gastric wall lesions group, as well as between poorly differentiated group and well-differentiated group. In particular, nICAP demonstrated a higher efficiency in the diagnosis of poorly differentiated gastric adenocarcinoma, with AUC, sensitivity and specificity of 0.896, 79.07 and 95.45%, respectively. Meanwhile, nICPP showed a higher efficacy for the detection of gastric cancer, with AUC, sensitivity and specificity of 0.923, 91.95 and 87.96%, respectively. These results can be partly explained by different functional roles of nICAP and nICPP. nICAP mainly reflects the capillary density and the blood supply of gastric carcinomas, while nICPP may indicate the flow of blood supply and the retention of contrast agent in intrasvasular and extravascular space following AP. It is noticeable that venous phase enhancement is more prominent in gastric cancer, suggesting that PP enhancement characteristics are more useful for the detection of gastric cancer. Besides, the reason why PP is less effective than AP in distinguishing histological types may be due to the influence of blood flow. In addition, nICPP has been reported to exert a high sensitivity in differentiating malignant gastric mucosal lesions from normal gastric mucosa [11]. Furthermore, studies on the diagnostic efficacy of tumor differentiation degree are inconsistent [35, 36], which may be due to the different biological behaviors of tumors and degrees of differentiation. A previous study has found that the values of IC and nIC of poorly differentiated adenocarcinoma are not significantly different compared to those of moderately and well-differentiated adenocarcinomas in AP [17]. These inconsistent results may be attributed to different patient populations and scan protocol. In that study, patients were subjected to triple-phase CT imaging, including AP at 25 s, which are different from ours. In sum, DESCT is more useful in evaluating gastric cancer with a delay AP scan protocol.

Apart from that, Karim et al. [37] reported that younger age is correlated with the histology grade of gastric cancer. However, the histology grade is not correlated with gender and tumor location [38]. In addition, Wang et al. [38] demonstrated that tumour size is a prognostic factor in patients with advanced gastric cancer. In the present study, no significant differences were found in the values of ICAP, ICPP, nICAP and nICPP between age, gender, tumor thickness and tumor location.

There are some unavoidable limitations in this preliminary study. First, DESCT scans were performed on the first-generation Discovery CT750 HD scanner with a fixed mA value of 600 mA. This yielded a CTDIvol of 23.84 mGy, which is considerably high in current clinical practise settings. With the introduction of the second-generation CT750 HD scanner, the radiation dose has been reduced to 30% in GSI mode, and further dose reduction is forthcoming. Second, this is a retrospective study, and the sample size was relatively small, especially the number of patients with well-differentiated adenocarcinoma was too low to to allow a statistical comparison with moderately and poorly differentiated ones. Third, only patients with gastric adenocarcinoma were enrolled in this study, patients with other histological types of gastric cancer were not taken into account. Moreover, it was difficult to obtain pathologic confirmation of the entire gastric wall in non-cancer patients, and the patients with gastric inflammation and normal gastric wall were grouped together. Finally, since DESCT is a relatively new technique for gastric cancer, it may hinder the adaptation process based on these preliminary results.

Conclusions

In conclusion, this preliminary study compared the quantitative spectral CT parameters between benign lesion and gastric cancer groups, as well as different histological types of gastric adenocarcinoma. IC values can be used to accurately identify gastric cancer and quantitatively assess the degree of differentiation, without being affected by age, gender, tumor thickness and tumor location. These findings may improve the preoperative staging of gastric cancer, and lay the foundations for modern functional imaging in oncology. However, further studies with larger sample sizes are needed to draw a firm conclusion.

Abbreviations

AP: Arterial phase; AUC: Area under the curve; CT: Computed tomography; CTDIvol: CT dose index volume; DEsCT: Dual-energy spectral CT; IC: Iodine concentration; ICC: Intraclass correlation coefficient; MD: Material decomposition; MVD: Microvessel density; nIC: Normalized iodine concentration; PP: Portal venous phase; ROC: Receiver-operating characteristics analysis; ROI: Regions-of-interest; SD: Standard deviation; VEGF: Vascular endothelial growth factor

Acknowledgements
None.

Funding
National Natural and Science Fund of China (NO. 81271573).

Authors' contributions

RL: manuscript preparation, literature research, data analysis, statistical analysis and manuscript editing; JL: data acquisition and statistical analysis; PL: literature research and data analysis; XP W: data acquisition; JB G: study conception and design, manuscript review and guarantor of integrity of the entire study. All authors read and approved the final manuscript.

Competing interests

The authors declare that they have no competing interests.

Author details
[1]Department of Radiology, the First Affiliated Hospital of Zhengzhou University, No. 1, East Jianshe Road, Zhengzhou 450052, Henan, China. [2]Department of Radiology, the Affiliated Cancer Hospital of Zhengzhou University, Henan Cancer Hospital, No. 127, Dongming Road, Zhengzhou 450008, Henan, China.

References

1. Torre LA, Bray F, Siegel RL, et al. Global cancer statistics, 2012. CA Cancer J Clin. 2015;65:87–108.
2. Dicken BJ, Bigam DL, Cass C, et al. Gastric adenocarcinoma: review and considerations for future directions. Ann Surg. 2005;241:27–39.
3. Wong BC, Lam SK, Wong WM, et al. Helicobacter pylori eradication to prevent gastric cancer in a high-risk region of China: a randomized controlled trial. JAMA. 2004;291:187–94.
4. Yan SY, Hu Y, Fan JG, et al. Clinicopathologic significance of HER-2/neu protein expression and gene amplification in gastric carcinoma. World J Gastroenterol. 2011;17:1501–6.
5. Bang YJ, Kang YK, Kang WK, et al. Phase II study of sunitinib as second-line treatment for advanced gastric cancer. Investig New Drugs. 2011;29:1449–58.
6. Sekiguchi M, Oda I, Taniguchi H, et al. Risk stratification and predictive risk-scoring model for lymph node metastasis in early gastric cancer. J Gastroenterol. 2016;51:961–70.
7. Sasaki T, Koizumi W, Higuchi K, et al. Therapeutic strategy for type 4 gastric cancer from the clinical oncologist standpoint. Gan To Kagaku Ryoho. 2007; 34:988–92.
8. Liu S, Liu Song, Ji C, et al. Application of CT texture analysis in predicting histopathological characteristics of gastric cancers. Eur Radiol. 2017;27:4951–9.
9. Shen Y, Kang HK, Jeong YY, et al. Evalution of early gastric cnncer at multidetector CT with multiplanar reformation and virtual endoscopy. Radiographics. 2011;31:189–99.
10. Lv P, Lin X, Gao J, Chen K. Spectral CT: preliminary studies in the liver cirrhosis. Korean J Radiol. 2012;13:434–42.
11. Meng X, Ni C, ShenY HX, et al. Differentiating malignant from benign gastric mucosal lesions with quantitative analysis in dual energy spectral computed tomography: Initial experience. Medicine (Baltimore). 2017;96:e5878.
12. Pan Z, Pang L, Ding B, et al. Gastric cancer staging with dual energy spectral CT imaging. PLoS One. 2013;8:e53651.
13. Li C, Shi C, Zhang H, et al. Computer-aided diagnosis for preoperative invasion depth of gastric Cancer with dual-energy spectral CT imaging. Acad Radiol. 2015;22:149–57.
14. Li C, Zhang S, Zhang H, et al. Using the K-nearest neighbor algorithm for the classification of lymph node metastasis in gastric cancer. Compu Math Methods Med. 2012;2012:876545.
15. Tang L, Li ZY, Li ZW, et al. Evaluating the response of gastric carcinomas to neoadjuvant chemotherapy using iodine concentration on spectral CT: a comparison with pathological regression. Clin Radiol. 2015;70:1198–204.
16. Li J, Fang M, Wang R, et al. Diagnostic accuracyof dual-energy CT-based nomograms to predict lymph node. Eur Radiol. 2018. https://doi.org/10.1007/s00330-018-5483-2 [Epub ahead of print].
17. Chen LH, Xue YJ, Duan Q. Spectral CT imaging in quantitative evaluation on histological degree of gastric cancers. Chin J Med Imaging Technol. 2013;29: 225–9 Chinese.
18. Hurrell MA, Butler AP, Cook NJ, et al. Spectral Hounsfield units: a new radiological concept. Eur Radiol. 2012;22:1008e13.
19. Tang L, Zhang XP, Sun YS, et al. Spectral CT in the demonstration of the gastrocolic ligament: a comparison study. Surg Radiol Anat. 2013;35:539e45.
20. Li XH, Zhao R, Liu B, et al. Determination of urinary stone composition using dual-energy spectral CT: initial in vitro analysis. Clin Radiol. 2013;68:e370e7.
21. Matsumoto K, Jinzaki M, Tanami Y, et al. Virtual monochromatic spectral imaging with fast kilovoltage switching: improved image quality as compared with that obtained with conventional 120-kVp CT. Radiology. 2011;259:257–62.

22. Silva AC, Morse BG, Hara AK, et al. Dual-energy (spectral) CT: applications in abdominal imaging. Radiographics. 2011;31:1031–46.

23. Lv P, Lin XZ, Li J, et al. Differentiation of small hepatic hemangioma from small hepatocellular carcinoma: recently introduced spectral CT method. Radiology. 2011;259:720–9.

24. Wang Q, Shi G, Qi X, et al. Quantitative analysis of the dual-energy CT virtual spectral curve for focal liver lesions characterization. Eur J Radiol. 2014;83:1759–64.

25. Kim JE, Kim HO, Bae K, et al. Differentiation of small intrahepatic mass-forming cholangiocarcinoma from small liver abscess by dual source dual-energy CT quantitative parameters. Eur J Radiol. 2017;92:145–52.

26. Zhang Y, Cheng J, Hua X, et al. Can spectral CT imaging improve the differentiation between malignant and benign solitary pulmonary nodules? PLoS One. 2016;11:e 0147537.

27. Liu X, Ouyang D, Li H, et al. Papillary thyroid cancer: dual-energy spectral CT quantitative parameters for preoperative diagnosisof metastasis to the cervical lymph nodes. Radiology. 2015;275:167–76.

28. Miles KA. Tumour angiogenesis and its relation to contrast enhancement on computed tomography: a review. Eur J Radiol. 1999;30:198–205.

29. Haist T, Pritzer H, Pauthner M, et al. Prognostic risk factors of early gastric cancer-a western experience. Langenbeck's Arch Surg. 2016;401:667–76.

30. Du JR, Jiang Y, Zhang YM, et al. Vascular endothelial growth factor and microvascular density in esophageal and gastric carcinomas. World J Gastroenterol. 2003;9:1604–6.

31. Chang Y, Niu W, Lian PL, et al. Endocan-expressing microvessel density as a prognostic factor for survival in human gastric cancer. World J Gastroenterol. 2016;22:5422–9.

32. Hu S, Huang W, Chen Y, et al. Spectral CT evaluation of interstitial brachytherapy in pancreatic carcinoma xenografts: preliminary animal experience. Eur Radiol. 2014;24:2167–73.

33. Chen XH, Ren K, Liang P, et al. Spectral computed tomography in advanced gastric cancer: can iodine concentration non-invasively assess angiogenesis? World J Gastroenterol. 2017;23:1666–75.

34. Lee DH, Kim SH, Joo I, et al. CT perfusion evaluation of gastric cancer: correlation with histologic type. Eur Radiol. 2018;28:487–95.

35. Lin LY, Zhang Y, Suo ST, et al. Correlation between dual-energy spectral CT imaging parameters and pathological grades of non-small cell lung cancer. Clin Radiol. 2018;73:412.e1–7.

36. Chuang-Bo Y, Tai-Ping H, Hai-Feng D, et al. Quantitative assessment of the degree of differentiation in colon cancer with dual-energy spectral CT. Abdom Radiol (NY). 2017;42:2591–6.

37. Karim S. Clinicopathological and p53 gene alteration comparison between young and older patients with gastric cancer. Asian Pac J Cancer Prev. 2014; 15:1375–9.

38. Wang HM, Huang CM, Zheng CH, et al. Tumor size as a prognostic factor in patients with advancer gastric cancer in the lower third of the stomach. World J Gastroenterol. 2012;18:5470–5.

29

Castleman disease versus lymphoma in neck lymph nodes: a comparative study using contrast-enhanced CT

Jie Li[1], Jia Wang[2], Zhitao Yang[1], Hexiang Wang[1], Junyi Che[3] and Wenjian Xu[1*]

Abstract

Background: The purpose of this study was to determine the contrast-enhanced CT characteristics for differentiating between Castleman disease (CD) and lymphoma in neck lymph nodes.

Methods: This retrospective study evaluated the number (solitary or multiple), strength of contrast-enhancement, type of contrast-enhancement, surrounding vessels, contrast-enhanced Hounsfield unit (HU) values, and anatomical distributions of lymph nodes in 34 patients with confirmed CD and 55 patients with newly diagnosed untreated lymphoma. Independent t-tests, receiver operating characteristic (ROC) curve analysis, and chi-square tests were used to evaluate the variables and CT features.

Results: Several significant differences were found between CD and lymphoma. The interval between first contrast-enhanced CT and biopsy/surgery was significantly longer in the CD group (mean 72 ± 105 days, median 60 days) than in the lymphoma patients (mean 30 ± 2 days, median 12 days; $p = 0.015$). The lymphoma patients presented significantly more often with fatigue and fever ($p = 0.023$ and $p = 0.016$ respectively) than did the CD subjects. HU values of nodules after enhancement were significantly higher in the CD patients than in the lymphoma patients. In cases involving multiple lymph nodes, in all the CD cases, all affected nodes were located in only the left or right side of the neck, not bilaterally. ROC analysis showed a significant difference in contrast-enhanced CT attenuation values between lymphoma and CD ($p < 0.001$, area under the curve = 0.954), with a cut-off value of 92.5 HU. We constructed a decision tree according to these imaging characteristics.

Conclusions: Contrast-enhanced CT can be useful for differentiating between CD and lymphoma.

Keywords: Neck, Castleman disease, Lymphoma, Contrast-enhanced CT

Background

The incidence of Castleman disease (CD) has increased in recent years, with this phenomenon having been attributed to factors such as an increase in acquired immunodeficiency syndrome (AIDS), serum interleukin-6 (IL-6) levels, and/or human herpes virus-8 (HHV-8) [1–3].

CD can mimic other pathology, and especially when it is located in the neck, it often shares similar clinical presentations and imaging characteristics to lymphoma, such as a progressive growing lesion and enlarged lymph nodes on imaging [4, 5]. In addition, because of the low incidence of

CD, it can be easy for the radiologist to misdiagnose it as lymphoma, without raising suspicion of CD. Although the two conditions share some similar clinical presentations and imaging characteristics, the treatments for lymphoma and CD are quite different [6, 7]. Surgical resection is suitable for patients with non-multicentric type CD [6, 8–10], while the treatment of choice for lymphoma is chemotherapy and radiotherapy [7].

To achieve an accurate diagnosis and appropriate treatment, it would be helpful if these two conditions could be accurately differentiated on imaging. To our knowledge, very few studies have assessed the diagnostic performance of contrast-enhanced CT for differentiating CD from lymphoma [11–13]. Therefore, the purpose of this study was to compare the characteristics of CD and

* Correspondence: 13963952822@163.com
[1]Department of Radiology, The Affiliated Hospital of Qingdao University, 16 Jiangsu Road, Qingdao, Shandong, China
Full list of author information is available at the end of the article

lymphoma on contrast-enhanced CT, to promote appropriate treatment.

Methods
Patients
This retrospective study was approved by our institutional review boards and the requirement for informed consent was waived. The pathology database of our institution was searched for cases of CD and cases of lymphoma occurring between December 2012 and May 2018. A total of 44 patients with CD in the neck were retrieved, although 4 cases were excluded because of the absence of a contrast-enhanced CT exam, and 6 cases were excluded because of neoplastic disease. A total of 113 patients with lymphoma were retrieved, but 58 cases were excluded from the study because of the lack of a contrast-enhanced CT exam, previous treatments, or other neoplasms occurring in other parts of the body. A final total of 89 patients were therefore included in this retrospective study, with 34 patients with CD forming a CD group, and 55 patients with newly diagnosed lymphomas involving neck lymph nodes forming a lymphoma group. All of the 89 patients were confirmed by pathological examination.

The 34 patients with CD showed no evidence of neoplastic disease or infection. All of the 34 CD patients underwent a contrast-enhanced CT exam, and 30 patients also received an ultrasound examination.

The 55 patients with newly diagnosed and untreated lymphoma all underwent a contrast-enhanced CT exam, and 46 patients also received an ultrasound examination.

Imaging technique
CT imaging was performed using a 64-row multidetector CT scanner (Sensation 64; Siemens, Erlangen, Germany) or a 128-row CT scanner (Discovery 750 HDCT; GE Healthcare, Milwaukee, WI, USA). All of the patients were scanned using the same parameters: 3-mm slice-thickness reconstruction, 23–25-cm field of view, 120-kV voltage, 200–300-mA current, and 256 × 256 matrix. An iodinated contrast agent (Ultravist 370; Bayer HealthCare LLC, Leverkusen, Germany; 2.0 ml/kg) was administered via the antecubital vein by an automated injector system (CT 9000; LiebeleFlarsheim, Cincinnati, OH, USA) at a rate of 2.5 ml/s. The contrast-enhanced imaging phase was started 30 s after injection of the iodinated contrast agent.

Image analysis
Two head and neck radiologists with 15 years and 11 years of experience blinded to the final diagnosis independently reviewed all CT images on a picture archiving and communication system (PACS), and recorded the number of nodules (solitary or multiple),

and their size, location, degree of enhancement, and average contrast-enhanced Hounsfield unit (HU) value. On the contrast-enhanced CT imaging, the degree of enhancement was categorized as mild, moderate, or marked enhancement, with the standard used for assessment of enhancement being: mild enhancement, the enhancement of the nodule was close to that of adjacent muscles; moderate enhancement, enhancement slightly higher than the adjacent muscles; marked enhancement, enhancement markedly higher than in the muscles. The average HU value was measured from a small region of interest (ROI) placed in the middle of a node and areas of necrosis were avoided. Any discrepancies in interpretation between the observers were resolved by consensus.

Statistical analysis
The anatomical distributions and enhancement features of the involved lymph nodes of the two patient groups were analyzed statistically using the SPSS statistical package (version 13.0; SPSS Inc., Chicago, IL, USA). Age at the time of diagnosis and interval from the first contrast-enhanced CT to stereobiopsy or surgery were expressed as the mean ± standard deviation and compared using independent t-tests. Receiver operating characteristic (ROC) curve analysis was used to assess the diagnostic value of the CT attenuation values, including determination of an appropriate cut-off value. Differences in the categorical variables between the CD and lymphoma groups were analyzed using chi-square tests. Sensitivity, specificity, positive predictive value (PPV), negative predictive value (NPV), and Youden Index were also analyzed. The Youden index was calculated as (sensitivity + specificity – 1). A p value of less than 0.05 was considered statistically significant.

Results
Patient and clinical data
The patient recruitment data are summarized in Table 1. The interval between the first contrast-enhanced CT and biopsy/surgery was significantly longer in the CD group (mean 72 ± 105 days, median 60 days) than in the

Table 1 Patient recruitment data

	CD	lymphoma
NO. of patients	34	55
Sex	12 female,	33 female,
	22 male	22 male
Age	38 ± 9 years (median 35 years)	43 ± 8 years (median 39 years)
Interval from the first contrast-enhanced CT to stereobiopsy or surgery	72 ± 105 days (median 60 days)	30 ± 2 days (median 12 days)
	min. 5 day	min. 1 day
	max. 250 days	max. 30 days

Table 2 Clinical presentation

Clinical symptoms	CD (NO. of patients)	lymphoma (NO. of patients)
progressive growing mass or masses	29	40
fatigue	2	45
fever	6	35
neck pain	24	6
anemia	0	15

NO. number

lymphoma patients (mean 30 ± 2 days, median 12 days; $p = 0.015$), while there was no statistically significant difference in sex and age between the two groups.

Table 2 lists the various clinical manifestations presented by the CD and lymphoma patients. The most common manifestation in the two subject groups was a progressive growing mass or masses in the neck. Lymphoma patients presented with fatigue and fever significantly more often ($p = 0.023$, $p = 0.016$ respectively) than CD subjects. CD patients presented with neck pain significantly more often than lymphoma patients ($p = 0.009$).

Contrast-enhanced CT findings

The diagnostic contrast-enhanced CT characteristics of both groups are summarized in Table 3. At the time of the initial contrast-enhanced CT, 82.4% of CD patients

Table 3 Contrast-enhanced CT findings in CD and lymphoma at the time of initial evaluation

Characteristics	CD	lymphoma	P value
Type of lesions, No. (%)			< 0.001
solitary nodule	28(82.4%)	12(21.8%)	
multiple nodules	6(17.6%)	43(78.2%)	
Vessel(s) entering nodule(s)	23(67.6%)	0(0.0%)	< 0.001
Dilated and tortuous vessels in the periphery of nodule(s)	12(35.3%)	1(1.8%)	< 0.001
Type of enhancement, No. (%)			0.684
homogeneous	30(88.2%)	50(90.9%)	
nonhomogeneous	4(11.8%)	5(9.1%)	
presence of necrosis	1(2.9%)	2(3.6%)	
Degree of enhancement, No. (%)			< 0.001
mild enhancement	0(0.0%)	12(21.8%)	
moderate enhancement	5(14.7%)	43(78.2%)	
marked enhancement	29(85.3%)	0(0.0%)	
Hounsfield units (HU)	108.6 ± 20.5	75.6 ± 13.2	0.033
Margin, No. (%)			0.233
well-defined margin	28(82.1%)	50(90.9%)	
ill-defined margin	6(17.6%)	5(9.1%)	
Calcification	1(2.9%)	1(1.8%)	0.621

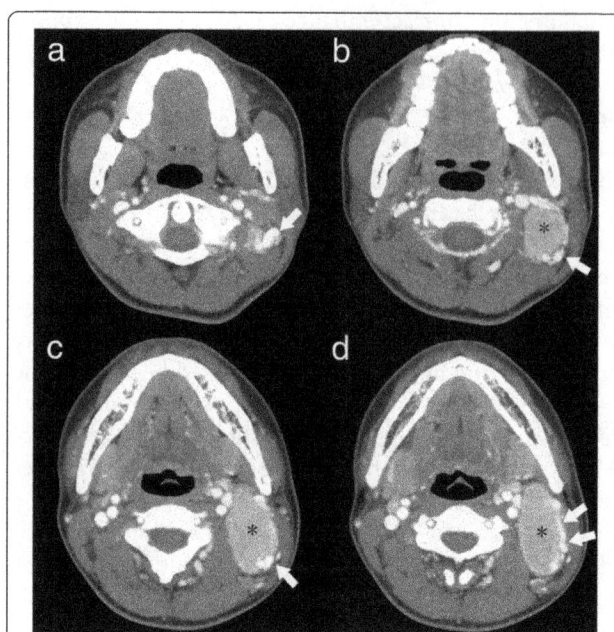

Fig. 1 A 29-year-old man who presented with hyaline vascular type Castleman disease. **a-d** Contrast-enhanced CT images of the neck show a solitary nodule (black *) with a marked enhancement pattern and dilated and tortuous vessels in the periphery of the nodule (white arrows)

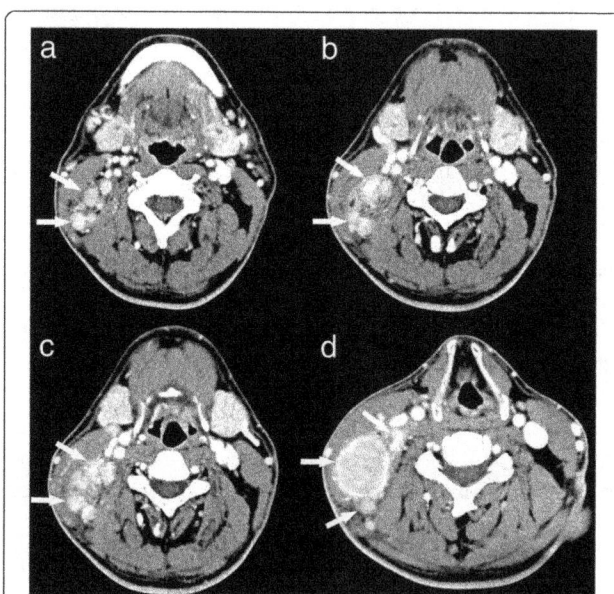

Fig. 2 A 37-year-old man who presented with hyaline vascular type Castleman disease. **a-d** Contrast-enhanced CT images of the neck show multiple nodules with a marked enhancement pattern (white arrows), with all of the nodules located on the right side of the neck. There are no enlarged lymph nodes on the left side of the neck

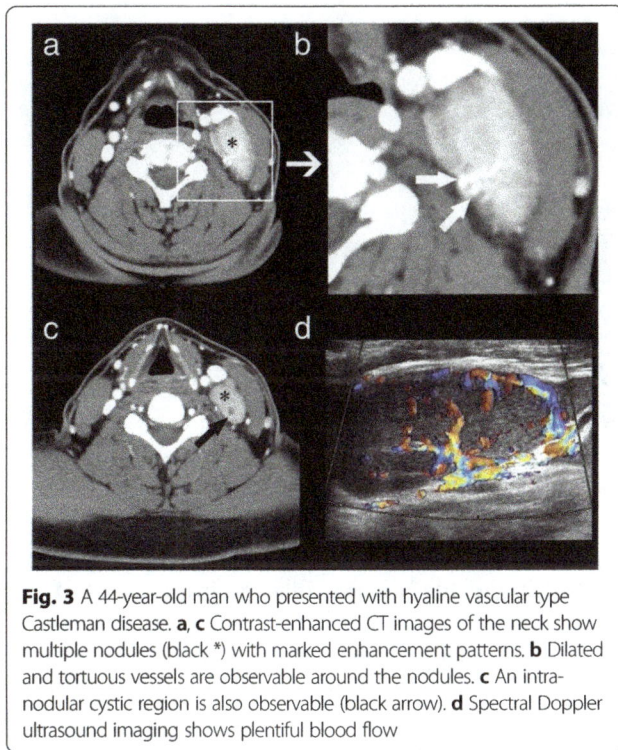

Fig. 3 A 44-year-old man who presented with hyaline vascular type Castleman disease. **a**, **c** Contrast-enhanced CT images of the neck show multiple nodules (black *) with marked enhancement patterns. **b** Dilated and tortuous vessels are observable around the nodules. **c** An intra-nodular cystic region is also observable (black arrow). **d** Spectral Doppler ultrasound imaging shows plentiful blood flow

enhancement in 21.8% (Fig. 4a, b). In 38 of 43 lymphoma cases presenting with multiple nodules, the multiple nodules were located bilaterally in the sides of the neck (Fig. 5a, b). The lymphomas mostly showed homogeneous enhancement (90.9%), with non-homogeneous enhancement being detected in only 9.1% of cases. The presence of necrosis was rare (3.6%; Fig. 6). Ill-defined margins were more often detected in CD (17.6%) than in lymphoma (9.1%; Fig. 2a–d).

The involvement of the neck lymph nodes showed several significant differences between the two conditions (Table 3). Notably, no marked enhancement was found in lymphoma patients, in contrast to marked enhancement being detected in 85.3% of CD cases ($p < 0.001$). Vessels entering a nodule were detected in 67.6% of CD cases (Fig. 3a–d), but none were detected in lymphoma cases. Dilated and tortuous vessels in the periphery of a nodule were significantly more frequent in CD than in lymphoma ($p < 0.001$; Fig. 1a–d). ROC analysis (Fig. 7) showed a significant difference in contrast-enhanced CT values between lymphoma and CD ($p < 0.001$, area under curve = 0.954), with an estimated cut-off value of 92.5 HU. HU values of nodules after enhancement were significantly higher in the CD patients than in the lymphoma patients. In addition, we constructed decision trees according to these imaging characteristics (Figs. 8 and 9).

Indicators of the diagnostic value of contrast-enhanced CT for CD are listed in Table 4.

Discussion

CD is a rare neoplasm involving the lymph nodes, which may involve the mediastinum, abdomen, and neck, and accounts for approximately 8–12% of primary neck tumors. In the present study, we compared the contrast-enhanced CT characteristics of CD and lymphoma. At initial evaluation, CD usually presented as a

presented with a solitary nodule (Fig. 1a–d). CD typically appeared as marked enhancement in 85.3% of cases (Fig. 2a–d), with moderate enhancement being observed in 14.7% of cases. CD presented as multiple nodules in 6 (17.6%) cases, with all of the multiple nodules being located in only the left or right side of the neck (Fig. 2a–d), not bilaterally. Homogeneous enhancement was present in 88.2% of cases, with only one case of CD showing the presence of necrosis (Fig. 3c).

In the lymphoma subjects, multiple nodules were present in 78.2% of cases and solitary nodules in 21.8%. Moderate enhancement was detected in 43 cases (46.3%) and mild

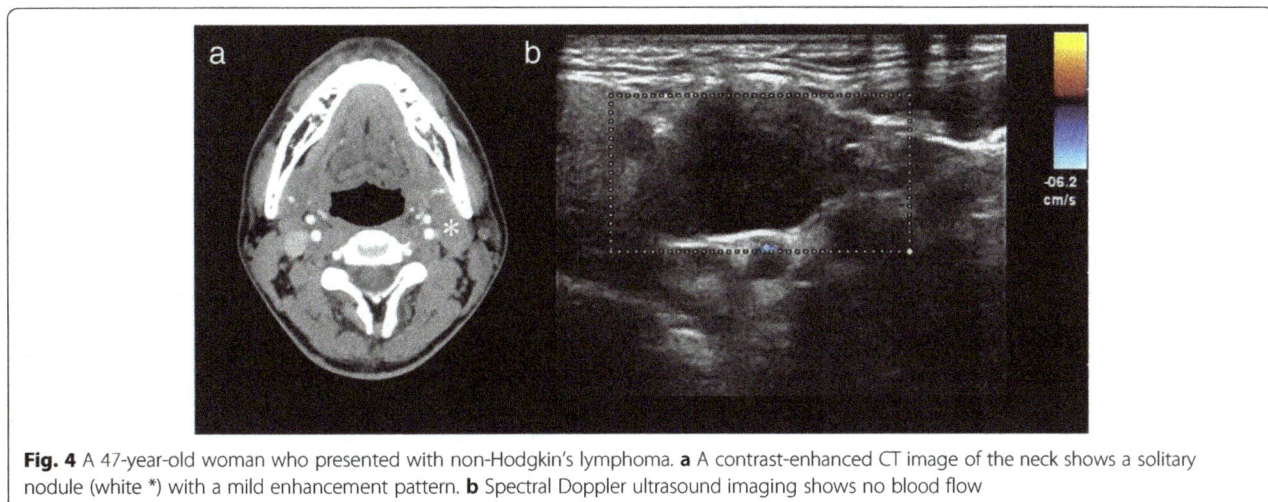

Fig. 4 A 47-year-old woman who presented with non-Hodgkin's lymphoma. **a** A contrast-enhanced CT image of the neck shows a solitary nodule (white *) with a mild enhancement pattern. **b** Spectral Doppler ultrasound imaging shows no blood flow

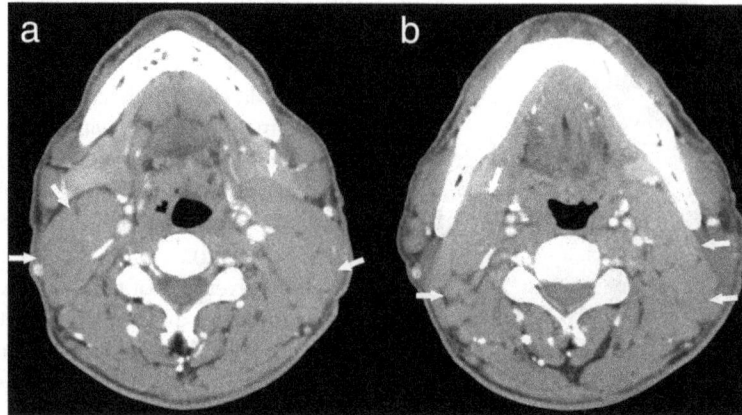

Fig. 5 A 35-year-old man who presented with non-Hodgkin's lymphoma. **a-b** Contrast-enhanced CT images of the neck show multiple nodules with mild enhancement patterns (white arrows), with the nodules being located on both sides of the neck (white arrows)

solitary enlarged lymph node or nodule(s) with homogenous enhancement, while lymphoma typically manifested as multiple enlarged lymph nodes with moderate enhancement (78.2% of cases). Calcification and the presence of necrosis were rare in either condition.

We also detected several striking differences between CD and lymphoma, and in patients with CD or lymphoma manifesting as a solitary mass, the most significant difference was the degree of enhancement; while marked enhancement was not detected in lymphoma, most CD nodules (85.3%) showed marked enhancement. For CD and lymphoma patients presenting with multiple

enlarged lymph nodes, the most striking difference was the location of the nodules. Bilateral involvement of the sides of the neck was not detected in any CD case. This single-sided location may be a striking characteristic of CD in patients with multiple nodules. Additionally, vessels entering nodules (67.6%) were frequently observed in CD, but were rare in lymphoma. Dilated and tortuous vessels in the periphery of a nodule were also more common in CD than in lymphoma.

Several reports have attempted to distinguish CD from benign nodules on CT imaging [4, 9, 11], with marked enhancement having been suggested as a meaningful CT feature for CD. On contrast-enhanced CT imaging, CD usually manifested as marked enhancement and occasionally as intermediate enhancement, with cysts and necrosis in the nodules being rare. Jiang et al. reported on 21 cases of CD [5], with 15 cases (71.4%) showing marked enhancement. Hill et al. reported on 26 patients

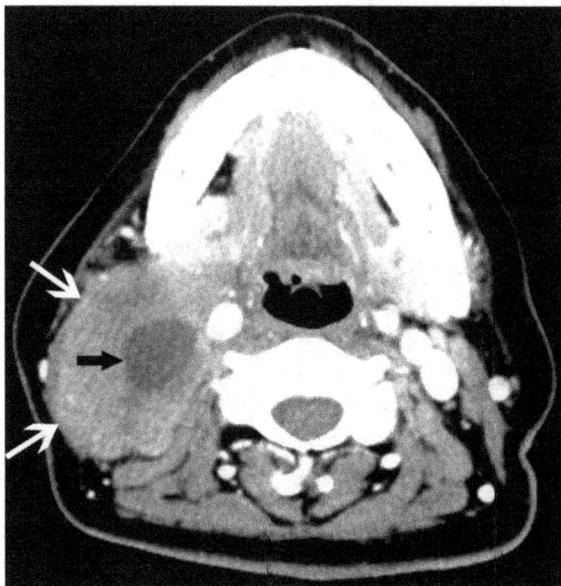

Fig. 6 A 47-year-old woman who presented with non-Hodgkin's lymphoma. A contrast-enhanced CT image of the neck shows an ill-defined margin (white arrow) and a region of liquefaction and necrosis with a mild enhancement pattern in the interior of the mass (black arrow)

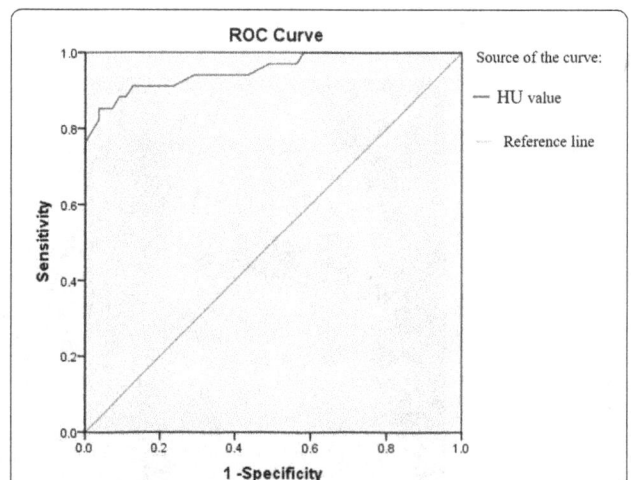

Fig. 7 Receiver operating characteristic curves for attenuation values in differentiating CD from lymphoma

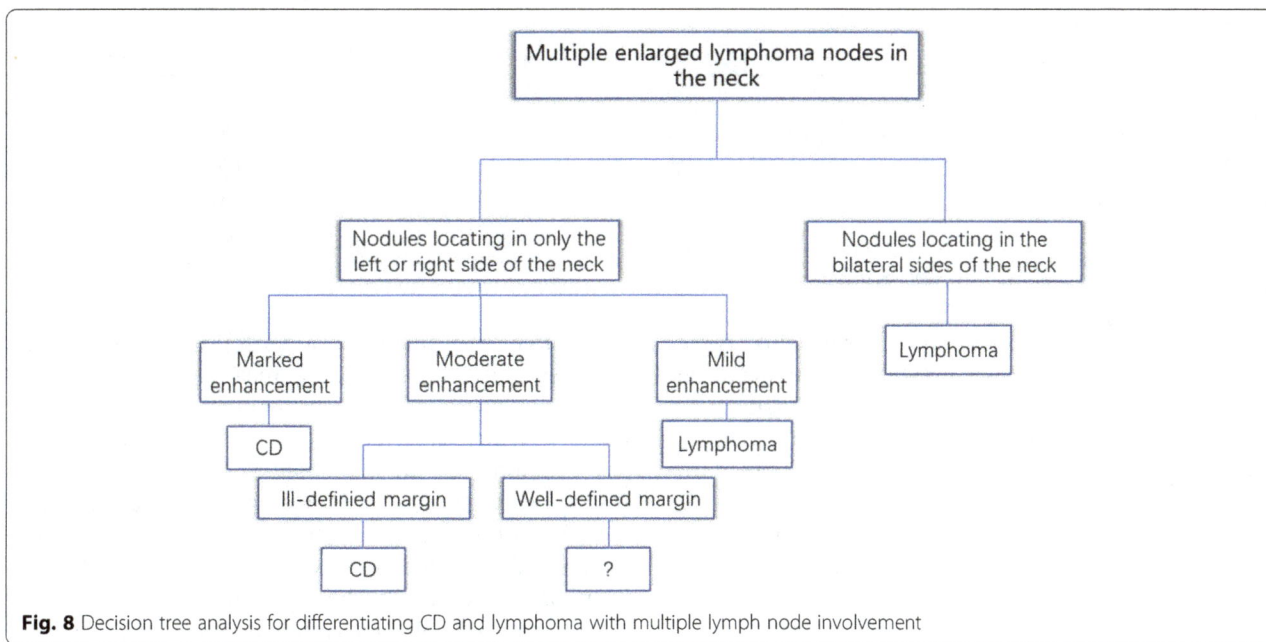

Fig. 8 Decision tree analysis for differentiating CD and lymphoma with multiple lymph node involvement

with CD, with 21 (80.7%) of the patients demonstrating these typical CT imaging findings [14]. Our imaging findings of CD are in agreement with these previous reports, with the proportion of marked enhancement and intermediate enhancement in CD being 85.3% and 14.7% respectively in the present study. Only one CD case manifested as a non-homogeneous nodule with a central non-enhancing area of mild hypodensity. The imaging characteristics of this case were similar to one of the four Castleman disease cases reported by Park et al., who also reported a CD lesion with a central non-enhancing low-density area, which was attributed to a dense fibrous scar [15].

Lymphomas are primary neoplasms of the lympho-reticular system [16] and may be divided into two types according to their histopathologic classification: Hodgkin's disease (HD) and non-Hodgkin's lymphoma (NHL) [17]. HD often occurs in younger patients, while NHL is commonly seen in the Chinese population and occurs in a greater range of ages than HD [18]. In our series of lymphoma patients, most of the cases were NHL. In published articles, lymphoma generally presents as an isolated mass or enlarged lymph nodes, with homogeneous mild or moderate contrast-enhancement [19, 20]. Intra-nodular necrosis or cysts are only occasionally discovered in untreated lymphomas with a large diameter [21]. Our

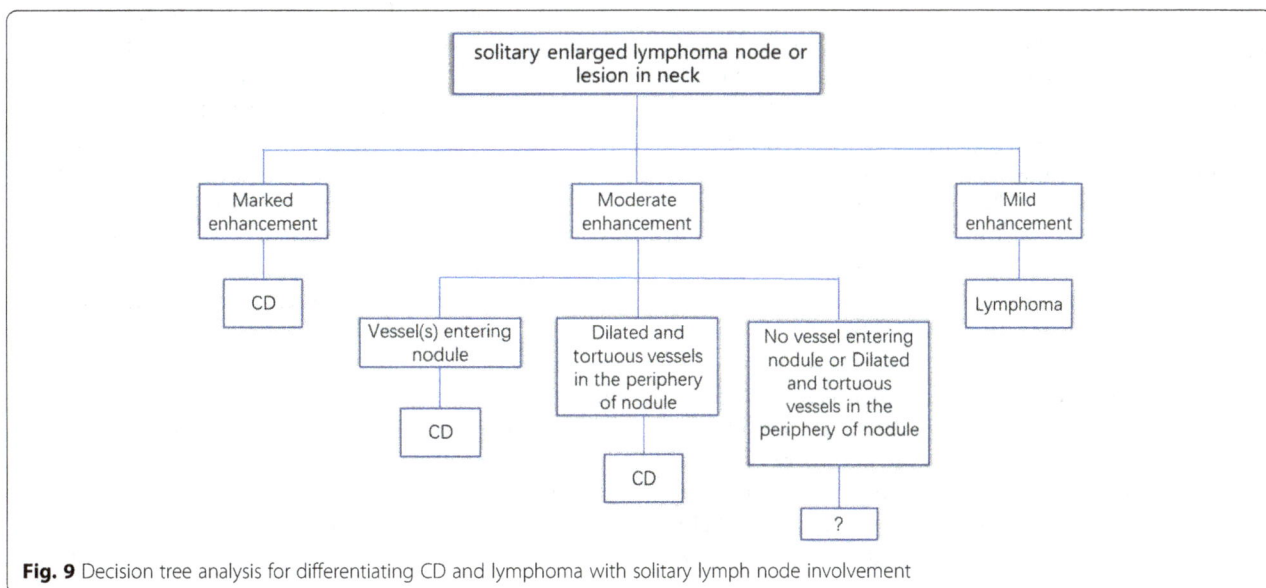

Fig. 9 Decision tree analysis for differentiating CD and lymphoma with solitary lymph node involvement

Table 4 Diagnostic Value of CT Indicators for CD

Contrast-enhanced CT features	Sensitivity	Specificity	PPV	NPV	Youden Index
vessel(s) entering nodule (1)	75%	74%	55%	84%	0.49
Dilated and tortuous vessels in the periphery of nodule (2)	67%	79%	61%	92%	0.46
(1) + (2)	78%	93%	79%	91%	0.71
Degree of enhancement (3)	85%	78%	53%	93%	0.63
(1) + (2) + (3)	89%	94%	89%	94%	0.83

Abbreviations: PPV positive predictive value, *NPV* negative predictive value

lymphoma subjects demonstrated similar imaging characteristics, with 43 (78.2%) cases presenting as moderate enhancement and 12 (21.8%) cases as mild enhancement. The presence of central necrosis was detected in only 2 (3.6%) cases with a large diameter, and was attributed to a lack of blood supply in the center of the lesions.

The presentation of patients with CD is variable, and depends on the subtype; CD can present along a spectrum ranging from an asymptomatic localized nodal mass, which is often discovered incidentally, to multifocal adenopathy with B-symptoms and hematological derangements that clinically mimic lymphoma. In our study, the patients with lymphoma presented significantly more frequently with systemic symptoms such as fatigue and fever [22], and the interval between the first contrast-enhanced CT and biopsy or surgery was significantly shorter in the lymphoma group than in the CD patients. The absence of systemic symptoms was more often detected in patients with the hyaline vascular (HV) subtype of CD, and CD is typically of the diffuse HV-CD type, only rarely presenting as other types such as plasma cell, HHV-8-associated, and multicentric type CD. Those may illustrate the phenomenon.

There are few reports on CT imaging of the vessels which surround or enter nodules of the two conditions. Although previous CT studies have focused on the degree of enhancement to distinguish CD from lymphoma [4, 16, 23, 24], the enhancement extent of the two entities sometimes overlaps. In our study, 5 (14.7%) cases with CD and 43 (78.2%) cases with lymphoma demonstrated moderate enhancement on initial contrast-enhanced CT. This study showed that dilated and tortuous vessels surrounding or entering nodules were significantly more often observed in CD than in lymphoma. The presence of these vessels can therefore be taken as suggesting the possibility of CD. In our study, 23 (67.6%) cases with CD showed arteries entering nodules and 12 (35.3%) cases demonstrated dilated and tortuous vessels surrounding nodules. The combination of dilated and tortuous vessels in the periphery of a nodule, and vessels entering a nodule, yielded high capability in the differential diagnosis, with sensitivity, specificity, and Youden index of 78%, 93%, and 0.71 respectively. In the lymphoma group, we also detected vessels

surrounding the nodules in a small proportion of cases; however, most of the vessels were slender with a smaller diameter. Furthermore, no lymphoma case showed evidence of vessels entering nodules on CT imaging.

We found that an additional feature for helping to distinguish CD from lymphoma was the anatomical distribution of the nodules. In cases involving multiple lymph nodes, all the nodes were located in only the left or right side of the neck in CD cases, not bilaterally. Unilaterality of enlarged lymph nodes may help reach the correct diagnosis of CD on imaging.

Few articles have evaluated the CT attenuation values for differentiation of CD and lymphoma. In this study, ROC curves were used to compare the diagnostic performance of the attenuation values, with the area under the curve being 0.954; this value demonstrated good validity for the diagnosis of CD. The optimal cut-off point for differentiating CD from lymphoma was 92.5 HU, with values above this threshold being likely to represent CD.

The present study has several limitations. Because of its retrospective nature and the radiation dose to the patients, there was insufficient data available to evaluate advanced CT techniques such as CT perfusion. Second, the analysis of the degree of enhancement in neck nodules was partially performed by visual assessment. Two experienced head and neck radiologists reviewed all CT images to reduce bias in these visual assessments. We must also emphasize the general incidence of both conditions, with CD occurring less frequently than lymphoma. This makes the diagnosis of the two conditions more complex, as few contrast-enhanced CT features are able to make a clear differentiation between the conditions. We therefore attempted to combine relevant contrast-enhanced CT features to facilitate the differentiation and provide radiological clues for further work-up.

Conclusions

Our findings suggest that at initial presentation, contrast-enhanced CT is suitable for differentiating between CD and lymphoma of the neck in many cases, with the differentiation being performed on the basis of enhancement patterns, nodule locations, attenuation values, and the presence of tortuous vessels in enlarged lymph nodes.

Abbreviations
AIDS: Acquired immunodeficiency syndrome; CD: Castleman disease; HD: Hodgkin's disease; HHV-8: Human herpes virus-8; HU: Hounsfield unit; HV-CD: Hyaline vascular CD; IL-6: Interleukin-6; NHL: Non-Hodgkin's lymphoma; NPV: Negative predictive value; PPV: Positive predictive value; ROC: Receiver operating characteristic; ROI: Region of interest

Authors' contributions
Guarantor of integrity of the entire study: WX, JL; study concepts and design: WX; literature research: JL, JW; clinical studies: JW; data analysis: JL, HW; manuscript preparation: JL, JW manuscript editing: JL, ZY, JC. All authors read and approved the final manuscript.

Competing interests
The authors declare that they have no competing interests.

Author details
[1]Department of Radiology, The Affiliated Hospital of Qingdao University, 16 Jiangsu Road, Qingdao, Shandong, China. [2]Department of Ultrasound, Qingdao Women and Children Hospital, Qingdao, Shandong, China. [3]Department of Radiology, Qingdao Municipal Hospital, Qingdao, Shandong, China.

References
1. Kligerman S, Auerbach A, Franks T, Galvin J. Castleman disease of the thorax: clinical, radiologic, and pathologic correlation: from the radiologic pathology archives. Radiographics. 2016;36(5):1309–32.
2. Ooi CC, Cheah FK, Wong SK. Castleman's disease of the kidney: sonographic findings. J Clin Ultrasound. 2015;43(7):438–42.
3. Ottaviani F, Galli J, Di Girolamo S, Almadori G. Castleman's disease restricted to the parapharyngeal space. J Otolaryngol. 1999;28(2):95–8.
4. Bonekamp D, Hruban RH, Fishman EK. The great mimickers: Castleman disease. Semin Ultrasound CT MR. 2014;35(3):263–71.
5. Jiang XH, Song HM, Liu QY, Cao Y, Li GH, Zhang WD. Castleman disease of the neck: CT and MR imaging findings. Eur J Radiol. 2014;83(11):2041–50.
6. Chan KL, Lade S, Prince HM, Harrison SJ. Update and new approaches in the treatment of Castleman disease. J Blood Med. 2016;7:145–58.
7. Deng XW, Wu JX, Wu T, Zhu SY, Shi M, Su H, et al. Radiotherapy is essential after complete response to asparaginase-containing chemotherapy in early-stage extranodal nasal-type NK/T-cell lymphoma: a multicenter study from the China lymphoma collaborative group (CLCG). Radiother Oncol. published online, https://doi.org/10.1016/j.radonc.2018.04.026
8. Zhang J, Li C, Lv L, Yang C, Kong XR, Zhu J, et al. Clinical and experimental study of Castleman disease in children. Pediatr Blood Cancer. 2015;62(1):109–14.
9. Gossios K, Nikolaides C, Bai M, Fountzilas G. Widespread Castleman disease: CT findings. Eur Radiol. 1996;6(1):95–8.
10. Xiao J, Chen L, Chen W, Zhou L, Li X, Chen Y, et al. Clinical characteristics and surgical treatment for localized Castleman's disease. Zhonghua Zhong Liu Za Zhi. 2012;34(1):61–4.
11. Yamashita Y, Hirai T, Matsukawa T, Ogata I, Takahashi M. Radiological presentations of Castleman's disease. Comput Med Imaging Graph. 1993;17(2):107–17.
12. Wen L, Zhang D, Zhang Z. CT characteristics of cervical Castleman's disease. Clin Imaging. 2005;29(2):141–3.
13. Mangini M, Aiani L, Bertolotti E, Imperatori A, Rotolo N, Paddeu A, et al. Parapancreatic Castleman disease: contrast-enhanced sonography and CT features. J Clin Ultrasound. 2007;35(4):207–11.
14. Hill AJ, Tirumani SH, Rosenthal MH, Shinagare AB, Carrasco RD, Munshi NC, et al. Multimodality imaging and clinical features in Castleman disease: single institute experience in 30 patients. Br J Radiol. 2015;88(1049):20140670.
15. Park J, Hwang J, Kim H, Choe H, Kim Y, Kim H, et al. Castleman disease presenting with jaundice: a case with the multicentric hyaline vascular variant. Korean J Intern Med. 2007;22(2):113–7.
16. Pantoja Pachajoa DA, Bruno MA, Alvarez FA, Viscido G, Mandojana F, Doniquian A. Multiple primary tumors: colorectal carcinoma and non-Hodgkin's lymphoma. Int J Surg Case Rep. 2018;48:92–4.
17. Mettler J, Muller H, Voltin CA, Baues C, Klaeser B, Moccia A, et al. Metabolic Tumour Volume for Response Prediction in Advanced-Stage Hodgkin Lymphoma. J Nucl Med. published online, https://doi.org/10.2967/jnumed.118.210047.
18. Lenga L, Czwikla R, Wichmann JL, Leithner D, Albrecht MH, D'Angelo T, et al. Dual-energy CT in patients with abdominal malignant lymphoma: impact of noise-optimised virtual monoenergetic imaging on objective and subjective image quality. Clin Radiol. published online, https://doi.org/10.1016/j.crad.2018.04.015
19. Choi EJ, Jin GY, Chung MJ. Serial chest CT findings of intravascular large B-cell lymphoma of the lungs. J Thorac Dis. 2018;10(3):E218–20.
20. Zhang J, Fan Y, Liu M, Li Q, Wang R. Newly diagnosed primary gum lymphoma on FDG PET/CT. Clin Nucl Med. 2018;43(6):466–7.
21. Reinert CP, Kloth C, Fritz J, Nikolaou K, Horger M. Discriminatory CT-textural features in splenic infiltration of lymphoma versus splenomegaly in liver cirrhosis versus normal spleens in controls and evaluation of their role for longitudinal lymphoma monitoring. Eur J Radiol. 2018;104:129–35.
22. Bernstine H, Domachevsky L, Nidam M, Goldberg N, Abadi-Korek I, Shpilberg O, et al. 18F-FDG PET/MR imaging of lymphoma nodal target lesions: comparison of PET standardized uptake value (SUV) with MR apparent diffusion coefficient (ADC). Medicine (Baltimore). 2018;97(16):e0490.
23. Ma Y, Li F, Chen L. Widespread hypermetabolic lesions due to multicentric form of Castleman disease as the cause of fever of unknown origin revealed by FDG PET/CT. Clin Nucl Med. 2013;38(10):835–7.
24. Delgado A, Mesa J, Guayambuco S, Rodriguez T, Fernandez I, Rodeno E. PET/CT imaging with 18F-FDG in Castleman disease. Rev Esp Med Nucl Imagen Mol. 2016;35(3):200–1.

30

Fat-suppressed gadolinium-enhanced isotropic high-resolution 3D-GRE-T1WI for predicting small node metastases in patients with rectal cancer

Yan Chen[1†], Xinyue Yang[1†], Ziqiang Wen[1†], Baolan Lu[1], Xiaojuan Xiao[2], Bingqi Shen[1] and Shenping Yu[1*]

Abstract

Background: To investigate the application value of fat-suppressed gadolinium-enhanced isotropic high-resolution 3D-GRE-T1WI in regional nodes with different short-axis diameter ranges in rectal cancer, especially in nodes ≤5 mm.

Methods: Patients with rectal adenocarcinoma confirmed by postoperative histopathology were included, and all the patients underwent preoperative 3.0 T rectal magnetic resonance imaging (MRI) and total mesorectal excision (TME) within 2 weeks after an MR scan. The harvested nodes from specimens were matched with nodes in the field of view (FOV) of images for a node-by-node evaluation. The maximum short-axis diameters of all the visible nodes in the FOV of images were measured by a radiologist; the morphological and enhancement characteristics of these nodes were also independently evaluated by two radiologists. The χ^2 test was used to evaluate differences in morphological and enhancement characteristics between benign and malignant nodes. The enhancement characteristics were further compared between benign and malignant nodes with different short-axis diameter ranges using the χ^2 test. Kappa statistics were used to describe interobserver agreement.

Results: A total of 441 nodes from 70 enrolled patients were included in the evaluation, of which 111 nodes were metastatic. Approximately 85.5 and 95.6% of benign nodes were found to have obvious enhancement and homogeneous or mild-heterogeneous enhancement, respectively, whereas approximately 89.2 and 85.1% of malignant nodes showed moderate or mild enhancement and obvious-heterogeneous or rim-like enhancement, respectively. The area under the receiver operating characteristic (ROC) curve (AUC) values of the enhancement degree for identifying
the overall nodal status, nodes ≤5 mm and nodes > 5 mm and ≤ 10 mm were 0.887, 0.859 and 0.766 for radiologist 1 and 0.892, 0.823 and 0.774 for radiologist 2, respectively. The AUCs of enhancement homogeneity were 0.940, 0.928 and 0.864 for radiologist 1 and 0.944, 0.938 and 0.842 for radiologist 2, respectively. Nodal border and signal homogeneity were also of certain value in distinguishing metastatic nodes.

Conclusions: Enhancement characteristics based on fat-suppressed gadolinium-enhanced isotropic high-resolution 3D-GRE-T1WI were helpful for diagnosing metastatic nodes in rectal cancer and were a reliable indicator for nodes ≤5 mm.

Keywords: Gadolinium-enhanced, 3D-GRE-T1WI, Rectal cancer, Small lymph nodes

* Correspondence: yushp@mail.sysu.edu.cn
†Yan Chen, Xinyue Yang and Ziqiang Wen contributed equally to this work.
[1]Department of Radiology, Sun Yat-sen University First Affiliated Hospital, Guangzhou 510080, China
Full list of author information is available at the end of the article

Background

Colorectal cancer is the third most common cancer and the fourth leading cause of cancer deaths globally, with rectal cancer accounting for the vast majority of cases [1]. Regional node involvement is associated with local and distant recurrence, along with poor prognosis in rectal cancer [2], and is generally considered an indication for neoadjuvant chemoradiotherapy (CRT) in these patients [3]. Neoadjuvant CRT provides decreased local recurrence and improved general survival, along with less extensive surgery [4]. Therefore, accurate prediction of the regional node status of rectal cancer prior to surgery is closely tied to treatment decisions and prognosis.

The imaging detection of node metastases in rectal cancer is primarily performed with endoluminal ultrasound (EUS), computed tomography (CT) or magnetic resonance imaging (MRI). However, these three modalities have low discriminant accuracy, particularly for nodes smaller than 5 mm [5]. Although high-resolution T2-weighted imaging (T2WI) allows the evaluation of nodal border and signal homogeneity, the diagnostic efficiency has not improved significantly since the majority of metastatic rectal cancer nodes are smaller than 5 mm, making them difficult to evaluate accurately based on morphological changes alone [6]. It is generally believed that gadolinium-enhanced T1-weighted imaging (T1WI) provides minimal benefit for the accurate determination of metastatic nodes in rectal cancer [7]; however, consistent with results of other studies [8–10], gadolinium-enhanced three-dimensional gradient recalled-echo T1-weighted imaging (3D-GRE-T1WI) has shown high accuracy and repeatability in distinguishing malignant from benign nodes in rectal cancer. This technique has been widely used for the head and neck, spine, joints, abdomen, and pelvis [11–15]. However, the discrimination of nodal status in rectal cancer using gadolinium-enhanced 3D-GRE-T1WI has seldom been reported, and a comparative analysis of the diagnostic value of different short-axis diameter ranges has not yet been performed. This study evaluated the enhancement characteristics in lymph nodes and aimed to assess the value of 3.0 T MR fat-suppressed gadolinium-enhanced isotropic high-resolution 3D-GRE-T1WI in the diagnosis of regional node metastases in different short-axis diameter ranges, especially for small nodes in rectal cancer.

Methods

Study population

This prospective study was conducted from January 2016 to December 2016. Inclusion criteria consisted of (1) postoperative histopathology confirming primary rectal adenocarcinoma and (2) the existence of 3.0 T rectal MR scans performed with identical imaging parameters within 2 weeks of their curative resection.

Exclusion criteria included (1) postoperative histopathology confirming a special histopathological type, such as mucous adenocarcinoma or signet ring cell carcinoma; and (2) history of prior radiotherapy, chemotherapy or other rectal tumor therapies.

Patient preparation and MR image acquisition

According to the tumor location on colonoscopy, an appropriate amount (20-80 mL) of ultrasonic gel was poured into the rectum but was not used for low or large rectal tumors. To prevent intestinal peristaltic artifacts, a dose of 20 mg of raceanisodamine hydrochloride was injected intramuscularly approximately 10 min prior to the MR examination unless contraindicated.

Imaging was performed using a 3.0 T unit (Magnetom Verio, Siemens, Germany) with a 6-channel phased-array wrap-around surface coil. The coil center was placed on the level of the pubic symphysis and adjusted according to the tumor location. All the patients were placed in the supine position with the feet first. Rectal MRI protocols included high-resolution two-dimensional turbo spin-echo T2-weighted imaging (2D-TSE-T2WI) sequences in the sagittal, coronal and oblique axial planes that were orthogonal to the base of the tumor. In addition, a fat-suppressed gadolinium-enhanced isotropic high-resolution 3D-GRE-T1WI sequence in the coronal plane was applied. Details of the protocols are listed in Table 1. The technique for water excitation normal was employed to suppress fat. Gadolinium (Gadopentetate Dimeglumine Injection, Consun, Guangzhou) was administered at a dose of 0.2 mL/kg bodyweight and a rate of 3.0 mL/sec by a bolus injection with a power injector through the cubital vein. Then, a dose of 25 mL of 0.9% saline was injected at the same rate.

Image evaluation

Two radiologists (R1: YC, R2: XY), who were experienced in reading MR images of rectal cancer and were blind to the histopathological results, analyzed all the rectal MR images at the MRI workstation.

First, each visible node was carefully identified in the field of view (FOV) of MR images by one radiologist (R1). Meanwhile, the maximum short-axis diameters (millimeters) of the nodes were measured three times with a workstation electronic caliper, and the average readings were reported. Then, two radiologists independently evaluated and recorded the nodal border and signal homogeneity on high-resolution 2D-TSE-T2WI images, in addition to the enhancement degree and homogeneity on fat-suppressed gadolinium-enhanced isotropic high-resolution 3D-GRE-T1WI images.

These evaluation parameters were defined specifically as follows: (1) the nodal border was categorized as either smooth or irregular; (2) the signal homogeneity was classified as homogeneous, mild-heterogeneous or

Table 1 Rectal high-resolution MRI protocols for 2D and 3D sequences

Sequences	TR/TE (msec)	Slice thickness/Gap (mm)	No. of slices	Frequency direction	Flip angle (°)	Matrix	FOV (cm)	Voxel size (mm)	Acquisition time
2D-TSE-T2WI									
Sagittal	3000/87	3/0	19	H to F	150	320 × 256	18	0.7 × 0.6 × 3.0	2 min 30 s
Coronal	4000/77	3/0	25	F to H	137	384 × 308	22	0.7 × 0.6 × 3.0	2 min 52 s
Oblique axial	3000/84	3/0	24	R to L	150	320 × 320	18	0.6 × 0.6 × 3.0	3 min 18 s
3D-GRE-T1WI									
Coronal	10/4.9	1/0	144	R to L	10	384 × 384	38	1.0 × 1.0 × 1.0	3 min 10 s

Notes: *TR* repetition time, *TE* echo time, *FOV* field of view, *H* head, *F* feet, *R* right, *L* left

obvious-heterogeneous; (3) the enhancement degree was categorized into three subtypes by comparison to the vessels at the same level, and obvious enhancement was recorded if the node appeared to be equal in signal intensity, mild enhancement was recorded if the node appeared to have significantly low signal intensity, and intermediate enhancement was recorded if the signal intensity was between obvious and mild enhancement. When a node appeared to have heterogeneous enhancement, the enhancement degree of the main region in the node was evaluated; (4) the enhancement homogeneity was classified as homogeneous, mild-heterogeneous, obvious-heterogeneous or rim-like enhancement [10, 16] (Fig. 1).

Histopathologic assessment and nodal comparison

All the enrolled patients underwent total mesorectal excision (TME) of the rectum within 2 weeks after MR scans (median duration: 5 days; range: 1-14 days). On the basis of localized nodes that were all visible in the FOV on preoperative MR images, a surgeon with expertise in colorectal cancer successively localized and recorded regional nodes in different groups during surgery. Then, these nodes were removed from the specimen and taken to the pathology department promptly placed in individual trays marked according to each node identified by MR images. All the nodes were analyzed by a dedicated gastrointestinal pathologist and reported as malignant when tumor cells were observed in the node under a light microscope. To provide an accurate node-by-node comparison of MR images and histopathologic findings, special attention was paid to the nodal size and morphology, in addition to the position of the node relative to the tumor, rectal wall, mesorectal fascia, vessels and adjacent nodes. The nodes were matched with MR images in corresponding groups and were excluded if they could not be matched. The pathological staging of rectal cancer referred to the rules for TNM staging of the American Joint Committee on Cancer (AJCC)/ Union for International Cancer Control (UICC) [17].

Statistical methods

Statistical analysis was performed using SPSS 20.0 software. All quantitative data were tested for a normal distribution with the one-sample Kolmogorov-Smirnov test. Quantitative data with a non-Gaussian distribution were expressed as the medians with the ranges. Correlation analysis was performed with the Spearman rank correlation test. The χ^2 test was used to compare the correlated qualitative factors (nodal border, signal homogeneity, enhancement degree and homogeneity) between benign and malignant nodes. Kappa statistics (0.00-0.20 poor, 0.21-0.40 fair, 0.41-0.60 moderate, 0.61-0.80 good and 0.81-1.00 excellent agreement) were calculated for the evaluation of interobserver agreement. Clinical pathological features were also compared between node-negative and node-positive patients using the χ^2 test or the Mann-Whitney U test. A two-tailed P value < 0.05 was considered to indicate a statistically significant difference. Receiver operating characteristic (ROC) analyses were performed to assess the diagnostic utility of the enhancement characteristics for the detection of metastatic nodes in different short-axis diameter ranges, and the area under the ROC curve (AUC) and 95% confidence interval (CI) were calculated. Each AUC value was interpreted as having no (< 0.5), low (0.5-0.7), moderate (0.7-0.9) or high (> 0.9) diagnostic value. As mentioned above, the morphological characteristics of small nodes are currently difficult to observe well on high-resolution MRI. Therefore, the morphological characteristics of nodes in different short-axis diameter ranges (≤5 mm, > 5 mm and ≤ 10 mm, and > 10 mm) were not further analyzed in this study.

Results

General and histopathological findings

A total of 70 patients (36 males and 34 females; median age: 60 years; range: 31-80 years) were enrolled in this study. Of the 70 patients, 36 (51.4%) were confirmed to have metastatic regional nodes. Histopathology of 1004 nodes harvested from the rectal specimens in 70 patients (median: 13; range: 7-45) indicated that 176 (17.5%) contained metastases. Lymph node metastases

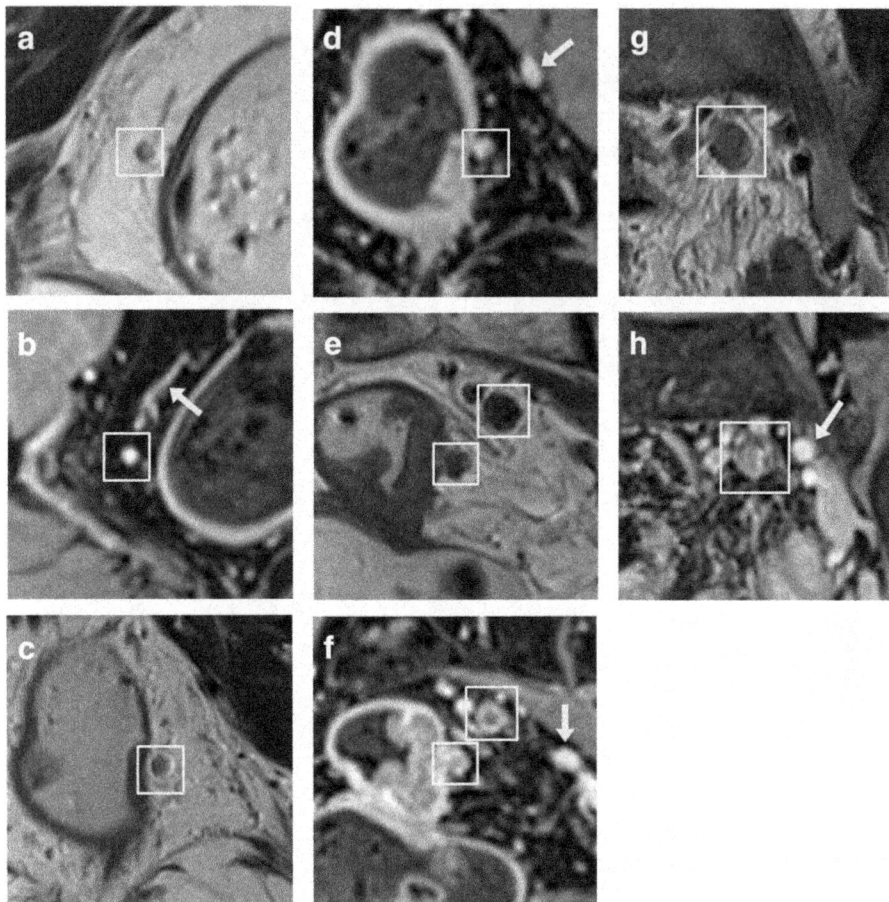

Fig. 1 The white boxes indicate lymph nodes, and the white arrows indicate vessels. (**a**, **c**, **e** and **g**), coronal high-resolution 2D-TSE-T2WI; (**b**, **d**, **f** and **h**), coronal fat-suppressed gadolinium-enhanced isotropic high-resolution 3D-GRE-T1WI. **a-b**, Benign node 3.0 mm in diameter with a smooth border, homogeneous signal, and obvious and homogeneous enhancement. **c-d**, Benign node 3.6 mm in diameter with a smooth border, mild-heterogeneous signal, and obvious and mild-heterogeneous enhancement. **e-f**, Node 4.2 mm in diameter adjacent to the rectal wall that was malignant with an irregular border, mild-heterogeneous signal, and intermediate and rim-like enhancement. The superior node 6.2 mm in diameter was also malignant, with a smooth border, obvious-heterogeneous signal, and mild and rim-like enhancement. **g-h**, Malignant node 8.2 mm in diameter with an irregular border, mild-heterogeneous signal, and mild and obvious-heterogeneous enhancement

were more likely occur in pT3-4 patients ($P < 0.001$). The location and differentiation of rectal cancer were not related to whether the patient had metastatic nodes ($P = 0.055, 0.052$, respectively) (Table 2).

For the node-by-node evaluation, a correlation between the results of MR images and histopathology was feasible for 441 (43.9%) nodes, including 111 metastatic nodes. According to the MR measurements, the median short-axis diameter 3.8 mm (range: 1.2-18.1 mm) for all the nodes; 3.4 mm (range: 1.2-8.4 mm) for the benign nodes; and 7.0 mm (range: 3.1-18.1 mm) for the malignant nodes. Of 313 nodes with short-axis diameter ≤ 5 mm, 23 (7.3%) contained metastases; of 111 nodes > 5 mm and ≤ 10 mm, 71 (64.0%) contained metastases; and all 17 nodes > 10 mm contained metastases.

Relationship between nodal status and its morphological and enhancement characteristics (Table 3)

Malignant nodes mostly demonstrated an irregular border (R1: 73.9%, R2: 70.3%) and a mild-heterogeneous or obvious-heterogeneous signal (R1: 92.8%, R2: 90.1%). Additionally, 83.9 and 87.0% of benign nodes showed obvious enhancement according to the two radiologists; conversely, only 10.8% of metastases were found to have obvious enhancement, and most (89.2% for both radiologists) had mild or intermediate enhancement. Regarding enhancement homogeneity, benign nodes were more commonly (R1: 96.7%, R2: 94.5%) found to have homogeneous or mild-heterogeneous enhancement, whereas 84.7 and 85.5% of malignant nodes were detected to have obvious-

Table 2 Relationship between clinical pathological features and nodal metastases in 70 patients

Parameters	Patients with nodal metastases			P
	Total (n = 70)	Negative (n = 34)	Positive (n = 36)	
Age,median (range)	60 (31-80)	60 (31-76)	61 (42-80)	0.155
Gender				0.469
Male	36 (51.4%)	19 (55.9%)	17 (47.2%)	
Female	34 (48.6%)	15 (44.1%)	19 (52.8%)	
Location				0.055
Low	33 (47.1%)	21 (61.8%)	12 (33.3%)	
Middle	27 (38.6%)	10 (29.4%)	17 (47.2%)	
High	10 (14.3%)	3 (8.8%)	7 (19.4%)	
Differentiation				0.052
Well	2 (2.9%)	2 (5.9%)	0 (0.0%)	
Moderately	56 (80.0%)	29 (85.3%)	27 (75.0%)	
Poorly	12 (17.1%)	3 (8.8%)	9 (25.0%)	
T stage				< 0.001
pT1	5 (7.1%)	5 (14.7%)	0 (0.0%)	
pT2	16 (22.9%)	13 (38.2%)	3 (8.3%)	
pT3	22 (31.4%)	9 (26.5%)	13 (36.1%)	
pT4	27 (38.6%)	7 (20.6%)	20 (55.6%)	

Notes: According to the distance from the most caudal border of the rectal tumor to the anal verge on MRI: low, < 5 cm; middle, 5-10 cm; high, > 10 cm; p pathological

heterogeneous or rim-like enhancement by the two radiologists. The larger nodes were, the more heterogeneous the signal (R1: $r_s = 0.639$, $P < 0.001$, R2: $r_s = 0.720$, $P < 0.001$) and enhancement were (R1: $r_s = 0.757$, $P < 0.001$, R2: $r_s = 0.785$, $P < 0.001$). The interobserver

agreement values for nodal border, signal homogeneity, enhancement degree and homogeneity were good ($\kappa = 0.633$, 0.611, 0.703 and 0.744, respectively). The ROC curve of enhancement characteristics for the prediction of nodal status is shown in Fig. 2a.

Table 3 Rectal cancer nodal morphological and enhancement characteristics on MR images versus histopathological findings in 440 nodes

Radiologist	Radiologist 1			Radiologist 2			κ
Histopathologic Findings	Benign (330)	Malignant (111)	P	Benign (330)	Malignant (111)	P	
Border			< 0.001			< 0.001	0.633
Smooth	319 (96.7%)	29 (26.1%)		305 (92.4%)	33 (29.7%)		
Irregular	11 (3.3%)	82 (73.9%)		25 (7.6%)	78 (70.3%)		
Signal homogeneity			< 0.001			< 0.001	0.611
Homogenous	230 (69.7%)	8 (7.2%)		225 (68.2%)	11 (9.9%)		
Mild-heterogeneous	99 (30.0%)	46 (41.4%)		104 (31.5%)	59 (53.2%)		
Obvious-heterogeneous	1 (0.3%)	57 (51.4%)		1 (0.3%)	41 (36.9%)		
Enhancement degree			< 0.001			< 0.001	0.703
Obvious	277 (83.9%)	12 (10.8%)		287 (87.0%)	12 (10.8%)		
Intermediate	46 (13.9%)	57 (51.4%)		32 (9.7%)	55 (49.5%)		
Mild	7 (2.1%)	42 (37.8%)		11 (3.3%)	44 (39.6%)		
Enhancement homogeneity			< 0.001			< 0.001	0.747
Homogeneous	223 (67.6%)	5 (4.5%)		210 (63.6%)	2 (1.8%)		
Mild-heterogeneous	96 (29.1%)	12 (10.8%)		102 (30.9%)	14 (12.6%)		
Obvious-heterogenous	2 (0.6%)	36 (32.4%)		3 (0.9%)	42 (37.8%)		
Rim-like	9 (2.7%)	58 (52.3%)		15 (4.5%)	53 (47.7%)		

Relationship between nodal status and its enhancement characteristics in subgroups (Table 4)

Among nodes with short-axis diameter ≤ 5 mm, 87.9 and 91.4% of benign nodes showed obvious enhancement, compared with 82.6 and 73.9% of malignant nodes showed mild or intermediate enhancement. Additionally, 98.3 and 97.3% of benign nodes showed homogeneous or mild-heterogeneous enhancement, and 65.2% of malignant nodes were found to have obvious-heterogeneous or rim-like enhancement. The interobserver agreement value for enhancement homogeneity was good ($\kappa = 0.699$), whereas that for enhancement degree was moderate ($\kappa = 0.593$).

Among nodes with short-axis diameter > 5 mm and ≤ 10 mm, 55.0% of benign nodes showed obvious enhancement, and 88.7 and 91.6% of metastatic nodes showed mild or intermediate enhancement. Additionally, 85.0 and 75.0% of benign nodes manifested homogeneous or mild-heterogeneous enhancement, while 88.7 and 90.2% of malignant nodes showed obvious-heterogeneous or rim-like enhancement. The interobserver agreement values for enhancement degree and homogeneity were good ($\kappa = 0.627$ and 0.651, respectively).

The nodes > 10 mm were all metastatic and all showed mild or intermediate enhancement, and 94.1% showed obvious-heterogeneous or rim-like enhancement. The interobserver agreement value for enhancement homogeneity was good ($\kappa = 0.783$), whereas that for enhancement degree was moderate ($\kappa = 0.521$).

Subgroup ROC curves of the enhancement characteristics for the prediction of nodal status are shown in Fig. 2b, c.

Discussion

High-resolution pelvic MRI is widely considered the optimal imaging method for rectal cancer [3], and it enables precise identification of high-risk factors, such as the extent of tumor invasion, extramural vascular invasion (EMVI) and the potential circumferential resection margin (CRM) [18]; however, the prediction of regional node metastases remains a challenge. Size is the usual criterion for metastatic nodes using MRI; however, the considerable size overlap between benign and malignant nodes affects the overall predictive value [19]. We found similar results in this study. The short-axis diameters of benign and malignant nodes ranged from 1.2 to 8.4 mm and from 3.1 to 18.1 mm, respectively. Discrimination between benign and malignant nodes by high-resolution MRI may be more reliable than that by nodal size when morphologic features such as border and signal homogeneity are also considered [16, 20]. However, due to the limitation of image acquisition resolution and differences in image feature interpretation, the consistency between observers may be poor [21]; moreover, the ability to resolve such small nodes is apparently suboptimal [22]. Most studies [7, 23] have suggested that MRI with an intravenous gadolinium-based contrast agent did not improve the accuracy of metastatic nodal diagnosis in rectal cancer. However, Beets-Tan's [8–10] team reported that assessing nodes using gadolinium-enhanced 3D-GRE-T1WI with a 1.5 T unit not only found a better nodal detection rate and better observation of nodal characteristics but also produced a powerful predictor of nodal status that showed satisfactory reproducibility.

Fat-suppressed gadolinium-enhanced isotropic high-resolution 3D-GRE-T1WI serves as a promising technique for rectal metastatic node detection. This technique adopts multiple approaches of fast acquisition to cover the entire pelvis, contributing to a decrease in the risk of motion artifacts. In addition, this technique maintains a higher signal-to-noise ratio (SNR) despite its thinner slice thickness due to the lack of interlayer interference and phase-encoding direction oversampling in all three sections. Moreover, this technique provides much higher spatial resolution than a 2D high-resolution sequence and can provide multiplanar reconstruction (MPR) images at an arbitrary angle from a no-interval volumetric interpolated examination of

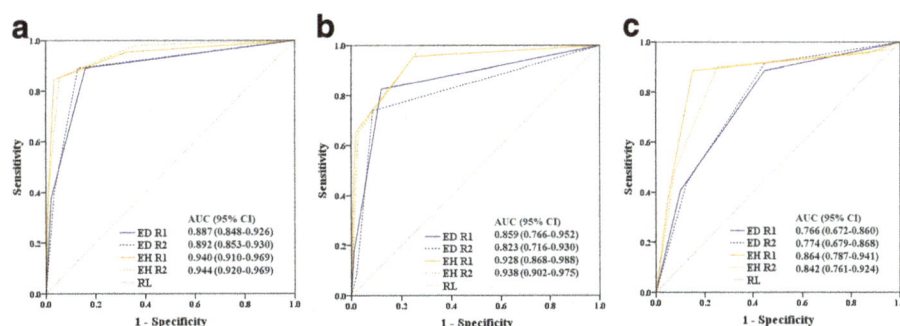

Fig. 2 ROC curves and AUCs of enhancement characteristics for determining nodal status for nodes (**a**), overall; (**b**), ≤5 mm; and (**c**), > 5 mm and ≤ 10 mm. Notes: *ED* enhancement degree; *EH* enhancement homogeneity; *RL* reference line; *R* radiologist

Table 4 Rectal cancer nodal enhancement characteristics on MR images versus histopathological findings in subgroups with different short-axis diameter ranges

Radiologist	Radiologist 1			Radiologist 2			κ
Histopathologic Findings	Benign	Malignant	P	Benign	Malignant	P	
≤5 mm	290	23		290	23		
Enhancement degree			< 0.001			< 0.001	0.593
Obvious	255 (87.9%)	4 (17.4%)		265 (91.4%)	6 (26.1%)		
Intermediate	32 (11.0%)	15 (65.2%)		19 (6.6%)	15 (65.2%)		
Mild	3 (1.0%)	4 (17.4%)		6 (2.1%)	2 (8.7%)		
Enhancement homogeneity			< 0.001			< 0.001	0.699
Homogeneous	218 (75.2%)	1 (4.3%)		209 (72.1%)	0 (0.0%)		
Mild-heterogeneous	67 (23.1%)	7 (30.4%)		73 (25.2%)	8 (34.8%)		
Obvious-heterogenous	0 (0.0%)	3 (13.0%)		0 (0.0%)	1 (4.3%)		
Rim-like	5 (1.7%)	12 (52.2%)		8 (2.8%)	14 (60.9%)		
> 5 mm and ≤ 10 mm	40	71		40	71		
Enhancement degree			< 0.001			< 0.001	0.627
Obvious	22 (55.0%)	8 (11.3%)		22 (55.0%)	6 (8.5%)		
Intermediate	14 (35.0%)	34 (47.9%)		13 (32.5%)	34 (47.9%)		
Mild	4(10.0%)	29 (40.8%)		5 (12.5%)	31 (43.7%)		
Enhancement homogeneity			< 0.001			< 0.001	0.651
Homogeneous	5 (12.5%)	3 (4.2%)		1 (2.5%)	2 (2.8%)		
Mild-heterogeneous	29 (72.5%)	5 (7.0%)		29 (72.5%)	5 (7.0%)		
Obvious-heterogenous	2 (5.0%)	27 (38.0%)		3 (7.5%)	34 (47.9%)		
Rim-like	4 (10.0%)	36 (50.7%)		7 (17.5%)	30 (42.3%)		
> 10 mm*	0	17		0	17		
Enhancement degree			–			–	0.521
Obvious	0	0 (0.0%)		0	0		
Intermediate	0	8 (47.1%)		0	6 (35.3%)		
Mild	0	9 (52.9%)		0	11 (64.7%)		
Enhancement homogeneity			–			–	0.783
Homogeneous	0	1 (5.9%)		0	0		
Mild-heterogeneous	0	0 (0.0%)		0	1 (5.9%)		
Obvious-heterogenous	0	6 (35.3%)		0	7 (41.2%)		
Rim-like	0	10 (58.8%)		0	9 (52.9%)		

Notes: *The χ^2 test was not used in the subgroup with > 10 mm nodes because all were metastatic; that is, the dependent variable was constant

thinner thicknesses. Additionally, the sequential symmetric k-space filling technique can ensure its centric contrast and retain the surrounding datum, which not only provides better-detailed anatomical structures but also increases the vessel contrast. Furthermore, lymph nodes are generally distributed along vessels and embedded in fat tissue around the vessels. The above-mentioned advantages not only can provide easier detection of small nodes and differentiation from surrounding vessels but can also yield higher contrast than either high-resolution T2WI or the common enhanced sequence; therefore, nodal enhancement characteristics can be easily depicted [12, 24, 25]. This study found that fat-suppressed gadolinium-enhanced isotropic high-resolution 3D-GRE-T1WI could ensure more accurate identification of rectal metastatic from benign nodes ≤5 mm than an assessment using high-resolution T2WI based on morphology (AUC: 0.72-0.77) or the common enhanced scan (AUC: 0.70-0.80) [7]. Enhancement degree and homogeneity were satisfactory criteria for evaluating the status of such small nodes, with moderate to high AUCs (R1: 0.859 and 0.928, respectively, R2: 0.823 and 0.938, respectively), and the results were comparable to those of Zhang et al. [26], who assessed nodes ≤5 mm using high-resolution T2WI on the strength of the chemical shift effect (AUC: 0.845-0.879).

Enhancement characteristics were proven to be highly reliable predictors of nodal positivity, with a significant difference between benign and malignant nodes in different short-axis diameter ranges. These characteristics tended to show obvious enhancement in benign nodes (R1: 83.9%, R2: 87.0%) and mild or intermediate enhancement in malignant nodes (89.2% for both radiologists). Nearly all (R1: 96.7%, R2: 94.5%) the benign nodes manifested homogeneous or mild-heterogeneous enhancement; in contrast, quite a few (R1: 84.7%, R2: 85.5%) metastatic nodes showed obvious-heterogeneous or rim-like enhancement. The larger nodes became prone to necrosis and liquefaction; hence, they had a tendency toward a more heterogeneous signal. Thus, obvious-heterogeneous or rim-like enhancement was usually (94.1% for both radiologists) observed in nodes > 10 mm. These results essentially met the pathophysiological basis of contrast material uptake by lymph nodes. Normal and reactive nodes would take up gadolinium-based medium, resulting in an intense enhancement comparable to that of the surrounding vessels. Conversely, in metastatic nodes, normal lymphatic tissue and macrophages within sinuses were replaced by the tumor to varying degrees, hindering the medium uptake. Therefore, malignant nodes had a significantly longer time to peak and showed mild and heterogeneous enhancement [27–29].

However, it should be noted that some of the nodes had atypical enhancement characteristics. (1) For example, 10.8% of metastatic nodes showed obvious enhancement. This finding likely occurred because intravenously injected contrast medium entered medullary sinuses directly via capillary interendothelial channels. However, if the contrast medium nonspecifically permeated into the interstitial space through fenestrated capillaries and was then transported to nodes via lymphatic vessels, the medium would be prevented from entering nodes by tumor cells in the interstitial spaces or nodes [28]. (2) More than half of the nodes located in the presacral space along the superior rectal vessels contained dilated vessels, thus possibly causing rapid gadolinium washout [8]. This situation could be responsible for the benign nodes in this area showing low enhancement. (3) The homogeneous or mild-heterogeneous enhancement in 15.3 and 14.4% of malignant nodes may be related to an inability to discern nodal micrometastases, although our study employed the isotropic 3D technique with 1 mm slice thickness without interslice spacing. (4) Some benign nodes were detected with mild-heterogeneous enhancement, probably because of the limitation of partial volume averaging effects or the non-uniform distribution of capillary density within nodes [30].

Our results showed that 26.1 and 29.7% of metastatic nodes exhibited a smooth border. However, most of these malignant nodes showed mild or intermediate and/or obvious-heterogeneous or rim-like heterogeneous features. This finding may have occurred because the tumor within a node that had not yet infiltrated the peripheral capsule into extranodal fat would have smooth nodal borders, whereas tumor cells inside the nodes influenced the uptake of gadolinium, leading to their enhancement characteristics differing from those of benign nodes. It was suggested that enhancement characteristics seem to be more sensitive than border status for identifying nodal status. A relatively large number of nodes with a mild-heterogeneous signal were found for each of the two nodal statuses (R1: 30.0% vs. 41.1%, R2: 31.5% vs. 53.2%). This finding might be correlated with the use of high-resolution MRI, which shows different signal intensities of the anatomic structures inside a benign node rather than showing uniform signal intensity on non-high-resolution images. Most of the nodes were ≤ 5 mm, which may have led to the misinterpretation of internal signal characteristics due to the limited spatial resolution.

The result showing increased risk of nodal metastases with higher tumor stages was in line with previous studies [21]. This finding may be due to lymphatic vessels being mainly located in the submucosa; thus, deeper infiltration of the tumor will correspond to a greater likelihood that the nodes will be affected [31].

There are some potential limitations of this study. First, the nodal match rate was not very high. This rate was mainly affected by the presence of a degree of specimen distortion and the harvesting of some nodes from specimens out of the FOV of MR images. Second, the number of metastatic nodes was relative lower than that of benign nodes, and for patients with definite metastatic nodes, neoadjuvant CRT is usually recommended. Third, the numbers of nodes in different short-axis diameter ranges was a far cry, especially such little nodes > 10 mm. Statistical analyses could not be conducted for all the evaluated malignant nodes. Fourth, iliac nodes were not assessed because TME is not typically performed for an extended pelvic lymphadenectomy. Finally, a multicenter study should be conducted to further evaluate the clinical significance of the gadolinium-enhanced isotropic high-resolution 3D sequence. Confirming the value of this sequence in a large patient cohort would make a crucial impact on the patient selection for personalized treatment. Patients with node-positive disease will benefit from neoadjuvant CRT, whereas true node-negative patients may undergo immediate surgery [3, 4].

Conclusions

Enhancement characteristics based on fat-suppressed gadolinium-enhanced isotropic high-resolution 3D-GRE-T1WI yielded better predictive power for regional nodes in rectal cancer and hold considerable promise for determining the status of nodes ≤5 mm. Nodal border and signal homogeneity also provided some contribution but were not as powerful as enhancement characteristics. These findings suggest prospects for the broad application of these enhanced observations to 3D sequence.

Funding
The funding source was Science and Technology Planning Project of Guangdong Province.

Authors' contributions
SY contributed the study concept, and YC designed the study. Data acquisition was performed by YC and XY. YC and ZW performed the statistical analysis. All the authors contributed to the data analysis and interpretation. YC, XY and ZW were major contributors and contributed equally to writing the manuscript. All the authors read and approved the final manuscript.

Competing interests
The authors declare that they have no competing interest.

Author details
[1]Department of Radiology, Sun Yat-sen University First Affiliated Hospital, Guangzhou 510080, China. [2]Department of Radiology, Peking University Shenzhen Hospital, Shenzhen 518036, China.

References
1. Brenner H, Kloor M, Pox CP. Colorectal cancer. Lancet. 2014;383:1490–502.
2. Peng J, Wu H, Li X, Sheng W, Huang D, Guan Z, Wang M, Cai S. Prognostic significance of apical lymph node metastasis in patients with node-positive rectal cancer. Color Dis. 2013;15:e13–20.
3. Benson AR, Venook AP, Bekaii-Saab T, Chan E, Chen YJ, Cooper HS, Engstrom PF, Enzinger PC, Fenton MJ, Fuchs CS, et al. Rectal Cancer, version 2.2015. J Natl Compr Cancer Netw. 2015;13:719–28. 728
4. Blazic IM, Campbell NM, Gollub MJ. MRI for evaluation of treatment response in rectal cancer. Br J Radiol. 2016;89:20150964.
5. Li XT, Sun YS, Tang L, Cao K, Zhang XY. Evaluating local lymph node metastasis with magnetic resonance imaging, endoluminal ultrasound and computed tomography in rectal cancer: a meta-analysis. Color Dis. 2015;17:O129–35.
6. Langman G, Patel A, Bowley DM. Size and distribution of lymph nodes in rectal Cancer resection specimens. Dis Colon rectum. 2015;58(4):406–14.
7. Jao SY, Yang BY, Weng HH, Yeh CH, Lee LW. Evaluation of gadolinium-enhanced T1-weighted magnetic resonance imaging in the preoperative assessment of local staging in rectal cancer. Color Dis. 2010;12:1139–48.
8. Heijnen LA, Lambregts DMJ, Martens MH, Maas M, Bakers FCH, Cappendijk VC, Oliveira P, Lammering G, Riedl RG, Beets GL, Beets-Tan RGH. Performance of gadofosveset-enhanced MRI for staging rectal cancer nodes: can the initial promising results be reproduced? Eur Radiol. 2014;24:371–9.
9. Lambregts DMJ, Heijnen LA, Maas M, Rutten IJG, Martens MH, Backes WH, Riedl RG, Bakers FCH, Cappendijk VC, Beets GL, Beets-Tan RGH. Gadofosveset-enhanced MRI for the assessment of rectal cancer lymph nodes: predictive criteria. Abdom Imaging. 2013;38:720–7.
10. Lambregts DMJ, Beets GL, Maas M, Kessels AGH, Bakers FCH, Cappendijk VC, Engelen SME, Lahaye MJ, de Bruïne AP, Lammering G, et al. Accuracy of Gadofosveset-enhanced MRI for nodal staging and restaging in rectal Cancer. Ann Surg. 2011;253:539–45.
11. Cho H, Choi YH, Cheon J, Lee SM, Kim WS, Kim I, Paek M. Free-breathing radial 3D fat-suppressed T1-weighted gradient-Echo sequence for contrast-enhanced pediatric spinal imaging: comparison with T1-weighted Turbo spin-Echo sequence. Am J Roentgenol. 2016;207:177–82.
12. Yu X, Lin M, Ye F, Ouyang H, Chen Y, Zhou C, Su Z. Comparison of contrast-enhanced isotropic 3D-GRE-T1WI sequence versus conventional non-isotropic sequence on preoperative staging of cervical cancer. PLoS One. 2015;10:e122053.
13. Wu X, Raz E, Block TK, Geppert C, Hagiwara M, Bruno MT, Fatterpekar GM. Contrast-enhanced radial 3D fat-suppressed T1-weighted gradient-recalled echo sequence versus conventional fat-suppressed contrast-enhanced T1-weighted studies of the head and neck. AJR Am J Roentgenol. 2014;203:883–9.
14. Reiner CS, Neville AM, Nazeer HK, Breault S, Dale BM, Merkle EM, Bashir MR. Contrast-enhanced free-breathing 3D T1-weighted gradient-echo sequence for hepatobiliary MRI in patients with breath-holding difficulties. Eur Radiol. 2013;23:3087–93.
15. Kudo H, Inaoka T, Kitamura N, Nakatsuka T, Kasuya S, Kasai R, Tozawa M, Nakagawa K, Terada H. Clinical value of routine use of thin-section 3D MRI using 3D FSE sequences with a variable flip angle technique for internal derangements of the knee joint at 3T. Magn Reson Imaging. 2013;31:1309–17.
16. Kim JH, Beets GL, Kim M, Kessels AGH, Beets-Tan RGH. High-resolution MR imaging for nodal staging in rectal cancer: are there any criteria in addition to the size? Eur J Radiol. 2004;52:78–83.
17. Edge SB, Compton CC. The American joint committee on Cancer: the 7th edition of the AJCC Cancer staging manual and the future of TNM. Ann Surg Oncol. 2010;17:1471–4.
18. Dieguez A. Rectal cancer staging: focus on the prognostic significance of the findings described by high-resolution magnetic resonance imaging. Cancer Imaging. 2013;13:277–97.
19. Horne J, Bateman AC, Carr NJ, Ryder I. Lymph node revealing solutions in colorectal cancer: should they be used routinely? J Clin Pathol. 2014;67:383.
20. Brown G, Richards CJ, Bourne MW, Newcombe RG, Radcliffe AG, Dallimore NS, Williams GT. Morphologic predictors of lymph node status in rectal cancer with use of high-spatial-resolution MR imaging with histopathologic comparison. Radiology. 2003;227:371–7.
21. Park JS, Jang YJ, Choi GS, Park SY, Kim HJ, Kang H, Cho SH. Accuracy of preoperative MRI in predicting pathology stage in rectal cancers: node-for-node matched histopathology validation of MRI features. Dis Colon rectum. 2014;57:32–8.
22. Beets-Tan RG. Pretreatment MRI of lymph nodes in rectal cancer: an opinion-based review. Color Dis. 2013;15:781–4.
23. Okizuka H, Sugimura K, Yoshizako T, Kaji Y, Wada A. Rectal carcinoma: prospective comparison of conventional and gadopentetate dimeglumine enhanced fat-suppressed MR imaging. J Magn Reson Imaging. 1996;6:465–71.
24. Bratis K, Henningsson M, Grigoratos C, Omodarme MD, Chasapides K, Botnar R, Nagel E. Clinical evaluation of three-dimensional late enhancement MRI. J Magn Reson Imaging. 2017;45:1675–83.
25. Kaur H, Choi H, You YN, Rauch GM, Jensen CT, Hou P, Chang GJ, Skibber JM, Ernst RD. MR imaging for preoperative evaluation of primary rectal cancer: practical considerations. Radiographics. 2012;32:389–409.
26. Zhang H, Zhang C, Zheng Z, Ye F, Liu Y, Zou S, Zhou C. Chemical shift effect predicting lymph node status in rectal cancer using high-resolution MR imaging with node-for-node matched histopathological validation. Eur Radiol. 2017;27(9):3845–3855.
27. Misselwitz B. MR contrast agents in lymph node imaging. Eur J Radiol. 2006;58:375–82.
28. Lee KC, Moon WK, Chung JW, Choi SH, Cho N, Cha JH, Lee EH, Kim SM, Kim HS, Han MH, Chang K. Assessment of lymph node metastases by contrast-enhanced MR imaging in a head and neck Cancer model. Korean J Radiol. 2007;8:9–14.
29. Choi SH, Moon WK. Contrast-enhanced MR imaging of lymph nodes in Cancer patients. Korean J Radiol. 2010;11:383–94.
30. Willard-Mack CL. Normal structure, function, and histology of lymph nodes. Toxicol Pathol. 2006;34:409–24.
31. Sitzler PJ, Seow-Choen F, Ho YH, Leong APK. Lymph node involvement and tumor depth in rectal cancers: an analysis of 805 patients. Dis Colon rectum. 1997;40(12):1472–6.

31

Evaluation of pancreatic tumor development in *KPC* mice using multi-parametric MRI

Ravneet Vohra[1], Joshua Park[1], Yak-Nam Wang[2], Kayla Gravelle[2], Stella Whang[2], Joo-Ha Hwang[3] and Donghoon Lee[1*] ⓘ

Abstract

Background: Pancreatic ductal adenocarcinoma (PDA) is a fatal disease with very poor prognosis. Development of sensitive and noninvasive methods to monitor tumor progression in PDA is a critical and unmet need. Magnetic resonance imaging (MRI) can noninvasively provide information regarding underlying pathophysiological processes such as necrosis, inflammatory changes and fibrotic tissue deposition.

Methods: A genetically engineered *KPC* mouse model that recapitulates human PDA was used to characterize disease progression. MR measures of T_1 and T_2 relaxation times, magnetization transfer ratio (MTR), diffusion and chemical exchange saturation transfer were compared in two separate phases i.e. slow and rapid growth phase of tumor. Fibrotic tissue accumulation was assessed histologically using Masson's trichrome staining. Pearson correlation coefficient (r) was computed to assess the relationship between the fibrotic tissue accumulation and different MR parameters.

Results: There was a negative correlation between amide proton transfer signal intensity and tumor volume ($r = -0.63$, $p = 0.003$) in the slow growth phase of the tumor development. In the terminal stage of rapid growth phase of the tumor development MTR was strongly correlated with tumor volume ($r = 0.62$, $p = 0.008$). Finally, MTR was significantly correlated with % fibrosis ($r = 0.87$; $p < 0.01$), followed by moderate correlation between tumor volume ($r = 0.42$); T_1 ($r = -0.61$), T_2 ($r = -0.61$) and accumulation of fibrotic tissue.

Conclusions: Here we demonstrated, using multi-parametric MRI (mp-MRI), that MRI parameters changed with tumor progression in a mouse model of PDA. Use of mp-MRI may have the potential to monitor the dynamic changes of tumor microenvironment with increase in tumor size in the transgenic *KPC* mouse model of pancreatic tumor.

Keywords: Pancreatic ductal adenocarcinoma, Tumor microenvironment, *KPC*, Multi-parametric MRI

Background

Pancreatic ductal adenocarcinoma (PDA) is the most lethal form of human cancer [1]. Desmoplasia, a hallmark pathologic feature of PDA, is characterized by the presence of a robust stroma containing fibroblasts and inflammatory cells [2]. Diagnosis of pancreatic cancer is usually made at later stages of the disease making it even more difficult to treat. Clear understanding of tumor progression may help in identifying PDA at an early stage. Therefore, in order to characterize the tumor progression,

we need 1) to investigate tumor development in an effective preclinical model that closely mimics human disease progression and 2) a sensitive, non-invasive monitoring tool that would provide detailed information regarding the disease progression and can be used in future clinical studies.

As an experimental model for pancreatic cancer, tumors have been implanted subcutaneously and within the pancreas [3–5]. However, both of these models do not parallel the human disease progression. A genetically engineered mouse model, having genetic alterations in genes K-ras^{LSL-G12D/+}; Trp53^{LSL-R172H/+}; Cre (KPC) offers an alternative to transplantation models for preclinical therapeutic evaluation as it expresses mutations similar to

* Correspondence: dhoonlee@uw.edu
[1]Department of Radiology, University of Washington, Seattle, USA
Full list of author information is available at the end of the article

human pancreatic cells [6] and develops pancreatic tumors in which pathophysiology and molecular features resemble those of human PDA [7]. There is a dire need to develop non-invasive techniques to monitor disease progression as well as study the therapeutic effects of existing and novel chemotherapeutic agents.

Magnetic resonance imaging (MRI) has been proven to be extremely useful in clinical trials for monitoring tumor development [8] and assessing therapeutic effects of novel therapeutic strategies [9–11]. Currently, management decisions in almost all phases of diagnosis, treatment, and follow-up rely on gold standard magnetic resonance (MR) measures i.e. spin-lattice relaxation time (T_1) and spin-spin relaxation time (T_2) [12, 13]. However, T_1 and T_2 measures alone may not be sensitive enough to investigate the entire spectrum of tumor properties. Recently, diffusion weighted imaging (DWI) [14, 15] and magnetization transfer imaging (MTI) [16–18] have been used as complementary imaging techniques to conventional MR measures to characterize adenocarcinoma. Finally, amide proton transfer (APT) imaging based on the chemical exchange saturation transfer (CEST) approach, which provides valuable information regarding the tumor microenvironment, has drawn considerable attention as a novel MRI contrast agent in the field of molecular imaging [19, 20]. To monitor the dynamic microenvironment of the tumor as in PDA, we need to employ mp-MRI to understand the disease progression, and the tumor environment thereby helping to plan the appropriate therapeutic regimen. In fact, several studies have demonstrated that multiparameteric MR based approach enables better quantitation of pathological processes in abdominal solid organs [21–23].

Based on the promising results of these studies, we hypothesized the mp-MRI may enable to accurately quantify the disease progression in *KPC* mice. In this study, we conducted MRI at a high field strength of 14 Tesla (T) utilizing the T_1, T_2, DWI, MTI and CEST imaging sequences to monitor the progression of pancreatic ductal adenocarcinoma in *KPC* mice. Additionally, we compared MR parameters with the histologic markers of fibrotic tissue accumulation in pancreatic tumors in the *KPC* mouse model.

Methods
Animal handling and care
The study was conducted with the approval from our institutional animal care and use committee (IACUC). *KPC* mice (*n* = 16) were enrolled in the study when they had a small palpable mass, which was confirmed by ultrasound imaging and MR imaging. All mice were imaged upon enrollment and at the final time point when the tumor reached terminal size (10 mm in any one direction). A subgroup of *KPC* mice (*n* = 9) were

imaged weekly between the baseline and final time points. All mice were euthanized at the terminal time point and the tumor and associated pancreatic tissue was excised and prepared for histological evaluation.

MR data acquisition
MRI experiments were performed on a 14 T Bruker Avance 600 MHz/89 mm wide-bore vertical MR spectrometer (Bruker Corp., Billerica, MA). A birdcage coil (inner diameter 25 mm) was used to image the animal mounted on a cradle with a respiratory monitoring probe. Animals were anesthetized before being secured to the custom-built cradle. The coil was then inserted vertically into the scanner. For the entire duration of the experiment core body temperature of mice was maintained at 37 °C. The entire MR data acquisition took 50–60 min during which the animals were continuously monitored for respiratory rate. All the images were gated to respiration of the animal. Following the MR acquisition, mice were removed from the coil and allowed to recover. Longitudinal MRI was implemented to measure pancreatic tumor growth in *KPC* mice (*n* = 9) over a period of 6 weeks. Mice included in longitudinal MRI had a palpable mass at the baseline measurement, which was measured by ultrasound (US) and later corroborated using MRI.

Anatomical images
The multi-slice MRI protocol, covering the whole tumor, started with fat-suppressed T_1 weighted coronal images (repetition time (TR) = 2000 ms, echo time (TE) = 5.49 ms, number of averages (NA) = 1, field of view (FOV) = 30×30 mm^2, rare factor = 8, matrix size = 128×256; yielding spatial resolution of 0.234×0.117 mm/pixel) for anatomical reference. Subsequently, 20 axial images were acquired to calculate tumor volume.

T_1 mapping
Multiple images using rapid acquisition with refocused echoes (RARE) were acquired using following parameters: TE = 9.66 ms, TR = 5500, 3000, 1500, 1000, 385.8 ms, NA = 1, FOV = 30×30 mm^2, rare factor = 2, matrix size = 256×128 (reconstructed phase encoding steps = 128; acquisition phase encoding steps = 96) yielding spatial resolution of 0.117×0.234 mm/pixel. The data acquisition time was approximately 9 min.

T_2 mapping
Multiple spin-echo data were acquired in coronal orientation covering the area from liver to kidneys. The quantitative T_2 maps were generated using a multi-slice multi echo sequence, with fat signal suppressed, utilizing following parameters: TR = 4000 ms; TE = 12 echoes equally spaced from 6.28 ms to 75.4 ms; NA = 1; FOV = 30×30 mm^2; matrix size =

256 × 128 (reconstructed phase encoding steps = 128; acquisition phase encoding steps = 91) yielding spatial resolution of 0.117 × 0.234 mm/pixel. To cover the entire abdominal region, 10 contiguous slices were acquired without any inter slice gap. The data acquisition time was approximately 6 min.

Magnetization transfer (MT)

MT ratios (MTR) were acquired using a gradient echo sequence (TR/TE = 625/2 ms, flip angle = 30°) with an off-resonance frequency of 7000 Hz and a saturation pulse block pulse shape, 50 ms width, and 10 μT amplitude. A series of 10 images were acquired with FOV = 30 × 30 mm^2, matrix size = 256 × 256 yielding spatial resolution of 0.117 × 0.117 mm/pixel. The acquisition time for data acquisition was approximately 3 min.

Diffusion weighted imaging (DWI)

An echo planar imaging (EPI) diffusion measurement (echo train length = 16, pulse duration = 3.0 ms and diffusion time = 7.46 ms) was performed to acquire series of 10 slices using following parameters: TR = 2500 ms; TE = 17.7 ms; NA = 1; FOV = 30 × 30 mm^2; matrix size = 128 × 128 yielding spatial resolution of 0.234 × 0.234 mm/pixel. Diffusion weighted measurements were acquired with 8 different b values (0, 30, 60, 100, 150, 200, 300, 500 s/mm^2). The data acquisition time was 2 m 40s.

Chemical exchange transfer saturation (CEST) imaging

On a single 1 mm slice, delineating tumor, amide proton transfer (APT) imaging was performed with respiratory gating using small animal monitoring device (SA instruments, Inc., Stony Brook, NY). CEST imaging data were acquired using RARE sequence (continuous-wave block pulse, B1 = 0.5 μT, duration = 2 s), which was applied at 25 frequency offsets from – 360 Hz to 360 Hz with an interval of 0.5 ppm to estimate a center frequency shift (water saturation shift referencing (WASSR) approach) [24–26]. Other imaging parameters were: TR/TE = 2200/ 7 ms, FOV = 30 × 30 mm^2, matrix size = 128 × 128, flip angle = 180°, and number of excitations = 1. For saturation a single slice was acquired with 6 frequency offsets at ±3.0, ±3.5, ±4.0 ppm, with an off-resonance RF pulse applied for 3 s at a power level of 2 μT. Other parameters were: TR/TE = 5000/7 ms, matrix = 128 × 128 (reconstructed phase encoding steps = 128; acquisition phase encoding steps = 96), FOV = 30 × 30 mm^2, rare factor = 8. Finally, a control image with the saturation offset at 300 ppm was also acquired. Total acquisition time for each animal was approximately 19 min.

Ultrasound (US) data acquisition

The animal was anaesthetized, placed in the supine position and images of the whole tumor were acquired (550 s probe, Vevo 2100, Fujifilm Visualsonics, Toronto, Canada). Ultrasound images were taken every 0.5 mm, in the transverse plane, throughout the whole tumor. The area of the tumor in each image was determined using Vevo LAB v2.1.0. The tumor volume was calculated by multiplying the area with the inter-slice distance.

Image analyses

All raw MR images were processed using Image-J software (http://imagej.nih.gov/ij/), to measure mean values of the different tumors. Regions of interest (ROI) were drawn to circumscribe the entire tumor (Additional file 1: Figure S1). *Anatomical Images* were used to measure tumor volume. Tumor volume was measured and reconstructed using Amira (Visualization Sciences Group, Burlington, MA), a 3-D software platform [18]. T_1 *and* T_2 *maps*: Maps were generated using T_1 and T_2 weighted images. *MTR maps*: The MTR was measured using the following ratio: (SI$_0$ - SI$_s$/SI$_0$), where SI$_0$ represents the tissue signal intensity without saturation pulse applied while SI$_s$ represents the tissue signal intensity with saturation pulse. *Diffusion maps*: Diffusion weighted MR signal decay was analyzed using mono-exponential model: S$_b$/S$_0$ = exp.(–b·ADC). Where S$_b$ is the MRI signal intensity with diffusion weighting b, S$_0$ is the non-diffusion-weighted signal intensity and ADC is the apparent diffusion coefficient. In addition to mono-exponential model, a bi-exponential model was used to estimate intra voxel incoherent motion (IVIM) related parameters of perfusion fraction (or pseudo-diffusion) and diffusion [27]. Three lowest b values of 0, 30 and 60 s/mm^2 were used to calculate perfusion component (or pseudo-diffusion) whereas rest of the 5 b values of 100, 150, 200, 300 and 500 s/mm^2 were used to calculate tissue diffusivity component. Finally, *APT-MR* images were quantified using the following equation: [S$_{sat}$ (– 3.5 ppm) – S$_{sat}$ (3.5 ppm)]/S$_0$ where S$_{sat}$ and S$_0$ are the water signal intensities measured with and without saturation pulse.

Histogram analyses

Regions of interest were selected across consecutive three slices having greatest tumor area to increase the coverage and improve the reliability. For each tumor, values from each slice were combined to generate a single histogram. Histograms were then normalized by plotting the percentage of pixels remaining above the specific measurement in the x-axis, generating a cumulative histogram. Finally, the area under curve (AUC) with units of % pixels x parameter on x-axis was used to compare values in two different groups.

Histological analysis

After extracting the tumor, it was immediately embedded in optimum cutting temperature (OCT) medium. Three serial, 8-μm thick sections were cut every 1 mm through the entire tumor (CM1950, Leica Biosystems Inc., Buffalo Grove, Illinois) and the sequential sections at each level were stained with Masson's trichrome to visualize fibrotic tissue deposition. The three sections, matching with MR images, were used for fibrotic tissue quantification. All sections were examined using a Nikon 80i upright microscope (Nikon, Melville, New York). Images of whole sections stained with Masson's trichrome were acquired with a 10 x objective lens. Fibrotic tissue, identified by blue staining, was separated by thresholding of the hue (130–190), saturation (20–255), and brightness (10–240) values using ImageJ (ImageJ 1.42 National Institutes of Health, Bethesda, MD). The fibrotic tissue content is presented as the percent area of fibrosis over the whole tumor area. High resolution, 40 μm thick, cryo-images of one of the tumor bearing mice were acquired at Bioinvision® (www.bioinvision.com).

Statistical analysis

Statistical analysis was performed using Graph Pad prism version 6.0 (GraphPad, La Jolla, CA, USA). Tumor volume was compared between baseline and final time points using paired t test. Pearson correlation coefficient (r) with Bonferroni correction was computed to assess the relationship between the tumor volume and different MR parameters. All data were presented as means and standard deviations (SD). Statistical significance was accepted for $p < 0.05$.

Results

Increase in pancreatic tumor volume with age in *KPC* mice

Longitudinal MRI demonstrated two distinct phases existed in tumor progression in *KPC* mice i.e. slow phase and rapid phase. Tumor growth, measured by MRI, in 6 out of 9 *KPC* mice increased exponentially once it surpassed a threshold value of 250 mm^3 (Fig. 1a). Overall, there was a significant increase in tumor mass from baseline measurements (205.5 ± 154.4 mm^3, mean ± SD) to the 6-week time point (455.9 ± 137.3 mm^3). A moderate correlation was found between volume measurement by US and MRI ($r = 0.59$) (Fig. 1b). Finally, a high-resolution MR coronal section was compared with a whole body cryo-image (Fig. 1c) and MR axial section was compared with axial US image (Fig. 1d) to compare spatial resolution of different modalities.

MR parameters correlate with tumor volume

Multi-parametric data was analyzed based on the size of the tumor i.e. < 250 mm^3 and > 250 mm^3 as shown in Figs. 2 and 3. We chose a threshold value of 250 mm^3 to differentiate between a slow and rapid growth phase in tumor development. Tumor size is an important prognostic factor in various cancers. Indeed, studies have documented

a certain cut off size in various tumors enhance the prognosis [28–30]. Furthermore, there was a strong correlation between tumor volume and amide proton transfer (APT) signal intensity ($r = -0.63$, $p = 0.003$) in < 250 mm^3 whereas no correlation was present between APT signal intensity and tumor volume ($r = -0.03$) when the tumor size was > 250 mm^3. When the tumor size surpassed the threshold value i.e. 250 mm^3, magnetization transfer ratio (MTR) displayed strong positive correlation with the tumor volume ($r = 0.62$, $p = 0.008$). Based on intravoxel incoherent motion (IVIM) model, [27, 31, 32] pseudo-diffusion or perfusion component (using low-b value) showed a strong negative correlation with the tumor volume ($r = -0.70$, $p = 0.003$) whereas we did not find any correlation between diffusion (high-b values) and tumor volume ($r = 0.12$; < 250mm^3, $r = 0.11$; > 250 mm^3).

Histogram analyses of tumor progression

To assess pixel-pixel changes in MR parameters regionally, histogram analysis was implemented in the tumor area of *KPC* mice. Histograms were generated for T_1, T_2, MTR, and apparent diffusion coefficient (ADC) by combining values from 3 different slices for the pancreatic tumor. There was a general shift toward higher values for MTR and lower values for ADC in a larger tumor group i.e. > 250 mm^3 (Fig. 4a). Additionally, the difference between smaller and larger tumor groups was better visualized in a cumulative histogram, which was produced by plotting the percentage of pixels remaining above the x-axis values (Fig. 4b). Finally, area under curve (AUC) was calculated from cumulative histograms for mp-MRI did not show any significant difference between < 250 mm^3 and > 250 mm^3 (Fig. 5).

Histological analysis

Fibrotic tissue deposition was identified by Masson's trichrome stained tumors and compared to mp-MR maps (Fig. 6). There was a significant correlation between MTR and % fibrosis ($r = 0.87$; $p < 0.01$), followed by moderate correlation between tumor volume ($r = 0.42$; $p = 0.30$), T_1 ($r = 0.59$, $p = 0.13$), T_2 ($r = -0.61$, $p = 0.10$) and fibrotic tissue deposition (Fig. 7).

Discussion

The present study evaluated multi-parametric MRI (mp-MRI) to monitor pancreatic tumor progression in the *KPC* mouse model. MR measurements consisted of T_1, T_2, ADC, MTR and APT imaging. The results from the present study revealed that 1) the tumor size increases exponentially once it crosses a threshold value i.e. 250 mm^3; 2) MTR (%) and ADC (pseudo-diffusion) demonstrated higher correlation with tumor volume

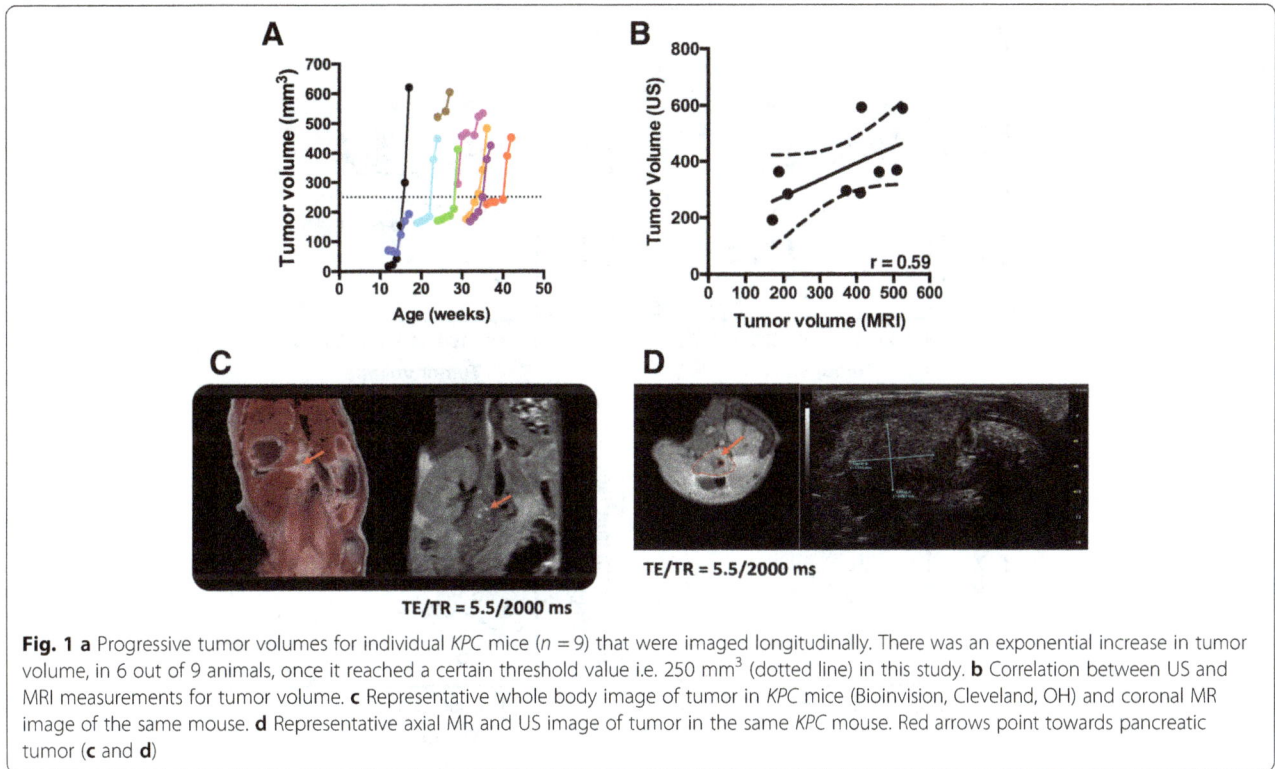

Fig. 1 a Progressive tumor volumes for individual *KPC* mice (*n* = 9) that were imaged longitudinally. There was an exponential increase in tumor volume, in 6 out of 9 animals, once it reached a certain threshold value i.e. 250 mm³ (dotted line) in this study. **b** Correlation between US and MRI measurements for tumor volume. **c** Representative whole body image of tumor in *KPC* mice (Bioinvision, Cleveland, OH) and coronal MR image of the same mouse. **d** Representative axial MR and US image of tumor in the same *KPC* mouse. Red arrows point towards pancreatic tumor (**c** and **d**)

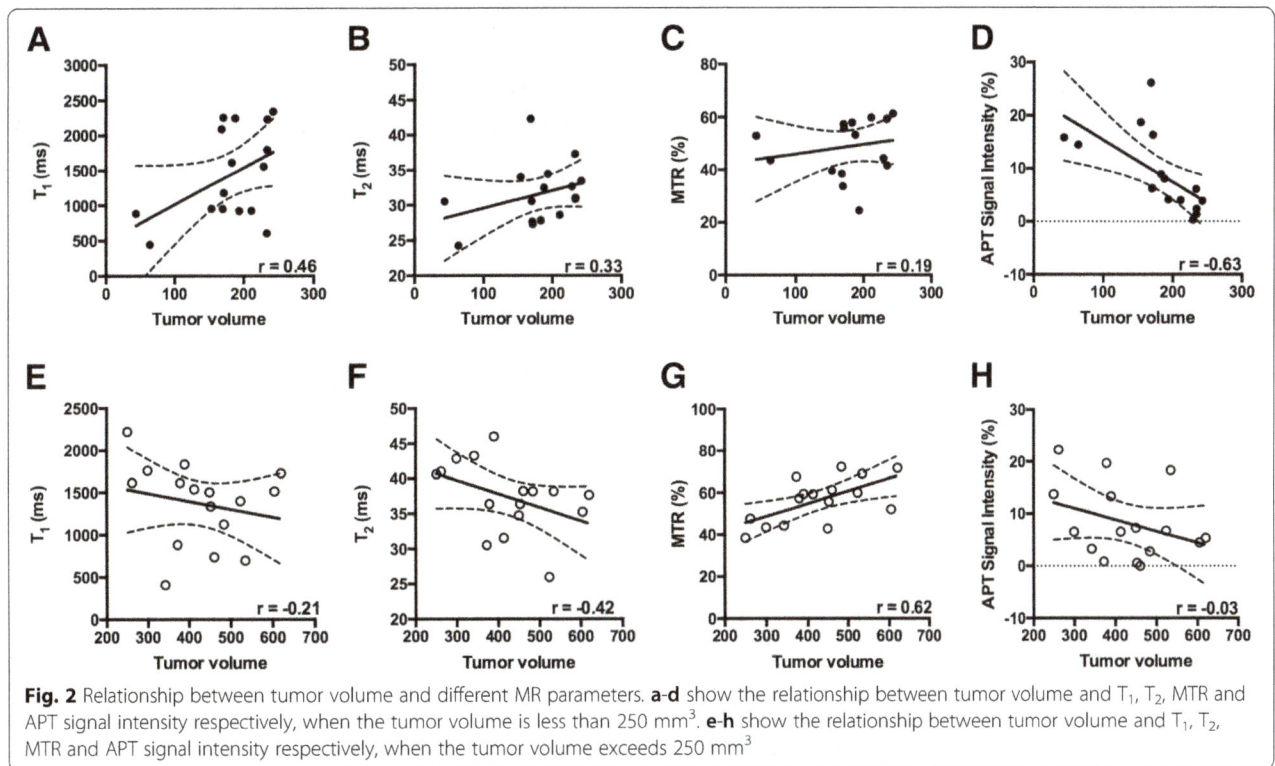

Fig. 2 Relationship between tumor volume and different MR parameters. **a-d** show the relationship between tumor volume and T_1, T_2, MTR and APT signal intensity respectively, when the tumor volume is less than 250 mm³. **e-h** show the relationship between tumor volume and T_1, T_2, MTR and APT signal intensity respectively, when the tumor volume exceeds 250 mm³

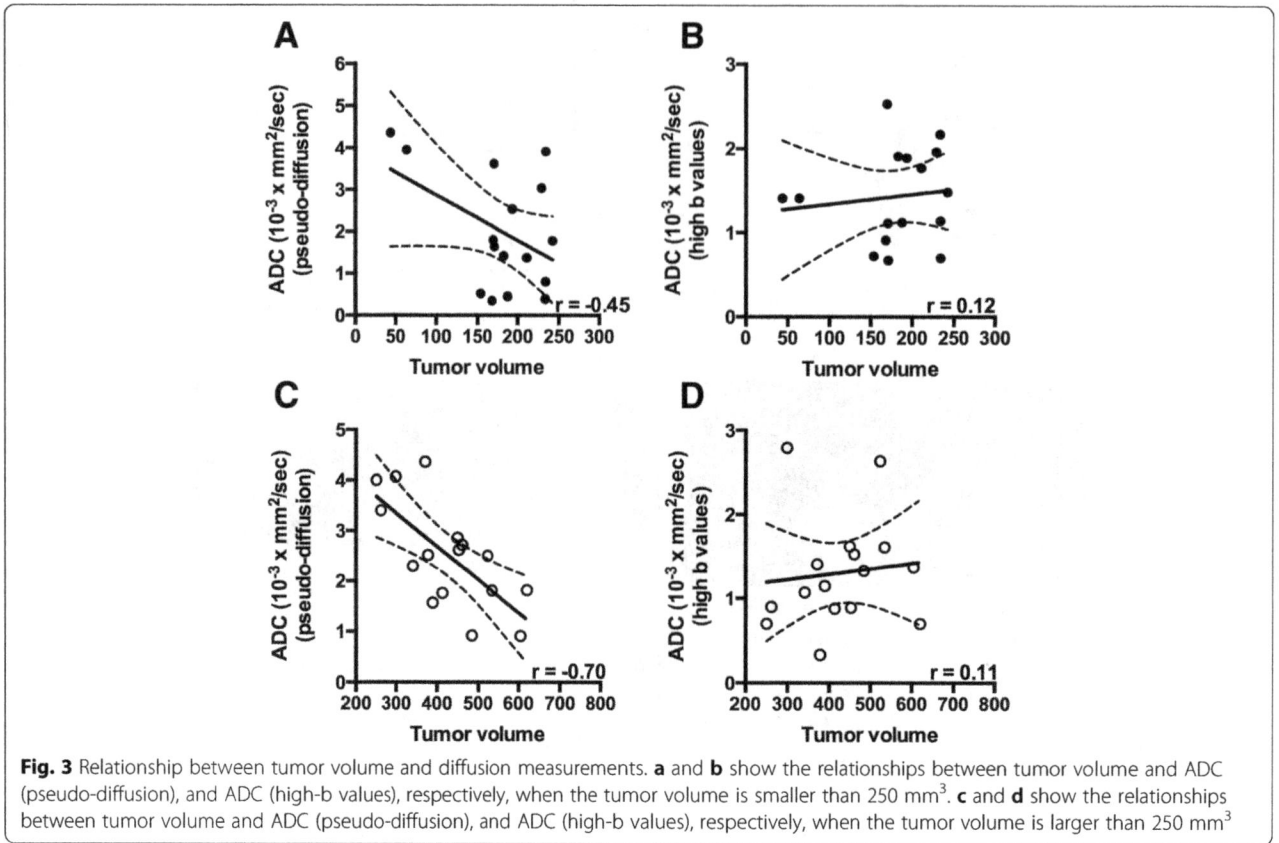

Fig. 3 Relationship between tumor volume and diffusion measurements. **a** and **b** show the relationships between tumor volume and ADC (pseudo-diffusion), and ADC (high-b values), respectively, when the tumor volume is smaller than 250 mm³. **c** and **d** show the relationships between tumor volume and ADC (pseudo-diffusion), and ADC (high-b values), respectively, when the tumor volume is larger than 250 mm³

compared to other measures especially during the later stages of tumor development; and 3) MTR was significantly correlated with increase in fibrotic tissue accumulation.

We have demonstrated a moderate correlation between US and MRI measures of tumor volume. Although US has

been used extensively as an imaging tool in small animals, poor signal-to-noise ratio (SNR) images is one of the major limitations to ultrasound use. On the other hand, MRI has the ability to provide images in great anatomic detail. Decreased SNR could be one of the reasons that explains a moderate correlation between tumor volume measurements

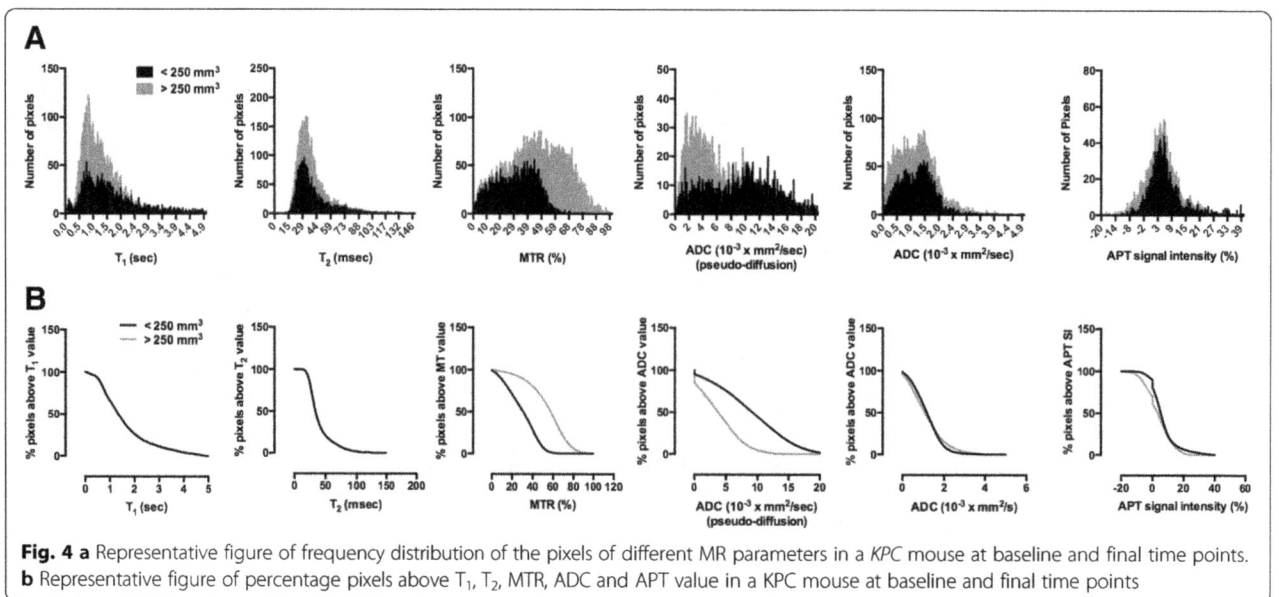

Fig. 4 a Representative figure of frequency distribution of the pixels of different MR parameters in a *KPC* mouse at baseline and final time points. **b** Representative figure of percentage pixels above T_1, T_2, MTR, ADC and APT value in a KPC mouse at baseline and final time points

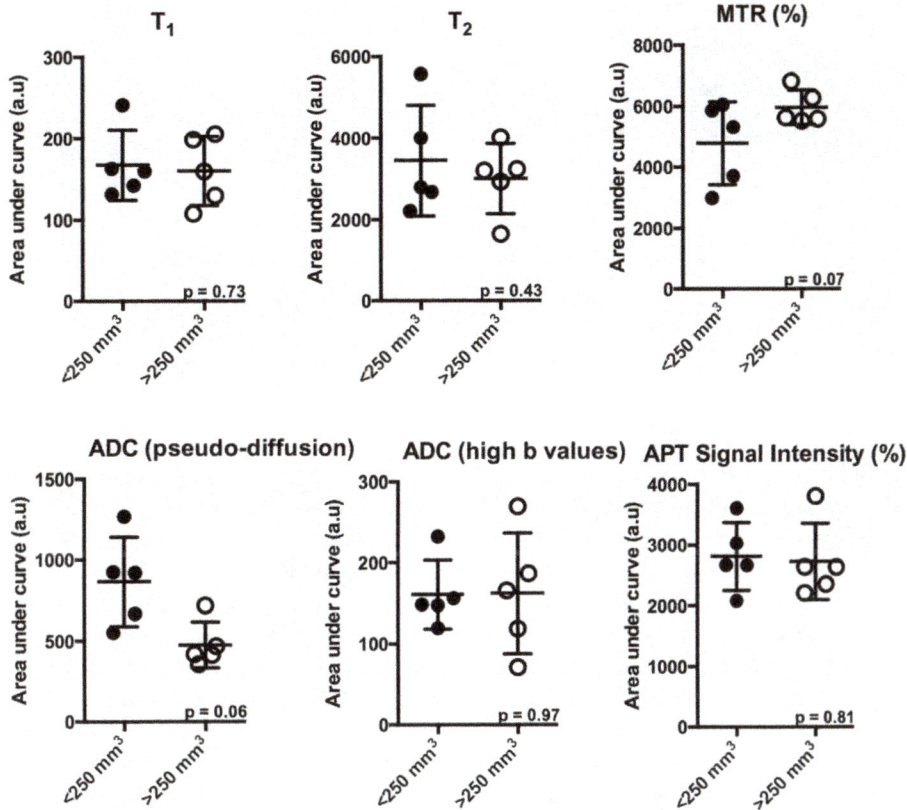

Fig. 5 Area under curve (AUC) demonstrating differences in multi-parametric MR measures in PDA of < 250 mm^3 and > 250 mm^3 in 5 *KPC* mice

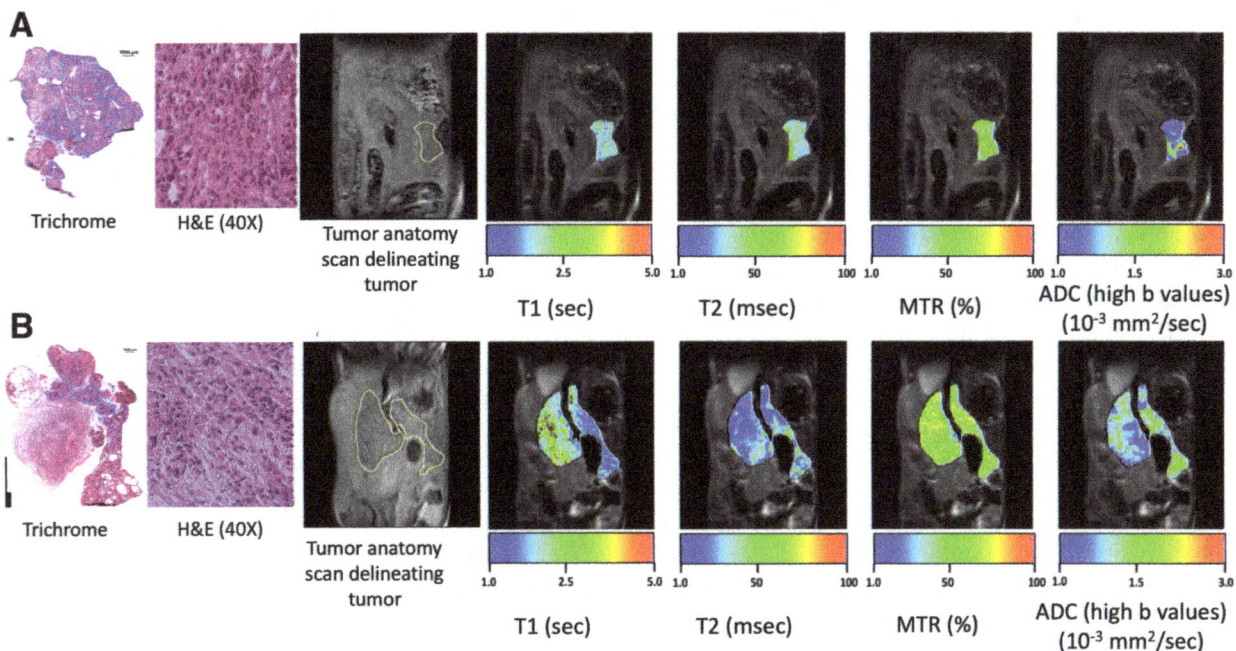

Fig. 6 Representative Masson's Trichrome and H&E stains for a smaller tumor (**a**) and larger tumor (**b**) from *KPC* mice and corresponding anatomic images and colored maps with T$_1$, T$_2$, MTR and ADC measures for pancreatic tumor

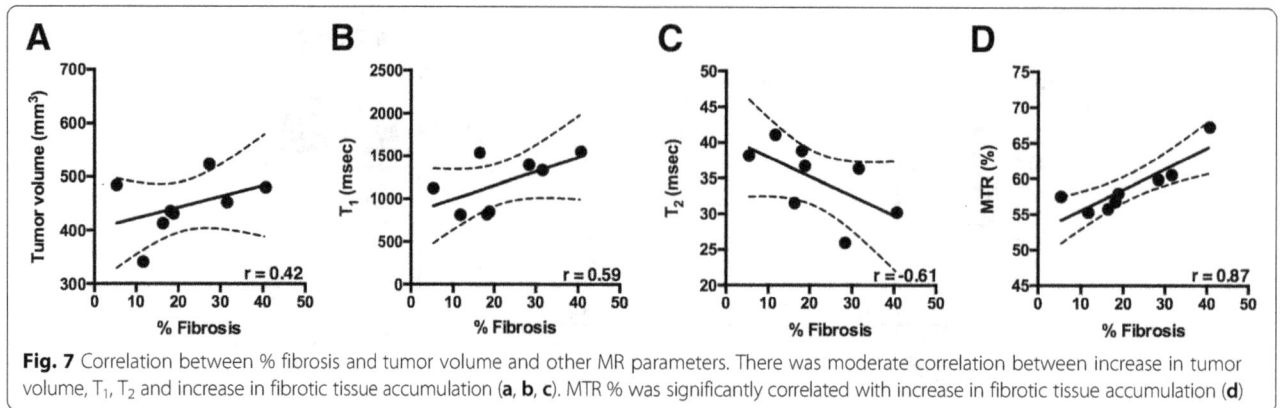

Fig. 7 Correlation between % fibrosis and tumor volume and other MR parameters. There was moderate correlation between increase in tumor volume, T_1, T_2 and increase in fibrotic tissue accumulation (**a**, **b**, **c**). MTR % was significantly correlated with increase in fibrotic tissue accumulation (**d**)

using US and MRI. Additionally, tumor burden or size has been demonstrated to be an important prognostic factor among patients with different types of carcinomas [28–30]. Furthermore, it has been suggested that tumors grow in a non-linear fashion [33]. Similarly, in the present study we have demonstrated that the growth of tumors follows a non-linear trend i.e. in two separate phases i.e. slow and rapid. Finally, we found that a cut off size of 250 mm³ in the *KPC* mouse model may provide enhanced prognosis.

The measurement of any MR parameter in isolation may undermine the dynamic nature of tumor microenvironment. However, the use of mp-MRI enables the evaluation of multiple parameters to give a more representative picture of the tumor microenvironment. Methods such as quantitative T_1, T_2, ADC and MTR are well established methods used to characterize tumor progression [8, 34–36]. T_1 and T_2 relaxation times of water molecules in tissue have been demonstrated as sensitive indicators of tumor progression as well as responses to different therapeutic agents [35, 37]. T_1 is sensitive to factors such as the amount of 1) water in the extracellular space and 2) protein in the water [38]. Similarly, the results of our study demonstrate a moderate positive correlation between T_1 and tumor volume in the smaller tumor group (< 250 mm³) suggesting increased water and protein content especially during the earlier stages of tumor development. Conversely, when the tumor size increased beyond the threshold value (250 mm³), T_1 failed to provide detailed information regarding the tumor development. In advanced tumor stages there is more fibrotic tissue deposition when compared to earlier stages [39], which can be demonstrated by a decrease in T_2 relaxation time. Similarly, in the present study, we revealed a moderate negative correlation between T_2 and tumor volume in the larger tumor group and a decrease in T_2 relaxation time was also correlated to an increase in fibrotic tissue content. These findings suggested that fibrotic tissue accumulated during later stages of disease progression and

that T_2 is more sensitive than T_1 to tumor progression, especially in terms of fibrotic tissue accumulation.

DWI is sensitive to the thermally driven motion of water molecules along the orientation of additional diffusion sensitizing gradients applied during MR sequence. The signal attenuation coefficient, known as apparent diffusion coefficient (ADC) can be derived from diffusion weighted images. ADC has been shown to be sensitive to tissue structure at the cellular level [40, 41]. Results from the present study revealed only moderate correlation between tumor volume and ADC in larger tumor group suggesting that tumor environment becomes more restrictive as tumor size increases. Moreover, a study by Muraoka et al. demonstrated significant differences in ADC between areas of sparse and dense fibrotic area [8]. Furthermore, ADC is a combined measure of thermally driven molecular movement of water i.e. diffusion and microcirculation of blood in capillaries i.e. perfusion [42] as demonstrated by intravoxel incoherent motion (IVIM) model. Indeed, the IVIM model has been used to study various cancer types [31, 32]. The signal from blood flow is rapidly attenuated at low b values (b < 100–150 s/mm²), whereas higher b values are required to suppress the perfusion contribution [43, 44].

One of the most sensitive measures to monitor the tumor progression, in our animal model, was MTR (%). Previous studies have demonstrated that the transgenic *KPC* mouse model has the highest degree of fibrotic tissue accumulation as compared to other mouse models evaluated [45]. Furthermore, studies have demonstrated that MTR values are sensitive to fibrotic tissue deposition and have been used to study liver fibrosis and PDA [17, 18, 34]. Additionally, a study by Farr et al. has demonstrated a significant correlation between MTR and fibrotic tissue deposition in the *KPC* mouse model [18]. Furthermore, using a xenograft mouse model, Li et al. have demonstrated a significant correlation between MTR and fibrotic tissue deposition in different cell lines when the tumor size was close to 10 mm [17]. Similarly, in our study, we have demonstrated a significant correlation between MTR and tumor volume especially when the tumor volume exceeded 250 mm^3. Whereas when the tumor volume was less than 250 mm^3, we did not find any correlation between MTR and tumor volume. Additionally, we found that there was a moderate correlation between an increase in tumor volume and fibrotic tissue deposition and a strong correlation between MTR and accumulation of fibrotic tissue suggesting that with an increase in tumor volume there is increase in fibrotic tissue deposition and that MTR changes are sensitive to accumulation of fibrotic tissue in the tumor. Therefore, MTR may be a valuable measure in evaluation of novel treatments and more importantly, in determining the stage of cancer and planning the treatment regimen accordingly.

Finally, APT imaging has been used to measure the concentration of endogenous mobile proteins and peptides which are increased in high-grade brain tumors compared with low-grade tumors [46]. We, however, did not find any significant increase in APT signal intensity when comparing tumor in small and large tumor groups. Surprisingly, in the smaller tumor group, we found a significant decrease in the amide proton group with an increase in tumor volume suggesting that these protons have an important role during early stages of tumor development. Once a threshold value is reached, the concentration of amide protons remained unchanged, suggesting a role of other chemical constituents in higher tumor volumes. Indeed, studies of PDA have suggested that there is increased accumulation of hyaluronic acid (HA) rather than an increase in tumor cellularity, which may be one of the major factors leading to an increase in tumor volume [47, 48].

The multi-parametric approach has been utilized before to characterize various tumors and therapeutic effects [18, 49]. To the best of our knowledge this is the first study to characterize the *KPC* mouse model using a host of MR measurements. Our study has a few limitations that need to be acknowledged. First, due to the dynamic nature of the tumor microenvironment, a host of pathological processes such as necrosis and fibrotic tissue accumulation occur simultaneously with tumor development and future studies need to be conducted in *KPC* mice at various stages of tumor development. Additionally, MR results need to be correlated with histological measurements in detail. In this study, we did not validate the MR measures with the pathological events at different stages of tumor development. Second, we did not quantify HA accumulation, which correlates with high tumor interstitial fluid pressure (IFP) which in turn collapses the surrounding capillaries. Future studies looking at these features and corroboration with histological measurements are warranted.

Conclusions

We believe that quantitative mp-MRI has a potential role in the monitoring of disease progression and therapeutic evaluation of tumors. In our study, we have demonstrated that MR parameters such as T_1 and APT are sensitive to changes in the tumor microenvironment during the early stages of tumor development whereas parameters such as T_2, MTR and ADC are sensitive to pathology during the later stages of tumor development. Additionally, our multi-parametric data suggests that changes in advanced MR techniques such as MTR, ADC and APT imaging have the potential to be used in both preclinical and eventually in clinical models to document the underlying pathophysiological processes and thereby initiating tumor targeting therapy.

Abbreviations
APT: amide proton transfer; AUC: area under curve; CEST: chemical exchange saturation transfer; DWI: diffusion weighted imaging; MTR: magnetization transfer ratio; PDA: pancreatic ductal adenocarcinoma

Acknowledgements
Not applicable.

Funding
This work is supported by NIH R01CA188654 and NIH R01CA154451.

Author's contributions
DL contributed the study concept, and RV and DL designed the study. Data acquisition was performed by RV, JP, YNW, KG, SW. RV performed the statistical analysis. All authors contributed to data analysis, interpretation and approval of final manuscript.

Competing interests
The authors declare that they have no competing interest.

Author details
[1]Department of Radiology, University of Washington, Seattle, USA. [2]Applied Physics Laboratory, University of Washington, Seattle, USA. [3]Department of Medicine, University of Washington, Seattle, USA.

References
1. Siegel RL, Miller KD, Jemal A. Cancer statistics, 2017. CA Cancer J Clin. 2017;67(1):7–30.
2. Yang S, Wang X, Contino G, Liesa M, Sahin E, Ying H, Bause A, Li Y, Stommel JM, Dell'antonio G, Mautner J, Tonon G, Haigis M, Shirihai OS, Doglioni C, Bardeesy N, Kimmelman AC. Pancreatic cancers require autophagy for tumor growth. Genes Dev. 2011;25(7):717–29.
3. Grimm J, Potthast A, Wunder A, Moore A. Magnetic resonance imaging of the pancreas and pancreatic tumors in a mouse orthotopic model of human cancer. Int J Cancer. 2003;106(5):806–11.

4. Cui JH, Kruger U, Vogel I, Luttges J, Henne-Bruns D, Kremer B, Kalthoff H. Intact tissue of gastrointestinal cancer specimen orthotopically transplanted into nude mice. Hepatogastroenterology. 1998;45(24):2087–96.

5. Tan MH, Chu TM. Characterization of the tumorigenic and metastatic properties of a human pancreatic tumor cell line (AsPC-1) implanted orthotopically into nude mice. Tumour Biol. 1985;6(1):89–98.

6. Hingorani SR, Wang L, Multani AS, Combs C, Deramaudt TB, Hruban RH, Rustgi AK, Chang S, Tuveson DA. Trp53R172H and KrasG12D cooperate to promote chromosomal instability and widely metastatic pancreatic ductal adenocarcinoma in mice. Cancer Cell. 2005;7(5):469–83.

7. Hruban RH, Adsay NV, Albores-Saavedra J, Anver MR, Biankin AV, Boivin GP, Furth EE, Furukawa T, Klein A, Klimstra DS, Kloppel G, Lauwers GY, Longnecker DS, Luttges J, Maitra A, Offerhaus GJ, Perez-Gallego L, Redston M, Tuveson DA. Pathology of genetically engineered mouse models of pancreatic exocrine cancer: consensus report and recommendations. Cancer Res. 2006;66(1):95–106.

8. Muraoka N, Uematsu H, Kimura H, Imamura Y, Fujiwara Y, Murakami M, Yamaguchi A, Itoh H. Apparent diffusion coefficient in pancreatic cancer: characterization and histopathological correlations. J Magn Reson Imaging. 2008;27(6):1302–8.

9. Ansari C, Tikhomirov GA, Hong SH, Falconer RA, Loadman PM, Gill JH, Castaneda R, Hazard FK, Tong L, Lenkov OD, Felsher DW, Rao J, Daldrup-Link HE. Development of novel tumor-targeted theranostic nanoparticles activated by membrane-type matrix metalloproteinases for combined cancer magnetic resonance imaging and therapy. Small. 2014;10(3):566–75 417.

10. Baron P, Deckers R, Knuttel FM, Bartels LW. T1 and T2 temperature dependence of female human breast adipose tissue at 1.5 T: groundwork for monitoring thermal therapies in the breast. NMR Biomed. 2015;28(11):1463–70.

11. Hectors SJ, Jacobs I, Heijman E, Keupp J, Berben M, Strijkers GJ, Grull H, Nicolay K. Multiparametric MRI analysis for the evaluation of MR-guided high intensity focused ultrasound tumor treatment. NMR Biomed. 2015;28(9):1125–40.

12. Shami VM, Mahajan A, Loch MM, Stella AC, Northup PG, White GE, Brock AS, Srinivasan I, de Lange EE, Kahaleh M. Comparison between endoscopic ultrasound and magnetic resonance imaging for the staging of pancreatic cancer. Pancreas. 2011;40(4):567–70.

13. Kinney T. Evidence-based imaging of pancreatic malignancies. Surg Clin North Am. 2010;90(2):235–49.

14. Ma C, Li Y, Wang L, Wang Y, Zhang Y, Wang H, Chen S, Lu J. Intravoxel incoherent motion DWI of the pancreatic adenocarcinomas: monoexponential and biexponential apparent diffusion parameters and histopathological correlations. Cancer Imaging. 2017;17(1):12.

15. De Robertis R, Tinazzi Martini P, Demozzi E, Dal Corso F, Bassi C, Pederzoli P, D'Onofrio M. Diffusion-weighted imaging of pancreatic cancer. World J Radiol. 2015;7(10):319–28.

16. Li W, Zhang Z, Nicolai J, Yang GY, Omary RA, Larson AC. Quantitative magnetization transfer MRI of desmoplasia in pancreatic ductal adenocarcinoma xenografts. NMR Biomed. 2013;26(12):1688–95.

17. Li W, Zhang Z, Nicolai J, Yang GY, Omary RA, Larson AC. Magnetization transfer MRI in pancreatic cancer xenograft models. Magn Reson Med. 2012;68(4):1291–7.

18. Farr N, Wang YN, D'Andrea S, Gravelle KM, Hwang JH, Lee D. Noninvasive characterization of pancreatic tumor mouse models using magnetic resonance imaging. Cancer Med. 2017;6(5):1082–90.

19. Sagiyama K, Mashimo T, Togao O, Vemireddy V, Hatanpaa KJ, Maher EA, Mickey BE, Pan E, Sherry AD, Bachoo RM, Takahashi M. In vivo chemical exchange saturation transfer imaging allows early detection of a therapeutic response in glioblastoma. Proc Natl Acad Sci U S A. 2014;111(12):4542–7.

20. Zhou JY, Payen JF, Wilson DA, Traystman RJ, van Zijl PCM. Using the amide proton signals of intracellular proteins and peptides to detect pH effects in MRI. Nat Med. 2003;9(8):1085–90.

21. Watanabe H, Kanematsu M, Tanaka K, Osada S, Tomita H, Hara A, Goshima S, Kondo H, Kawada H, Noda Y, Tanahashi Y, Kawai N, Yoshida K, Moriyama N. Fibrosis and postoperative fistula of the pancreas: correlation with MR imaging findings--preliminary results. Radiology. 2014;270(3):791–9.

22. Hwang I, Lee JM, Lee KB, Yoon JH, Kiefer B, Han JK, Choi BI. Hepatic steatosis in living liver donor candidates: preoperative assessment by using breath-hold triple-echo MR imaging and 1H MR spectroscopy. Radiology. 2014;271(3):730–8.

23. Taouli B, Tolia AJ, Losada M, Babb JS, Chan ES, Bannan MA, Tobias H. Diffusion-weighted MRI for quantification of liver fibrosis: preliminary experience. AJR Am J Roentgenol. 2007;189(4):799–806.

24. Kim M, Gillen J, Landman BA, Zhou J, van Zijl PC. Water saturation shift referencing (WASSR) for chemical exchange saturation transfer (CEST) experiments. Magn Reson Med. 2009;61(6):1441–50.

25. Jin T, Wang P, Zong X. Kim SG. MR imaging of the amide-proton transfer effect and the pH-insensitive nuclear overhauser effect at 9.4 T. Magn Reson Med. 2013;69(3):760–70.

26. Desmond KL, Moosvi F, Stanisz GJ. Mapping of amide, amine, and aliphatic peaks in the CEST spectra of murine xenografts at 7 T. Magn Reson Med. 2014;71(5):1841–53.

27. Kim S, Decarlo L, Cho GY, Jensen JH, Sodickson DK, Moy L, Formenti S, Schneider RJ, Goldberg JD, Sigmund EE. Interstitial fluid pressure correlates with intravoxel incoherent motion imaging metrics in a mouse mammary carcinoma model. NMR Biomed. 2012;25(5):787–94.

28. Chen L, Ma X, Li H, Gu L, Li X, Gao Y, Xie Y, Zhang X. Influence of tumor size on oncological outcomes of pathological T3aN0M0 renal cell carcinoma treated by radical nephrectomy. PLoS One. 2017;12(3):e0173953.

29. Gao Z, Wang C, Xue Q, Wang J, Shen Z, Jiang K, Shen K, Liang B, Yang X, Xie Q, Wang S, Ye Y. The cut-off value of tumor size and appropriate timing of follow-up for management of minimal EUS-suspected gastric gastrointestinal stromal tumors. BMC Gastroenterol. 2017;17(1):8.

30. Su X, Fang D, Li X, Xiong G, Zhang L, Hao H, Gong Y, Zhang Z, Zhou L. The influence of tumor size on oncologic outcomes for patients with upper tract urothelial carcinoma after radical Nephroureterectomy. Biomed Res Int. 2016;2016:4368943.

31. Lemke A, Laun FB, Klauss M, Re TJ, Simon D, Delorme S, Schad LR, Stieltjes B. Differentiation of pancreas carcinoma from healthy pancreatic tissue using multiple b-values: comparison of apparent diffusion coefficient and intravoxel incoherent motion derived parameters. Investig Radiol. 2009;44(12):769–75.

32. Le Bihan D, Breton E, Lallemand D, Aubin ML, Vignaud J, Laval-Jeantet M. Separation of diffusion and perfusion in intravoxel incoherent motion MR imaging. Radiology. 1988;168(2):497–505.

33. Liu X, Johnson S, Liu S, Kanojia D, Yue W, Singh UP, Wang Q, Wang Q, Nie Q, Chen H. Nonlinear growth kinetics of breast cancer stem cells: implications for cancer stem cell targeted therapy. Sci Rep. 2013;3:2473.

34. Aisen AM, Doi K, Swanson SD. Detection of liver fibrosis with magnetic cross-relaxation. Magn Reson Med. 1994;31(5):551–6.

35. Beall PT, Asch BB, Chang DC, Medina D, Hazlewood CF. Distinction of normal, preneoplastic, and neoplastic mouse mammary primary cell cultures by water nuclear magnetic resonance relaxation times. J Natl Cancer Inst. 1980;64(2):335–8.

36. Yin T, Peeters R, Feng Y, Liu Y, Yu J, Dymarkowski S, Himmelreich U, Oyen R, Ni Y. Characterization of a rat orthotopic pancreatic head tumor model using three-dimensional and quantitative multi-parametric MRI. NMR Biomed. 2017;30(2).

37. Gullino PM. Considerations on blood supply and fluid exchange in tumors. Prog Clin Biol Res. 1982;107:1–20.

38. Rofstad EK, Steinsland E, Kaalhus O, Chang YB, Hovik B, Lyng H. Magnetic resonance imaging of human melanoma xenografts in vivo: proton spin-lattice and spin-spin relaxation times versus fractional tumour water content and fraction of necrotic tumour tissue. Int J Radiat Biol. 1994;65(3):387–401.

39. Li W, Hong L, Hu L, Magin RL. Magnetization transfer imaging provides a quantitative measure of chondrogenic differentiation and tissue development. Tissue Eng Part C Methods. 2010;16(6):1407–15.

40. Le Bihan D, Delannoy J, Levin RL. Temperature mapping with MR imaging of molecular diffusion: application to hyperthermia. Radiology. 1989;171(3):853–7.

41. Latour LL, Svoboda K, Mitra PP, Sotak CH. Time-dependent diffusion of water in a biological model system. Proc Natl Acad Sci U S A. 1994;91(4):1229–33.

42. Le Bihan D, Breton E, Lallemand D, Grenier P, Cabanis E. Laval-Jeantet M. MR imaging of intravoxel incoherent motions: application to diffusion and perfusion in neurologic disorders. Radiology. 1986;161(2):401–7.

43. Le Bihan D, Turner R. The capillary network: a link between IVIM and classical perfusion. Magn Reson Med. 1992;27(1):171–8.

44. Le Bihan D, Breton E, Lallemand D, Desbleds MT, Aubin ML, Vignaud J, Roger B. Contribution of intravoxel incoherent motion (IVIM) imaging to neuroradiology. J Neuroradiol. 1987;14(4):295–312.

45. Olive KP, Jacobetz MA, Davidson CJ, Gopinathan A, McIntyre D, Honess D, Madhu B, Goldgraben MA, Caldwell ME, Allard D, Frese KK, Denicola G, Feig C, Combs C, Winter SP, Ireland-Zecchini H, Reichelt S, Howat WJ, Chang A, Dhara M, Wang L, Ruckert F, Grutzmann R, Pilarsky C, Izeradjene K, Hingorani SR, Huang P, Davies SE, Plunkett W, Egorin M, Hruban RH, Whitebread N, McGovern K, Adams J, Iacobuzio-Donahue C, Griffiths J, Tuveson DA. Inhibition of hedgehog signaling enhances delivery of chemotherapy in a mouse model of pancreatic cancer. Science. 2009;324(5933):1457–61.

46. Wen Z, Hu S, Huang F, Wang X, Guo L, Quan X, Wang S, Zhou J. MR imaging of high-grade brain tumors using endogenous protein and peptide-based contrast. Neuroimage. 2010;51(2):616–22.

47. DuFort CC, DelGiorno KE, Carlson MA, Osgood RJ, Zhao C, Huang Z, Thompson CB, Connor RJ, Thanos CD, Scott Brockenbrough J, Provenzano PP, Frost GI, Michael Shepard H, Hingorani SR. Interstitial pressure in pancreatic ductal adenocarcinoma is dominated by a gel-fluid phase. Biophys J. 2016;110(9):2106–19.

48. Provenzano PP, Cuevas C, Chang AE, Goel VK, Von Hoff DD, Hingorani SR. Enzymatic targeting of the stroma ablates physical barriers to treatment of pancreatic ductal adenocarcinoma. Cancer Cell. 2012;21(3):418–29.

49. Hectors SJ, Jacobs I, Strijkers GJ, Nicolay K. Multiparametric MRI analysis for the identification of high intensity focused ultrasound-treated tumor tissue. PLoS One. 2014;9(6):e99936.

Permissions

The contributors of this book come from diverse backgrounds, making this book a truly international effort. This book will bring forth new frontiers with its revolutionizing research information and detailed analysis of the nascent developments around the world.

We would like to thank all the contributing authors for lending their expertise to make the book truly unique. They have played a crucial role in the development of this book. Without their invaluable contributions this book wouldn't have been possible. They have made vital efforts to compile up to date information on the varied aspects of this subject to make this book a valuable addition to the collection of many professionals and students.

This book was conceptualized with the vision of imparting up-to-date information and advanced data in this field. To ensure the same, a matchless editorial board was set up. Every individual on the board went through rigorous rounds of assessment to prove their worth. After which they invested a large part of their time researching and compiling the most relevant data for our readers.

The editorial board has been involved in producing this book since its inception. They have spent rigorous hours researching and exploring the diverse topics which have resulted in the successful publishing of this book. They have passed on their knowledge of decades through this book. To expedite this challenging task, the publisher supported the team at every step. A small team of assistant editors was also appointed to further simplify the editing procedure and attain best results for the readers.

Apart from the editorial board, the designing team has also invested a significant amount of their time in understanding the subject and creating the most relevant covers. They scrutinized every image to scout for the most suitable representation of the subject and create an appropriate cover for the book.

The publishing team has been an ardent support to the editorial, designing and production team. Their endless efforts to recruit the best for this project, has resulted in the accomplishment of this book. They are a veteran in the field of academics and their pool of knowledge is as vast as their experience in printing. Their expertise and guidance has proved useful at every step. Their uncompromising quality standards have made this book an exceptional effort. Their encouragement from time to time has been an inspiration for everyone.

The publisher and the editorial board hope that this book will prove to be a valuable piece of knowledge for researchers, students, practitioners and scholars across the globe.

Contributors

Felipe Couñago, Elia del Cerro, Ana Aurora Díaz-Gavela and Francisco José Marcos
Department of Radiation Oncology, Hospital Universitario Quiron Madrid, Calle Diego de Velazquez, 1, 28223, Pozuelo de Alarcón, Madrid, Spain

Manuel Recio
Department of Radiology, Hospital Universitario Quiron, Madrid, Spain

Antonio Maldonado
Department of Nuclear Medicine, Hospital Universitario Quiron, Madrid, Spain

Israel J. Thuissard and David Sanz-Rosa
School of Doctoral Studies and Research, Universidad Europea de Madrid, Madrid, Spain

Karmele Olaciregui
Clinical Department, School of Biomedical Sciences, Universidad Europea de Madrid, Madrid, Spain

María Mateo
Hospital Universitario Quiron, Madrid, Spain

Laura Cerezo
Department of Radiation Oncology, Hospital Universitario La Princesa, Madrid, Spain

Jana Taron, Konstantin Nikolaou, Mike Notohamiprodjo and Rüdiger Hoffmann
Department of Diagnostic and Interventional Radiology, University Hospital of Tuebingen, Hoppe-Seyler-Str. 3, 72076 Tuebingen, Germany

Jonas Johannink
Department of Visceral Surgery, University Hospital of Tuebingen, Tuebingen, Germany

Michael Bitzer
Department of Internal Medicine, University Hospital of Tuebingen, Tuebingen, Germany

Jonathon Willatt, Julie A. Ruma, Shadi F. Azar, Nara L. Dasika and F. Syed
Veterans Administration, University of Michigan, Ann Arbor, MI, USA

Y. N. Shen, X. L. Bai, G. G. Li and T. B. Liang
Department of Hepatobiliary and Pancreatic Surgery, Second Affiliated Hospital of Zhejiang University School of Medicine, Zhejiang University, Jiefang Road, Shangcheng District, Hangzhou, China
Zhejiang Provincial Key Laboratory of Pancreatic Disease, Hangzhou, China

José Hugo Mendes Luz, Henrique Salas Martin, Hugo Rodrigues Gouveia, Roberto Romulo Souza, Igor Murad Faria and Tiago Nepomuceno de Miranda
Department of Interventional Radiology, Radiology Division, National Cancer Institute, INCA, Praça Cruz Vermelha 23, Centro, Rio de Janeiro CEP 20230-130, Brazil

Paula Mendes Luz
National Institute of Infectious Disease EvandroChagas, Oswaldo Cruz Foundation, Rio de Janeiro, Brazil

Tiago Bilhim, Élia Coimbra and Filipe Veloso Gomes
Department of Interventional Radiology, Centro Hepato-Bilio-Pancreático e de Transplantação. Hospital Curry Cabral, CHLC, Lisbon, Portugal.

Erik Rollvén and Lennart Blomqvist
Department of Molecular Medicine and Surgery, Karolinska Institutet, Department of Radiology, Karolinska University Hospital, Solna SE - 171 76, Stockholm, Sweden

Mirna Abraham-Nordling and Torbjörn Holm
Department of Molecular Medicine and Surgery, Karolinska Institutet, Center for Digestive Diseases, Karolinska University Hospital, Stockholm, Sweden

Jennifer Sammon, Ravi Menezes, Hooman Hosseini-Nik and Kartik Jhaveri
Toronto Joint Department of Medical Imaging, University Health Network, Sinai Health System and Women's College Hospitals, University of Toronto, Toronto, Canada

Sandra Fischer
Department of Pathology, University Health Network, University of Toronto, Toronto, Canada

Sara Lewis and Bachir Taouli
Department of Radiology, Mount Sinai New York, New York, USA

Catherine Guezennec, Nathalie Keromnes, Philippe Robin, Ronan Abgral, David Bourhis, Solène Querellou, Romain de Laroche, Alexandra Le Duc-Pennec, Pierre-Yves Salaün and Pierre-Yves Le Roux
Service de Médecine Nucléaire, EA3878 (GETBO) IFR 148, CHRU de Brest, Brest, France

Viktoria Palm
Department of Diagnostic and Interventional Radiology, Heidelberg University Hospital, INF 110, 69120 Heidelberg, Germany

Philipp Mayer, Hans-Ulrich Kauczor and Tim Frederik Weber
Department of Diagnostic and Interventional Radiology, Heidelberg University Hospital, INF 110, 69120 Heidelberg, Germany
Liver Cancer Center Heidelberg, Heidelberg University Hospital, INF 224, 69120 Heidelberg, Germany

Ruofan Sheng
Department of Radiology, Zhongshan Hospital, Fudan University, 180 Fenglin Road, Shanghai 200032, China

Karl-Heinz Weiss
Department of Gastroenterology, Infectious Diseases, Intoxication, Heidelberg University Hospital, INF 410, 69120 Heidelberg, Germany
Liver Cancer Center Heidelberg, Heidelberg University Hospital, INF 224, 69120 Heidelberg, Germany

Anne Katrin Berger
Department of Medical Oncology, National Center for Tumor Diseases (NCT), Heidelberg University Hospital, INF 460, 69120 Heidelberg, Germany

Christoph Springfeld
Department of Medical Oncology, National Center for Tumor Diseases (NCT), Heidelberg University Hospital, INF 460, 69120 Heidelberg, Germany
Liver Cancer Center Heidelberg, Heidelberg University Hospital, INF 224, 69120 Heidelberg, Germany

Arianeb Mehrabi
Department of General, Visceral and Transplantation Surgery, Heidelberg University Hospital, INF 110, 69120 Heidelberg, Germany
Liver Cancer Center Heidelberg, Heidelberg University Hospital, INF 224, 69120 Heidelberg, Germany

Thomas Longerich
Division Translational Gastro-intestinal Pathology, Institute of Pathology, Heidelberg University Hospital, INF 224, 69120 Heidelberg, Germany

Liver Cancer Center Heidelberg, Heidelberg University Hospital, INF 224, 69120 Heidelberg, Germany

Natalia Goldberg, Meital Nidam, Dan Stein, Ifat Abadi-Korek and Liran Domachevsky
Department of Nuclear Medicine, Assuta Medical Center, 20 habarzel st., 6971028 Tel-Aviv, Israel

David Groshar and Hanna Bernstine
Department of Nuclear Medicine, Assuta Medical Center, 20 habarzel st., 6971028 Tel-Aviv, Israel
Sackler Faculty of Medicine, Tel Aviv University, Tel-Aviv, Israel

Sven Schneeweiß, Marius Horger, Anja Grözinger, Konstantin Nikolaou, Dominik Ketelsen, Roland Syha and Gerd Grözinger
Department of Diagnostic Radiology, Eberhard-Karls-University, Hoppe-Seyler-Str.3, 72076 Tübingen, Germany

Babina Gosangi
Thoracic Radiology, Brigham and Women's Hospital, 45 Francis Street, Boston, MA 02115, USA

Matthew Davids
Harvard Medical School, 25 Shattuck Street, Boston, MA 02115, USA
Chronic Lymphocytic Leukemia, Dana Farber Cancer Institute, 450 Brookline Avenue, Boston 02284, USA

Bhanusupriya Somarouthu
Radiology, Massachusetts General Hospital, 55 Fruit Street, Boston, MA 02114, USA

Francesco Alessandrino
Emergency Radiology, Brigham and Women's Hospital, 45 Francis Street, Boston, MA 02115, USA

Angela Giardino, Nikhil Ramaiya and Katherine Krajewski
Department of Radiology, Dana Farber Cancer Institute, Boston, MA 02284, USA

Chao Ma, Yanjun Li, Li Wang, Shiyue Chen and Jianping Lu
Department of Radiology, Changhai Hospital of Shanghai, The Second Military Medical University, No.168 Changhai Road, Shanghai 200433, China

Yang Wang
Department of Pathology, Changhai Hospital of Shanghai, The Second Military Medical University, No.168 Changhai Road, Shanghai, China

Yong Zhang and He Wang
MR Group, GE Healthcare, No. 1 Huatuo Road, Shanghai, China

Marcos Duarte Guimarães
Department of Imaging, AC Camargo Cancer Center, Rua Prof. Antônio Prudente, 211, Liberdade, São Paulo/SP 01509-010, Brazil
Universidade Federal do Vale do São Francisco (UNIVASF), Av. José de Sá Maniçoba, Petrolina, PE 56304-917, Brazil

Julia Noschang and Alex Dias Oliveira
Department of Imaging, AC Camargo Cancer Center, Rua Prof. Antônio Prudente, 211, Liberdade, Sao Paulo/SP 01509-010, Brazil

Sara Reis Teixeira and Marcel Koenigkam Santos
Division of Radiology, Department of Internal Medicine, Ribeirao Preto Medical School, University of Sao Paulo, Av. Bandeirantes, 3900, Ribeirao Preto/ SP 14049-090, Brazil

Henrique Manoel Lederman
Universidade Federal de São Paulo, Departamento de Diagnóstico Por Imagem, Disciplina de Diagnóstico por Imagem em Pediatria, Rua Napoleão de Barros, 800, Vila Clementino, Sao Paulo/SP 04024002, Brazil

Vivian Tostes
Universidade Federal de São Paulo, Centro de Diagnóstico por Imagem do Instituto de Oncologia Pediátrica e Médica Radiologista do Centro de Diagnóstico por Imagem do Instituto de Oncologia Pediátrica, Rua Napoleão de Barros, 800, Vila Clementino, Sao Paulo/SP 04024002, Brazil

Vikas Kundra
Department of Diagnostic Radiology, The University of Texas MD Anderson Cancer Center, 1515 Holcombe Blvd, Houston, TX 77030, USA

Bruno Hochhegger
Department of Radiology, Universidade Federal de Ciências da Saúde de Porto Alegre, Rua Professor Anes Dias, 285, Centro Histórico, Porto Alegre/RS 90020-090, Brazil

Edson Marchiori
Department of Radiology, Universidade Federal do Rio de Janeiro, Rua Thomaz Cameron, 438, Valparaíso, Petrópolis/RJ 25685-129, Brazil

Amir Iravani, Tony Mulcahy and Bimal K. Parameswaran
Centre for Molecular Imaging, Department of Cancer Imaging, Peter MacCallum Cancer Centre, 305 Grattan Street, Melbourne, Australia.

Michael S. Hofman and Rodney J. Hicks
Centre for Molecular Imaging, Department of Cancer Imaging, Peter MacCallum Cancer Centre, 305 Grattan Street, Melbourne, Australia Sir Peter MacCallum Department of Oncology, University of Melbourne, 305 Grattan Street, Melbourne, Australia

Scott Williams
Sir Peter MacCallum Department of Radiation Oncology, University of Melbourne, 305 Grattan Street, Melbourne, Australia

Declan Murphy
Sir Peter MacCallum Department of Surgical Oncology, University of Melbourne, 305 Grattan Street, Melbourne, Australia

Jose Hugo Mendes Luz, Henrique S. Martin, Hugo R. Gouveia and Tiago Nepomuceno de Miranda
Department of Interventional Radiology, Radiology Division, National Cancer Institute, INCA, Praça Cruz Vermelha 23, Centro, Rio de Janeiro CEP 20230-130, Brazil

Paula M. Luz
National Institute of Infectious Disease Evandro Chagas, Oswaldo Cruz Foundation, Avenida Brasil 4365, Manguinhos, Rio de Janeiro 21040-360, Brazil

Raphal Braz Levigard and Felipe Diniz Nogueira
Department of Interventional Radiology, Radiology Division, Hospital Federal de Bonsucesso, Avenida Londres, 616, Bonsucesso, Rio de Janeiro 21041-030, Brazil

Bernardo Caetano Rodrigues
Department of Interventional Radiology, Radiology Division, Hospital Federal de Ipanema, Rua Antônio Parreiras, 67, Ipanema, Rio de Janeiro 22411-020, Brazil

Marcelo Henrique Mamede
Department of Anatomy and Radiology, Full Professor, Medicine School – UFMG, Avenida Presidente Antônio Carlos, 6627 Pampulha, Belo Horizonte, Minas Gerais 31270-901,Brazil

Meng Li, Li Zhang and Lv Lv
Department of Diagnostic Radiology, National Cancer Center/Cancer Hospital, Chinese Academy of Medical Sciences and Peking Union Medical College, Beijing, China

Ning Wu
Department of Diagnostic Radiology, National Cancer Center/Cancer Hospital, Chinese Academy of Medical Sciences and Peking Union Medical College, Beijing, China

PET-CT Center, National Cancer Center/Cancer Hospital, Chinese Academy of Medical Sciences and Peking Union Medical College, Beijing, China

Ying Liu
PET-CT Center, National Cancer Center/Cancer Hospital, Chinese Academy of Medical Sciences and Peking Union Medical College, Beijing, China

Dongmei Lin and Wei Sun
Department of Pathology, Beijing Cancer Hospital, Beijing, China

Jiansong Ren
National Office for Cancer Prevention and Control, National Cancer Center/ Cancer Hospital, Chinese Academy of Medical Sciences and Peking Union Medical College, Beijing, China

Cheng-Gong Yan, Ze-Long Cheng, Yuan-Kui Wu, Peng Hao, Bing-Quan Lin and Yi-Kai Xu
Department of Medical Imaging Center, Nanfang Hospital, Southern Medical University, #1838 Guangzhou Avenue North, Guangzhou City 510515, Guangdong Province, China

Li Yuan
Department of Medical Imaging Center, Nanfang Hospital, Southern Medical University, #1838 Guangzhou Avenue North, Guangzhou City 510515, Guangdong Province, China Department of Radiology, Hainan General Hospital, Haikou 570311, Hainan Province, China

Jian-Jun Li and Chang-Qing Li
Department of Radiology, Hainan General Hospital, Haikou 570311, Hainan Province, China

Lei Deng, Qiu-ping Wang, Lu Bai, You-min Guo and Quan-xin Yang
Department of Radiology, the First Affiliated Hospital, Xi'an Jiaotong University Xi'an, #277, Yanta West Road, Xi'an 710061, Shaanxi, China

Rui Yan
Department of Radiology, the Northwest Women and Children Hospital, #1616, Yanxiang Road, Xi'an 710054, Shaanxi, China

Xiao-yi Duan
Department of Nuclear Medicine, the First Affiliated Hospital, Xi'an Jiaotong University Xi'an, #277, Yanta West Road, Xi'an 710061, Shaanxi, China

Nan Yu
Department of Radiology, The Affiliated Hospital of Shaanxi University of traditional Chinese Medicine, #2. Wei Yang West Road, Xian Yang 712000, Shaanxi, China

Sung Uk Bae, Woon Kyung Jeong and Seong Kyu Baek
Department of Surgery, Keimyung University Dongsan Medical Center, Daegu, Republic of Korea

Kyoung Sook Won, Bong-Il Song and Hae Won Kim
Department of Nuclear Medicine, Keimyung University Dongsan Medical Center, 56 Dalseong-ro, Jung-gu, Daegu 41931, Republic of Korea

Chuangen Guo, Qidong Wang, Wenbo Xiao and Zhan Feng
Department of Radiology, the First Affiliated Hospital, College of Medicine Zhejiang University, 79 Qingchun road, Hangzhou 310003, China

Xiaoling Zhuge
Department of Laboratory Medicine, the First Affiliated Hospital, College of Medicine Zhejiang University, 79 Qingchun road, Hangzhou 310003, China

Xiao Chen, Zhonglan Wang and Zhongqiu Wang
Department of Radiology, the Affiliated Hospital of Nanjing University of Chinese Medicine, 155 Hanzhong road, Nanjing 210029, China

Lisa C. Adams, Yi-Na Y. Bender, Keno Bressem, Bernd Hamm, Jonas Busch and Marcus R. Makowski
Department of Radiology, Charité, Charitéplatz 1, 10117 Berlin, Germany

Bernhard Ralla
Department of Urology, Charité, Charitéplatz 1, 10117 Berlin, Germany

Florian Fuller
Department of Urology, Charité, Hindenburgdamm 30, 12200 Berlin, Germany

Hong-Zhi Zhang, Jie Pan, Jing Sun, Yu-Mei Li, Kang Zhou, Yang Li, Jin Cheng, Ying Wang and Dong-Lei Shi
Department of Radiology, Peking Union Medical College Hospital, Peking Union Medical College, Chinese Academy of Medical Sciences, No. 1 Shuaifuyuan, Dongcheng District, Beijing 100730, China

Shao-Hui Chen
Department of Anesthesiology, Peking Union Medical College Hospital, Peking Union Medical College, Chinese Academy of Medical Sciences, Beijing, China

Sungmin Jun
Department of Nuclear Medicine, Kosin University Gospel Hospital, Kosin University College of Medicine, Busan 49297, South Korea

Jung Gu Park
Department of Radiology, Kosin University Gospel Hospital, Kosin University College of Medicine, Busan 49297, South Korea

Youngduk Seo
Department of Nuclear Medicine, Busan Seongso Hospital, Suyeong-ro, Nam-gu, Busan 48453, Republic of Korea

Ronit Gill and Natalia Pirmisashvili
Department of Nuclear Medicine, Rambam Health Care Campus, Haifa, Israel

Zohar Keidar and Ora Israel
The Bruce Rappaport Faculty of Medicine, Technion – Israel Institute of Technology, Haifa, Israel

Elinor Goshen
Department of Nuclear Medicine, Wolfson Medical Center, Holon, Israel
Sackler School of Medicine, Tel Aviv University, Tel Aviv, Israel

Tima Davidson and Maryna Morgulis
Department of Nuclear Medicine, Chaim Sheba Medical Center, Ramat Gan, Israel

Simona Ben-Haim
Department of Medical Biophysics and Nuclear Medicine, Hadassah University Hospital, Ein Kerem, Jerusalem, Israel
University College London and UCL Hospitals, NHS Trust, London, UK

Daniele Paixão and Amanda França Nóbrega
Department of Oncogenetics, A.C. Camargo Cancer Center, Professor Antonio Prudente Street, 211 – Liberdade, São Paulo, SP 01509-900, Brazil

Marcos Duarte Guimarães and Rubens Chojniak
Department of Imaging, A.C. Camargo Cancer Center, São Paulo, SP, Brazil

Kelvin César de Andrade
Clinical Genetics Branch, Division of Epidemiology and Cancer Genetics, National Cancer Institutes, National Institutes of Health, Bethesda, MD, USA
International Research Center, A.C. Camargo Cancer Center, São Paulo, SP, Brazil

Maria Isabel Achatz
Centro de Oncologia, Hospital Sírio-Libanês, São Paulo, Brazil

T. Beyer
QIMP Group, Centre Medical Physics and Biomedical Engineering, Medical University Vienna, Währinger Str 18-20/4L, 1090 Vienna, Austria

R. Hicks
The Sir Peter MacCallum Department of Oncology, the University of Melbourne, Melbourne 3000, Australia

C. Brun
European Society for Hybrid Medical Imaging, Neutorgasse 10, 1010 Vienna, Austria

G. Antoch
Department of Diagnostic and Interventional Radiology, University Düsseldorf, Medical Faculty, Moorenstrasse 5, 40225 Düsseldorf, Germany

L. S. Freudenberg
ZRN Rheinland, Ueberseite 88, 41352 Korschenbroich, Germany

Rui Li, Xiaopeng Wang, Pan Liang and Jianbo Gao
Department of Radiology, the First Affiliated Hospital of Zhengzhou University, No. 1, East Jianshe Road, Zhengzhou 450052, Henan, China

Jing Li
Department of Radiology, the Affiliated Cancer Hospital of Zhengzhou University, Henan Cancer Hospital, No. 127, Dongming Road, Zhengzhou 450008, Henan, China

Jie Li, Zhitao Yang, Hexiang Wang and Wenjian Xu
Department of Radiology, The Affiliated Hospital of Qingdao University, 16 Jiangsu Road, Qingdao, Shandong, China

Jia Wang
Department of Ultrasound, Qingdao Women and Children Hospital, Qingdao, Shandong, China

Junyi Che
Department of Radiology, Qingdao Municipal Hospital, Qingdao, Shandong, China

Yan Chen, Xinyue Yang, Ziqiang Wen, Baolan Lu, Bingqi Shen and Shenping Yu
Department of Radiology, Sun Yat-sen University First Affiliated Hospital, Guangzhou 510080, China

Xiaojuan Xiao
Department of Radiology, Peking University Shenzhen Hospital, Shenzhen 518036, China

Ravneet Vohra, Joshua Park and Donghoon Lee
Department of Radiology, University of Washington, Seattle, USA

Yak-Nam Wang, Kayla Gravelle and Stella Whang
Applied Physics Laboratory, University of Washington, Seattle, USA

Joo-Ha Hwang
Department of Medicine, University of Washington, Seattle, USA

Index

www.ingramcontent.com/pod-product-compliance
Lightning Source LLC
Chambersburg PA
CBHW061330190326
41458CB00011B/3953